Methods of
Immunological Analysis

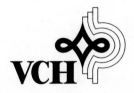

© VCH Verlagsgesellschaft mbH, D-69451 Weinheim (Federal Republic of Germany), 1993

Distribution

VCH, P.O.Box 10 11 61, D-69451 Weinheim (Federal Republic of Germany)

Switzerland: VCH, P.O.Box, CH-4020 Basel (Switzerland)

United Kingdom and Ireland: VCH (UK) Ltd., 8 Wellington Court, Wellington Street, Cambridge CB1 1HZ (England)

USA and Canada: VCH, Suite 909, 220 East 23rd Street, New York, NY 10010-4606 (USA)

Japan: VCH, Eikow Building, 10-9 Hongo 1-chome, Bunkyo-hu, Tokyo 113 (Japan)

ISBN 3-527-27908-3 (VCH, Weinheim)   ISBN 0-89573-904-6 (VCH, New York)

Methods of Immunological Analysis

Editor-in-Chief: René F. Masseyeff
Editors: Winfried H. Albert and Norman A. Staines

Volume 3
Cells and Tissues

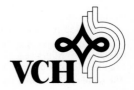

VCH

Editor-in-chief

Prof. René F. Masseyeff
Labs
57, Route de Canta-Gallet
F-06200 Nice
France

Language Editor

Prof. Donald W. Moss
Royal Postgraduate Medical School
University of London
Hammersmith Hospital
Du Cane Road
London W12 ONN
United Kingdom

Editors

Dr. Winfried H. Albert
Boehringer Mannheim GmbH
Res. Centre Tutzing, ST-B
Bahnhofstraße 9–15
D-82327 Tutzing
Germany

Editorial Dept. at VCH

Dr. Hans F. Ebel
and
N. Banerjea-Schultz

Prof. Norman A. Staines
Infection and
Immunity Group
King's College London
Campden Hill Road
London W8 7AH
United Kingdom

Published jointly by
VCH Verlagsgesellschaft mbH, Weinheim (Federal Republic of Germany)
VCH Publishers Inc., New York, NY (USA)

Deutsche Bibliothek Cataloguing-in-Publication Data

Methods of immunological analysis / ed.-in-chief: René F. Masseyeff. Ed.: Winfried H. Albert and Norman A. Staines. – Weinheim ; Basel (Switzerland) ; Cambridge ; New York, NY : VCH.

NE: Masseyeff, René F. [Hrsg.]

Vol. 3. Cells and Tissues. – 1993
   ISBN 3-527-27908-3 (Weinheim ...)
   ISBN 0-89573-904-6 (New York)

Library of Congress Card No. 92-49344

British Library Cataloguing-in-Publication Data. A catalogue record for this book is available from the British Library.

Production Manager: L & J Publikations-Service GmbH, D-69469 Weinheim
Composition: Mitterweger Werksatz GmbH, D-68723 Plankstadt
Printing and Bookbinding: Graph. Betrieb Konrad Triltsch, D-97070 Würzburg
Printed in the Federal Republic of Germany

Preface to the Series

Analysis based on the principle of the specific reaction between an antigen and its complementary antibody is now a major technique in all fields of biological and chemical science; in human and veterinary medicine, in environmental science, and even in plant physiology and pathology. The inherent advantage of immunological analysis, its specificity for the target analyte with its consequences of minimum sample preparation and sensitivity, is so great that it is now almost impossible to ignore the possible use of this technique in any application requiring the detection or measurement of organic molecules.

Immunological analysis has its roots in the 19th century, in the agglutination reactions of red blood cells or bacteria, and in immune precipitation and complement fixation reactions. While these principles are still in use, their further development was limited by the low sensitivity of immune precipitation and the insufficient reproducibility of agglutination and complement fixation. The explosive growth of immunological analysis in the second half of the present century is the result of advances in fundamental understanding of the immune response and of the molecular nature of the antigen-antibody reaction, coupled with practical developments such as the ability selectively to introduce a signal-generating label into antigens or antibodies without affecting their immunological reactivity. Of particular relevance to immunological analysis, fundamental research has revealed the fine structure of the binding sites of antibodies, progressively disclosing the molecular basis of their astonishing variability and providing a clearer understanding of the determinants of specificity. Research has also demonstrated the importance of correct presentation of a potential antigen to the antibody-producing cell, while developments in organic synthesis, especially of peptides, have greatly expanded the range of putative antigens. The development of monoclonal antibodies has provided an almost limitless range of reagents of clearly defined specificities, capable of further refinement through genetic engineering. Great technical ingenuity has been expended on the practical aspects of immunological analysis, in developing methods of increased sensitivity and reliability for measuring the analytical signal, and in increasing the convenience and speed of analysis through mechanization and automation.

The result of these advances has been to present the analyst, whose background may not be in immunology, with an embarrassment of riches when faced with the selection of an immunoassay to meet his particular requirements. The need for a comprehensive source of reliable, practical information on immunological analysis is apparent, considering, for example, Bergmeyer's "Methods of Enzymatic Analysis". The importance of enzyme labels in immunoassay required four volumes for its treatment in that series: nevertheless, it was clear that the much wider scope of immunoassay in general demands its own series. Thus, "Methods in Immunological Analysis" was conceived. Its aim is to provide the analyst with a guidebook with which to set out confidently into the rich territory of immunological analysis.

The Editors retained some of the organizational features that made the success of "Methods of Enzymatic Analysis". A survey of the fundamental observations on which immunological analysis is based, namely, the nature of the immune response and physicochemical aspects of the structures of antigens and antibodies and their interaction, is followed by discussion of the strategies available in immunoassay. Tested and reliable methods for a wide range of analytes are described in a detailed and rigorously specified format that is intended to provide working protocols that obviate the need for reference to other sources. Furthermore, informed by the principles of analysis set out in the series, the analyst should be able to modify the protocols where necessary to meet his individual needs. In addition to this "cook-book" approach, the series contains papers on the various applications of immunoassays in different fields, with emphasis on medical aspects. The place of immunological assays in the context of other methods is discussed for each group of assays. Chapters on method comparison provide additional guidance. Special problems in standardization, disclosed by results of quality assessment surveys, are covered in specific papers. The editors' aim is not only to provide recipes for the assay of a variety of analytes, but also to assist the reader in the selection of the most suitable method for his needs, and thus to provide him with the knowledge needed for an optimal use of immunological methods and their interpretation.

Immunological analysis exploits the specificity of the reaction between differently-specific antibody molecules (possibly as many as ten million) and their ligands. The results of immunological analysis are method-dependent. This, however, is not well appreciated, even by experienced immunoassayists. Such problems in immunological analysis derive from the incomplete characterization of the reagent antigens and antibodies as well as from matrix effects, and lead to problems of standardization and comparability of results. The introduction of monoclonal antibodies in many applications has improved the reproducibility of immunological reagents, but formidable problems of standardization remain, and are fully discussed in this series.

As well as striking an appropriate balance between fundamental principles and practical descriptions, the Editors have endeavoured to make a systematic selection from the vast array of methodological principles and variations that are now represented in immunological analysis. This situation is rendered even more complex by the changing balance of method development, from the universities and research institutes towards industry, often with consequent patent protection and restricted availability of certain reagents. Fortunately, however, many procedural variations are of a minor nature, dictated in some cases only by the need to establish commercial novelty. By emphasizing the modular nature of assays and their classification in terms of the analytical principles involved, and by avoiding confusing abbreviations and acronyms, the Editors have attempted to bring some order into the potentially bewildering array of available methods.

The analytes for which assays are described have been chosen for their importance, e.g., the frequency with which their measurement is required, and also for their suitability for the demonstration of particular analytical approaches. Several types of methods are available for certain analytes with a long history of biomedical importance, such as a variety of drugs or hormones. In such cases alternative, reliable methods have been described so that an intending user should be able to select the one that is most appropriate to his available resources. However, less well-known methods and those which demonstrate original analytical principles have not been neglected. Methods subject to patent protection, or offered in the form of commercial reagent kits, have not been excluded, provided that the nature and composition of their reagents is disclosed in sufficient detail for them to be repeated with readily available substances. Authors of methods which depend on specific immunological reagents have been asked to state whether these reagents can be provided to intending users.

Throughout, the Editors' aim has been to provide a comprehensive handbook of value to the specialist and non-specialist alike.

All contributions are written in English. However, since the authors, as well as their potential readers, come from all over the world, a uniform style of grammar and spelling has been adopted to provide readers with a consistent and unambiguous text. Modern English spelling has been chosen which minimizes the differences between English and American usage, in the hope of making the volumes readily accessible to the widest possible readership.

The Editors' grateful thanks are due to the authors who placed their specialist knowledge so freely at the service of their colleagues, and who patiently accepted the editorial requirements of the series. The ultimate success of the volumes is entirely due to their willing cooperation. The Editors owe a special tribute to Professor H. U. Bergmeyer and to Professor D. Moss for contributing their immense experience. They are also grateful for the expert support of VCH, especially of Mrs. N. Banerjea-Schultz, while the technical assistance of L & J Publikations-Service has greatly facilitated the rapid production of the volumes.

Nice, July 1992   René F. Masseyeff

Preface to Volume 3

The detection and quantification of the component molecules of cells require an approach subtly different from that used to deal with analytes already present in solution. This volume, the Third in the "Methods of Immunological Analysis" series, is concerned with the approach to using immunological methods for the analysis of cells and tissues. The constituents of cells naturally do not exist or function in isolation of each other, and it is the very intimate relations these molecules have that makes their analysis such a challenge. Many, probably most, are inaccessible in normal circumstances, hidden by lipid membranes or inside organelles; others are relatively insoluble or buried beneath other molecules. So, in order to exploit the exquisite specificity of antibodies to analyse cells, the component analytes, for some purposes, have to be revealed or separated from their neighbours for accurate assessment. This is the starting point of this Volume.

In the first sections, the methods necessary for the isolation of cells from many different tissues are described. The emphasis is upon human cells, but many references are made to animal cells in acknowledgement of their importance in experimentation. Throughout, the common principles essential to handling cells from many varied sources are stressed.

The culture of cells, over both long and short periods, is an essential component of many experiments. Indeed, the availability of well-characterized and standardized cell lines has been central to the elucidation of cell structure and function. Thus, methods of tissue culture are dealt with here, not only with regard to mammalian cells but also those from arthropods and plants which both enjoy a new prominence in contemporary research. The propagation and characterization of bacterial cells are covered too. The importance of eukaryotic cell clones is exemplified by a section on the T-lymphocytes of the immune system which, because of their great heterogeneity of specificity and function, are ideal candidates for cloning. Because B-lymphocyte clones have been used extensively to make monoclonal antibodies, these were dealt with in Volume 2 of the series.

Aside from cell cloning, there are many ways in which cells can be physically separated from each other, and the systems involving gradient centrifugation, panning and magnetic beads are discussed critically. In a related way, the separation of sub-cellular fractions and components is necessary in many studies, and this too is discussed.

Using standardized immunoassay methods it is possible to quantify the amount of particular analytes in cell extracts, assuming of course a quantitative recovery in the extraction process. However, there are many situations where it is desirable to quantify the analyte *in situ* and to define precisely its subcellular location. For reasons mentioned earlier, there may be considerable problems in this but there has been much encouraging progress through the development and application of methods of, for example, image analysis, confocal microscopy, flow cytometry and immunocytochemistry. The importance and versatility of these technologies are dealt with in critical detail.

An important aspect of immunological analysis of cells is the use of antibody-based methods in immunocytochemistry. In a a major section, the various approaches to this most central of cell biological methods are described and their comparative uses and performance discussed. Precise protocols are given in the style established in Volume 2 of this series: the common features of immunocytochemical methods and their modular nature is emphasized and exploited in a step-by-step approach to setting up and applying them. These now can be used to localize with some precision the target antigens in cells and tissues when examined under light or electron microscopy, but the methods do not yet approach the quantitative accuracy of conventional immunoassays for soluble analytes. The reasons for this are discussed and the limitations of the cytochemical approach dealt with critically.

Immunocytochemical methods have found wide application in many areas of cell biology, and an authoritative commentary is provided on this by several different authors. The ways in which immunological methods have greatly facilitated the analysis of cells and tissue organization are exemplified by their use in unravelling the development of lymphocytes. Immunological methods have, however, been central to dissecting cell organelles and structures as well, and the ways in which immunochemical and immunocytochemical methods have been used to investigate nuclear and cytoplasmic structures are described so that they will enable the interested reader to undertake analysis of any tissue, cell or organelle by similar approaches.

Much of the value in the application of immunological methods has been in the study of cell phenotype, which in essence reflects the structural organization of the cell. From this can be inferred, for example, the means and circumstances of the regulation of gene expression. It is only now, however, that immune methods are applied successfully to analyse cell function. Two major approaches that are described critically here have been developed for primarily immunological purposes, but they clearly have applications in many other areas. The first of these is the ELISPOT method that allows the enumeration of cells secreting any particular molecule – an antibody, hormone or cytokine for example. This has great potential to be applied in many circumstances. The second is the use of immunocytochemical methods to identify cells making soluble secretable molecules such as cytokines. Here as elsewhere comparisons are made with other methods, in this case the use of nucleotide probes and PCR methods, in order that the value of immunological methods can be fairly appreciated. Judging from progress in developing these methods in recent years, there is justified optimism that they will be refined to the point where they will provide accurate quantitative data. Without doubt, other methods will be derived from them.

The title of this particular volume of this series might imply that it is devoted to the analysis of immune cells. As this account makes clear, this is not the case. Certainly, immune cells are mentioned in many places, but largely because they are the object of study by cell biologists in general, and not immunologists in particular. The criterion for inclusion of a particular approach or method here has been that it uses an immunological probe, almost always an antibody, to examine a cell. The last part of the volume nonetheless considers the ways in which immune cells can be analysed by methods conventionally understood by immunologists, but not necessarily using antibodies. The ways in which immune cells are examined nowadays would provide material for many volumes beyond the size and scope of this: here we confine ourselves to our brief to explain how immunological methods can be put to work in cell biology. Discussion and commentary form vital parts of the volume, but they are only the support for its main purpose which is to give precise laboratory protocols that can be established by the non-expert and applied without reference beyond this volume.

Many authors have contributed to this volume and to them, the editors express their sincere thanks. As in the other volumes of the series, the excellent help and cooperation of Professor H. U. Bergmeyer and Professor D. Moss have been especially valuable and appreciated.

March 1993   The Editors

Contents

List of Contributors XXXI

1   General Introduction 1

Immunological Methods of Analysis of Cell Structure and Function   2
G. Gordon MacPherson

Why Antibodies? 2

Cell-mediated Immunity in Immunoanalysis 3

Cell Quantitation 4

Cell Preparation and Separation 5

Immunocytochemistry 6

Antibody as a Probe of Function 8

Future Prospects 9

2   Preparation of Cells and Tissues 11

2.1   General Considerations 12
Anne S. Hamblin

2.1.1   Cells 12
2.1.1.1   Estimating Cell Numbers 13
2.1.1.2   Estimating Cell Viability 15
2.1.1.3   Handling Conditions 18

2.1.2   Tissues 20

2.2   Blood and Its Constituent Cells 22
Arne Bøyum

2.2.1   Reagents and Solutions 23

2.2.2   Cell Separation Procedures   24
2.2.2.1   Preparation of Unfractionated Leucocytes   24
2.2.2.2   Separation of MNC and Granulocytes from Whole Blood with One
           Layer of Gradient Medium   25
2.2.2.3   Separation of MNC and Granulocytes from Leucocyte-rich Plasma   27
2.2.2.4   Separation of MNC and Granulocytes from Animal Blood   28
2.2.2.5   One-step Separation of MNC and Granulocytes   30
2.2.2.6   Simultaneous Separation of MNC and Granulocytes with a
           Two-layer Technique   31
2.2.2.7   Separation of MNC and Granulocytes at 4°C, with 17% Plasma in
           the Gradient Medium   32
2.2.2.8   Separation of Lymphocytes   33
2.2.2.9   Separation of Monocytes   34
2.2.2.10   Separation of Erythrocytes and Reticulocytes   35
2.2.2.11   Separation of Platelets   36
2.2.2.12   Removal of Platelets   37

2.3   **Serous Cavity Cells**   39
           Derralynn A. Hughes and Siamon Gordon

2.3.1   Lavage of Cells From the Peritoneal Cavity   40
2.3.1.1   Adult Mice   40
2.3.1.2   Newborn Mice   41
2.3.1.3   Depletion of Peritoneal Macrophages by Lavage   41
2.3.1.4   Other Laboratory Species   42
2.3.1.5   Peritoneal Lavage of Non-mammals   42
2.3.1.6   Human Peritoneal Cells   42

2.3.2   Recruitment of Cells to the Peritoneal Cavity   42

2.3.3   Cell Purification from Peritoneal Lavage   46

2.3.4   *In-vivo* and *in-vitro* Labelling of Peritoneal Cells   47
2.3.4.1   Fluorescent Labelling   47
2.3.4.2   Phagocytic Labelling   48

2.3.5   Measurement of the Turnover of Peritoneal Cells   48

2.3.6   Cells From the Pleural Cavity   49

2.4   **Alveolar Cells**   52
           Allen G. Harmsen

2.4.1   Bronchoalveolar Lavage of Human Subjects   52

2.4.2   Bronchoalveolar Lavage of Animals   53
2.4.2.1   Large Animals   53
2.4.2.2   Rodents   54

2.4.3   Cell Yields of BAL   55
2.4.3.1   Humans   56
2.4.3.2   Large Animals   56
2.4.3.3   Rodents   56
2.4.3.4   Differential Phenotype Analysis   57
2.4.3.5   Recovery and Dilution of Cells and Fluid by BAL   57

2.4.4   Limitations   58

2.5   Lymphoid Tissue Cells   60
          Deborah J. Bevan and Norman A. Staines

2.5.1   General   60

2.5.2   Preparation of Cell Suspensions from Rodent Lymphoid Organs . .   61
2.5.2.1   Thymus   62
2.5.2.2   Bone Marrow   62
2.5.2.3   Spleen   63
2.5.2.4   Lymph Nodes   65
2.5.2.5   *Peyer's* Patches   65
2.5.2.6   Blood   66

2.5.3   Preparation of Human Lymphoid Cells   66
2.5.3.1   Tonsil   67
2.5.3.2   Blood   67

2.6   Arthropod Tissues and Cells   68
          Klaus-Peter Sieber

2.6.1   General Properties   68

2.6.2   Preparation of Tissues and Cells   69
2.6.2.1   General   69
2.6.2.2   Dissection   70
2.6.2.3   Purification   70
2.6.2.4   Cell Culture   71
2.6.2.5   Buffers and Media   72

2.6.3   Assay Methods   73
2.6.3.1   Principle   73
2.6.3.2   Quantitative Determination of *in-vitro* Synthesized Vitellogenin . .   73
2.6.3.3   Quantitative Determination of Prothoracicotropic Hormone
          (PTTH) *in vitro*   74

2.6.4   Preparation of Tissues for Immunocytochemistry   74
2.6.4.1   Insect Tissues   74
2.6.4.2   Crustacean Tissue (*Homarus americanus*)   75

2.6.5   Reagents and Solutions   76

2.7   **Plant Tissues and Cells**   79
Hans-Willi Krell

2.7.1   General Properties of Plant Tissue   79

2.7.2   Methods of Disintegration   80
2.7.2.1   Disruption of Tissues and Cells   80
2.7.2.2   Media for Cell and Tissue Disintegration   81
2.7.2.3   Post-treatment of Extracts   81

2.7.3   Histological Methods   82

2.7.4   Preparation of Plant Cell Constituents   83
2.7.4.1   Cell Wall   83
2.7.4.2   Protoplast   83
2.7.4.3   Nuclei   83
2.7.4.4   Plastids   84
2.7.4.5   Mitochondria   84
2.7.4.6   Microbodies (Glyoxisomes, Peroxisomes)   84
2.7.4.7   *Golgi* Apparatus and Related Cell Components   85
2.7.4.8   Vacuoles   85
2.7.4.9   Plant Cell Membranes   85

2.8   **Prokaryotic Cells**   89
Matthias C. C. Poetsch

2.8.1   Equipment   89

2.8.2   Sources of Microorganisms   90

2.8.3   Media   90
2.8.3.1   Composition   90
2.8.3.2   Preparation   91
2.8.3.3   Sterilization   91

2.8.4   Culture   92
2.8.4.1   Propagation   92
2.8.4.2   Harvest and Disruption of the Cells   93

3   **Cell Culture**   95

3.1   **General Principles**   96
Christopher B. Morris, Bryan J. Bolton and Jon M. Mowles

3.1.1   Laboratory Design   96

3.1.2   Equipment   98

3.1.2.1	Incubators	98
3.1.2.2	Microscope	99
3.1.2.3	Other Items	99
3.1.3	Good Laboratory Practice	100
3.2	**Long-term Cultures and Cell Lines**	103

Bryan J. Bolton, Christopher B. Morris and Jon M. Mowles

3.2.1	Types of Cell Lines	103
3.2.2	Media	104
3.2.2.1	Types, Choice and Preparation	104
3.2.2.2	Serum-free Media	105
3.2.3	Subculture and Maintenance	105
3.2.3.1	Attached Cell Lines	106
3.2.3.2	Suspension Cell Lines	106
3.2.3.3	Cell Counting	107
3.2.4	Cryopreservation	107
3.2.4.1	Equipment and Materials	107
3.2.4.2	Method	109
3.2.5	Microbiological Quality Control	110
3.2.5.1	Testing for Bacteria and Fungi	111
3.2.5.2	Testing for Mycoplasma	111
3.2.5.3	Elimination of Mycoplasma	115
3.2.6	Authenticity of Cell Lines	116
3.2.6.1	Isoenzyme Analysis	116
3.2.6.2	Cytogenetic Analysis	117
3.2.6.3	DNA Fingerprinting	117
3.3	**Lymphocyte Clones**	120

Robyn E. O'Hehir, Brigitte A. Askonas and Jonathan R. Lamb

3.3.1	Lymphocyte Cultures	121
3.3.1.1	Media	121
3.3.1.2	Lymphocyte Preparation	122
3.3.2	CD4+ T-Cell Growth *in vitro*	122
3.3.2.1	T-Cell Proliferative Assays	123
3.3.2.2	T-Cell Hybridization	125
3.3.2.3	Viral Transformation	125
3.3.2.4	Sources of IL-2	125
3.3.3	Cloning Techniques for Human CD4+ T-Cells	126
3.3.3.1	Primary Cultures	126

3.3.3.2   Established T-Cell Lines   127
3.3.3.3   Limiting Dilution Isolation of T-Cell Clones   128
3.3.4   CD8+ Cytotoxity T-Cell Growth *in vitro*   129
3.3.4.1   Background   129
3.3.4.2   The Generation of CTL and Their Culture   130

3.3.5   Cloning Techniques for CD8+ Cytotoxic T-Cells   130
3.3.5.1   Target Cells for Cytotoxicity Assay   131
3.3.5.2   Cytotoxicity Assay   132

3.3.6   Applications of T-Cell Clones   132

3.4   Arthropod Cells   139
          Klaus-Peter Sieber

3.4.1   Setting up Arthropod Cell Cultures   139
3.4.1.1   Starting Material   139
3.4.1.2   Primary Cell Culture   140
3.4.1.3   Cell Lines   141
3.4.1.4   Media   142
3.4.1.5   Cell Culture of *Spodoptera frugiperdis* Cells (SF9-cells)   143
3.4.1.6   Cloning Methods   144
3.4.1.7   Culture Parameters   144

3.4.2   Applications   144
3.4.2.1   Arthropod-transmitted Virus   145
3.4.2.2   Studies on Differentiation and Genetics   145
3.4.2.3   Gene Expression in Transfected Insect Cells   145

3.5   Plant Cells   148
          Hans-Willi Krell

3.5.1   Setting up Plant Tissue Cultures   149
3.5.1.1   Plant Material   149
3.5.1.2   Induction of a Callus Culture   150
3.5.1.3   Suspension Cultures   150
3.5.1.4   Haploid Cell Cultures   150
3.5.1.5   Media   151

3.5.2   Applications   153
3.5.2.1   Somaclonal Variation   153
3.5.2.2   Protoplast Fusion   153
3.5.2.3   Transformed (transgenetic) Plants   153
3.5.2.4   Plant Regeneration   153
3.5.2.5   Production of Secondary Metabolites   154

3.6   **Prokaryotic Cells**   156
Matthias C. C. Poetsch

3.6.1   Bioreactors   156
3.6.1.1   Mixing and Aeration   158
3.6.1.2   Temperature and pH Control   158
3.6.1.3   Foam Control   158
3.6.1.4   Sterilization   159

3.6.2   Characteristics of the Culture Procedure   159
3.6.2.1   Media   159
3.6.2.2   From Colony to Large Scale Culture   159
3.6.2.3   Monitoring and Control of Fermentation   160
3.6.2.4   Kinetics of Growth in Batch Culture   160
3.6.2.5   Kinetics of Growth in Continuous Culture   161
3.6.2.6   Harvest of Cells   162

4   **Cell Fractionation and Purification**   165

4.1   **General**   166
Norman A. Staines

4.2   **Differential Adherence and Antibody-based Methods**   167
Deborah J. Bevan

4.2.1   Methods Employing Cell Adherence to a Solid Matrix   167
4.2.1.1   Glass Bead Column Filtration for Removal of Adherent Cells   168
4.2.1.2   Gel Filtration for Removal of Adherent Cells   168
4.2.1.3   Affinity Chromatography   169
4.2.1.4   Nylon Wool Adherence   169
4.2.1.5   Sequential Adherence for Purification/Removal of Monocytes and
Dendritic Cells   170

4.2.2   Cell Separation Methods Utilizing Antibodies   171
4.2.2.1   Complement-mediated Cytolysis   172
4.2.2.2   Panning   173
4.2.2.3   Rosetting Methods Utilizing Erythrocytes   175
4.2.2.4   Immunomagnetic Rosetting Methods   180
4.2.2.5   Preparative Flow Cytometry   185

4.3   **Biopsy-based Methods**   190
Timothy J. Peters

4.3.1   Principles   190
4.3.1.1   Sample Variability   190

4.3.1.2   Sample Collection   191
4.3.1.3   Tissue Preservation   191

4.3.2   Cell Isolation Procedures   192

4.3.3   Subcellular Fractionation Techniques   193
4.3.3.1   Homogenization Assessments   193
4.3.3.2   Homogenization Procedures   194
4.3.3.3   Principles of Analytical and Preparative Techniques   195
4.3.3.4   Centrifugation Methods   196
4.3.3.5   Affinity Chromatography   198
4.3.3.6   Gel Permeation Chromatography   198
4.3.3.7   Phasepartition Chromatography   198
4.3.3.8   Electrophoretic Methods.............................   199

4.3.4   Enzyme Analysis of Biopsies and Fractions   199

5   **Methods of Phenotype Analysis**   203

5.1   **General Features of Immunocytochemistry**   204
          Susan Van Noorden

5.1.1   Principles   204

5.1.2   Choice of Reagents   205

5.1.3   Methodology   206

5.1.4   Applicability   208

5.1.5   Limitations   208

5.2   **Preparation of Specimens for Immunocytochemistry**   210
          Susan Van Noorden

5.2.1   Purpose of Fixation   210
5.2.2.1   Action of Fixatives   210

5.2.2   Processing for Paraffin Sections of Pre-fixed Material   211
5.2.2.1   Fixation   211
5.2.2.2   Washing   212
5.2.2.3   Dehydrating and Embedding in Paraffin   212
5.2.2.4   Processing to Epoxy Resin   213
5.2.2.5   Uses of Paraffin or Resin Sections   214

5.2.3   Preparation of Frozen Fixed Tissue Blocks   214
5.2.3.1   Sections of Frozen Fixed Tissue Blocks   215

5.2.3.2   Semithin or Ultrathin Frozen Fixed Tissue Sections   215
5.2.3.3   Uses of Pre-fixed Frozen Sections   216

5.2.4   Unembedded, Unfrozen Pre-fixed Material   216
5.2.4.1   Vibratome® Sections   216
5.2.4.2   Whole-Mount Material   216
5.2.4.3   Uses of Vibratome and Whole-Mount Preparations   127

5.2.5   Unfixed Material   217
5.2.5.1   Fresh Frozen Tissue   217
5.2.5.2   Fixatives for Frozen Sections   219

5.2.6   Freeze-dried Material   219
5.2.6.1   Procedure   219
5.2.6.2   Uses for Freeze-dried Vapour-fixed Sections   220

5.2.7   Live Cells   221
5.2.7.1   Use and Handling   221
5.2.7.2   Procedures   222
5.2.7.3   Limitations   223

5.2.8   Non-living Cells   223
5.2.8.1   Use and Handling   223
5.2.8.2   Preparing the Cells   224
5.2.8.3   Fixation and Storage   224
5.2.8.4   Immunostaining   225

5.2.9   Fixatives   225

5.2.10   Coating Slides with *Poly*-L-lysine   227
5.2.10.1   Procedure   227

5.3   Labels for Immunocytochemistry   229
Susan Van Noorden

5.3.1   Fluorescent Labels   229
5.3.1.1   General   229
5.3.1.2   Selected Labels   230

5.3.2   Enzyme Labels   231
5.3.2.1   Horseradish Peroxidase   231
5.3.2.2   Alkaline Phosphatase   232
5.3.2.3   Glucose Oxidase   233
5.3.2.4   β-D-Galactosidase   233

5.3.3   Radioactive Labels   234

5.3.4   Colloidal Gold   234
5.3.4.1   Properties and Use   234
5.3.4.2   Advantages and Disadvantages   236

5.3.5   Bridging Labels   236
5.3.5.1   Haptens   236
5.3.5.2   Biotin   237

5.3.6   Methods of Labelling Antibodies   237
5.3.6.1   Fluorescent Labels   237
5.3.6.2   Enzyme Labels   238
5.3.6.3   Adsorption of Protein to Colloidal Gold   240
5.3.6.4   Biotinylation of Ab   241
5.3.6.5   Further Labelling Methods   242

5.3.7   Visualization of Fluorescent Labels   242
5.3.7.1   Microscope   242
5.3.7.2   Mountants   242
5.3.7.3   Storage   243
5.3.7.4   Restoration of Fluorescence   243
5.3.7.5   Fluorescent Counterstains   243

5.3.8   Visualization of Peroxidase   244
5.3.8.1   Blocking Endogenous POD Reactions   244
5.3.8.2   Development Methods   246

5.3.9   Visualization of Alkaline Phosphatase   253
5.3.9.1   Blocking Endogenous Enzyme   253
5.3.9.2   Development Methods   254

5.3.10   Visualization of Glucose Oxidase   256

5.3.11   Visualization of β-D-Galactosidase   257

5.3.12   Visualization of Colloidal Gold Labels   257

5.3.13   Autoradiographic Development   259

5.4   Range and Scope of Immunocytochemical Methods   264
          Susan Van Noorden

5.4.1   Direct Method   264

5.4.2   Indirect Method   266

5.4.3   Three-layer Techniques   268
5.4.3.1   Unlabelled Enzyme Anti-enzyme Method   268
5.4.3.2   Avidin-Biotin Methods   271

5.4.4   Build-up Methods   275

5.4.5   Labelled Antigen   275

5.4.6   Multiple Immunostaining   281
5.4.6.1   Serial Sections   281

5.4.6.2   Mirror-Image Sections 281
5.4.6.3   Single Preparations 281
5.4.6.4   Double Direct Immunostaining 282
5.4.6.5   Double Indirect (2-Step) Immunostaining 283
5.4.6.6   Triple Immunostaining 285

5.4.7   Quantification 285
5.4.7.1   Limits to Quantification 285
5.4.7.2   Image Analysis 286
5.4.7.3   Antigen Concentrations and Antibody Dilution 286

5.5   **Immunostaining Procedures** 289
          Susan Van Noorden

5.5.1   General Aspects 289
5.5.1.1   Materials Needed 289
5.5.1.2   Application of Reagents 290
5.5.1.3   Hydrophobic Pen 290
5.5.1.4   Establishing Antibody Standard Working Dilutions 290

5.5.2   Cell Preparations and Frozen Sections 291
5.5.2.1   Direct Immunofluorescence 291
5.5.2.2   Indirect (2-Layer) Immunoperoxidase Staining 292
5.5.2.3   Alkaline Phosphatase Anti-Alkaline Phosphatase (APAAP)
          Staining 292

5.5.3   Paraffin Sections 293
5.5.3.1   Peroxidase Anti-Peroxidase (PAP) Staining 293
5.5.3.2   Avidin-Biotinylated POD Complex (ABC) Staining 294
5.5.3.3   Enzyme Digestion 295
5.5.3.4   Antigen Retrieval by Microwave Treatment 297

5.5.4   Pre-fixed Frozen Sections, Vibratome Sections, Whole-Mount
          Preparations 298
5.5.4.1   Pre-fixed Thick Preparations, PAP Method 298
5.5.4.2   Pre-fixed Thick Preparations, Immunofluorescence 299

5.5.5   Immunogold Staining with Silver Intensification (IGSS)
          (Paraffin Sections) 299

5.6   **Problem Solving and Practical Aspects** 300
          Susan Van Noorden

5.6.1   Unwanted Staining 300
5.6.1.1   Fc Receptors 301
5.6.1.2   Complement Binding 301
5.6.1.3   Hydrophobic or Charged Tissue Sites 301

5.6.1.4   Aldehyde Groups in Tissue   302
5.6.1.5   Endogenous Enzyme   302
5.6.1.6   Endogenous Biotin   302
5.6.1.7   Avidin Binding   303
5.6.1.8   Binding of Aggregated Igs to Basic Peptide Sequences   303
5.6.1.9   Free Label   303
5.6.1.10 Poorly Preserved Tissue   304
5.6.1.11 Contaminating Antibodies   304
5.6.1.12 Cross-reactions of Immunoglobulins   304
5.6.1.13 Cross-reactions of Primary Antibody   305
5.6.1.14 Method Factors   305

5.6.2   Lack of Staining   305
5.6.2.1   Unavailable Antigen   305
5.6.2.2   Incorrect Tissue Treatment   306
5.6.2.3   Prozone Effect   306

5.6.3   Controls   306
5.6.3.1   Specificity Controls   307
5.6.3.2   Importance of Antigen Purity   307
5.6.3.3   Receptor Sites for the Antigen May Be Present in the Same Tissue
          as the Stored Antigen   307
5.6.3.4   Destruction of the Antigen   308
5.6.3.5   Nonspecific Binding of Ig- or Ag-Ab Complexes   308
5.6.3.6   Cross-reacting Antibodies   308
5.6.3.7   Positive/Method Controls   309
5.6.3.8   Negative Controls   309

5.6.4   Other Important Factors   310
5.6.4.1   Concentration/Dilution of Antibodies   310
5.6.4.2   Temperature   311
5.6.4.3   Diluent for Antibodies   311
5.6.4.4   Storage of Antibodies   311

5.6.5   Apparatus   312
5.6.5.1   General   312
5.6.5.2   Automation   312

5.6.6   Photomicrography   313

5.7   **Immunogold Methods for Electron Microscopy**   314
          F. B. Peter Wooding and Marion D. Kendall

5.7.1   Special Considerations and Choice of Method   314

5.7.2   Antibody Labelling Regimes   316
5.7.2.1   Direct Labelling of the Primary Antibody with Colloidal Gold . . .   317
5.7.2.2   Indirect Labelling   317

5.7.2.3   Multilayer Techniques   318
5.7.2.4   Co-Localization of Antigens on the Same Section   318

5.7.3   Fixation   319

5.7.4   Processing of Tissues   321
5.7.4.1   Freezing   322
5.7.4.2   Cryosectioning   322
5.7.4.3   Resin Embedding   323

5.7.5   Colloidal Gold   324
5.7.5.1   Size Considerations   324
5.7.5.2   Variants of Gold Colloid Labels   326

5.7.6   Quantitation   327

5.7.7   Alternatives to Post-embedding Labelling   328
5.7.7.1   Pre-embedding Labelling   328
5.7.7.2   Scanning EM Labelling   329

5.7.8   Basic Indirect Method for K4M Acrylic Resin   329

5.7.9   Variations of Basic K4M Method   332
5.7.9.1   K4M Embedding at −20 °C   332
5.7.9.2   Cryoprocessing   332
5.7.9.3   Osmium-Fixed Epoxy Embedded Material   333
5.7.9.4   Light Microscopy Protocol   333
5.7.9.5   Absorption Control Protocols   333

5.8   **Quantitative Histochemistry**   338
          Joseph Chayen and Lucille Bitensky

5.8.1   Basic Procedures   339
5.8.1.1   Problems in Preparing the Specimen   339
5.8.1.2   Effect of Other Histochemical Procedures   339
5.8.1.3   Preparation of Sections   339
5.8.1.4   Reactions   340
5.8.1.5   Measurement   340

5.8.2   Procedures for Localizing the Antibody-Antigen Reaction   341
5.8.2.1   Immunological Methodology   341
5.8.2.2   Possible Pitfalls   342

5.9   **Image Analysis**   345
          Don-Carlos Abrams and David R. Springall

5.9.1   General Considerations   345
5.9.1.1   What is an Image?   346
5.9.1.2   What is Image Analysis?   348
5.9.1.3   Hardware Requirements   348

5.9.1.4 .Image Capture 348
5.9.1.5 Display 349
5.9.1.6 Storage 350
5.9.1.7 Networks 350
5.9.1.8 Software Requirements 350

5.9.2   Stages in Image Analysis 352
5.9.2.1 Sample Preparation 352
5.9.2.2 Image Quality 352
5.9.2.3 Segmentation 353
5.9.2.4 Mensuration 355

5.9.3   General Applications of Image Analysis 356

5.9.4   Quantification of Immunostaining 356
5.9.4.1 Area Measurement 357
5.9.4.2 Intensity of Staining 357

5.10   Confocal Microscopy 362
        Vyvyan Howard, Arlene Hall and Mark Browne

5.10.1   General Considerations 362
5.10.1.1 Conventional Light Microscopy 363
5.10.1.2 Scanning Optical Microscopy 366

5.10.2   Features of Confocal Microscopy 366

5.10.3   Applications of Confocal Microscopy 372

5.10.4   Measurement 373

5.11   Flow Cytometry 376
        Manfred Kubbies

5.11.1   Principles 376

5.11.2   Analytical Applications 377
5.11.2.1 General Aspects 377
5.11.2.2 Analysis of Surface Antigens 378
5.11.2.3 Analysis of Intracellular Antigens 383
5.11.2.4 Cell Proliferation and Cell Activation 384

6   Application of Phenotype Analysis 387

**6.1   Immunological Detection of Membrane-bound Antigens and
        Receptors** 388
        Philippe Poncelet, Françoise George and Thierry Lavabre-Bertrand

6.1.1   General   388

6.1.2   Technical Considerations   388

6.1.3   Basic Research Applications   392
6.1.3.1   Cell and Tissue Distribution of Antigens   393
6.1.3.2   Biochemistry of Antigens   394
6.1.3.3   Molecular Genetics   394
6.1.3.4   Biological Functions   394

6.1.4   Clinical Applications   396
6.1.4.1   Acquired and Congenital Immunodeficiency Disorders   396
6.1.4.2   Genetically Inherited Immunodeficiency Disorders   397
6.1.4.3   Infectious Diseases   398
6.1.4.4   Autoimmune Diseases   399
6.1.4.5   Transplantation Immunology   399
6.1.4.6   Platelet Immunology   400

6.1.5   Oncology   401
6.1.5.1   Solid Tumours   401
6.1.5.2   Immune Phenotype in Haemopoietic Malignancies   402

6.1.6   Other Applications   404
6.1.6.1   Therapy and Monitoring of Therapy   404
6.1.6.2   Detection of Rare Cells   405

6.2   **Development of the Immune System**   418
          Françoise Dieterlen-Lièvre and Josselyne Salaün

6.2.1   General Considerations of Developmental Biology   418

6.2.2   Primary Lymphoid Organ Differentiation   420

6.2.3   T-Cell Differentiation during Ontogeny Followed through
          Phenotype Analysis   422

6.2.4   Haemopoietic Stem Cells   423

6.2.5   Tolerance   427

6.3   **Immunological Detection of Intracellular Structures/Antigens**   431

6.3.1   Cytoskeleton, Filaments and Tubules   431
          Kay E. Foster and Keith Gull
6.3.1.1   Autoantibodies Against the Cytoskeleton   432
6.3.1.2   Organelle Shot-gun Approach to Making Antibodies   433
6.3.1.3   Purified and Expressed Proteins as Cytoskeletal Antigens   434
6.3.1.4   Peptides and Specific Isotype Probes   435
6.3.1.5   Antibodies and Function of the Cytoskeleton   436

6.3.2   Chromatin and Chromosomal Proteins 439
         Michael Bustin
6.3.2.1 Immunogens, Antigens, Antisera and Assays 441
6.3.2.2 The Specificity of Chromosomal Proteins and Chromatin 443
6.3.2.3 Localization and Organization of Components in Chromatin and
         Chromosomes 444
6.3.2.4 Immunofractionation of Chromatin and Nucleosomes 445
6.3.2.5 Functional Analysis 446

6.3.3   The Mitotic Apparatus and Chromosomes 451
         Claudio E. Sunkel
6.3.3.1 Organization of the Chromosome Scaffold 452
6.3.3.2 Centromeric DNA 453
6.3.3.3 The Kinetochore 453
6.3.3.4 The Centrosome 455
6.3.3.5 The Mitotic Spindle 456
6.3.3.6 The Control of Mitosis 458

6.3.4   Mitochondria 463
         *Timothy M. Lever, Sanya J. Sanderson, Anne E. Taylor and
         J. Gordon Lindsay*
6.3.4.1 Production of Polyclonal Antiserum and Assessment of Quality .. 463
6.3.4.2 Immune Electron Microscopy 464
6.3.4.3 Immunological Detection and Characterization of Mitochondrial
         Antigens: the Versatility of Immunoblotting (Western Blotting) ... 465
6.3.4.3 Peptide Antibodies 471
6.3.4.5 Immunological Detection of Mitochondrial Proteins Synthesized
         in vivo or *in vitro* 473
6.3.4.6 Concluding Remarks 475

6.4   Immunological Detection of Extracellular Matrix Antigens 479
         Robert G. Price and Sarah A. Taylor

6.4.1   Collagens 480
6.4.1.1 Type I Collagen 480
6.4.1.2 Type II Collagen 484
6.4.1.3 Type III Collagen 484
6.4.1.4 Type IV Collagen 532

6.4.2   Laminin 489

6.4.3   Proteoglycans 491

6.4.4   General Considerations 493

7   **Immunoanalysis of Cell Function** 503

7.1   **Enzyme-Linked Immunospot (ELISPOT)**
Assays for Detection of Specific Antibody-Secreting Cells 504
Cecil Czerkinsky and Jonathon Sedgwick

7.1.1   General Considerations 504
7.1.1.1   The Choice of Method 504
7.1.1.2   Application 505
7.1.1.3   Advantages of Enzyme Assays for Enumerating ASC 507

7.1.2   ELISPOT Assays 507
7.1.2.1   Method Design 507
7.1.2.2   Selection and Adaptation of Assay Conditions 510
7.1.2.3   Equipment 512
7.1.2.4   Reagents and Solutions 512
7.1.2.5   Procedure 515

7.1.3   Alternative Techniques 518
7.1.3.1   ELISPOT Assays Employing Plastic-based Vessels 518
7.1.3.2   Immunoenzyme Amplification Techniques for Use in ELISPOT
Assays 521
7.1.3.3   Two-colour Technique (Bichromatic ELISPOT Test) 529

7.1.4   Validation and Performance of Method 531
7.1.4.1   Precision, Accuracy, Sensitivity and Detection Limit 531
7.1.4.2   Sources of Error 531
7.1.4.3   Specificity 532
7.1.4.4   Assessment for *de novo* Protein Synthesis 534

7.1.5   Appendix 535
7.1.5.1   Preparation of Single Cell Suspensions from Mouse Spleen 535
7.1.5.2   Preparation of KLH-coated Nitrocellulose-bottomed Dishes 535
7.1.5.3   Preparation of KLH-coated Plastic Dishes 536
7.1.5.4   Preparation of Agarose Substrate Solutions for Plastic-based
ELISPOT Assays 536
7.1.5.5   Biotinylation of Antibodies 537

7.2   **Cytokine Analysis in Cells** 540
Anthony R. Mire-Sluis, Meenu Wadhwa, Christopher R. Bird,
M. Gisella Cavallo, Lisa A. Randall and Robin Thorpe

7.2.1   Analysis of Cell Extracts 541
7.2.1.1   Radioimmunoassays (RIA) 542
7.2.1.2   IRMA and ELISA 543
7.2.1.3   Detection by Immunoblotting 544

7.2.2   Analysis of Individual Cells 546

7.2.2.1   Reverse Haemolytic Plaque Assay   546
7.2.2.2   Immunocytochemical Analysis   547
7.2.2.3   Flow-Cytometric Analysis of Intracellular Cytokines   552

7.2.3   Detection of Cytokine mRNA   553

8   Analysis of Immune Cell Function   557
           Frank Emmrich and Andreas H. Guse

8.1   The Nature of Immunocytes   558

8.2   Cell Isolation, Phenotyping and Culture   560

8.3   Signal Transduction   562

8.3.1   Protein Phosphorylation   562

8.3.2   Metabolism of Phosphoinositides and Inositol Phosphates   564

8.3.3   Free Cytosolic Calcium Concentration   564

8.4   Effector Function   565

8.4.1   Polyclonal *versus* Antigen-Specific Stimulation   566

8.4.2   B-Cell Functions   567

8.4.3   T-Cell Functions   568

8.5   Regulatory Interactions   569

Appendix   573
I   List of Symbols, Quantities, Units and Constants   574
II   List of Abbreviations   577
III   List of Symbols Used for the Figures   580

Index   583

List of Contributors

Editor-in-chief

Prof. Dr. René Masseyeff
Laboratoire d'analyses
biologiques spécialisées
57, Route de Canta-Gallet
F-06200 Nice
France
Tel.: (93)97 15 15
Fax: (93)96 68 16

Editors

Dr. Winfried H. Albert
Boehringer Mannheim GmbH
Forschungszentrum Tutzing
Dept. ST-B
Bahnhofstraße 9–15
D-82327 Tutzing
Germany
Tel.: (8158)22 40 16
Fax: (8158)22 45 17

Prof. Norman A. Staines
King's College London
Infection and Immunity Group
Campden Hill Road
London W8 7AH
United Kingdom
Tel.: (71)33 34 461
Fax: (71)33 34 607

Authors

Abrams, Don-Carlos
Dept. of Medical Physics
Royal Postgraduate Medical School
Hammersmith Hospital
Du Cane Road
UK-London W12 ONN
United Kingdom

Askonas, Brigitte A.
Molecular Immunology Group
Institute of Molecular Medicine
John Radcliffe Hospital
Headington
UK-Oxford OX3 9DU
United Kingdom

Bevan, Deborah J.
Guy's Hospital
Tissue Typing
New Guy's House
St. Thomas' Street
UK-London SE1 9RT
United Kingdom

Bird, Christopher R.
NIBSC
Blanche Lane
South Mimms
Potters Bar
UK-Hertfordshire EN6 3QG
United Kingdom

Bitensky, Lucille
Robens Institute of Health and Safety
University of Surrey
UK-Guildford, Surrey GU2 5XH
United Kingdom

Bolton, Bryan J.
ECACC/PHLS
Porton Down
Salisbury
UK-Wiltshire SP4 OJG
United Kingdom

Bøyum, Arne
Norwegian Defense Res.
Establishment
Division of Environmental Toxicology
N-2007 Kjeller
Norway

Browne, Mark
Confocal Technologies Ltd.
South Harrington Building
Sefton Street
UK-Liverpool L3 4BQ
United Kingdom

Bustin, Michael
Chief, Protein Section
Laboratory of Molecular Carcinogenesis
NCI, NIH
Bethesda, Maryland 20892
USA

Cavallo, Gisella M.
Cattedra di Endocrinologica (I)
II Clinica Medica
University of Rome "La Sapienza"
I-Rome
Italy

Chayen, Joseph
Robens Institute of Health and Safety
University of Surrey
UK-Guildford, Surrey GU2 5XH
United Kingdom

Czerkinsky, Cecil C.
Dept. of Medical Microbiology and
Immunology
University of Göteborg
Guldhedsgatan 10A
S-41346 Göteborg
Sweden

Emmrich, Frank
Max-Planck-Gesellschaft
Klinische Arbeitsgruppen für
Rheumatologie und Immunologie
Schwabachanlage 10
D-91054 Erlangen
Germany

Foster, Kay E.
Biological Laboratory
University of Kent
Canterbury
Kent CT2 7NJ
United Kingdom

George, Françoise
Laboratoire d'Hématologie
Faculté de Pharmacie
27 Bd J. Moulin
F-13385 Marseille Cedex (F)
France

Gordon, Simon
Sir William Dunn School of Pathology
South Parks Road
UK-Oxford OX1 3RE
United Kingdom

Gull, Keith
Dept. of Biochemistry and
Molecular Biology
University of Manchester
Medical School
Oxford Road
UK-Manchester M13 9PT
United Kingdom

Guse, A. H.
Max-Planck-Gesellschaft
Klinische Arbeitsgruppen für
Rheumatologie und Immunologie
Schwabachanlage 10
D-91054 Erlangen
Germany

Hall, Arlene
Quantitative 3-D Microscopy
Research Group
Dept. of Fetal and Infant Pathology
University of Liverpool
P.O. Box 147
UK-Liverpool L69 3BX
United Kingdom

Hamblin, Anne S.
Dept. of Pathology and
Infectious Diseases
The Royal Veterinary College
Royal College Street
UK-London NW1 0TU
United Kingdom

Harmsen, Allen G.
Trudeau Institute, Inc.
Biomedical Research Labs.
P.O. Box 59
Saranac Lake
New York
New York 12983
USA

Howard, Vyvyan
Dept. of Fetal and Infant Pathology
Royal Liverpool
Children's Hospital
Alder Hey
Eaton Road
P.O. Box 147
UK-Liverpool L12 3AP
United Kingdom

Hughes, D. A.
Sir William Dunn School of Pathology
South Parks Road
UK-Oxford OX1 3RE
United Kingdom

Kendall, Marion D.
AFRC Institute of Animal Physiology
and Genetic Research
Babraham
UK-Cambridge CB2 4AT
United Kingdom

Krell, Hans-Willi
Boehringer Mannheim GmbH
Forschungszentrum Penzberg
Dept. BB-MA 3
Nonnenwald 2
D-82377 Penzberg
Germany

Kubbies, Manfred
Boehringer Mannheim GmbH
Forschungszentrum Penzberg
Dept. BB-ZS 1
Nonnenwald 2
D-82377 Penzberg
Germany

Lamb, Jonathan R.
Dept. of Immunology
St. Mary's Hospital Medical School
Norfolk Place
UK-London W2 1PG
United Kingdom

Lavabre-Bertrand, Thierry
Service des Maladies du Sang
CHU Lapeyronie
555 Route de Ganges
F-34059 Montpellier Cedex (F)
France

Lever, Timothy M.
University of Glasgow
Dept. of Biochemistry
Glasgow G12 8QQ
Scotland

Lindsay, J. Gordon
University of Glasgow
Dept. of Biochemistry
Glasgow G12 8QQ
Scotland

MacPherson, G. Gordon
Sir William Dunn School of Pathology
University of Oxford
South Parks Road
UK-Oxford OX1 3RE
United Kingdom

Mire-Sluis, Anthony R.
NIBSC
Blanche Lane
South Mimms
Potters Bar
UK-Hertfordshire EN6 3QG
United Kingdom

Morris, Christopher B.
ECACC/PHLS
Porton Down
Salisbury
UK-Wiltshire SP4 OJG
United Kingdom

Mowles, Jon M.
ECACC/PHLS
Porton Down
Salisbury
UK-Wiltshire SP4 OJG
United Kingdom

Van Noorden, Susan
Histopathology Section
Royal Postgraduate Medical School
Hammersmith Hospital
Du Cane Road
UK-London W12 ONN
United Kingdom

O'Hehir, Robyn E.
Dept. of Immunology
St. Mary's Hospital Medical School
Norfolk Place
UK-London W2 1PG
United Kingdom

Peters, T. J.
Dept. of Clinical Biochemistry
King's College School of
Medicine & Dentistry
Bessemer Road
UK-London SE5 9PJ
United Kingdom

Poetsch, Matthias C. C.
Boehringer Mannheim GmbH
Forschungszentrum Penzberg
Dpt. BN-FM
Nonnenwald 2
D-82377 Penzberg
Germany

Poncelet, Philippe
Laboratoire d'Hématologie
Faculté de Pharmacie
27 Bd J. Moulin
F-13385 Marseille Cedex (F)
France

Price, Robert G.
Division of Life Sciences
King's College London
Campden Hill Road
UK-London W8 7AH
United Kingdom

Randall, Lisa A.
NIBSC
Blanche Lane
South Mimms
Potters Bar
UK-Hertfordshire EN6 3QG
United Kingdom

Sanderson, Sanya J.
University of Glasgow
Dept. of Biochemistry
Glasgow G12 8QQ
Scotland

Sedgwick, Jonathon
Centenary Institute of
Cancer Medicine
and Cell Biology
University of Sydney
Sydney
New South Wales 2006
Australia

Sieber, Klaus-Peter
Boehringer Mannheim GmbH
Forschungszentrum Penzberg
Nonnenwald 2
D-82377 Penzberg
Germany

Springall, David R.
Dept. of Histochemistry
Royal Postgraduate Medical School
Hammersmith Hospital
Du Cane Road
UK-London W12 ONN
United Kingdom

Staines, Norman A.
Infection and Immunity Group
King's College London
Campden Hill Road
UK-London W8 7AH
United Kingdom

Sunkel, Claudio E.
Instituto Nacional de
Investigação Científica
Centro de Citologia Experimental
Universidade do Porto
Portugal

Taylor, Anne E.
University of Glasgow
Dept. of Biochemistry
Glasgow G12 8QQ
Scotland

Taylor, Sarah A.
Division of Life Sciences
King's College London
Campden Hill Road
UK-London W8 7AH
United Kingdom

Thorpe, Robin
NIBSC
Blanche Lane
South Mimms
Potters Bar
UK-Hertfordshire EN6 3QG
United Kingdom

Wadhwa, Meenu
NIBSC
Blanche Lane
South Mimms
Potters Bar
UK-Hertfordshire EN6 3QG
United Kingdom

Wooding, F. B. Peter
AFRC Institute of Animal Physiology
and Genetics Research
Babraham
UK-Cambridge CB2 4AT
United Kingdom

1 General Introduction

Immunological Methods of Analysis of Cell Structure and Function

G. Gordon MacPherson

This, the third volume in the series, is devoted to methods used in the immunological analysis of cells and tissues. It provides a comprehensive, practical guide for both the novice and the expert. Its subject matter is not confined to strictly immunological methods but also describes in detail methods of cell preparation, culture and fractionation that are essential components of the investigation of cellular structure and function. Although the bulk of the volume deals with mammalian, and especially human, tissues, there are individual sections covering plant and prokaryotic cells. The application of immunological techniques to cells and tissues is covered extensively and in sufficient detail to enable even the inexperienced investigator to use them quickly and productively.

This introduction is designed to give an overview which will stimulate the interest of readers who may be inexperienced in these areas. It gives examples which, it is hoped, will highlight the excitement felt by workers who have found that immunoanalysis has opened up novel approaches to their research. In addition it will point out some of the more general problems and pitfalls which face investigators when they consider the application of immunological techniques to their work. The examples chosen are largely based on cellular immunology but should be of general interest to workers outside this area.

In recent years, the use of antibodies to investigate cell and tissue phenotype and function has been one of the most rapidly growing and productive techniques available to medicine and biology. Until the advent of *in situ* hybridization, no other approach was similarly able to identify the presence of a variety of specific molecules expressed in cells and tissues. However, even with *in situ* hybridization, construction of the specific probe is usually consequent to the initial identification and characterization of a molecule by an antibody. Also, the identification of mRNA in a cell does not necessarily mean that the corresponding protein is being synthesized. Two additional major advantages that antibodies possess in comparison with other analytical approaches are that they may be used as probes of molecular and cellular function and that the development of an antibody to a molecule is not necessarily dependent on an understanding of the structure or function of that molecule.

Why Antibodies?

It is a fortunate accident of evolution that we have such useful reagents available. The immune system evolved to protect against infectious disease and, in order so to do, it has developed the capacity to recognize pathogens as foreign. In that pathogens are composed of molecules largely similar to those present in their host, the immune system has to "learn" to discriminate between self and foreign and, as the differences between molecules present on pathogens and their hosts may be minimal, the better the immune system is at discriminating between similar molecules, the more efficient it will be in protection. Thus evolution has selected for receptors whose affinity for their ligands can be dramatically altered by single amino acid substitutions in proteins or by the stereochemical disposition of side-groups on haptens. It is this specificity of an antibody for distinct epitopes that makes it such an excellent probe of cellular and molecular structure and function.

Monoclonal antibodies: the explosion in the use of immunoanalysis in recent years is largely due to the widespread introduction of monoclonal antibodies (mAbs). The preparation and properties of mAbs are dealt with in detail in Volume II of this series and will only be considered in this volume where there is particular relevance to cell and tissue analysis. It is, however, worthwhile to review briefly some of those properties which make mAbs such valuable reagents. Until the advent of mAbs the only antibodies available were components of polyclonal antisera produced by xeno- or allo-immunization, with the disadvantages of non-reproducibility and instability, lack of specificity and frequently of low affinity. In contrast, mAbs are stable reagents, available in bulk, with a constant, defined specificity and functional affinity for their ligands. It is possible that a mAb might have a higher affinity for a ligand other than the one it is used to define, and in this sense an antiserum might be more specific for an antigen than a mAb, but in practice this has not proved to be a problem. Antisera do, however, have valuable roles to play and there are several situations where they are of more use than mAbs. Thus antisera, recognizing multiple epitopes on an antigens, are more likely to inhibit or stimulate function than are mAbs and they are more likely to be cytotoxic in the presence of complement.

Despite the enormously valuable properties of mAbs, they are not always ideal reagents. They are large molecules which do not diffuse easily, they are foreign proteins and are thus immunogenic when introduced into the species from which the antigen was derived and they are relatively difficult to make (by intentional immunization) in species other than rodents. Several approaches have been identified to overcome these problems. Molecular engineering is in the forefront of these approaches and offers exciting possibilities, for example making domain or mini-antibodies consisting of variable regions only, and inserting by genetic engineering the Ag-binding site from a mouse mAb into the framework of a human mAb. These approaches are described in detail in Volume 2.

Cell-mediated Immunity in Immunoanalysis

Although the great bulk of immunoanalysis depends on the use of antibodies as the specific detection reagents, it is worth considering the potential roles of cell-mediated immunity (CMI). CMI depends on the recognition of antigen by T-lymphocytes and it is now clear that the Ag receptor on T cells does not recognize whole molecules: rather, it recognizes small peptides of eight to twenty amino acids in length, bound to a groove on the surface of major histocompatibility complex (MHC) molecules. In general, peptides bound to Class II MHC molecules are derived from exogenous proteins and those bound to Class I from endogenous proteins [1]. Thus, CMI cannot easily be used to identify individual molecules. However, it does have a role in the analysis of intracellular events occurring during protein synthesis and metabolism. Thus, the investigation of mechanisms involved in the killing of virus-infected cells has led to the definition of a pathway by which endogenous proteins are metabolized within the cytoplasm and their degradation peptides transported to the rough endoplasmic reticulum where they associate with MHC Class I molecules. Another example is the identification of tumour-specific transplantation antigens. Many tumours induced by chemical carcinogens or ultraviolet light express specific antigens which can be recognised by CMI but not by antibodies. It has recently been shown in some elegant experiments that many of these antigens are derived from mutated endogenous proteins, not expressed at the cell surface, which explains the difficulty in characterising them by antibodies [2].

Cell Quantitation

General considerations

It is often essential to be able to count the number of cells of a specific type in a population and, if a type-specific marker is available, an antibody to this can be used as a label. For the majority of molecules, antibody is the only satisfactory label. The binding of antibody can be detected by a variety of systems, discussed elsewhere in this volume. It is, however, critically important to realize that the ability to detect the expression of a molecule by a cell is dependent on both the sensitivity of the assay used and the number of molecules present in or on the cell. This has important implications. Thus, many cell-surface molecules may be present individually in too few copies to be detectable above background by current technologies, although their presence can be revealed by functional assays. Perhaps more importantly, for many assays the sensitivity threshold is a function of the assay itself: for example, complement-mediated lysis of a cell is dependent on the approximation of two or more Fc antibody regions on the cell surface and thus on the number of copies of a molecule present, and, in rosetting assays, the definition of a rosette is decided by the observer and cells expressing few molecules may be counted as negative. Similarly, in techniques dependent on adhesion of cells to a substrate (cf. 4.1.1) such as panning, magnetic beads and column techniques, the adhesion of cells to the substrate is dependent on the number of molecules of antigen present, the binding affinity and the vigour with which the substrate is washed! It follows that in many methods of this kind, the proportion of cells counted as positive may not equate with the absolute numbers expressing the molecule. It also follows that, when changes are seen in the proportion of positive cells, one has to be careful that they do reflect absolute changes and not changes in the number of molecules expressed per cell, leading to an increase in the proportion detected above the sensitivity threshold.

Flow cytometry

When considering cells in suspension, flow cytometry has many advantages over other methods, in particular in its ability to quantitate rapidly the amount of antibody bound to a cell and to process large numbers of cells in a short time (cf. 5.11). By using a suitable reference antigen, the number of molecules of antibody per cell can be estimated and thus populations can be defined, not just as positive or negative, but in terms of the actual amount of antigen expressed. When this quantitative approach is combined with the use of two or more antibodies for labelling different molecules, and with the measurement of other parameters such as cell size and granularity by light scattering, the sizes and relationships of different subpopulations of cells can be depicted graphically with an accessibility and clarity that is unattainable with any other techniques. The advent of flow cytometers which are purely analytical and thus considerably cheaper has made this technology much more widely available.

Quantitation in tissues

The quantitation of specific cell types within tissues is an important goal for many workers but one that is difficult to achieve in practice. Ideally, this can be achieved by sophisticated image analysis systems (cf. 5.9) but such systems are complex, expensive and generally require considerable expertise in setting up and running. Most investigators are forced to rely on a visual approach which limits the number of cells that can be counted. Available methods are discussed in Section 5. Apart from this, there are some other possible pitfalls to consider. Often, one is trying to determine if the frequency of cells of a particular type changes within a tissue. Stereological considerations need to be considered in these cases. If the size distribution of the cells changes, the probability of a cell profile appearing in a section will also change, leading to over- or underestimates of actual cell numbers. Quantitation of the absolute amount of antigen present in a tissue can be achieved relatively easily by binding or absorption assays but the measurement of the amount of antigen present on individual cells within a tissue is much more difficult, requiring quantitative histochemical methods (cf. 5.8). In general, only relative amounts can be estimated and often all that can be said is that a cell is more or less strongly stained than others in the same tissue.

Cell Preparation and Separation

One of the major uses of antibodies is in the preparation of defined subpopulations of cells expressing a particular surface antigen (positive selection) or, alternatively, selectively to deplete a subpopulation (negative selection). Although much separation is done as a single stage procedure, for example by rosetting or cell sorting, there are relatively few cell surface molecules so far characterized that identify a specific lineage of cells or a specific differentiation stage. Thus, to isolate a "pure" population it is often necessary to use a series of procedures to achieve the desired degree of purity. These may involve separation using physical properties such as size, density or adhesiveness, chemical properties such as lectin binding, and one or more stages involving selection with antibodies.

Some cell populations such as blood (cf. 2.2), lymph or peritoneal cells are already present as suspensions but for others it is necessary to dissociate tissues or aggregates (cf. 2.5 and 2.6) and these procedures give rise to a number of problems. A major danger is that the preparation technique itself may alter the characteristics of the isolated cells. Thus treatment of tissues with proteolytic enzymes may cleave cell-surface molecules or possibly reveal novel antigenic epitopes not present on native molecules. Similarly, even short times in culture *in vitro* may alter the expression of some molecules and, with cell types such as macrophages, may dramatically alter their functional properties. Thus, it is often difficult to relate the phenotypic and functional properties of isolated cells to their *in situ* state.

A general problem with all methods of cell preparation and separation is that of differential cell loss. This may occur for a variety of reasons, many unpredictable. Thus differences in nonspecific adhesiveness may cause losses of particular cell types, while some cells, such as lymphoblasts, are particularly sensitive to mechanical damage. It follows that good "housekeeping" at every stage of the separation procedure is essential if spurious results are to be avoided. An example of the kind of difficulties that can be encountered is given by the isolation of lymphoid dendritic cells. These Ag-presenting cells are extracted from spleen by a combination of adherence, density-gradient centrifugation and rosetting. Their *in situ* counterpoint was thought to be the interdigitating cell present in T-cell areas. However, a mAb made against isolated dendritic cells, which stained all such cells, did not stain interdigitating cells; rather, it stained a population of cells in the marginal zone [3]. The clear implication is that interdigitating cells are not being isolated by the techniques utilized, perhaps because they remain bound to lymphocytes.

Immunocytochemistry

From elegant studies of the cell biology of Ag-processing at the electron microscope level to the diagnosis of the histological origin of undifferentiated tumours, immuno-cytochemistry has come to play an increasingly important role in laboratory practice. For many purposes, immunocytochemistry is a well-standardized, reliable and routine procedure but, in considering novel applications and developments, thought must be given to some of the potential pitfalls. There is almost always conflict between two goals in immunocytochemistry, the preservation of adequate morphological detail and the retention of antigenicity. The preservation of detail involves chemical stabilization of components of cells and tissues and the inhibition of natural autolytic processes by fixation with denaturing or cross-linking reagents. Any such process is likely to alter the conformation of epitopes and thus the affinity of antibody for them. Antigens, or rather their epitopes, vary enormously in their sensitivity to fixation and, in general, fixatives which give the best preservation of morphology are most likely to alter antigenicity. Most, but not all, antigens are not significantly affected by ethanol or acetone while many are totally destroyed by glutaraldehyde. In most cases an intermediate position has to be aimed for which will give acceptable morphology while retaining sufficient antigenicity to permit specific localization. There do not seem to be any rules available to help in this and the optimal conditions have to be defined empirically.

Cells in suspension need to be immobilized on a microscope slide prior to processing and this can be achieved by centrifugation (Cytospin) or by adhesion to poly-L-lysine coated slides. The advantage of the latter is that fewer cells are needed and that all cells are retained, but it has the disadvantage that cells do not flatten as well as with cytospins. Cytospins have the potential problems of uneven distribution of cells and selective loss during centrifugation.

For solid tissues, sections need to be cut, involving the need for mechanical stabilization by embedding or freezing. Cryomicrotomy is a routine procedure for light microscopy but thought must always be given to specimen size and freezing techniques. For diagnostic histopathology, however, cryomicrotomy is not generally available, and a major goal in this area is the definition of informative antigen epitopic markers which are stable to standard fixation and wax embedding.

Electron microscope immunocytochemistry is still a very difficult technique. Ultracryomicrotomy is a sophisticated technique requiring specialized facilities beyond the range of many laboratories and is subject to technical difficulties. Labelling of thin sections has, however, become rather more straightforward since the introduction of colloidal gold as a marker and the availability of particles of defined sizes permits double labelling (cf. 5.2.6). Many groups have investigated the use of resins as embedding media with very varied results. Only when antigen is present at high concentration is the technique reliable and most attempts to label membrane antigens have proved unsuccessful. Most resins require etching with more or less fierce reagents in order to reveal Ab-binding sites and it is surprising and gratifying that so many epitopes survive such treatment. Often, antigens present in granules are relatively easy to detect and it is of interest that, by scanning electron microscopy, in etched sections of cells the granules stand out as roughened hillocks, suggesting that a large number of epitopes may be exposed [4].

An alternative procedure for electron microscopy is to cut slices (50–100 μm) of tissue using a tissue slicer. These can be stained immunocytochemically after mild fixation, then post-fixed and embedded in resins. This approach has been widely used in studies of the nervous system but there are always likely to be problemse with limited diffusion of antibody into the section.

Antibody as a Probe of Function

In many instances, it is sufficient to be able to ascertain whether a cell or tissue expresses a particular antigen; for instance, whether a cell line thought to be endothelium-derived expresses the Factor VIII-related Ag, or whether a suspected case of AIDS has an altered CD4+/CD8+ T cell ratio in peripheral blood. The introduction of monoclonal technology into immunoanalysis has resulted in the identification of vast numbers of cell and tissue molecules, for many of which no function has been described even though they may define specific cell populations. It seems improbable that molecules detectable by antibody do not have physiological functions and it follows that antibody ought to be utilizable as a probe of that function.

One problem with mAbs is that they may not recognize an epitope on a molecule which has a known physiological function and thus they are unable to block or stimulate functional activity directly. Some investigators have avoided this problem by devising screening techniques for monoclonals which rely on the inhibition or stimulation of function, for example *Springer* [5] has defined functional molecules on lymphocytes and other cells by screening for inhibition of stimulation and *Woodruff* [6] identified a lymphocyte-homing receptor by screening for inhibition of lymphocyte binding to endothelium. However, most mAbs have not been defined in this way and there is usually no easy way of discovering the function of the molecules they recognize. Some clues may be gained by using mAb to isolate the molecule and, by constructing a suitable probe, isolating and sequencing the gene. This may identify the molecule as belonging to a particular family or superfamily but, for example, to ascribe a molecule to the immunoglobulin superfamily reveals very little about its function.

Often, attempts to discover function are a hit-and-miss affair and often they do not succeed. In rare cases, it seems clear from the cellular distribution of a molecule that it has a very specialized function but the mAb has no effect on any of the functions known to be restricted to that cell. This might be explained if the mAb was not recognizing a functional epitope. In these cases it may be worthwhile to use the mAb to isolate the molecule and then to make an antiserum to the pure form; the idea is that an antiserum will bind to multiple epitopes, one of which might be functional. Occasionally, the mAb, although not directly affecting function, may be able to modulate the expression of the molecule, permitting assays for loss of function.

In some instances, clinical findings can lead to the identification of functional molecules. For example, an autoantibody found in the serum of patients suffering from pemphigus vulgaris, a disease in which the skin forms large blisters, has been found to dissociate epidermal cell sheets growing in culture. The molecule involved has been identified as a cell surface protein, $M_r = 210000$ [7]. However, it is still the case that for many molecules defined by antibodies, almost everything is known about them except their function.

How an antibody recognizing a functional epitope on a molecule can be used depends on the nature and distribution of the molecule. For cell surface molecules, the assays are generally well defined and straightforward but, for intracellular molecules, the development of functional assays is in its infancy. The central problem lies in delivering the antibody to the relevant internal compartment of the cell and this usually relies on micro-injection with the consequence that only small numbers of cells can be examined.

A second approach to function is to use the antibody to isolate a population of cells expressing a particular molecule and then to determine which specific functions are associated with that population. Function can be assayed *in vitro* or in some cases *in vivo,* following adoptive transfer into animals. These approaches have been central to the definition of functional lymphocyte subpopulations in man and other species.

A third approach is to use antibody to affect cell populations *in vivo*. In animal models, antibodies to CD4 and CD8 can deplete lymphocyte populations very effectively but the isotype of the antibody used is critical. In other examples, mAbs can be used to inhibit the function of a molecule *in vivo*. Thus mAbs against MHC Class II molecules inhibit the development of CD4-restricted T-cells and mAbs to the TSH receptor may cause hyperthyroidism. The experimental and clinical use of mAbs in this way is, however, limited because of their antigenicity and this is one area where engineering through genetic modification is of central importance.

Future Prospects

Immunoanalysis is here to stay. There is no prospect of finding other markers of molecules with similar characteristics of specificity and discrimination. Much work in the future will be devoted to refining the production of antibodies, including obviating the need for immunization and the use of animals. Having developed the specific antibody, how it is used will depend on the needs and the imagination of the worker. Many groups are involved in improving the technical aspects of immunoanalysis, in particular by improving the signal to noise ratios in different assays in order to facilitate the detection of antigens present at low densities. New approaches in microscopy include the development of confocal (cf. 5.10) and laser-scanning microscopes and the introduction of computer-based image-refining techniques giving higher resolution and permitting analysis of living cells. Novel methods of cell manipulation, for example magnetic bead sorting (cf. 4.1), are already coming into use and will offer alternatives to the flow cytometer. In clinical practice, the number of diagnostic tests and assays available will continue to increase. In almost every area of biomedical research and clinical practice a worker without the tools of immunoanalysis at hand will be at a severe disadvantage.

The quantitative immunological analysis of the structure and function of cells and tissues is an area that, in particular, will witness great developments. The need for precise methods for basic and clinical investigators is pressing: this volume describes the current state of the art and discusses future developments.

References

[1] *F. M. Brodsky, L. E. Guagliardi*, The Cell Biology of Antigen Processing and Presentation, Ann. Rev. Immunol. *9*, 707–744 (1991).

[2] *C. Sibille, P. Chomez, C. Wildman, A. van Pel, E. de Plaen, J. L. Maryanski, V. de Bergeyck, T. V. Boon*, Structure of the Gene of Tumour Transplantation Antigen P198: A Point Mutation Generates a New Antigenic Peptide, J. Exp. Med. *172*, 35–45 (1990).

[3] *J. P. Metlay, M. D. Witmer-Pack, R. Agger, M. T. Crowley, D. Lawless, R. M. Steinmann*, The Distinct Leukocyte Integrins of Mouse Spleen Dendritic Cells as Identified with New Hamster Monoclonal Antibodies, J. Exp. Med. *171*, 1753–1772 (1990).

[4] *S. Enestrom, B. Kniola*, Quantitative Ultrastructural Immunocytochemistry Using a Computerized Image Analysis System, Stain Technol. *65*, 263–278 (1990).

[5] *T. A. Springer, M. L. Dustin, T. K. Kishimoto, S. D. Marlin*, The Lymphocyte Function-associated LFA-1, CD2 and LFA-3 Molecules: Cell Adhesion Receptors of the Immune System. Ann. Rev. Immunol. *5*, 223–252 (1987).

[6] *J. J. Woodruff, L. M. Clarke, H. Y. Chin*, Specific Cell-adhesion Mechanisms Determine Migration Pathways of Recirculating Typhocytes. Ann Rev. Immunol. *5*, 201–222 (1987).

[7] *J. R. Stanley, L. Koulu, C. Thivolet*, Distinction between Epidermal Antigens Binding Pemphigus Vulgaris and Pemphigus Foliaceous Antigens, J. Clin Invest. *77*, 313–320 (1984).

2 Preparation of Cells and Tissues

2.1   General Considerations

Anne S. Hamblin

It may seem obvious to state that cells and tissues outside the body may not behave in the same way as those within the body. They are no longer subject to the homeostatic control mechanisms which influence the behaviour of the whole organism. Detached from their blood supply and innervation, they lack the vital signals which make the organism function as a whole. Nonetheless, scientists wishing to study the function of cells or tissues may often only be able to do so by removing them from the whole organism, and placing them under conditions of warmth and nutrition in which they can remain viable and functional. Under well controlled conditions, it is accepted that normal, or near normal, behaviour may be observed *ex vivo*.

Much has been learnt from *ex vivo* examination of cells and tissues that has contributed to our modern understanding of cell and molecular biology. By examination of the structure and function of normal healthy cells and tissues *in vitro*, in comparison with those which are abnormal or diseased, and by examination of the responses of cells and tissues to outside stimuli, our understanding of pathology and physiology has been much extended. Such advances can only be made with confidence when the quality of the cells and tissues is assured.

Clearly the choice of cells and of tissues depends on the nature of the experiment. However, there are some general considerations that apply to the preparation and handling of cells and tissues outside the body. Awareness of these considerations ensures that experimenters understand the quality of the material with which they work and thus the limitations of the conclusions that they may draw. This Section focuses on general considerations which should be applied to the preparation of cells for immunological analysis as well as those which apply to the use of immunological methods to prepare cells.

2.1.1   Cells

Cells may be recovered from organs or tissues in which they occur freely, such as blood, lymph, cerebrospinal fluid, lung (alveolar spaces) or the peritoneal cavity, and can be used as they are retrieved, with minimal *in vitro* manipulation. Alternatively, cells can be derived from tissues, the architecture of which is disrupted by mechanical or enzymatic means [1–4]. Generally cells from either of these sources represent a mixture of one or more different cell types, which may be further manipulated to obtain a particular cell type, or subpopulation of a cell type [2, 3, 5–7]. The desirability of the methods used will depend on a combination of their speed, and the recovery, viability and purity of the cells.

To bypass some of the preparative problems associated with the impurity of cells from primary tissues, standard cell lines may be obtained from tissue culture collections, or cell lines or clones can be derived from primary cultures in individual laboratories [3, 4, 8]. These may have the advantage of being homogeneous, but also the disadvantage, because of the extensive selection process necessary in producing them, of being far removed from "normality".

2.1.1.1   Estimating Cell Numbers

There is an obvious need to know the numbers of cells available for any experimental procedure. In addition, there is often a need to estimate cell growth and to estimate cell recovery after various *in vitro* manipulations. The two major methods of estimating cell numbers involve using either a haemocytometer or an electronic particle counter, such as the *Coulter* counter [1, 9, 10]. Whatever the method, it is vital that cells are thoroughly, but gently, mixed prior to sampling, since cells sediment very rapidly. Mix by shaking, pipetting or mechanical vortexing but avoid foaming since bubbles trap cells in a high-shear environment. The amount of tolerated physical abuse depends on the cell type being used and this is something with which the operator must become familiar. Finally, to get an accurate count it is essential that the cells are in a single cell suspension and that there are no clumps.

Counting cells with a haemocytometer

This has the advantage of being simple, cheap and informative; the experimenter is able to look at the cells directly. The disadvantage is that that the technique may have poor statistical precision because of the small number of cells counted. Counting cells by use of a light microscope can be facilitated by first staining the cells. This may be particularly important if there is a need to distinguish different types for example, on the basis of nuclear structure, as might be needed for a peripheral blood differential cell count. Cell stains such as crystal violet (0.1 % w/v in water, used at a one in ten dilution) or *Turk's* solution (0.1 % (w/v) solution of crystal violet in 3 % acetic acid) are appropriate. The latter solution is useful if contaminating red cells are a problem, since they are removed prior to counting by lysis by the acetic acid. Cells are mixed with the dye and allowed to stand for 1 min, before mixing thoroughly and putting in the haemocytometer.

Method

1. The counting chamber must be clean and dry. Wash the chamber thoroughly with water and then alcohol or acetone and finally dry it.
2. Moisten two parallel sides of the coverslip or haemocytometer, and press the coverslip firmly but gently down onto the haemocytometer. Look for the *Newton's* rings between the coverslip and the slide. These are the interference-generated rainbow colours.

3. Dilute the cells in tissue culture medium with or without a cell stain to give a suitable cell concentration for counting (in the range 10^5 to 10^7/ml) and mix well for about 2 min.

4. Smoothly transfer the cell suspension to one half of the chamber with a *Pasteur* pipette. Run in sufficient to cover the area, but not so much that fluid runs into the troughs.

5. Keep horizontal and allow the cells to settle for 1 min.

6. Using a $\times 10$ or a $\times 40$ objective count at least 200 cells according to a pattern (Fig. 1 b). Count only those cells which are inside or touching the bottom and left hand borders.

7. Calculate the concentration. The standard chamber depth is 0.1 mm and each small square (Fig. 1 a, squares 5A,B,C,D, or E) has sides of 0.2 mm. The area is therefore $0.04\ mm^2$. Count all of the cells in the central area (Fig. 1 a, square 5 contains 25 small squares) and multiply this value by 10^4 to calculate the cell concentration. Count 200–500 cells. If there are insufficient cells in this central square, count the four corner squares (Fig. 1 a, squares 1 to 4, each containing 16 small squares) as well. Five squares of equivalent area have now been counted. Divide the number by five before multiplying by 10^4.

8. Make an adjustment for the dilution made at the beginning with tissue culture medium or cell stain to obtain the final cell concentration.

9. Repeat the count to ensure accuracy.

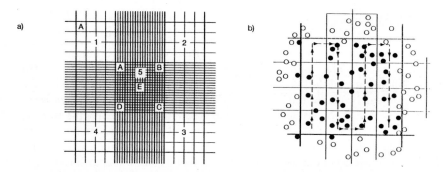

Fig. 1. Grid markings on an improved *Neubauer* haemocytometer and the method of counting cells.
a) All the markings are shown. The heavy lines are in fact triple lines. When cells are sparse they are counted in squares 1 to 5 inclusive. The concentration of cells is determined as described in the text. When cells are numerous they are counted in squares 5A,B,C,D and E. The area of square 1=2=3=4=5 and the area of square 5A=5B=5C=5D=5E.
b) The counting sequence to be followed. The figure shows an enlargement of square 5A. Cells indicated ● are included, those indicated ○ are excluded from the count.
From *L. B. Page, P. J. Culver*, Syllabus of Laboratory Examinations in Clinical Diagnosis, Harvard University Press. Reprinted by Permission.

Electronic particle counting

The particle counting equipment draws a known volume of diluted cell suspension through a hole across which an electric potential is maintained [9, 10]. Cells may be discriminated on the basis of size, and by setting the threshold, small debris and red cells may be gated out if necessary. Alternatively, red cells may be lysed with saponin solution available in commercial form (Zaponin, *Coulter*).

The advantage of this method is that a large number of events may be recorded and therefore that statistically accurate data may be rapidly accumulated. The disadvantage is that the cells are only recorded as particles and therefore there is no qualitative control of them as is possible with light microscopy.

2.1.1.2   Estimating Cell Viability

For the *in vitro* investigation of cell function it is essential to work with live cells [1, 2, 4]. In addition, investigation of the cell surface expression of molecules may require live-cell staining, since dead cells may take up dyes and stain differently. Cells teased from tissues will have a reduced cell viability compared with free cells derived from body fluids [2]. Once taken from their usual environment, cells start to die and the rapidity with which this occurs depends on the type of cell and the ways in which it is handled. Shear forces and mechanical stress, temperature changes, inappropriate handling media and time thus may all contribute to an unacceptable loss of viability [1]. Assessment of cell viability therefore forms an important component of cell processing *ex vivo*. It is hard to know when a cell is irrevocably dead, but a number of methods are available for estimating viability, each of which is appropriate for a different type of cell analysis. Each provides some estimate of the state of health of the general population under study.

Dye exclusion

The ability of a cell to exclude a dye is a reflection of intactness of the cell membrane. A number of dyes are therefore excluded by live cells and taken up by dead cells. These include dyes for light microscopy (Trypan blue, eosin Y and nigrosin) and for fluorescence microscopy and flow cytometry analysis (propidium iodide).

Trypan blue

This is the most commonly used dye for light microscopy and stains dead cells blue. These can be easily distinguished from live cells, which remain unstained. It is essential to operate within the times indicated below as cells will continue to die during the process.

Method

1. Mix 10 µl of cell suspension at approximately 10^6 cells/ml with 10 µl of trypan blue solution (0.1 % w/v in PBS, *Dulbecco's A, Oxoid,* pH 7.3).
2. Without delay, run suspension into a haemocytometer counting chamber and allow 1 min for the cells to settle.
3. Within 2–3 min count the numbers of blue and unstained cells and express the number of blue cells as a percentage of the total number of cells counted. This gives the percentage of dead cells. At total of at least 100 cells must be counted to give an accurate estimation.

Eosin Y

Unlike trypan blue the uptake of eosine Y [8] is affected by serum, so cells must be resuspended in protein-free medium for counting. Dead cells are stained red and viable cells remain unstained.

Method

Prepare a stock solution of 0.2 % eosin (w/v) in PBS. Be sure that the eosin is suitable for vital staining, and mix equal volumes of cells and dye as for trypan blue method above. Follow steps 2 and 3 as above but here count the number of red and unstained cells. Calculate the number of dead cells as in (3) above.

Nigrosin

This dye [2] is also excluded by live cells: dead cells appear black. The procedure is the same as for trypan blue above using a 0.2 % (w/v) solution of nigrosin in PBS.

Propidium iodide

Propidium iodide [11] is a fluorescent dye that intercalates double-stranded nucleic acids. It is unable to penetrate intact membranes, but when a cell dies the dye crosses the membrane and binds to the nucleic acid. In blue light dead cells fluoresce red and viable cells are unstained.

Method

Prepare a filtered stock solution of propidium iodide at a concentration of 2.5 g/l in PBS and add to cells at a final concentration of 25 mg/l. The concentration of the cells is determined by the counting method to be used but a concentration of around 10^7 cells/ml is appropriate for both fluorescence microscopy and flow cytometry [11, 12]. For fluorescence microscopy, score in a haemocytometer or as a wet preparation using a microscope set up for fluorescein optics. Dead cells fluoresce red.

For flow cytometry the sample is analysed for a gate set on negative red fluorescence, i.e. live cells. The proportion of red cells is the proportion of dead cells (Fig. 2). Flow cytometric methods have the advantage of analysing large numbers of cells, and therefore of being very accurate, and of being objective. They have the disadvantage of counting particles rather than permitting the direct visualization of cells (cf. 5.11).

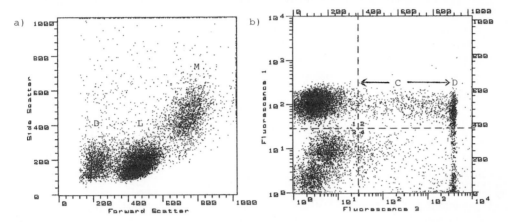

Fig. 2. Flow cytometry profiles of a mononuclear cell preparation obtained from Ficoll/Hypaque separation of human blood which had subsequently been frozen in liquid nitrogen and then thawed.
a) The axes are forward scatter (size) and side scatter (granularity).
The separation of lymphocytes (L), monocytes (M) and debris (D) is displayed.
b) The axes are: Fluorescence 1, detecting green FITC labelling; and Fluorescence 3, detecting red propidium iodide staining. Cells had been labelled with FITC-conjugated anti-CD3 antibody and propidium iodide. Quadrants 1 and 2 contain CD3 positive cells; cells in quadrant 3 and 4 are CD3 negative. The cells in quadrants 1 and 3 are not stained with propidium iodide and are alive. The cells in 2 and 4 are stained with propidium iodide; of these, the cells beneath the D are dead and those between D and the quadrant line (under region C) are showing some degree of breakdown in membrane integrity. A gate may be set to exclude dead cells.

Dye uptake

An alternative to staining dead cells as above is to stain the live cells and leave the dead cells unstained [1, 11]. The dye fluorescein diacetate stains intact cells green. The cells may, in addition, be stained simultaneously with propidium iodide as above, so that live cells appear green and dead cells red.

Method

Mix cells at a concentration of 10^6 cells/ml with an equal volume of fluorescein diacetate solution (100 µg/l) and/or propidium iodide (100 µg/l). Estimate the proportions of red and green cells by fluorescence microscopy or flow cytometry.

2.1.1.3   Handling Conditions

Cells removed from the body are subject to the stresses of physical handling, temperature change and an abnormal nutritional environment [1, 4]. These have the effect of reducing cell viability and cell recovery. By and large, the more cells are handled the less likely they are to survive intact. In addition, cells may be altered by their physical treatment. Antigenic epitopes may be lost and others may be upregulated. Different cells vary in their capacity to withstand the stress of these changes. Thus, whilst human peripheral blood lymphocytes withstand physical handling and survive well in culture for days, human polymorphs are very easily activated and start to die within hours of being removed from the body [9, 10]. What follows is a general description of the factors to be taken into consideration when dealing with cells *ex vivo*. However, it is important to realize that cells vary greatly in their resilience to abuse.

Handling medium

When handling cells *in vitro* [1, 4] it is necessary to maintain them at the correct pH: the normal pH of blood is 7.4 and cells deriving from that source need to be maintained at that pH. Cells may be maintained at the correct pH with simple media buffered with phosphate, which has strong buffering capacity on exposure to air. Phosphate-buffered saline (PBS) or modifications of it (*Dulbecco's A* or *B*) are satisfactory. High concentrations of phosphate cannot be tolerated for long and therefore hydrogen carbonate-buffered solutions, such as *Earle's* or *Hank's* balanced salt solutions (BSS), or tissue culture media such as RPMI 1640 or Minimal Essential Medium (MEM) are used for more protracted cell handling and culture. These gradually lose CO_2 to the air so that the solution becomes more alkaline. Generally, this alkalinity is obvious because a dye is incorporated into the culture medium which is orange at pH 7.4 and becomes purple at alkaline pH. The pH can be maintained by storing cells in an atmosphere of 5 % CO_2 in air. Alternatively, the solution can be buffered with HEPES (*N*-[2-hydroxy-ethyl]piperazine-*N*'-[2-ethanesulphonic acid]) which buffers over the pH range 6.8–8.2 in air.

A further factor critical to the handling of cells, particularly for extended periods of time, is the provision of nutritional support. This is provided by a number of synthetic media designed for different types of cells, each containing salts and amino acids required for maintenance and growth. The growth media usually come from the manufacturer unsupplemented and further additions of glutamine (a particularly labile amino acid), serum and antibiotics may be necessary. Growth nutrients which are not well defined are usually provided by serum, which may be autologous or heterologous, and which is present in media at concentrations of around 5–20 %. The choice of serum depends on the nature of cells and the experiment. However, it is important to realize that batches of serum may vary considerably in their growth-supporting activity. Some may be toxic and some may stimulate growth unacceptably. It is therefore wise to test serum in advance in the type of experiments to be undertaken, and then to acquire enough of an appropriate batch for all of the run of experiments. As an alternative to the addition of serum, commercial serum-free media are now available, again synthesized for specific purposes.

Finally, it is important to handle cells under sterile conditions if they are to be studied for extended periods *ex vivo,* since the culture conditions for cells also favour the growth of fungi, mycoplasma and bacteria. Sterility is usually ensured by handling cells in laminar flow conditions using sterile glassware and plastics, with sterile technique. Further insurance against infection may be obtained by adding antibiotics such as penicillin, streptomycin (anti-bacterial), gentamicin (anti-mycoplasma and anti-bacterial) and nystatin (anti-fungal) to tissue culture growth media. Particular care is needed when taking cells from experimental animals in which contact with fur and skin may result in contamination. A more extensive treatment of handling media is presented in 3.

The mechanical effects of cell separation

Cells are susceptible to shear forces, such as those that arise from centrifugation, pipetting and traumatic disruption from the tissues in which they normally reside, or from the surface on which they are attached, if they are growing in adherent culture [1, 3, 4]. Obviously, there is great variation between cells in their tolerance of shear forces. Thus, dendritic cells, with their long processes, are highly susceptible to shear forces and special measures must be adopted to recover them. It is advisable that centrifugation to pellet cells is at low g force (200–400 × g). When cells are cushioned on a density gradient, so that they do not form a pellet, higher g forces can be tolerated. Pipetting must be by gentle suction and expulsion with minimal air bubble formation.

Separation of cells from tissues requires unavoidable stress. Homogenization is the most brutal method and should be avoided in favour of teasing if possible. Enzymes which digest the proteins which attach cells to their matrix or physical support, such as trypsin, or which dissolve the matrix support, such as collagenase, provide a more gentle means of disruption. However, enzymes have the disadvantage of altering the expression of molecules on the cell surface. When cells grow attached to a glass or plastic surface they may be removed by physical scraping, but this can be physically very damaging. Gentler methods of detaching cells from their surface include EDTA and low temperature, although these may also cause cell disruption and may alter function.

Cells tend to stick to each other and to the vessel in which they are contained. This can lead to a loss of cells and to difficulties in accurately determining cell numbers. There is great variability in stickiness amongst different cells and thus the measures taken to avoid losses vary. Macrophages generally will adhere to surfaces available to them; cell losses may be avoided by working at 4 °C or by keeping cells in vessels made of polycarbonate or Teflon to which they adhere poorly. Sticking and clumping of cells tends to be much more pronounced when there is much cell death and therefore preservation of cell viability is likely to reduce cell losses due to adherence. Adherence of cells which are not normally particularly adherent can be reduced in the presence of protein, either in the form of serum or a small amount (0.2 %) of bovine serum albumin (BSA).

Temperature

The temperature at which mammalian cells live *in vivo* is accepted as being around 37 °C. Thus, the protracted maintenance of cells outside the body is usually at that temperature [1, 4].

The best temperature for manipulating cells *ex vivo* depends on the cell and the experiment but is usually 4 °C or room temperature. Cellular metabolism and membrane fluidity slow down when cells are cooled and this may be advantageous. For example, staining of live cells for immunofluorescent analysis with monoclonal or polyclonal antibodies against cell-surface antigens is usually undertaken at 4 °C, at which temperature cell-surface proteins remain evenly distributed [2, 3, 12]. At 37 °C the cell surface complex of cell-surface antigen and antibody may become polarized to one end of the cell to form a cap.

Although it is traditional and convenient to manipulate cells at temperatures lower than 37 °C outside the body, the very act of altering the temperature at which cells are maintained may bring about cellular changes which are experimentally important. Thus, human polymorphs cooled from 37 °C to 4 °C and then re-warmed increase their expression of various cell-surface antigens [13] which are important to polymorph functions.

2.1.2   Tissues

Some of the general considerations for the preparation of cells also apply to the preparation of tissues. However, there are also some special considerations in dealing with tissues for structural or functional analysis *in vitro*. Whilst estimating cell number does not arise, the handling conditions and viability of a tissue are important. Viability is particularly important if function is to be evaluated.

Tissues may be required in order to make sections for structural study by light or electron microscopy [14], for studying epitope expression by immunocytochemistry or fluorescence microscopy [12, 15, 16], or for studying gene expression by the polymerase chain reaction [17] or by *in situ* hybridization [18]. Here the major considerations are the preservation of antigenic epitopes or nucleic acid integrity, together with the preservation of an adequate morphology, so that interpretation of expression may be made in relation to structure. Such preservation is usually by fixation.

Tissues may be put into fixative immediately after removal from the body, thereby stopping the process of degeneration which starts at once. If this is impossible, the process can be slowed by storing the tissues at 4 °C. It must be remembered that time is needed for the fixative to penetrate the tissue: therefore, it is often preferable to use small pieces of tissue. Alternatively, the tissue may be preserved by snap freezing in isopentane at −70 °C, and the frozen sections can be cut before fixation. The range of fixatives available is wide and the choice depends on the nature of the subsequent experiment. The experimenter must choose with care, particularly if the interest is in the preservation of antigenic epitopes [11, 15]. Not all fixatives are suitable for all epitopes and new epitopes may be revealed by the fixation procedures.

Whole organs are sometimes required for transplantation and *in vitro* culture. Transplantation experience has indicated periods for which the organs may be kept cool at 4 °C, the so-called cold ischaemic time, and warm at room temperature or body temperature, the so-called warm ischaemic time, if they are to remain viable and functional for transplant [19]. Organs have a short life *ex vivo* which may be extended if they are perfused with, or immersed in, a suitable nutrient solution to replace the blood supply as a source of nutrients, and are kept at body temperature. Such organs may either be transplanted or may be cultured for hours or days, which may be sufficient time to allow their function or metabolic activity to be observed.

In conclusion, cells and tissues provide material with which to study the structure and function of living organisms *in vitro* in ways which are impossible *in vivo*. Additionally, they can also be manipulated *in vitro* and returned to the same or a different host for evaluation *in vivo*. Cells and tissues are therefore vital to many areas of biological research and clinical practice. The value of any information derived from these manipulations depends upon the quality of material used, and an understanding of the limitations of the investigative system.

References

[1] *S. Hunt*, Preparation of Lymphocytes and Accessory Cells, in: *G. G. B. Klaus* (ed.), Lymphocytes; a Practical Approach, IRL/Oxford University Press, Oxford 1987, pp. 1–34.

[2] *L. Hudson, F. C. Hay*, Practical Immunology, 3rd edition, Blackwell Scientific Publications, Oxford 1989.

[3] *D. M. Weir, L. A. Herzenberg, C. Blackwell, L. A. Herzenberg* (eds.), Handbook of Experimental Immunology, Volume 2; Cellular Immunology, 4th edition, Blackwell Scientific Publications, Oxford 1986.

[4] *R. I. Freshney*, Culture of Animal Cells: a Manual of Basic Technique, A. Liss, New York 1987.

[5] *D. W. Mason, W. J. Penhale, J. D. Sedgwick*, Preparation of Lymphocyte Subpopulations, in: *G. G. B. Klaus* (ed.), Lymphocytes; a Practical Approach, IRL/Oxford University Press, Oxford 1987, pp. 35–54.

[6] *S. Funderud, K. Nustad, T. Lea, F. Vartdal, G. Gaudernack, P. Stenstad, J. Ugelstad*, Fractionation of Lymphocytes by Immunomagnetic Beads, in: *G. G. B. Klaus* (ed.), Lymphocytes; a Practical Approach, IRL/Oxford University Press, Oxford 1987, pp. 55–65.

[7] *L. A. Herzenberg, R. G. Sweet, L. A. Herzenberg*, Fluorescence-activated Cell Sorting, Sci. Am. *234 (3)*, 108–116 (1976).

[8] *P. M. Taylor, D. B. Thomas, K. H. G. Mills,* In Vitro Culture of T Cell Lines and Clones, in: *G. G. B. Klaus* (ed.), Lymphocytes; a Practical Approach, IRL/Oxford University Press, Oxford 1987, pp. 133–147.

[9] *I. Chanarin* (ed.), Laboratory Haematology; an Account of Laboratory Techniques, Churchill-Livingstone, Edinburgh 1989.

[10] *J. V. Dacie, S. M. Lewis,* Practical Haematology, 6th edition, Churchill-Livingstone, Edinburgh 1984.

[11] *M. G. Ormerod* (ed.), Flow Cytometry; a Practical Approach, IRL/Oxford University Press, Oxford 1990.

[12] *G. Janossy, P. Amlot,* Immunofluorescence and Immunochemistry, in: *G. G. B. Klaus* (ed.), Lymphocytes; a Practical Approach, IRL/Oxford University Press, Oxford 1987, pp. 670–108.

[13] *K. D. Forsyth, R. J. Levinsky,* Preparative Procedures of Cooling and Rewarming Increase Leukocyte Integrin Expression and Function on Neutrophils, J. Immunol. Methods *128,* 159–163 (1990).

[14] *D. C. Pease, K. R. Porter,* Electron Microscopy and Ultramicrotomy, J. Cell Biol. *91,* 287s–292s (1981).

[15] *J. M. Polak, S. Van Noorden* (eds.), Immunocytochemistry, Butterworths-Heinemann, London 1986.

[16] *M. Spencer,* Fundamentals of Light Microscopy, Cambridge University Press, Cambridge 1982.

[17] *J. L. Marx,* Multiplying Genes by Leaps and Bounds, Science *240,* 1408–1410 (1988).

[18] *M. L. Pardue, J. G. Gell,* Molecular Hybridisation of Radioactive DNA to the DNA of Cytological Preparations. Proc. Natl. Acad. Sci. U.S.A. *64,* 600–604 (1969).

[19] *L. Brent, R. A. Sells,* Organ Transplantation; Current Clinical and Immunological Concepts, Ballieère Tindall, London 1989.

2.2   Blood and Its Constituent Cells

Arne Bøyum

Density gradient techniques for separation of white blood cells are based on differences in physical properties of cells. The sedimentation rate of cells depends strongly on cell size. Yet most techniques for separation of major subgroups are based on distinct density differences. For example, mononuclear cells (MNC) have a lower density than granulocytes and erythrocytes and efficient separation is achieved by using a separation fluid of intermediate density [1, 2]. However, it appears that the density distribution of MNC differs between species. Consequently it is not always possible to devise standard procedures that are applicable to all species. Thus, routine methods established with human blood do not necessarily yield satisfactory results with blood from other species. A common observation is that animal MNC (rat, rabbit) have a higher density than MNC in human blood. This may not only reduce the yield of MNC, but the granulocyte purity is reduced as well, due to contamination with MNC that move to the bottom during centrifugation. This problem may be overcome by increasing the density of the separation fluid, while the osmolality is kept constant. Another approach is to decrease the osmolality, at constant density of the separation fluid. The cells react promptly to a change of medium osmolality. In hypertonic medium the cells expel water, shrink, and the density increases. In a hypotonic environment the opposite effect is seen. For this purpose, Nycodenz, a non-ionic X-ray contrast medium is recommended. A favourable property of Nycodenz is that its osmolality and density can easily be varied over a broad range [3, 4].

The sections that follow describe routine procedure for separation of white blood cells by density gradient techniques. Furthermore, it will be demonstrated how improved cell purity may be obtained by fine adjustment of gradient medium density and osmolality.

2.2.1   Reagents and Solutions

Dextran 500 *(Pharmacia)*, 6% solution in 0.9% (w/v) NaCl, Hydroxy-ethyl starch (Plasmasteril, *Fresenius AG,* Bad Homburg, Germany), 6% solution in 0.9% (w/v) NaCl.

Iron particles in suspension, obtained as Lymphocyte Separating Reagent (*Technicon Instruments Co.* Tarrytown, N.Y.), or prepared as described [5].

Percoll *(Pharmacia)*. Mix 9 volumes stock solution with 1 volume 9% (w/v) NaCl. Measure the density and dilute with 0.9% NaCl, to desired density.

Lymphoprep (LP) 9.6% Isopaque, 5.6% Ficoll, density 1.077 g/ml) from *Nycomed,* Oslo, Norway.

Polyprep *(Nycomed)*. Density 1.113 g/ml, osmolality 460 mOsm/kg.

Histopaque *(Sigma)*. Density 1.119 g/ml, osmolality 490 mOsm/kg.

Preparation of Nycodenz solutions. Nycodenz (ND), *(Nycomed)* is a non-ionic, iodinated gradient medium, available as a 27.6% stock solution with density of 1.15 g/ml and osmolality of 290 mOsm/kg. A separation fluid of chosen density (d_2) is obtained by mixing V parts of Nycodenz stock solution with V_1 parts of a NaCl solution, V_1 being calculated from eqn. (a).

(a) $$V_1 = \frac{V\,(d - d_2)}{(d_2 - d_1)}$$

where d is the density of Nycodenz (1.15 g/ml) and d_1 the density of the NaCl solution, which is calculated as follows

(b) $$d_1 = 0.9982 + \frac{0.7\,m}{100}$$

where 0.9982 is the density of water (20°C), and m is the mass of NaCl in g per 100 ml solution. The best accuracy is obtained by using weighed fractions of the two components, rather than by measuring volumes. The desired osmolality is obtained by appropriate adjustment of the NaCl concentration. Table 1 gives recipes for a selection of Nycodenz-NaCl solutions. A computer program providing recipes for Nycodenz-NaCl solutions is available [4].

Table 1. Recipes for making Nycodenz-NaCl solutions, calculated by means of a computer programme

NaCl solutions to be mixed with 10 ml Nycodenz (27.6%)

Concentration (%)	Weight (g)[1]	Final density (g/ml)	Final osmolality (mOsm/kg)
0.96[2]	13.10	1.068	325
1.00[3]	13.13	1.068	335
0.62	9.82	1.077	260
0.65[4]	9.85	1.077	265
0.67	9.88	1.077	270
0.73	9.93	1.077	280
0.78[5]	9.99	1.077	290
0.78[6]	7.59	1.087	290
0.58	6.58	1.090	260
0.65	6.89	1.090	270
0.71	6.93	1.090	280
0.78	6.97	1.090	290
0.48[7]	4.64	1.103	260

[1]   The weight (g) of NaCl solutions of various concentration to be mixed with 10 ml (11.5 g) Nycodenz (27.6%) to obtain a separation fluid of desired density and osmolality.
[2, 3] Gradient media for separation of monocytes from human blood.
[4]   Nycodenz solution for separation of MNC and granulocytes from blood of rabbits, rats and mice.
[5]   Nycodenz solution for separation of MNC and granulocytes from human blood.
[6, 7] Nycodenz solutions (10 parts) to be mixed with plasma/serum (2 parts), for separation of human MNC and granulocytes with one solution[6], or a two-layer system[6,7].
[3, 4, 5] Commercially available gradient media.

2.2.2   Cell Separation Procedures

2.2.2.1   Preparation of Unfractionated Leucocytes

Unfractionated leucocytes may be obtained simply by leaving blood treated with anticoagulant in a test tube or beaker at room temperature. The leucocyte-rich plasma layer is collected after 1–2 h when the red cells have settled. The sedimentation is more rapid if an erythrocyte-aggregating agent is added.

Method

1. Mix 10 volumes of anticoagulated or defibrinated blood with 1 (or 2) parts 6% (w/v) dextran, or 2 parts hydroxy-ethyl starch (HES).
2. Collect the cell-rich plasma layer ($\sim$ 50% of total volume) when the red cells have settled.

The sedimentation of erythrocytes takes 15–40 min, depending upon individual variations and the height of the blood cell column. The sedimentation is independent of the diameter of the tube, except that it tends to slow down with diameters less than 10 mm – 12 mm. The differential distribution of the leucocytes apparently does not differ from that found in whole blood. Usually there is an admixture of 2–3 erythrocytes per leucocyte. This procedure may be used as a first step in techniques designed to separate subgroups of white blood cells.

2.2.2.2 Separation of MNC and Granulocytes from Whole Blood with One Layer of Gradient Medium

MNC have a lower density than granulocytes and erythrocytes. Thus after centrifugation of blood cells loaded on a separation fluid of appropriate density (1.077 g/ml), the MNC remaining at the top are easily collected. The granulocytes in the bottom fraction may next be separated from the erythrocytes by dextran sedimentation.

Method

1. Mix 1 part anticoagulated blood with 1 (or 0.7–0.8) part 0.9% NaCl.
2. Layer 6 ml (or 30 ml) mixture onto 3 ml (or 15 ml) LP (Lymphoprep), in a 12–13 ml (or 50 ml) tube, by keeping the pipette against the tube wall, 3–5 cm above the fluid meniscus.
3. Centrifuge for 15 min at $600 \times g$ at room temperature (or 4°C).
4. After centrifugation, remove the supernatant down to 3–4 mm above the white band of MNC (Fig. 1). Then collect the MNC with a *Pasteur* pipette, together with the upper part of the separation fluid. Make sure that no visible part of the white band is left. It is possible to collect the MNC without first removing the supernatant.
5. Dilute the collected cell suspension 1:1 with 0.9% NaCl (or culture medium) and centrifuge for 6 min at $600 \times g$. Remove the supernatant and resuspend the cell button in medium. Include additional centrifugations and washings if necessary.
6. Collect the granulocytes in the bottom fraction as follows: Remove the separation fluid down to 2–3 mm above the erythrocyte mass. Add 6–8 ml 0.9% NaCl, resuspend the cells and centrifuge for 6 min at $600 \times g$.

7. Remove the supernatant and add 2.5 ml medium and 0.4 ml 6% dextran and mix. Collect the supernatant containing the granulocytes when the red cells have settled.

   At this stage the cells from 2–3 tubes (6–9 ml) may be combined in one 12 ml tube prior to addition of dextran solution.

The upper fraction should contain approximately 80% lymphocytes and 20% monocytes and the bottom fraction predominantly granulocytes (> 97%). The granulocyte fraction is contaminated by erythrocytes, 2–4 per cell. If these erythrocytes influence subsequent functional studies, they may be removed by one of the following alternative procedures:

1. Centrifuge the cells for 5 min at $600 \times g$. Remove the supernatant and resuspend the cell button in 3–5 ml 0.83% (w/v) NH_4Cl. After 7 min at room temperature (or 37°C) centrifuge and remove the supernatant containing the lysed red cells.

   It has been reported that this treatment may cause a transient functional defect of lymphocytes [6], but it appears not to have permanent effects on the phagocytic

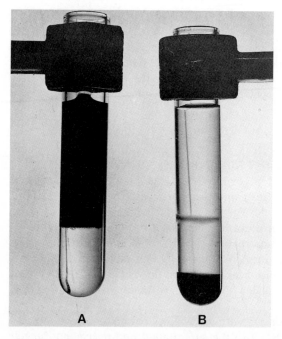

A   B

Fig. 1. Separation of mononuclear cells, MNC, (lymphocytes and monocytes) from human blood.

(a) Equal parts of anticoagulated or defibrinated blood are mixed well and 6–8 ml layered over 3 ml Isopaque-Ficoll (LP) or Nycodenz (ND) separation fluid and centrifuged at room temperature (or at 4°C) for 20 (or 15) min at $600 \times g$. (b) After centrifugation the MNC (and platelets) band at the top of the separation fluid, and can easily be collected with a pipette. The granulocytes in the bottom fraction can be separated from the erythrocytes as described in the text.

capacity of granulocytes or the respiratory activity of these cells, or erythrocytes when used as described.

2. Resuspend the cell pellet in one volume water. After 20–30 s add one volume double strength medium or 1.8% (w/v) NaCl, to restore osmolality. Remove the supernatant after centrifugation.

Centrifugation of undiluted blood leads to some loss (10–20%) of lymphocytes, which move to the bottom of the tube and thereby reduce the purity of the granulocyte fraction. In terms of purity, yield and viability, the following three gradient media (density 1.077 g/ml) yielded similar results: LP, Nycodenz (ND) and Percoll. LP which is widely used, contains a polysaccharide (Ficoll) in addition to the X-ray contrast medium. ND is a pure substance (X-ray contrast medium), and may be the choice if it is desirable to avoid exposure of cells to the polysaccharide. The X-ray contrast medium passes slowly [7] into cells, but apparently the exposure to contrast medium does not affect the viability of washed cells suspended in culture medium. Excellent viability has also been demonstrated for cells separated with Percoll as gradient medium [8]. However, the silica particles in Percoll may be engulfed by monocytes [9], which could lead to their activation. It should be noted that after dilution with NaCl, Percoll can no longer be autoclaved.

Any type of anticoagulant can be used. The MNC fraction is heavily contaminated by platelets. This can be avoided by using defibrinated blood. This involves a 30–40% reduction of the cell yield, with a selective loss of monocytes, thus yielding a purer lymphocyte suspension. Otherwise the majority of platelets can be removed by differential centrifugation (cf. 2.2.2.11).

2.2.2.3   Separation of MNC and Granulocytes from Leucocyte-rich Plasma

Blood as starting material

For separation of cells from large volumes of blood (> 50 ml) it is preferable to remove the erythrocytes by dextran sedimentation in an initial step, although this entails about a 30% loss of leucocytes. The practical advantage is that the volume to be separated is reduced by approximately 75%, as compared to diluted blood.

Method

1. Mix 10 volumes blood with 1 volume 6% dextran, and collect the cell-rich plasma layer when the erythrocytes have settled (cf. 2.2.2.1).
2. Small volumes: Layer 2–8 ml leucocyte-rich plasma over 2.5–3 ml LP (or ND) in a 12–15 ml tube and centrifuge at room temperature (or 4°C) for 15 min at 600 × g.

Larger volumes: Separate 30–40 ml leucocyte-rich plasma with 12–15 ml LP in larger tubes. The most convenient procedure is to add the separation fluid to the bottom of the tube, beneath the leucoccyte-rich plasma, by means of a syringe to which a long needle is attached. Centrifuge for 15 min at $600 \times g$.

3. Collect the MNC from the interface region, and wash as described (cf. 2.2.2.2). The granulocytes are found at the bottom, together with remaining erythrocytes.

Occasionally there may be some granulocytes (3–10%) in the MNC fraction, which will not be seen in parallel separations with whole blood. This granulocyte admixture has repeatedly been seen with blood from certain individuals, 3 out of approximately 50 donors. The granulocyte contamination can be abrogated by increasing the osmolality of the separation fluid by 3–5%. The osmolality can be adjusted by adding dry NaCl to the spearation fluid. Thirty mg NaCl per 100 ml will increase the osmolality by about 10 mOsm/kg.

Fresh leucocyte concentrates from the blood bank, usually amounting to 50–60 ml, represent a considerable supply of MNC and granulocytes.

Method

1. Mix the leucocyte concentrate with a slightly larger volume (60–70 ml) of 0.9% NaCl.
2. Add 6% dextran (1/10 volume) to enhance sedimentation of red cells.
3. Transfer leucocyte-rich plasma (30–35 ml) to a 50 ml tube.
4. Layer 12–15 ml of LP underneath the cell-rich plasma and centrifuge for 15 min at $600 \times g$.
5. Collect the MNC from the interface region and the granulocytes from the bottom.

2.2.2.4   Separation of MNC and Granulocytes from Animal Blood

The LP technique may be used for separation of blood lymphocytes in most species. However, in some animals the lymphocytes have a broader density distribution profile than in humans. Consequently some of the lymphocytes move to the bottom of the separation fluid during centrifugation, which leads to reduced yield. Furthermore, these high-density lymphocytes contaminate the granulocyte fraction. This is demonstrated in Fig. 2, which shows that with LP the granulocyte fraction contains 40–50% lymphocytes. The sedimentation of lymphocytes to the bottom may be prevented by increasing the density or reducing the osmolality of the separation fluid. The latter principle can be used successfully for separation of lymphocytes and granulocytes from rats (Fig. 2) and rabbits. The purity of the granulocyte suspension will improve as the osmolality is decreased.

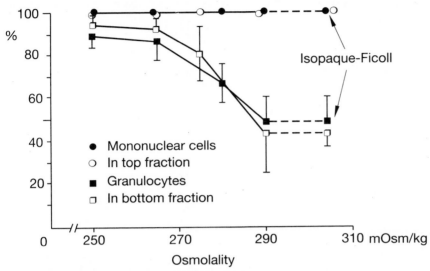

Fig. 2. Separation of MNC and granulocytes from rat blood.
Blood was collected from inferior vena cava in anaesthetized animals, into syringes containing 1 ml 2.7% EDTA (pH 7.4). Equal parts of EDTA-blood and 0.9% NaCl were mixed and 3 (up to 6) ml of the mixture was separated with Nycodenz (1.077 g/ml) solutions of different osmolalities (250–290 mOsm/kg), and with LP. Leucocyte-rich plasma obtained by dextran sedimentation was also separated. The Figure shows the percentage of MNC in the top fraction and of granulocytes in the bottom fraction. Closed symbols signify whole blood and open symbols leucocyte-rich plasma. Mean values ± SD (standard deviation) from 5 separations.

Routine method

1. a) Dilute whole blood with an equal volume 0.9% NaCl and layer 4–6 ml over 3 ml of ND separation fluid with density of 1.077 g/ml and osmolality of 265 mOsm/kg and centrifuge for 15 min at 600 × g.
   b) Layer 2–6 ml of leucocyte-rich plasma over the ND separation fluid and centrifuge for 15 min at 600 × g (cf. 2.2.2.3).
2. After centrifugation, collect MNC from the interface region and granulocytes from the bottom.

Use procedure a) when only lymphocytes are needed, and procedure b) for granulocyte separation. MNC from rabbits are less pure than MNC from rats due to contamination (~ 5%) with basophils. Inevitably reduced osmolality will lead to increased erythrocyte contamination in the MNC fraction (Table 2). Rat MNC separated from whole blood contain a significant number of red cells, which can be avoided if dextran sedimentation is included, whereas the reverse will occur with rabbit blood. Largely, the use of LP ensures a low erythrocyte contamination, and may be used for routine separation of lymphocytes, if a certain loss (15–30%) during the initial centrifugation is acceptable.

Table 2. Erythrocyte admixture (%) among mononuclear cells from rat and rabbit blood separated with ND solutions of different osmolalities, and with LP

		Osmolality of separation fluid (mOsm/kg)				
		ND				LP
		250	265	280	290	305
Rats	Whole blood	92 ± 3	88 ± 6	77 ± 10	65 ± 13	45 ± 13
	Dextran-sed.	9 ± 8	3 ± 3	2 ± 1	~ 1	~ 1
Rabbits	Whole blood	33 ± 6	19 ± 10	11 ± 5	7 ± 5	7 ± 5
	Dextran-sed.	82 ± 8	47 ± 12	45 ± 14	39 ± 18	6 ± 3

The erythrocyte contamination was calculated as the number of erythrocytes in percentage of the total number of erythrocytes and leucocytes. The ND solutions had a density of 1.077 g/ml with osmolality from 250 to 290 mOsm/kg. An LP solution (1.077 g/ml) with osmolality of 305 mOsm/kg was included for comparison. Mean values (± SD) from 5 separations.

2.2.2.5   One-step Separation of MNC and Granulocytes

In this method, EDTA-blood is layered over a hypertonic (460–490 mOsm/kg) separation fluid of high density and centrifuged [10]. As the red cells pass into the separation fluid they expel water and a density and osmolality gradient is created. Due to their different densities, MNC and granulocytes band at different levels and can be collected separately.

Method

1. Layer 5 ml blood over 3 ml Polyprep or Histopaque in 12–13 ml tubes and centrifuge for 20 min (Polyprep) or 30 min (Histopaque) at 600 × g.
2. Collect MNC and granulocytes separately with a *Pasteur* pipette. Dilute with 0.9% NaCl immediately, centrifuge and resuspend the cell button in buffered medium, to minimize the exposure time for the cells to the hypertonic gradient medium.

Separate larger volumes in tubes of larger size. Make sure that the height of the blood column corresponds to that in the 5 ml procedure. As shown in Table 3 this procedure yields fairly pure suspensions of MNC and granulocytes. The erythrocyte contamination in the granulocyte fraction is lower than with LP, but is still substantial. This appears to be a convenient technique for simultaneous separation of MNC and granulocytes from small blood volumes. It should be noted however, that hypertonicity may enhance protein leakage from cells [11]. For separation of granulocytes from large blood volumes, dextran sedimentation and LP separation appears more convenient, in particular for buffy coat samples from the blood bank.

Table 3. One-step procedure for separation of MNC and granulocytes.

		Differential counts (%)			Erythr./	Yield of MNC
		Granulocytes	Basophils	MNC	100 cells	or GR (%)
Histopaque	T	1.5 ± 1	0.1	98.4 ± 2	2 ± 2	> 95
30 min	M	97.8 ± 1	0.22	2.0 ± 1	39 ± 9	59 ± 20
Polyprep	T	2.8 ± 3	0.4	96.8 ± 2	4 ± 2	> 90
20 min	M	98.4 ± 1	0.2	1.4 ± 2	39 ± 11	69 ± 33

5 ml EDTA-blood were layered over 3 ml Histopaque (density 1.119 g/ml, 490 mOsm/kg) or Polyprep (density 1.114 g/ml, 460 mOsm/kg) and centrifuged for 20 (Polyprep) or 30 min (Histopaque) at 600 × g. After centrifugation two bands were visible. The top band (T) at the sample/medium interface consisted of MNC and the lower band (M) of granulocytes (neutrophils + eosinophils). The cells were collected with a *Pasteur* pipette. Mean values (± SD) from 5 separations.

2.2.2.6 Simultaneous Separation of MNC and Granulocytes with a Two-layer Technique

The granulocyte suspension obtained by routine procedures with LP or ND (1.077 g/ml) is contaminated by 2–3 erythrocytes per cell. The erythrocyte admixture may be reduced with a two-layer technique, thereby avoiding possible harmful effects of hypotonic lysis or NH_4Cl lysis. Two different procedures may be used.

Method

1. Layer 2.5 ml high-density (1.090 g/ml) ND beneath 2.5 ml ND (1.077 g/ml, 290 mOsm/kg) or LP by means of a syringe attached to a long needle. Recipes are given in Table 1.

2. Layer 5 ml leucocyte-rich plasma (cf. 2.2.2.3) on top of the gradient medium and centrifuge for 15 min at 600 × g.
3. Collect MNC from the top, and granulocytes from the intermediate layer.

As shown in Fig. 3 the highest granulocyte yield and the lowest erythrocyte contamination will be obtained with an osmolality of 270–280 mOsm/kg of the high density ND solution.

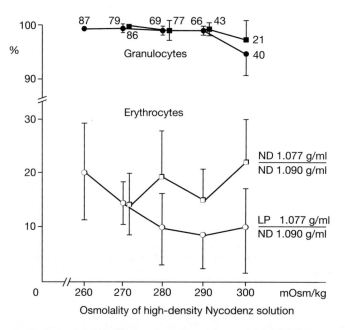

Fig. 3. Separation of MNC and granulocytes from whole blood.
Two-layer system composed of i) two ND solutions of different density, or ii) LP together with a high density ND solution. 2.5 ml ND (1.090 g/ml) of different osmolality were underlayered with 2.5 ml ND or LP (1.077 g/ml). Then 5 ml of leucocyte-rich human plasma was layered on the top and centrifuged for 15 min at 600 × g. The figure shows the granulocyte percentage in the intermediate layer, and the granulocyte yield is given at each experimental point. The erythrocyte contamination is given as % of the total number of erythrocytes and granulocytes in the intermediate layer. Mean values and SD from 5 separations.

2.2.2.7   Separation of MNC and Granulocytes at 4°C, with 17% Plasma in the Gradient Medium

It has been suggested that separation of cells should be carried out at 4°C, preferably with plasma in the gradient medium, to maintain good viability and avoid activation prior to functional studies. The procedures described above yield approximately the same result when done at 4°C. Otherwise gradient media containing 17% plasma can be made as follows: a) 10 parts ND, 1.087 g/ml, 290 mOsm/kg (cf. Table 1) + 2 parts autologous plasma. b) 10 parts ND, 1.103 g/ml, 260 mOsm/kg + 2 parts plasma.

Method

1. Centrifuge blood in a refrigerated centrifuge for 10 min at 1200 $\times$ g. Collect the plasma and keep it at 4°C.
2. Add 1 part dextran (or 2 parts HES) to whole blood, and collect leucocyte-rich plasma after sedimentation of red cells. This procedure should be done at 4°C, but the sedimentation with HES may be slow at this temperature.
3. Layer 2.5 ml solution (b) beneath 2.5 ml solution (a) in a 12–15 ml tube. Layer 5 ml of leucocyte-rich plasma on top of the gradient. The ND solutions should be precooled to 4°C.
4. Centrifuge for 15 min at 600 $\times$ g. Collect MNC from the plasma/ND interface region and granulocytes from the (a)/(b) interface region.

This procedure is convenient for separation of cells from rather small volumes. Solution (a) can be used alone for separation of MNC and granulocytes.

2.2.2.8   Separation of Lymphocytes

Lymphocytes and monocytes co-purify when blood is separated with the LP or ND procedure. By capitalizing on the ability of monocytes to engulf carbonyl iron particles, their density can be increased sufficiently to enable them to sediment through the gradient medium, whereas the lymphocytes remain at the top. Alternatively the monocytes can be removed with a magnet.

Method

1. Centrifuge heparinized blood (10 ml) for 10 min at 600 $\times$ g.
2. Collect the leucocyte layer ($\sim$ 1 ml) resting on top of the erythrocyte pellet and mix with 1 ml colloidal iron suspension.
3. Incubate the mixture in a shaking bath at 37°C for 30 min. If needed, cells from several 10 ml tubes can be mixed, but the height of the mixture should not exceed 8–10 mm, to ensure close contact between cells and iron particles.
4. After incubation, mix equal parts of the cell suspension and 0.9% NaCl. Layer 6 ml of the mixture over 3 ml LP and centrifuge for 15 min at 600 $\times$ g. Collect the lymphocytes from the top.

By this procedure the monocyte contamination may be reduced from 15–21% to 1%. Alternatively the iron-loaded monocytes may be removed with a magnet. It is difficult to completely remove the monocytes, but even better purity may be obtained with anti-monocyte mAbs and magnetic beads [4].

2.2.2.9   Separation of Monocytes

Monocytes have a slightly lower average density than lymphocytes. The osmolality of the medium is another important parameter in a separation procedure, since it appears that lymphocytes are slightly more sensitive to a change of osmolality than monocytes. A separation fluid for monocytes should therefore combine density and osmolality in such a way that all cells loaded on the gradient medium, except the monocytes, move to the bottom during centrifugation.

Method

1. Collect blood in tubes with EDTA. Other anticoagulants cannot be used.
2. Add 1 part dextran solution to 10 parts blood to enhance sedimentation of erythrocytes.
3. Layer 6–8 ml leucocyte-rich plasma over 3 ml ND with density of 1.068 g/ml and osmolality of 335 mOsm/kg. It is critical that no appreciable mixing between the plasma phase and the separation fluid takes places before centrifugation, because this will inevitably reduce the yield.
4. Centrifuge for 15 min at $600 \times g$. Remove the clear plasma down to 4–5 mm above the interface. Then collect the remaining plasma together with half the volume of the separation fluid. The interface band is less sharp than after centrifugation with LP.
5. Dilute the cells from 2 (or 3) tubes (4 ml) with 5–6 ml 0.9% NaCl or a buffered medium and centrifuge for 7 min at $600 \times g$ to pellet the monocytes. Wash repeatedly if needed.
6. Dilute 25 µl cell suspension 1/5 (or 1/10) with a staining fluid (0.05% methyl violet, 0.5% acetic acid). With some experience, differential counts can be made directly in the counting chamber.

As shown in Fig. 4, at a constant density (1.068 g/ml) the monocyte purity improves as the osmolality of the gradient medium is increased. Unfortunately the monocyte yield decreases with increasing osmolality. Thus an osmolality of 335 mOsm/kg is recommended for routine use (solution is commercially available). If a lower purity is acceptable, the osmolality can be reduced to 325 mOsm/kg (cf. Table 1), which will ensure a higher monocyte yield.

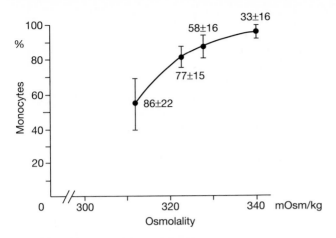

Fig. 4. Monocyte separation with ND solutions.
All with density of 1.068 g/ml, but with varying osmolality. Leucocyte-rich plasma (6–7 ml) was layered over 3 ml gradient medium and centrifuged for 15 min at $600 \times g$. Erythrocytes and granulocytes sedimented to the bottom whereas the upper part of the ND solution was composed of lymphocytes and monocytes. First the clear plasma down to to 3–4 mm above the interface between plasma and the ND solution was removed. Next, the remaining plasma together with half the volume of the separation fluid was collected. The figure shows the monocyte percentage for each osmolality of the ND solution. Mean values ($\pm$ SD) from 10–15 separations. The monocyte yield ($\pm$ SD) is indicated at each experimental point.

Use of this gradient medium may cause problems with regard to monocyte yield. Individual variations of monocyte density and concentration in blood may certainly contribute to variable results. Certain individual donors consistently give a high yield of monocytes. Mixing of the two phases should be avoided (cf. above pt. 3). It is important to use a smoothly running centrifuge. In establishing the procedure it is advisable to count the cells before and after washing to determine the cell loss in the washing procedure. In case of substantial cell loss, try washing at 4°C with 0.1–0.3% EDTA, and at least 0.1% serum albumin or 5% autologous plasma in the medium. A significant loss of monocytes not only reduces the yield, but also leads to an increase in the proportion of lymphocytes.

2.2.2.10 Separation of Erythrocytes and Reticulocytes

Leucocytes and platelets have a lower density than erythrocytes and after centrifugation most of the platelets and approximately 70% of the leucocytes form a white layer on top of the erythrocyte pellet.

Method

1. Centrifuge anticoagulated blood (10 ml) for 7 min at $1000 \times g$. Remove the supernatant and the leucocyte/platelet layer, together with 2–3 mm of the erythrocyte mass.
2. Resuspend the cells in buffered saline or medium and centrifuge for 7 min at $600 \times g$. Remove the supernatant and upper 2–4 mm of the cell mass.
3. Repeat this procedure. Count the remaining leucocytes under the microscope. Automated particle counting is unsatisfactory at these low cell concentrations. Include additional washing if the cell number is too high.

The majority of reticulocytes will be removed by this procedure, since they have a lower density than mature red cells. The density of erythrocytes increases with ageing, and the procedure may thus to some extent select for older erythrocytes. An alternative procedure is to remove platelets and leucocytes by filtration of blood through cotton or cellulose [12].

Different types of density gradient procedures have been used for separation of erythrocytes according to age [13–15]. With such procedures considerable enrichment of reticulocytes (10–30% of all cells) may be obtained in the top layers [13, 15–17]. To minimize leucocyte admixture it is advisable to include cellulose filtration as a first step [12]. Reticulocytes exhibit a large number of transferrin receptors, and by means of monoclonal antibodies to the receptor it has been possible to obtain pure reticulocyte suspensions by immunomagnetic separation [18]. However, the reticulocytes are attached to the beads.

2.2.2.11 Separation of Platelets

Due to their small size platelets can be separated from blood cells by differential centrifugation. For functional studies sodium citrate (or ACD) is used as anticoagulant [19], but EDTA can also be used in particular for biochemical studies of platelet components [20].

Method

1. Draw venous blood (9 volumes) into syringes each containing 1 volume 3.2% (w/v) sodium citrate.
2. Centrifuge the tubes for 15 min at $120 \times g$.
   Some investigators use stronger centrifugation, for instance $200 \times g$ for 12 min.
3. Collect platelet-rich plasma and centrifuge for 10 min at $600 \times g$ to pellet the platelets.
   Washing fluid and suspending fluids are described elsewhere [19].

The separation procedure is influenced by the height of the blood column, which should be standardized. In establishing the procedure, count leucocytes in the platelet-rich plasma. If there is a substantial leucocyte admixture it may be necessary to increase centrifugal force or time.

A gel filtration technique for separation of platelets from plasma constituents has been described [21]. Platelets can also be obtained by a centrifugation of human blood [22] through Nycodenz (NycoPrep 1.063).

2.2.2.12 Removal of Platelets

The MNC and monocyte suspension contains a considerable admixture of platelets. This can be avoided by using defibrinated blood. However, defibrination generally leads to a loss ($\sim 30\%$) of a cell types, and especially a selective loss of monocytes. Platelets can be removed by two different procedures:

Method of differential centrifugation

1. Collect MNC or monocytes from the interface band in 2–5 tubes, dilute with 0.9% NaCl and pellet the cells by centrifugation for 7 min at $600 \times g$.
2. Resuspend the cells in 6 ml (~ 5 cm height) saline or medium, preferably in conical tubes, and centrifuge for 10 min at $60 \times g$.
3. Remove the supernatant with the majority ($\sim 70\%$) of the platelets. Most of the cells will have sedimented to the bottom. Repeat the procedure if a more complete removal of platelets is necessary.

Method of centrifugation through plasma/serum

1. Centrifuge EDTA-blood for 10 min at $1000 \times g$ and collect the plasma.
2. Collect MNC or monocytes from 2–3 tubes, dilute with 0.9% NaCl or medium and pellet the cells by centrifugation for 7 min at $600 \times g$.
3. Resuspend the cells in 1 ml saline and layer the suspension over 3 ml autologous EDTA-plasma (or fetal calf serum) in a conical tube and centrifuge for 10 min at $60 \times g$.
4. Remove the plasma supernatant with most of the platelets, and retrieve the cells from the bottom.

Plasma obtained after dextran sedimentation and centrifugation may also be used for platelet removal. However, dextran itself may cause some aggregation of platelets and thereby enhance their sedimentation. Therefore plasma without dextran is preferred.

References

[1] A. Bøyum, Isolation of Mononuclear Cells and Granulocytes from Human Blood. Isolation of Mononuclear Cells by One Centrifugation, and of Granulocytes by Combining Centrifugation and Sedimentation at 1 G, Scand. J. Clin. Lab. Invest. 21, Suppl. 97, 77–89 (1968).

[2] A. Bøyum, Isolation of Lymphocytes, Granulocytes and Macrophages, Scand. J. Immunol. 5, Suppl. 5, 9–15 (1976).

[3] A. Bøyum, Isolation of Human Blood Monocytes with Nycodenz, a New Iodinated Density Gradient Medium, Scand. J. Immunol. 17, 429–436 (1983).

[4] A. Bøyum, D. Løvhaug, L. Tresland, E. M. Nordlie, Separation of Leucocytes. Improved Cell Purity by Fine Adjustments of Gradient Medium Density and Osmolality, Scand. J. Immunol. 34, 697–712 (1991).

[5] D. M. Wong, L. Varesio, Depletion of Macrophages from Heterogeneous Cell Populations by the Use of Carbonyl Iron, in: G. di Sabato, J. J. Langone, H. van Vunakes (eds.), Methods in Enzymology, Immunochemical Techniques, Part G, Separation and Characterization of Lymphoid Cells, Academic Press Inc., New York 1984, 108, pp. 307–313.

[6] I. Yust, R. W. Smith, J. R. Wunderlich, D. L. Mann, Temporary Inhibition of Antibody-dependent, Cell-mediated Cytotoxicity by Pretreatment of Human Attacking Cells with Ammonium Chloride, J. Immunol. 116, 1170–1172 (1976).

[7] A. Nordby, K. E. Tvedt, J. Halgunset, G. Kopstad, O. A. Haugen, Incorporation of Contrast Media in Cultured Cells, Invest. Radiol 24, 703–710 (1989).

[8] J. T. Kurnick, L. Østberg, M. Stegagno, A. K. Kimura, A. Ørn, O. Sjøberg, A Rapid Method for the Separation of Functional Lymphoid Cell Populations of Human and Animal Origin on PVP-silica (Percoll) Density Gradients, Scand. J. Immunol. 10, 563–573 (1979).

[9] J. S. J. Wakefield, J. S. Gale, M. V. Berridge, T. W. Jordan, H. C. Ford, Is Percoll Innocuous to Cells?, Biochem. J. 202, 795–797 (1982).

[10] A. Ferrante, Y. H. Thong, A rapid One-step Procedure for Purification of Mononuclear and Polymorphonuclear Leukocytes from Human Blood Using a Modification of the Hypaque-Ficoll Method, J. Immunol. Methods. 24, 389–393 (1978).

[11] A. Nordby, J. Halgunset, K. Thorstensen, O. A. Haugen, Short-term Effects of Radiographic Contrast Media on Monolayer Cell Cultures and Hepatocytes. Invest. Radiol. 22, 603–607 (1987).

[12] E. Beutler, C. West, K. G. Blume, The Removal of Leukocytes and Platelets from Whole Blood, J. Lab. Clin. Med. 88, 328–333 (1976).

[13] C. M. Rennie, S. Thompson, A. C. Parker, A. Maddy, Human Erythrocyte Fractionation in "Percoll" Density Gradients, Clin. Chim. Acta. 98, 119–125 (1979).

[14] L. Vettore, M. C. D. Matteis, P. Zampini, A New Density Gradient System for the Separation of Human Red Blood Cells, Am. J. Hematol. 8, 291–297 (1980).

[15] M. E. M. Pierpoint, Erythrocyte Carnitine: A Study of Erythrocyte Fractions Isolated by Discontinuous Density Gradient Centrifugation, Biochem. Med. 40, 237–246 (1988).

[16] P. I. Kelley, D. M. Feinberg, S. Segal, Galactose-1-phosphate Uridyl Transferase in Density-fractionated Erythrocytes, Hum. Gent. 82, 99–103 (1989).

[17] D. Rushing, V. Vengelen-Tyler, Evaluation and Comparison of Four Reticulocyte Enrichment Procedures, Transfusion Philadelphia 27, 86–89 (1987).

[18] A. Brun, G. Gaudernack, S. Sandberg, A New Method for Isolation of Reticulocytes: Positive Selection of Human Reticulocytes by Immunomagnetic Separation, Blood 76, 2397–2403 (1990).

[19] J. F. Mustard, D. W. Perry, N. G. Ardie, M. A. Packham, Preparation of Suspensions of Washed Platelets from Humans, Brit. J. Haematol. 22, 193–204 (1972).

[20] N. O. Solum, T. M. Olsen, Glycoprotein Ib in the Triton-insoluble (Cytoskeletal) Fraction of Blood Platelets, Biochim. Biophys. Acta. 799, 209–220 (1984).

[21] B. Lages, M. C. Scrutton, H. Holmsen, Studies on Gel-filtered Human Platelets: Isolation and Characterization in a Medium Containing no Added Ca^{2+}, Mg^{2+}, or K^+, J. Lab. Clin. Med. 85, 811–825 (1975).

[22] T. C. Ford, J. Graham, D. Rickwood, A New, Rapid One-step Method for the Isolation of Platelets from Human Blood, Clin. Chim. Acta. 192, 115–120 (1990).

2.3   Serous Cavity Cells

Derralynn A. Hughes and Siamon Gordon

The mammalian serous cavities, peritoneal, pleural and pericardial, are cell- and fluid-laden spaces resulting from folding of the embryo during early development. The pericardial cavity is enclosed by a transparent serous membrane (the pericardium) and contains the heart. The thoracic cavity is lined by, and divided into, right and left pleural sacs by the serous pleura which encloses the pleural cavity and contains the lungs. The peritoneal cavity, lined by the serous peritoneum, is the largest and most easily accessible of the cavities and thus provides a suitable example for discussion of sampling and manipulation of the cells, mainly leucocytes, obtained from such cavities. Historically, peritoneal leucocytes have been used in studies of both cell biology and immunology; e.g., early descriptions of macrophage differentiation [1–3] and particulate hydrolases [4].

The resting serosal cavity populations consist mainly of lymphocytes, loosely adherent macrophages and macrophages strongly adherent to the peritoneal mesothelium. In addition, minor populations of PMN, dendritic cells, natural killer cells, eosinophils and mast cells influence the immunological state of the cavity. Whilst the lymphocytes are part of a recirculating pool derived from the secondary lymphoid organs, the sub-serosal lymphoreticular masses (milk spots) of the peritoneum and pleura [5] have been suggested as the origin of the free macrophages of serosal cavities. There is evidence that resident peritoneal macrophages (RPM) are not continually replaced by recruitment of bone marrow-derived monocytes: the resting population is stable for at least 49 days without influx of monocytes [6] and RPM are resistant to the myeloablation resulting from a single dose of 5-fluorouracil [7] or strontium-89 [8]. Furthermore, only a small fraction of resident macrophages are dividing at any one time [9].

The serous cavities may be perturbed using nonspecific inflammatory or specific immune stimuli to induce exudation of bone marrow-derived PMN, monocytes and lymphocytes. Depending on the stimulus, serous cavity cells can be phenotypically diverse. For example, serous macrophages express three functionally distinct but to some extent interconvertible phenotypes: resident resting cells, inflammatory elicited cells, or immunogically activated cells [10, 11]. These differ in size, adherence and spreading on substrata, as well as in plasma membrane and secretory properties such as Ia expression and plasminogen activator release, and in microbicidal, cytotoxic and respiratory burst activity.

Leucocytes are obtained from the serous cavities without the requirement for tissue disaggregation or enzymatic digestion, which may alter cell surface phenotype in other isolated populations. They are therefore appropriate for applications in culture and adoptive transfer systems requiring unperturbed cells. The resident cells of the peritoneal cavity express phenotypic properties different from those of macrophages and lymphoid cells in other lymphohaemopoietic organs. Manipulation of the inflammatory status of the cavity using immunologically specific or other inflammatory stimuli results in a phased exudation of bone-marrow-derived PMN and macrophages, thus providing a convenient source of variously activated cells and a tool for investigating the pro-inflammatory and migratory signals of the leucocyte response.

The sections below deal with methods of obtaining normal adult and newborn serous cavity cells, various perturbations to modify the composition and nature of serous cavity populations, exemplified by the peritoneal cavity, and some standard protocols to evaluate the viability and phenotype of the cells.

2.3.1   Lavage of Cells from the Peritoneal Cavity

2.3.1.1   Adult Mice

Materials

Mice (12–16 weeks old). An unstimulated cavity yields approximately 5×10^6 total cells comprising 20–40% macrophages, 60–80% lymphocytes and a few mast cells [9].

Covered dissection board and pins,
Blunt (curved) and fine scissors,
CO_2 chamber,
20-ml syringe with 19-g needle,
Sterile glass *Pasteur* pipette with rubber 1 ml bulb,
Ice-cold PBS,
50 ml *Falcon* tube,
70% ethanol.

Method [12]

1. Kill the mouse by CO_2 asphyxiation rather than cervical dislocation to avoid leakage of blood into the peritoneal cavity.
2. Pin the mouse supine onto a dissection board and soak the skin with 70% ethanol.
3. Lift the skin and using the blunt curved scissors snip back into the iliac fossae without piercing the anterior abdominal wall. Reflect the flap of skin over the rib cage to expose the anterior abdominal wall from the inguinal regions to the thorax.

4. Inject up to 4–6 ml cold PBS through the fat in the right iliac fossa using a 20-ml syringe and 19-g needle. Lubricate the abdominal wall with PBS and gently agitate the cavity with a sterile *Pasteur* pipette.
5. Quickly withdraw around 4 ml fluid using a sterile syringe inserted horizontally into cavity and aspirate the remaining fluid using a *Pasteur* pipette, inserted directly through the abdominal wall, to recover up to 90% of the injected fluid.

To maintain cellular viability the "peritoneal lavage" should be stored in a capped polystyrene *(Falcon)* tube at 4°C for a minimum period before resuspension in RPMI 1640 containing 10% FCS (R10). As mononuclear phagocytes are sensitive to alkaline pH it is advantageous to lavage cells directly into a buffered medium such as Optimem-2 (*Gibco Life Laboratories*, Paisley, Scotland).

Samples from individual mice should be checked macroscopically for gut bacterial contamination; samples with obvious blood contamination should also be discarded before pooling others.

2.3.1.2   Newborn Mice

Materials

1–7 day old mouse,
Dissection board and pins,
2 × 1-ml syringe with 32-g needles,
Ice-cold PBS,
15 ml *Falcon* tube.

Method

1. Kill mouse by decapitation overdose and pin supine to the board.
2. Insert a 1-ml syringe with 27-g needle through the right iliac fossa into the peritoneal cavity (it is not necessary to remove the skin covering the anterior abdominal wall) and inject 0.5 ml PBS. Leave this syringe in position.
3. Insert a second syringe superiorly and exchange the total fluid between the syringes five times. Finally aspirate the fluid into the second syringe and store on ice in a 15 ml *Falcon* tube.

2.3.1.3   Depletion of Peritoneal Macrophages by Lavage

In addition to obtaining cells for *in-vitro* manipulation the living peritoneal cavity can be depleted of suspended and loosely adherent cells [13].

Method

1. Anaesthetize the mouse.
2. Insert two 22-g hypodermic needles into the inguinal regions and one near the sternum. Inject 5 ml of sterile saline into the peritoneal cavity *via* the sternal needle.
3. Massage the peritoneal cavity for one minute. Collect the peritoneal fluid by the two inguinal needles and repeat the operation three times to remove around 90% of the peritoneal macrophages.

2.3.1.4   Other Laboratory Species

The above methods are suitable for the lavage of most small laboratory mammals and birds provided the quantity of fluid used is varied appropriately: e. g., 25 ml PBS for a rat; 50 ml for a rabbit; and in larger mammals a silastic catheter may be surgically implanted into the cavity to permit serial sampling of leucocyte accumulation *in vivo* [14]. Sacrifice (e. g. of rabbits) by the intraperitoneal injection of barbiturates should be avoided since this has been found to alter cellular viability and characteristics.

2.3.1.5   Peritoneal Lavage of Non-mammals

Serous cavity cells can be obtained by lavage from small amphibians e. g. *Xenopus*. Pith the animal and expose the peritoneum by cutting the skin away from the anterior abdominal wall. Inject fluid and aspirate as for the mouse. However, since the diaphragm is absent the cells are not strictly analogous to those obtained from the mammalian peritoneal cavity.

2.3.1.6   Human Peritoneal Cells

They can be obtained from patients undergoing Continuous Ambulatory Perfusion Dialysis (CAPD) [15] and during infectious peritonitis may comprise 89% macrophages [16]. Paediatric patients undergoing CAPD often develop eosinophilia with more than 10^9 eosinophils per litre of fluid (up to 30% of leucocytes) [17].

2.3.2   Recruitment of Cells to the Peritoneal Cavity

Particulate and soluble stimuli can be used to recruit cells differentially to the serous cavities. Since the abundance of a cell within the recruited population depends not only on the eliciting factor but also on the duration of the response, the serous cavity exudate may be selectively enriched for a desired cell type. Elicited cells can be harvested as detailed above or sampled using implanted nitrocellulose filters or glass coverslips which are removed and stained at various times [18].

The details of stimuli summarized here and in Table 1 are appropriate for recruitment into the mouse peritoneal cavity but the same stimuli have been used to provoke similar inflammatory responses in the rat [19], hamster [20] and chicken [21]. Mouse strains vary in their response to irritants and poorly digestible substances such as mineral oil and starch may persist and act as continuous phagocytic stimuli in culture; therefore, check recruitment parameters for each strain and stimulus, and wash cells free of the stimulating agent before use.

Table 1. Agents used to stimulate monocyte recruitment to the peritoneal cavity
See text for further details. One ml of stated material is injected intraperitoneally per mouse

Elicited phenotype	Activated phenotype
Brewers' complete thioglycollate broth	
NaIO$_4$, 5mmol/l	IFNγ 10 U
Proteose peptone broth	Living *T. cruzi*
Concanavalin A, 50 µg	Pyridine extract *C. parvum*
PHA, 3µg	Pyran copolymer 25mg/kg
Pristane mineral oil	*BCG*
LPS	
Sodium caseinate, 1% (w/v)	
Biogel polyacrylamide beads	

Brewers' complete thioglycollate broth

Dissolve 40.5 g thioglycollate broth (*Difco*) in 1 l distilled water and boil until golden yellow. Store the autoclaved aliquots in the dark for two weeks before use.

Inject 0.5–1.0 ml intraperitoneally (0.05 ml for a neonatal mouse) to elicit peak PMN influx at around 18 h followed by increasing numbers and proportions of phagocytically active macrophages from 2–7 days: e. g. at day 2, 13×10^6 total cells comprising 86% macrophages and 7% PMN, 7% lymphocytes and, at 4–5 days, when there is a peak response, $10–20 \times 10^6$ macrophages. Thioglycollate-elicited macrophages contain agar inclusion vacuoles which may be visualized using phase contrast microscopy.

Biogel polyacrylamide beads

Use biogel (*Biorad*, California USA) [22] 200–400 mesh at 150 g/l and 100–200 mesh at 35 g/l in PBS. Heat to 90°C, allow to swell for 1 h, degas, autoclave and wash three times in PBS. After settling overnight read the volume and adjust the concentration.

Inject 1 ml into a mouse intraperitoneally to elicit PMN on day 1–2; the influx of macrophages becomes significant on day 3.

In contrast to thioglycollate-elicited macrophages, biogel-elicited macrophages have not encountered a phagocytic stimulus and lack inclusion bodies.

BCG and C. parvum

The intraperitoneal injection of ca. $1-2 \times 10^7$ live *BCG* organisms results in the dissemination of the bacillus and granuloma formation. After an initial PMN influx, there is recruitment of immunologically activated macrophages to the cavity (ca. 5×10^6 after 5–12 days) which can be boosted up to several months later by the intraperitoneal injection of heat-killed *BCG* (1 mg per mouse in 1 ml PBS).

Similarly, intraperitoneal injection of 1 mg whole *C. parvum* or 1 mg pyridine extract of *C. parvum* results in an influx of $3-5 \times 10^6$ immunologically activated macrophages after 4–10 days [23].

Further nonspecific stimuli, e.g. proteose peptone broth, or specific antigen challenge, e.g. with PPD, enhance the exudation of macrophages and sensitized lymphocytes; however, macrophage viability may be reduced by specific antigen.

Pristane (mineral oil)

1 ml elicits 3×10^6 total cells (50% inflammatory macrophages, 20% PMN, 20% lymphocytes) 3 days after intraperitoneal injection.

LPS

Inject 10–30 µg endotoxin, e.g. from phenol extracted *S. typhimurium,* to recruit 5×10^6 macrophages of the elicited phenotype at day 4.

Cytokines

Use of recombinant and purified cytokines facilitates rapid and targeted recruitment of a leucocyte population enriched for a particular cell type into the serosal cavity. Examples are cited here from the literature although variables such as species or preparation, and effects *via* resident or recruited cells on the host, should be checked.

PMN: Migration into rat cavities can be elicited by purified human IL-1 β [24], rIL-1 or rTNF [25], rIFN-γ or HuIFN-γ [26], GM-CSF, IL-3 and G-CSF [27] and is thought to depend on the release of a proinflammatory cytokine (IL-8) from macrophages [28]. The administration of muramyl dipeptide (MDP) to a guinea pig peritoneal cavity previously prepared with thioglycollate broth also induces a PMN accumulation by way of a macrophage chemotaxin [29].

Macrophages: GM-CSF is the most potent of the colony stimulating factors in inducing a cellular peritoneal response with macrophage levels of 100×10^6 being observed after 6 days compared to 20×10^6, 10×10^6 and 4×10^6 for IL-3, G-CSF and CSF-1 [27, 30]. These macrophages are phagocytically active and exhibit heightened mitotic activity *in situ* unlike CSF-recruited PMN which are entirely post-mitotic.

NK cells: Sayers et al. [31] elicited intraperitoneal NK activity, measured by ^{51}Cr release from YAC cells, by the injection of IFN-γ or IL-2. The increase in activity corresponded to an increase in both percentage and total number of NK cells detected by LGL-1, a rat mAb specific for NK cells [32].

Mast cells: Injection of IL-3 or 5-fluorouracil (3 mg/mouse in warm PBS) recruits mast cells to the peritoneal cavity [33].

The principle of introducing a foreign material into the human peritoneal cavity has traditionally been used to promote entry of leucocytes into the cavity prior to soilage resulting from surgery of the colon [34]. More recently, the intraperitoneal administration of recombinant IFN-γ has activated tumour-associated defence mechanisms (NK cells and lymphocytes) in patients with recurrent ovarian carcinoma [35].

General considerations for the quantification of serous cavity cells

For quantification, lavage the cavity using a divalent cation-free medium, e.g. Hepes-buffered EDTA, 3 mmol/l, in PBS (to release cells adhering to the serosal membranes by divalent cation-dependent mechanisms). Heparin, 10 I.U./ml, reduces clot obstruction. Repeat the lavage three to five times, finally incising the peritoneum to expose all remaining fluid. (Alternatively, standard lavage volumes can be compared.) Quantify total cells using a haemocytometer, and *Turk*'s white cell counting fluid to differentiate mononuclear phagocytes from other nucleated cells and use Trypan blue to determine viability (cf. 2.1.1.2). For more detailed numerical parameters of the inflammatory response, perform total and differential cell counts; stain Cytospin preparations immunocytochemically or with *May-Grünwald Giemsa* stain for phenotypic discrimination of cells. Phase contrast microscopy also permits subjective assessment of viability and cell type.

***Turk's* white cell counting fluid**

1 ml glacial acetic acid,
1 ml gentian violet, 1% aqueous solution,
make up to 100 ml in distilled water.

2.3.3   Cell Purification from Peritoneal Lavage

Cell separation will vary depending on the physical properties and surface phenotype of the cell to be recovered. Fluorescence- and magnetic-activated cell sorting (cf. 4.1.2.4 and 4.1.2.5) are efficient and allow recovery of both positive and negative cell populations but are limited by the availabilities of lineage-specific antibodies for a given species. Cell densities and osmolarities are not identical among species but the following physical methods should give good selection of a required serosal cell type.

PMN

PMN and macrophages may be separated on the basis of the density and osmolarity of the extracellular medium [36] (cf. 2.2).
1. Wash the lavage and resuspend 6×10^7 cells in 7 ml *Krebs-Ringer* solution pH 7.4 containing BSA 10 g/l.
2. Layer 3 ml Nycodenz gradient under the cells with a long needle.
3. Centrifuge at $700 \times g$ for 20 min at 20°C.
4. Aspirate the interface and wash the top and bottom fractions which contain mononuclear cells and PMN respectively.

Macrophages

Adherence to bacteriological plastic *via* a divalent cation-dependent mechanism provides a rationale for their selection from other serosal cells which fail to adhere to this matrix [37]. Macrophages adhere to other matrices such as glass, tissue culture plastic or fibrinogen coated plastics by additional divalent cation-independent and dependent mechanisms that modulate plasma membrane and secretory properties profoundly depending on the substratum. Detachment of viable macrophages can result in membrane damage and poor yields ($< 50\%$) (cf. 4.1.1, for full discussion of methods).
For selection of macrophages by adherence to bacteriological plastic:
1. Resuspend the serous cavity lavage in R10 at 5×10^6 cells/ml. Culture 12 ml suspension in a 9 cm bacteriological plastic *Petri* dish for 1 h at 37°C in 5% CO_2 in air.
2. Wash the adhered cells three times with R10, finally replacing the medium in the *Petri* dish with Hepes-buffered PBS EDTA, 3 mmol/l, for 10 min at 37°C.
3. Recover adherent macrophages by vigorous pipetting. Wash and resuspend.

Lymphocytes

These are mainly non-adherent and may be separated from strongly adherent cells on tissue culture plastic. T-cells may be further purified by filtration through nylon wool which retains other cell types (cf. 4.1.1).

Mast cells

Cells of the connective tissue lineage [38] may be recovered from a serous cavity lavage by density gradient centrifugation [39].
1. Resuspend the lavage in RPMI 2% FCS at 5×10^6 cells/ml.
2. Centrifuge 2×10^7 cells through 5 ml Percoll (1.075 g/ml in Hepes-buffered R10) at 400 x g for 30 min.
3. Mast cells account for more than 95% of the cell pellet since the low density cells including fibroblasts and macrophages have been removed.

Eosinophils

1. Layer $2–4 \times 10^8$ cells in 3 ml PBS over a discontinuous Percoll gradient (3 ml each of 45%, 55%, 65%, and 75% Percoll) in a 15 ml polystyrene tube.
2. Centrifuge 400 x g for 15 min at room temperature.
3. Erythrocytes pellet at the bottom with peritoneal leucocytes at the interfaces and the highest concentration of eosinophils is found above the 75% Percoll layer [17].

2.3.4   *In vivo* and *in vitro* Labelling of Peritoneal Cells

2.3.4.1   Fluorescent Labelling

Macrophages of the reticuloendothelial system have been classically labelled by the injection of vital dyes [40] or colloidal carbon [41] and recently by the sterile injection of fluorescent endocytic markers. A number of fluorescent dyes injected into the resting peritoneal cavity allow resting cells to be discriminated from those subsequently recruited [41]. Lipophilic dyes label the cells by incorporation into the plasma membrane and populations of serous cavity cells label differentially depending on rates of membrane turnover. This has proved useful in the *in-vitro* labelling of macrophages prior to adoptive transfer into syngeneic animals [42] and for *in-vitro* studies of plasma membrane flow throughout the cell [43, 44].

Di-1,1′-dioctadecyl-3,3,3′,3′-tetramethylindo carbocyanine
(*Molecular Probes, Eugene, Oregon, USA*)

Excitation 540 nm, Emission 556 nm.

1. Store at −20°C as a stock solution of 2 mg/ml in DMSO. Use the stock at 0.1% in serum free medium. Sonicate for 10 s and vortex vigorously.
2. Resuspend the cells at 10^7/ml in dye-containing medium and incubate at 37°C for 10 min to label mononuclear phagocytes preferentially.
3. Wash the cells three times in warm medium suplemented with 10% FCS and resuspend appropriately.

Labelling of longer duration will result in the incorporation of the dye into other less endocytically active cell populations.

PKH-1 (*Zynaxis Cell Science Inc., Malvern, PA, USA*)

Excitation 470–500 nm, Emission 500–525 nm.
According to *Melnicoff* et al., this dye is selectively taken up and retained by resident peritoneal macrophages but not by elicited macrophages [41].
 Store as a 40 μmol/l stock solution in 95% ethanol and dilute to 0.5% in HBSS for use. The intraperitoneal injection of 0.5 ml per animal labels resident peritoneal macrophages bright green compared to faint labelling of lymphocytes.

2.3.4.2   Phagocytic Labelling

Early studies of the phagocytic activity of the reticuloendothelial system involved the intravenous injection of particulate materials such as thorium hydroxide (Thorotrast) or finely divided carbon (*Pelican* ink) [45].
1. Inject 4×10^8 Hema (2-hydroxy ethyl methacrylate) microspheres per mouse.
2. Lavage the cavity 20 min after injection.
3. Phagocytically active cells are easily identified in a *May-Grünwald Giemsa* stained cytospin [33].

2.3.5   Measurement of the Turnover of Peritoneal Cells

The division of serous cavity cells under various inflammatory and immunological conditions may be assessed by the incorporation of tritiated thymidine (^{3}H-dT) [9] or bromodeoxyuridine (BrdU) [46].

1. Label cells *in vivo* by one i.v. injection of ^{3}H-dT (3.7 kBq/g body weight) before lavage of the cavity at a specific time. Pulse cells *in vitro* by incubating in medium containing 3.7 kBq/ml ^{3}H-dT or BrdU, 10 µmol/l, with fluorodeoxycytidine, 1 µmol/l.
2. Detect proliferating cells which have incorporated ^{3}H-dT or BrdU by scintillation counting, autoradiography or immunocytochemistry.

2.3.6   Cells from the Pleural Cavity

The cavity normally contains fluid sufficient only for lubrication; however, in some pathological states excessive quantities of exudates and transudates arise.

To lavage a mammalian pleural cavity [47]:
1. Prepare the animal (e.g. dog) as for surgery. To avoid puncturing the lung insert the needle in the 4th or 5th intercostal space on the left side near the sternum or dorsally in the 11th intercostal space.
2. Attach a syringe to the needle *via* a three-way stop-cock and manipulate to give negative pressure. Hold the animal in an erect position to allow fluid to drain into the sinus.

References

[1] *Z. A. Cohn, B. Benson*, The Differentiation of Mononuclear Phagocytes, J. Exp. Med. *121*, 153–169 (1965).
[2] *Z. A. Cohn, B. Benson*, The in vitro Differentiation of Mononuclear Phagocytes, I. The Influence of Inhibitors and the Results of Autoradiography, J. Exp. Med. *121*, 279–288 (1965).
[3] *Z. A. Cohn, B. Benson*, The in vitro Differentiation of Mononuclear Phagocytes, II. The Influence of Serum on Granule Formation, Hydrolase Production and Pinocytosis, J. Exp. Med. *122*, 835–848 (1965).
[4] *Z. A. Cohn, E. Weiner*, The Particulate Hydrolases of Macrophages, I. Comparative Enzymology, Isolation and Properties, J. Exp. Med. *118*, 991–1020 (1963).
[5] *M. Aronson, M. Shahar*, Formation of Histiocytes by the Omentum in vitro, Exp. Cell Res. *38*, 133–143 (1965).
[6] *M. J. Melnicoff, P. K. Horan, E. W. Breslin, P. S. Morahan*, Maintenance of Peritoneal Macrophages in the Steady State, J. Leukocyte Biol. *44*, 367–375 (1988).
[7] *J. S. Wakefield, J. S. Gale, M. V. Berridge, T. W. Jordan, H. C. Ford*, Is Percoll Innocuous to Cells? Biochem. J. *202*, 795–797 (1982).

[8] *Y. Shibata, W. L. Dempsey, P. S. Morahan, A. Volkman,* Selectively Eliminated Blood Monocytes and Splenic Suppressor Macrophages in Mice depleted of Bone Marrow by Strontium 89, J. Leukocyte Biol. *38,* 659–669 (1985).

[9] *R. Van-Furth, Z. A. Cohn,* The Origin and Kinetics of Mononuclear Phagocytes, J. Exp. Med. *128,* 415–433 (1968).

[10] *Z. Werp, M. J. Banda, R. Takemura, S. Gordon,* Secreted Proteins of Resting and Activated Macrophages, in: *D. M. Weir, L. A. Herzenberg, C. Blackwell, L. A. Herzenberg* (eds.), Handbook of Experimental Immunology (Volume 2), Cellular Immunology, Blackwell, Oxford 1986, pp. 47.1–47.29.

[11] *R. J. North,* The Concept of the Activated Macrophage, J. Immunol. *121,* 806–809 (1978).

[12] *A. E. Stuart,* Techniques for the Study of Phagocytes, in: *D. M. Weir, L. A. Herzenberg, C. Blackwell, L. A. Herzenberg* (eds.), Handbook of Experimental Immunology, Blackwell Scientific Publications, Oxford 1967, pp. 1034–1053.

[13] *G. E. Souza, F. Q. Cunha, R. Mello, S. H. Ferreira,* Neutrophil Migration Induced by Inflammatory Stimulation is Reduced by Macrophage Depletion, Agents Actions *24,* 377–380 (1988).

[14] *A. E. Postlethwaite, A. S. Townes, A. H. Kang,* Characterisation of Macrophage Migration Inhibitory Factor Activity Produced in vivo by a Cell Mediated Immune Reaction in the Guinea Pig, J. Immunol. *117,* 1716–1720 (1976).

[15] *Y. Maddox, M. Foegh, B. Zelig, M. Zmudka, J. Bellanti, P. Ramell,* A Routine Source of Human Peritoneal Macrophages, Scan. J. Immunol. *19,* 23–29 (1989).

[16] *M. N. J. A. Fieren, G. J. G. M. Van Dem Bend, I. L. Bonta,* Endotoxin Stimulated Peritoneal Macrophages Obtained from Continuous Ambulatory Perfusion Dialysis Patients Show Increased Capacity to Release IL-1 beta During Infectious Peritonitis, Eur. J. Clin. Invest. *20,* 453–457 (1990).

[17] *R. L. Roberts, B. J. Ank, I. B. Salusky, E. R. Strehm,* Purification and Properties of Peritoneal Eosinophils from Paediatric Dialysis Patients, J. Immunol. Methods *126,* 205–211 (1990).

[18] *G. F. Ryan, W. G. Spector,* Macrophage Turnover in Inflamed Connective Tissue, Proc. R. Soc. London B *175,* 269–292 (1970).

[19] *S. J. Norman, J. Cornelius,* Concurrent Depression of Tumour Macrophage Infiltration and Systemic Inflammation by Progressive Cancer Growth, Cancer Res. *38,* 3453–3459 (1978).

[20] *H. S. Lin, C. Kuhn, C. C. Stewart,* Peritoneal Exudate Cells, V. Influence of Age, Sex, Strain and Species on the Induction and Growth of Macrophage Colony Forming Cells, J. Cell. Physiol. *96,* 133–138 (1988).

[21] *T. Sabet, W. C. Hsla, H. Staniz, A. E. I. Donieiri, P. Van Aiten,* A Simple Method for Obtaining Peritoneal Macrophages from Chickens, J. Immunol. Methods *14,* 103–110 (1977).

[22] *R. M. Fauve, H. Jusforgues, B. Hevin,* Maintenance of Granuloma Macrophages in Serum Free Medium, J. Immunol. Methods *64,* 345–351 (1983).

[23] *Z. Werb, J. R. Chin,* Apoprotein E is Synthesized and Secreted by Resident and Thioglycollate Elicited Macrophages but not Pyran Copolymer or Bacillus Calmette Guerin Activated Macrophages, J. Exp. Med. *158,* 1272–1293 (1983).

[24] *F. Q. Cunha, S. H. Ferreira,* The Release of a Neutrophil Chemotactic Factor, An "in vivo" Demonstration, Braz. J. Med. Biol. Res. *19,* 775–779 (1986).

[25] *L. H. Faccioli, G. E. P. Souza, F. Q. Cunha, S. I. Poole, S. H. Ferreira,* Recombinant Interleukin-1 and Tumour Necrosis Factor Induce Neutrophil Migration "in vivo" by Indirect Mechanisms, Agents Actions *30,* 344–349 (1990).

[26] *R. A. Ribeiro, F. Q. Cunha, S. H. Ferreira,* Recombinant Gamma Interferon Causes Neutrophil Migration Mediated by the Release of a Macrophage Neutrophil Chemotactic Factor, Int. J. Exp. Pathol. *71,* 717–725 (1990).

[27] *D. Metcalf,* Actions of the CSFs *in vivo,* in: *D. Metcalf* (ed.), The Molecular Control of Blood Cells, Harvard Univ. Press, Harvard 1988, pp. 100–109.

[28] *E. J. Leonard, T. Yoshimura,* Neutrophil Attractant Activation Protein-1 (NAD-1[IL-8]), Am. J. Respir. Cell Mol. Biol. *2,* 479–486 (1990).

[29] *S. Nagao, M. Nakanishi, H. Kutsukake, K. Yagawa, S. Kusumoto, T. Shiba, A. Tanaka, S. Kotani*, Macrophages Are Stimulated by Muramyl Dipeptide to Induce Polymorphonuclear Leucocyte Accumulation in the Peritoneal Cavities of Guinea Pigs, Infect. Immun. *58*, 536–542 (1990).

[30] *D. A. Hume, P. Pavli, R. E. Donahue, I. J. Fidler*, The Effect of Human Recombinant Colony Stimulating Factor (CSF-1) on the Murine Mononuclear Phagocyte System in vivo, J. Immunol. *141*, 3405–3409 (1988).

[31] *T. J. Sayers, L. H. Mason, T. A. Witrout*, Trafficking and Activation of Murine Natural Killer Cells: Differing Roles For IFN-Gamma and IL-2, Cell. Immunol. *127*, 311–326 (1990).

[32] *L. H. Mason, S. L. Giardina, T. Hecht, J. Ortaldo, B. J. Mathieson*, LGL-1: a Non-polymorohic Antigen Expressed on a Major Population of Mouse Natural Killer Cells, J. Immunol. *140*, 4403–4412 (1988).

[33] *V. Vetvicka, M. Bilej, P. W. Kincade*, Resistance of Macrophages to 5-Fluorouracil Treatment, Immunopharmacol. *19*, 131–138 (1990).

[34] *F. W. Rankin, J. A. Bargen*, Vaccination against Peritonitis in Surgery of the Colon, Arch. Surg. *22*, 98–105 (1931).

[35] *P. Allavena, F. Peccaton, D. Maggiori, A. Erroi, M. Sironi, N. Colombo, A. Lissoni, A. Galazka, W. Miers, C. Mangioni, A. Mantovani*, Intraperitoneal Interferon Gamma in Patients with Recurrent Ascitic Ovarian Carcinoma; Modulation of Cytotoxicity and Cytokine Production in Tumour Associated Affectors and of Major Histocompatibility Antigen Expression on Tumour Cells, Cancer Res. *50*, 7318–7323 (1990).

[36] *S. Fisker, K. Kudahl Ole Sonne*, Isolation of Rat Mononuclear and Polymorphonuclear Leucocytes on Discontinuous Gradients of Nycodenz, J. Immunol. Methods *133*, 31–38 (1990).

[37] *H. Rosen, S. Gordon*, Monoclonal Antibody to the Murine Type Three Complement Receptor Inhibits Adhesion of Myelomonocytic Cells in vitro and Inflammatory Cell Recruitment in vivo, J. Exp. Med. *166*, 1655–1701 (1987).

[38] *R. L. Stevens, K. F. Austen*, Recent Advances in Cellular and Molecular Biology of Mast Cells, Immunol. Today *10*, 381–386 (1989).

[39] *A. G. Gibbons, P. Price, T. A. Roberton, J. M. Papadimitriou, G. R. Shellam*, Replication of Murine Cytomegalovirus in Mast Cells, Arch. Virol. *115*, 299–307 (1990).

[40] *A. Schoff*, Lectures in Pathology, Hoeber, New York 1924, pp. 1–33.

[41] *G. Biozzi, B. Benacerraf, B. N. Halpern*, Quantitative Study of the Granulopectic Activity of the Reticuloendothelial System, II. A Study of the Kinetics of the Granulopectic Activity of the Reticuloendothelial System in Relation to the Dose of Carbon Injected. Relationship between the Weight of the Organs, and Their Activity, Brit. J. Exp. Pathol. *34*, 441–457 (1953).

[42] *M. J. Melnicoff, P. S. Morahan, B. D. Jencen, E. W. Breslin, P. K. Horan*, In vivo Labelling of Resident Peritoneal Macrophages, J. Leukocyte Biol. *43*, 387–397 (1988).

[43] *H. Rosen, S. Gordon*, Adoptive Transfer of Fluorescence Labelled Cells Shows that Resident Peritoneal Macrophages Are Able to Migate into Specialised Lymphoid Organs and Inflammatory Sites in the Mouse, Eur. J. Immunol. *20*, 1251–1258 (1990).

[44] *D. L. Lucas, P. Dragsten, D. M. Robinson, C. A. Bowles*, Increased Lateral Diffusion of a Lipid Probe in the Plasma Membrane of Elicited Macrophages, J. Reticuloendothel. Soc. *30*, 107–114 (1981).

[45] *H. W. Florey, M. A. Jennings*, Chemotaxis, Phagocytosis and the Formation of Abscesses, The Reticuloendothelial System, in: *H. Florey* (ed.), General Pathology 2, Saunders, London 1970, pp. 124–174.

[46] *H. Gratzner*, Monoclonal Antibody to 5-Bromo, 5-Iododeoxyuridine. A new Reagent for Detection of DNA Replication, Science *218*, 474–475 (1982).

[47] *A. F. Moreland*, Collection and Withdrawal of Body Fluids and Infusion Techniques, in: *W. I. Gay* (ed.), Methods of Animal Experimentation, Vol. 1, Academic Press, New York 1965, pp. 1–42.

2.4   Alveolar Cells

Allen G. Harmsen

The respiratory tract is a frequent portal of entry for infectious and toxic materials. Defence against these insults by lung alveolar cells is critical for the maintenance of host homeostasis. Much of what we understand about these defence mechanisms has stemmed from studies of lung alveolar cells that have been obtained from the host. The lung alveolar cells are located in the lumina of alveoli on an epithelium that is continuous with that of the trachea. Because of the location of these cells, they can readily be obtained by instilling saline into the airways and aspirating back the fluids that then contain the alveolar cells. This procedure is termed bronchoalveolar lavage (BAL) and it can be performed in humans and animals with few side effects. However, for practical reasons, BAL of small laboratory animals is generally done after the animals are killed.

Because alveolar cells can be easily obtained by BAL, host pulmonary responses can readily be studied. Resident and inflammatory cells that accumulate in the lung can be isolated directly without the need for tissue digestion procedures which can alter cell surface molecules. This ease of obtaining alveolar cells makes the lung a particularly convenient organ for study of the accumulation of cells that contribute to host resistance.

2.4.1   Bronchoalveolar Lavage of Human Subjects

Human BAL is now routinely performed utilizing a flexible bronchoscope with tip diameters ranging from 4 to 5.9 mm. The bronchoscope contains three channels with separate channels being utilized for light source, viewing, and biopsy. The light source and viewing ports allow the operator visually to guide the tip of the bronchoscope into selected airways. The biopsy channel can be used for lavage, transbronchial biopsy, or obtaining a brush biopsy.

Although BAL is considered a safe procedure, it is nevertheless an invasive procedure. It should only be done by, and under the supervision of, qualified physicians. For this reason, only a brief description of the technique of BAL in human subjects will be given here.

Normally, the person undergoing BAL is awake and usually atropine and mild sedation is used as premedication. Spray topical anaesthetic into the upper airways to minimize discomfort and insert the fibre-optic bronchoscope through the nose into the respiratory tree. Visually examine the respiratory tract and wedge the tip of the bronchoscope into a subsegmental bronchus. Usually the lingula or right middle lobe of the lung are utilized. Other lung lobes can be utilized, but lavage of the upper or lower lobes is more difficult because of either the tight bend required to enable the bronchoscope to enter the lobe bronchi, or the inferior fluid recovery when utilizing the upper and lower lobes [1]. The seal produced by wedging the tip of the bronchoscope into the bronchus allows saline to be instilled into the lung and subsequently recovered. Routinely, two subsegmental lobe lavages are carried out in different areas of the lung.

The medium used for lavage is usually sterile buffered saline. Infuse in 50 ml aliquots to a cumulative amount of 200 to 300 ml [2]. After each aliquot is infused, withdraw lavage fluid by hand suction into a syringe. Use of too much suction can cause airways distal to the tip of the bronchoscope to collapse resulting in reduced volume of fluid return. In the first few aliquots recovered, the lavage fluid is usually frothy from the presence of surfactant. Fluid return from the first aliquot is usually minimal: however, the volume of fluid returned increases with subsequent aliquots. In general, when lavaging normal airways, about 50 to 60% recovery is expected; though with certain diseased lungs the return can drop significantly to the 10 to 40% range [3–5].

The aspirated fluids of the different aliquots can be kept separate or pooled and are usually immediately placed on ice. However, apparently, neither significant loss of viability in the cells nor overgrowth from contaminating bacteria occurs if the fluids are kept at room temperature for up to one hour [6]. The ability of the saline lavage fluid to support short-term cell viability may be due to the presence of protein and glucose picked up from the extracellular lining secretions in the lower airways and alveoli [2].

In general, the risk associated with BAL is not much greater than that associated with routine bronchoscopy [7, 8]. Following BAL, many patients have a troublesome cough that resolves quickly, and 10–50% of subjects have a transient fever that is not associated with infection [9]. Hypoxaemia has been observed in patients after BAL but is usually not clinically significant in normal individuals [9]. As reviewed elsewhere [9], BAL can be carried out safely in many patients with lung diseases such as asthma, sarcoidosis, hypersensitivity pneumonitis, pneumonia, emphysema, and interstitial pulmonary fibrosis. In fact, BAL has proved to be valuable in the diagnosis and investigation of numerous chronic lung diseases.

2.4.2 Bronchoalveolar Lavage of Animals

2.4.2.1 Large Animals

The lungs of large laboratory animals can be lavaged by the use of a fibre-optic bronchoscope in much the same way as human BAL is accomplished. In the dog, induce anaesthesia by halothane gas in oxygen given by face mask [10, 11]. After the dog reaches light surgical anaesthesia, place a latex endotracheal tube in the trachea, and inflate the balloon. Maintain anaesthesia using 1.5% halothane in oxygen gas through the endotracheal tube. Pass the end of a fibre-optic bronchoscope through the endotracheal tube and wedge in a selected airway. Then lavage the lung with 5 aliquots of 10 ml each of saline. Recover lavage fluid by gentle aspiration into disposable syringes. If sequential lavages are planned of the same lung areas, drawings depicting the branching of the airways should be made to assure re-entry into selected airways. After each bronchoscopy, turn off the halothane gas and disconnect the anaesthetic machine. When the swallow reflex returns, remove the endotracheal tube and return the dog to its recovery cage.

For BAL of sheep, animals can be physically restrained and topical anaesthesia obtained by nebulizing a 1% solution of lidocaine [12]. Alternatively, restrain the animals by general anaesthesia induced with halothane using a closed circuit anaesthesia machine [13]. Insert an endotracheal tube and pass the end of a long (80 cm) fibre-optic bronchoscope through the endotracheal tube and wedge in a selected airway [12, 13]. Perform lavage using 3–5 aliquots of 30–50 ml saline each.

Other laboratory animals such as rabbits, ferrets, and cats can be lavaged utilizing procedures similar to those described above except that a paediatric-sized fibre-optic bronchoscope should be used.

Use of a fibre-optic bronchoscope greatly enhances the ease and reproducibility of BAL. However, these bronchoscopes are very expensive. An alternative is to use a double lumen catheter, made by joining 3 *Foley* catheters [14], to lavage anaesthetized pigs. A piano wire may be inserted into the catheter to stiffen it and the catheter then passed through an endotracheal tube and wedged into an airway. The wire is then removed and the lung is lavaged as when using a bronchoscope. Although this method can be used, its one disadvantage is that airways to be lavaged can not be selected.

The lungs of large animals can also be lavaged after the animals are killed. For greatest ease remove the lungs and trachea from the animal in block, and lavage the explanted lungs through the trachea, by filling the lungs with saline and subsequently draining the fluid, by gravity, into a container.

2.4.2.2   Rodents

It is possible to do multiple BAL on living laboratory rodents [15], although the procedure is technically very involved. Normally, it is more practical to kill groups of rodents at different time points rather than to do sequential lavages. Anaesthetize laboratory rodents and kill by exsanguination [16]. Killing rats or mice by either CO_2 inhalation or cervical dislocation can cause haemorrhage into the lung alveoli. Expose the trachea of the animals by a small transverse cut made in the ventral wall of the trachea just posterior to the larynx and intubate it. For mice, use 1.56 mm O. D. tubing and for rats, 2.29 mm O. D. tubing. These sizes of tubing will work for most adult animals, but for smaller animals draw the ends of the tubing to decrease their diameter.

The tubing should fit snugly, but if it is too large it will tear the trachea. If the tubing is too small, it can be tied into the trachea with silk thread. Insert a properly sized hypodermic needle into the free end of the tubing and attach to a three-way stopcock with two syringes fitted to it. Fill one syringe with the lavage fluid and use the second syringe to aspirate the lavage fluids from the lungs. The three-way stopcock eliminates the need to connect and disconnect different syringes for instilling and aspirating the fluid.

Sterile PBS can be used as a lavage fluid but *Hanks* balanced salt solution without Ca^{++} and Mg^{++} is recommended. The addition of EDTA to a final concentration of 3 mmol/l increases yields of cells. How the EDTA increases cell yield is not known but it may be by either decreasing cell adherence or helping to keep lower airways open. Lavage mice with 5 aliquots of 1 ml each and rats with 5 aliquots of 5 to 10 ml each [15]. Occasionally, instilled fluid will not aspirate easily. This can be caused by the tubing twisting, resulting in the trachea itself twisting shut. Normally, moving the end of the tubing inside the trachea slightly or lightly massaging the thorax will increase fluid yield. In addition, too much suction applied by the syringe plunger when aspirating fluid can cause the airways to collapse resulting in decreased fluid yield.

2.4.3   Cell Yields of BAL

Collect lavage fluids into tubes placed on ice. Polypropylene tubes are the most satisfactory because adherent cells do not stick easily to them. Cell numbers in consecutive washes decrease as does the concentration of alveolar lining fluids and this is consistent with a general dilution model [2]. Therefore, pool lavage fluid aliquots or keep separate depending on need.

Cell counts of BAL fluids can be done on the unconcentrated lavage fluid. Count cells in lavage fluids before the cells have been centrifuged to avoid the problem of counting clumped cells that have been aggregated during centrifugation. Make a differential count from a cytocentrifuged cell preparation stained with a *Wright-Giemsa* type stain such as Diff-Quik (*American Scientific Products*, McGaw Park, IL) which gives consistent results and is stable, while the procedure used is very rapid. Alternatively, use a filtration method that captures the cells on a membrane which is then stained [17]. This is said to determine lymphocyte numbers more accurately, which can be underestimated on cytocentrifuge preparations [2] as a result of the lymphocytes being too spread out and therefore being mistaken for monocytes. However, the use of a slower speed on the cytocentrifuge and careful observation when doing differential counts can result in lymphocyte counts that correlate with counts done by an independent method such as cytofluorimetric analysis.

2.4.3.1   Humans

Yields of total cells in BAL fluids of normal humans ranges from 5–15×10^6 [1, 2]. The cells are composed of about 85–93% macrophages, 0–2% neutrophils, 7–12% lymphocytes, 0–1% eosinophils and basophils, and 1–5% ciliated cells [1, 2, 9]. The numbers of cells in BAL as well as the types of cells represented with change markedly with diseases of the lung. Many of these changes have been reviewed elsewhere [1, 2, 9].

2.4.3.2   Large Animals

The yields of cells in BAL fluids collected from large animals by fibre-optic bronchoscopy lavage is similar to that described for human subjects. In the chimpanzee, 1–6×10^6 total cells may be recovered composing about 90% alveolar macrophages, 6% lymphocytes and 4% neutrophils [18]. For the dog, about 10–20×10^6 total cells are recovered and consist of about 90% alveolar macrophages, 2% neutrophils and 8% lymphocytes [10, 11]. Similarly, sheep will yield 10–20×10^6 total cells by BAL of which approximately 74% are alveolar macrophages, 5% neutrophils, 8% eosinophils and 12% lymphocytes [12, 13].

2.4.3.3   Rodents

The yield of alveolar cells by lavage of rat lungs is between 2 and 5×10^6 cells. The cells consist of about 96% alveolar macrophages, 2% eosinophil and 2% neutrophils [15]. In mice, approximately 0.5×10^6 total cells are recovered. The cells consist of nearly 100% alveolar macrophages with few epithelial cells also present [16, 19]. Cells recovered by lavage can vary greatly in number and composition in mice, or any animal, depending on the age, general health, and husbandry conditions of the animals. In general, older mice yield more cells than younger mice of similar size. The increase in cell numbers is caused by increases in numbers of macrophages as well as of neutrophils and lymphocytes. This increase could be the result of protracted exposure of the mice to dust and potential infectious agents. Lavage cell yields are increased in animals experimentally exposed to dust and infectious agents [9]. Indeed, lung lavage yields containing small numbers of pure populations of alveolar macrophages are a good indicator that mice have not been exposed to potential pathogens.

2.4.3.4   Differential Phenotype Analysis

Cells in lung lavage fluids can be further characterized by the presence of specific antigens on their surface. This has been shown to be particularly useful for identifying lymphocyte subsets [20, 21, 22], by staining with mAbs specific for phenotypic markers and detection by flow cytometric analysis (cf. 5.11). One difficulty with this procedure used on BAL cells is the large amount of autofluorescence of alveolar macrophages. Because these cells can constitute the majority of alveolar cells, their presence can make it difficult to detect specific fluorescence caused by small populations of stained lymphocytes. Minimize this overlap in fluorescence by gating out macrophages through the use of forward and side scatter detection on the flow cytometer to separate the larger and more granular macrophages from the lymphocytes [23].

2.4.3.5   Recovery and Dilution of Cells and Fluid by BAL

In human BAL the volume of lung lavaged is not consistent from patient to patient. In addition, the volume of fluid recovered can vary between 40–80% of the instilled fluid [9]. Because of these differences, comparisons of quantities of cells and noncellular material in BAL fluids are difficult to make between subjects or even between different lavages acquired at different times from the same individual. For this reason there have been attempts to determine the extent of dilution of instilled fluid with lung fluid in order to standardize yields. Exogenous and endogenous markers have been used for this purpose. Of the endogenous markers, albumin or total protein have been most commonly used [9], in that results of BAL are corrected to milligrams of protein or albumin. However, in inflammatory states such as asthma, sarcoidosis, or oxygen toxicity [9], there is an increase in protein transfer across the alveolar capillary barrier. This makes the use of proteins as a marker for standardization unsatisfactory if inflammation is present. Urea has also been used as a marker because it readily crosses the alveolar capillary membrane and therefore is present in the same concentration in the lung fluid as in the peripheral blood. However, because urea passes rapidly from blood into the alveoli, the longer the dwell-time of the lavage fluid in the alveolus, the more urea will go into the fluid [24]. Apparently, though, if care is taken to have a short, consistent dwell-time, the concentration of urea in the BAL fluid can be used to estimate lung fluid dilution [25].

Two exogenous markers used to standardize BAL yields are methylene blue [26] and inulin [27]. Both these substances cross the alveolar-epithelial barrier very slowly and thus are useful for calculating the dilution of instilled fluid by lung fluid. However, care must be taken that the presence of these substances does not interfere with the measurement of other substances in the BAL fluid [28].

2.4.4   Limitations

Utilizing BAL to analyse a pulmonary response has the distinct advantage over biopsy in that a much larger area of the lung is sampled. Of course, in cases where the whole lung is lavaged this advantage is even greater. However, it must be remembered that both involved and uninvolved areas of the lung may exist and that BAL may yield cells from either of those two types of areas. In addition, it is possible that the area lavaged includes both involved and uninvolved areas so that cells collected by lavage can be a mixture of resident and elicited cells.

Cells collected by BAL are washed out from the lumina of the alveoli and lower airways of the lung and the composition of BAL cells is similar to that observed in the alveoli by biopsy [20, 29]. However, results of functional studies have suggested that cells collected by BAL differ from those found in the interstitium [30]. Further, although B-cells do not accumulate in the lumina of the lungs of mice resolving *Pneumocystis* pneumonia [22], they do accumulate in the insterstitium of the lung. Thus, cells collected by BAL may not represent all cells in the lungs.

References

[1] *G. W. Hunninghake, J. E. Gadek, O. Kawanami, V. J. Ferrans, R. G. Crystal,* Inflammatory and Immune Processes in the Human Lung in Health and Disease: Evaluation by Bronchoalveolar Lavage, Am. J. Pathol. *97,* 149–198 (1979).

[2] *H. Reynolds,* Bronchoalveolar Lavage, Am. Rev. Respir. Dis. *135,* 250–263 (1987).

[3] *T. N. Finley, E. W. Swenson, W. S. Curran, G. L. Huber, A. J. Ladman,* Bronchopulmonary Lavage in Normal Subjects and Patients with Obstructive Lung Disease, Ann. Intern. Med. *66,* 651–658 (1977).

[4] *T. R. Martin, G. Raghu, R. J. Maunder, S. C. Springmeyer,* The Effects of Chronic Bronchitis and Chronic Air Flow Obstruction on Lung Cell Populations Recovered by Bronchoalveolar Lavage, Am. Rev. Respir. Dis. *132,* 254–260 (1985).

[5] *G. W. Hunninghake, J. D. Fulmer, R. C. Young, J. E. Gadek, R. G. Crystal,* Localization of the Immune Response in Sarcoidosis, Am. Rev. Respir. Dis. *120,* 49–57 (1979).

[6] *J. A. Rankin, G. P. Naegel, H. Y. Reynolds,* Use of a Central Laboratory for Analysis of Bronchoalveolar Lavage Fluid, Am. Rev. Respir. Dis. *133,* 186–190 (1986).

[7] *R. Cole, C. Turton, H. Lanyon, J. Collins,* Bronchoalveolar Lavage for the Preparation of Free Lung Cells: Technique and Complications, Br. J. Dis. Chest *74,* 273–278 (1980).

[8] *I. J. Strumpf, M. K. Feld, M. J. Cornelius, B. A. Keogh, R. G. Crystal,* Safety of Fiberoptic Bronchoalveolar Lavage in Evaluation of Interstitial Lung Disease, Chest *80,* 268–271 (1981).

[9] *N. Grossblatt, L. R. Paulson* (eds.), Biologic Markers in Pulmonary Toxicology, National Academy Press, Washington, D. C. 1989.

[10] *D. E. Bice, D. L. Harris, J. O. Hill, B. A. Muggenburg, R. K. Wolff,* Immune Responses after Localized Lung Immunization in the Dog, Am. Rev. Respir. Dis. *122,* 755–760 (1980).

[11] *A. G. Harmsen, D. E. Bice, B. A. Muggenburg,* The Effect of Local Antibody Responses on *In Vivo* and *In Vitro* Phagocytes by Pulmonary Alveolar Macrophages, J. Leukocyte Biol. *37,* 483–492 (1985).

[12] *M. Rola-Pleszczynski, P. Sirois, R. Begin,* Cellular and Humoral Components of Bronchoalveolar Lavage in the Sheep, Lung *159,* 91–99 (1981).

[13] *A. D. Chanana, P. Chandra, D. D. Joel,* Pulmonary Mononuclear Cells: Studies of Pulmonary Lymph and Bronchoalveolar Cells of Sheep, J. Reticuloendothel. Soc. *29,* 127–135 (1981).

[14] *A. G. Harmsen, J. R. Birmingham, R. L. Engen, E. J. Jeska,* A Method for Obtaining Swine Alveolar Macrophages by Segmented Pulmonary Lavage, J. Immunol. Methods *27,* 199–202 (1979).

[15] *J. L. Mauderly,* Bronchopulmonary Lavage of Small Laboratory Animals, Lab. Anim. Sci. *27,* 255–261 (1977).

[16] *A. G. Harmsen,* Role of Alveolar Macrophages in Lipopolysaccharide-Induced Neutrophil Accumulation, Infect Immun. *56,* 1858–1863 (1988).

[17] *C. Saltini, A. J. Hance, V. J. Ferrans, J. Basset, P. B. Bitterman, R. G. Crystal,* Accurate Quantification of Cells Recovered by Bronchoalveolar Lavage, Am. Rev. Respir. Dis. *130,* 650–658 (1984).

[18] *B. A. Muggenburg, F. F. Hahn, J. A. Bowen, D. E. Bice,* Flexible Fiberoptic Bronchoscopy of Chimpanzees, Lab. Anim. Sci. *32,* 534–536 (1982).

[19] *A. G. Harmsen, E. A. Havell,* Roles of Tumor Necrosis Factor and Macrophages in Lipopolysaccharide-Induced Accumulation of Neutrophils in Cutaneous Air Pouches, Infect. Immun. *58,* 297–302 (1989).

[20] *R. G. Crystal, W. C. Roberts, G. W. Hunninghake, J. E. Gadek, J. D. Fulmer, B. R. Line,* Pulmonary Sarcoidosis: A Disease Characterized and Perpetuated by Activated Lung T-Lymphocytes, Ann. Intern. Med. *94,* 73–94 (1981).

[21] *J. W. Leatherman, A. F. Michael, B. A. Schwartz, J. R. Hoidal,* Lung T Cells in Hypersensitivity Pneumonitis, Ann. Intern. Med. *100,* 390–392 (1984).

[22] *A. G. Harmsen, M. Stankiewicz,* Requirement for CD4+ Cells in Resistance to *Pneumocystis carinii* Pneumonia in Mice, J. Exp. Med. *172,* 937–945 (1990).

[23] *L. C. Ginns, P. D. Goldenheim, R. C. Burton, R. B. Colvin, L. G. Miller, G. Goldstein, C. Hurwitz, H. Kazemi,* T-Lymphocyte Subsets in Peripheral Blood and Lung Lavage in Idiopathic Pulmonary Fibrosis and Sarcoidosis: Analysis by Monoclonal Antibodies and Flow Cytometry, Clin. Immunol. Immunopathol. *25,* 11–20 (1982).

[24] *T. W. Marcy, W. W. Merrill, J. A. Rankin, H. Y. Reynolds,* Limitations of Using Urea to Quantify Epithelial Lining Fluid Recovered by Bronchoalveolar Lavage, Am. Rev. Respir. Dis. *135,* 1276–1280 (1987).

[25] *S. I. Rennard, G. Basset, D. Lecossier, F. M. O'Donnell, P. Pinkston, P. G. Martin, R. G. Crystal,* Estimation of Absolute Volume of Epithelial Lining Fluid Recovered by Lavage Using Urea as a Marker of Dilution, J. Appl. Physiol. *60,* 532–538 (1986).

[26] *R. P. Baughman, C. H. Bosken, R. G. Loudon, P. Hurtubise, T. Wesseler,* Quantitation of Bronchoalveolar Lavage with Methylene Blue, Am. Rev. Respir. Dis. *128,* 266–270 (1983).

[27] *I. C. Normand, R. E. Oliver, E. O. Reynolds, L. B. Strang,* Permeability of Lung Capillaries and Alveoli to Non-Electrolytes in Foetal Lamb, J. Physiol. London *219,* 303–330 (1971).

[28] *A. M. Richter, R. T. Abboud, S. S. Johal,* Methylene Blue Decreases the Functional Activity of Alpha-1-Protease Inhibitor in Bronchoalveolar Lavage, Am. Rev. Respir. Dis. *134,* 326–327 (1986).

[29] *I. L. Paradis, J. H. Dauber, B. S. Rabin,* Lymphocyte Phenotypes in Bronchoalveolar Lavage and Lung Tissue in Sarcoidosis and Idiopathic Pulmonary Fibrosis, Am. Rev. Respir. Dis. *133,* 855–860 (1986).

[30] *J. C. Weissler, C. R. Lyons, M. F. Lipscomb, G. B. Toews,* Human Pulmonary Macrophages: Functional Comparison of Cells Obtained from Whole Lung and by Bronchoalveolar Lavage, Am. Rev. Respir. Dis. *133,* 473–477 (1986).

2.5   Lymphoid Tissue Cells

Deborah J. Bevan and Norman A. Staines

2.5.1   General

Lymphoid cells may be obtained from several sites in the body, the choice of which will be influenced by the type of cells required and the purpose to which they will be put. The absolute and relative numbers of immature, mature, B-cells, T-cells and non-lymphoid cells vary from tissue to tissue. A secondary consideration is the availability of the requisite organ(s), and this is particularly relevant with human tissues where access to solid organs is severely limited.

In order to obtain single cell suspensions of lymphoid tissue cells, solid organs are disrupted by various methods which inevitably produce cell mixtures containing live cells, dead cells, debris and often contaminating connective tissue and red blood cells (RBC). These contaminants may be removed by several methods which are detailed in this section. It is particularly important to remove debris in the cell suspension because viable cells become trapped as large clumps and reduce the cell yield. Once the cells have been obtained in single cell suspension their number and viability must be assessed.

The methods described here are suitable for the preparation of cells from mice and rats. They may also be applied in principle to the recovery of cells from other animal species. In general, human and non-human primate tissues can be processed similarly, and special mention is made of these.

Primary lymphoid organs: These are the bone marrow and thymus. The majority of cells in these organs, in the adult, are immature cells which will either mature or die. In the thymus, most are destined to die rather than migrate to the secondary tissues. Therefore, these organs are primarily used for the study of cell maturation processes.

Secondary lymphoid organs and tissues: They include the spleen, lymph nodes, *Peyer's* patches and tonsils. The ratio of T:B-cells varies with the organ. All these organs are sources of mature lymphocytes and accessory cells.

Small lymphocytes continuously recirculate from the blood to the tissues then to the peripheral lymphoid organs finally returning, in the efferent lymph *via* the thoracic duct, to the blood. Lymphocytes are sequestered from this recirculating pool when they encounter their specific antigens. Blood and lymph are correctly classified as secondary lymphoid tissues.

Anaesthesia: Before tissues are removed from animals, humane killing is necessary. Methods used must comply with local and national, ethical and legal restrictions. An overdose of an inhaled (e.g., ether, chloroform or halothane) or injected (e.g., sodium pentabarbitone) anaesthetic may be used but it is emphasized that agents of this type will be present in the cell suspension subsequently prepared. In consequence it may be necessary to control for their presence: some anaesthetics are known to affect the function of various cell types. Rapid physical stunning or cervical dislocation are therefore preferred methods except that they may cause internal bleeding and are not suitable for all applications (indicated later). Asphyxiation by inhalation of Gaseous CO_2 is an acceptable alternative that is widely used.

Handling of cell suspensions: The general conditions discussed in section 2.1 should be applied. It is particularly important, if lymphoid cells are to be recovered in good condition, that rapid changes of temperature are avoided. Therefore, if manipulations take a long time, maintain cell suspensions and handling solutions on melting ice. For washing, run the centrifuge at $+5\,°C$. Take care to avoid foaming of suspensions of lymphoid cells: this is especially damaging to them.

Cell yields and viability: The viability of a cell suspension should be ascertained before any experiment with the cells is carried out: a total cell count alone is insufficient. Methods of measuring viability by the exclusion of non-electrolyte dyes, for example, trypan blue or eosin, by viable cells are described in section 2.1.1.2.

Note: If trypan blue is used, the cells must be counted within 5 min as live cells will begin to take up this dye after that time.

Viability of lymphoid cells may be measured by the uptake of FDA (fluorescein diacetate) which is taken up by all cells but only hydrolysed by live cells which then fluoresce green.

2.5.2 Preparation of Cell Suspensions from Rodent Lymphoid Organs

In all procedures it is recommended to use a handling medium which is a balanced salt solution (BSS) containing 2 % (v/v) fetal or newborn calf serum. A suitable formulation [1] is based on two 10 times concentrated stock solutions that should be stored at $4\,°C$.

Solution (A):
Dissolve 10.00 g dextrose, 0.60 g KH_2PO_4, 3.58 g $Na_2HPO_4 \cdot 7H_2O$ and 20.0 ml 0.5 % (w/v) phenol red solution to 1 l with doubly distilled water.

Solution (B):
Dissolve 1.86 g $CaCl_2 \cdot 2H_2O$, 4.00 g KCl, 80.00 g NaCl, 1.04 g $MgCl_2$, 2.00 g (anhydrous) $MgSO_4 \cdot 7H_2O$ to 1 l doubly distilled water. For use, mix equal volumes of solns. (A) and (B); the resulting buffer should be at pH 7.2 to 7.4 and have a conductivity of 14–16 mS. If sterilized by passage through a 0.22 μm sterile filter, the BSS can be stored at room temperature, in the dark, with a very long shelf-life. To prepare handling medium, calf serum is added immediately before use as described above.

2.5.2.1   Thymus

The thymus is a bilobed organ, ventral and anterior to the heart. Kill animals by a method other than cervical dislocation to avoid bleeding in the thorax. Care should also be taken that the parathymic lymph nodes are not incorporated into the preparation by mistake. The thymus yields an almost pure preparation of T-cells (>90 % based on the cell surface expression of CD2).

1. Place the animal on its back and flood the neck/upper body with 70 % ethanol (this is necessary to sterilize the area), and allow to evaporate.
2. Pinch up the skin over the diaphragm and make an incision. Pull back the skin to reveal the rib cage; cut this at both sides so that by lifting the sternum the thymus may be easily accessed.
3. Free the organ by cutting around it. Avoid removing the parathymic lymph nodes, and avoid haemorrhage until the end of the surgery.
4. Place the organ in a 60 mm diameter *Petri* dish containing 10 ml of handling medium (BSS and 2 % calf serum). Hold the organ with blunt forceps and gently 'scrape' a scalpel blade across the thymus until all the cells are released. Transfer the cell suspension to a 10 ml centrifuge tube and allow debris to settle out by standing the tube for a few min in melting ice.
5. Remove the cells to a fresh tube, avoiding the debris, and wash them twice by centrifugation ($200 \times g$, 10 min). Resuspend the cell pellet in a small volume (<1 ml) of handling medium by repeated aspiration into and out of a *Pasteur* pipette or alternatively, 'flick' the tube to resuspend the cell pellet. Avoid air bubbles and foaming in the cell suspension.

2.5.2.2   Bone Marrow

The bone marrow consists of a heterogenous population of stem cells, blood cells and their precursors and also mature lymphocytes and macrophages. Therefore, if lymphocytes are required as a pure population, they must be separated from the myeloid cells by density gradient centrifugation or other appropriate method (cf. 2.2.2). The long bones of the hind limbs are most commonly used, the femora, occasionally the tibiae are used. If a large number of bone marrow cells are required the humeri of the forelimbs may be included.

1. Place the dead animal on its back, head facing away from you. Raise one hind limb by the foot to extend the limb. Make a V-shaped incision above the ankle and pull the skin down to above the knee. Cut the muscle away.
2. Remove the foot and break the knee joint.
3. Remove the tibia and place in a 60 mm diameter *Petri* dish, kept on ice, containing cold handling medium (BSS + 2 % calf serum).
4. Cut the skin up to the hip and reflect it.

5. Remove the muscle from the femur and cut the ligaments. Twist the femur to remove it from the hip joint.
6. Transfer the femur to the *Petri* dish.
7. Repeat the dissection process with the other hind leg.
8. Cut the ends off the tibiae and femora with strong scissors or animal nail clippers and, holding the bone with forceps, insert a 0.8 mm diameter (rat) or 0.6 mm diameter (mouse) hypodermic needle attached to a syringe containing 5 ml of cold handling medium. Flush the bone marrow through with the medium and collect into the *Petri* dish. Repeat the flushing process to remove all the marrow.
9. Gently break up any clumps of cells by repeated aspiration into a fine-bore *Pasteur* pipette.
10. Wash the cells twice by centrifugation ($220 \times g$, 10 min).

2.5.2.3   Spleen

The spleen is a good source of B-cells, T-cells and macrophages. The ratio of T-: B-cells is approximately 3:2 in this organ.

1. Place the dead animal on its right side, head to the left, and swab the left flank with 70 % ethanol.
2. Pinch up the skin over the abdomen, make a long median incision (using scissors or scalpel). At both ends of the incision make two further cuts at right angles to the original incision, pull the skin back to expose the peritoneal wall.
3. Cut through the peritoneal wall. The spleen lies on the left side of the peritoneal cavity, below the stomach and up against the cavity wall. The organ is recognized by it deep red colour and long thin shape.
4. Gently lift the spleen with blunt-ended forceps and cut away its vascular and connective tissue attachments using scissors.
5. Place the spleen in a sieve/tea strainer (domestic nylon strainers are suitable) over a 60 mm diameter *Petri* dish containing handling medium and coarsely chop the organ using scissors.
6. Push the spleen pulp through the sieve using the rubber-ended plunger from a 5 ml syringe. *Do not* scrape the plunger from side to side as the shearing forces will rupture many of the cells.

   Wash the cells through the sieve with 10 ml of handling medium. Alternatively, place the whole spleen in a 90 mm diameter *Petri* dish with about 20 ml of handling medium, the cells may be released from the spleen by gentle teasing with two 0.8 mm diameter hypodermic needles.
7. Aspirate the cell suspension from the *Petri* dish and transfer to a suitable number of tubes. Allow the debris to settle for 5 min and carefully remove the cell suspension avoiding the debris.
8. Transfer the cells to fresh tubes and wash the cells by centrifugation ($200 \times g$, 10 min). Remove the supernatant and gently resuspend the cell pellet in less than

1 ml of handling medium by either 'flicking' the tube or by gentle and repeated aspiration using a *Pasteur* pipette. Adjust the volume of the cell suspension to about 10 ml. Repeat the centrifugation wash step.

9. At this stage the RBC may be removed either by density gradient centrifugation or RBC lysis with isotonic ammonium chloride or by hypotonic shock using distilled water.

   The normal mononuclear cell yield from a spleen is approximately 1 to 2×10^8 for the mouse and up to 10^9 for the rat.

RBC lysis by hypotonic shock

1. To the packed cell pellet add an equal volume of BSS (at a 1:10 dilution in sterile doubly distilled water), mix and incubate for 10 s.
2. Immediately add $\times 50$ volume of BSS (normal concentration), centrifuge at $200 \times g$ for 10 min.
3. Wash the cells twice (as above) in BSS by centrifugation.
4. Repeat steps 1–3 if there are any RBC remaining.

RBC lysis with tris-buffered ammonium chloride

(This protocol is based on the method of *Mishell & Shiigi* [2])

1. Prepare the Tris ammonium chloride buffer by adding 90 ml ammonium chloride solution (0.856 g/100 ml) to 10 ml Tris (2.059 g/100 ml, pH 7.65). Adjust the final pH to 7.2.
2. Add 1 ml Tris ammonium chloride buffer to 0.1 ml packed cells. Mix and leave for 4 min at room temperature. Add 9 ml PBS or BSS to the mixture and centrifuge at $200 \times g$ for 10 min.
3. Wash the cells in BSS twice by centrifugation. Repeat steps 1, 2 and 3 if necessary to remove residual RBC.
4. Resuspend in BSS to the required concentration.

Removal of dead cells and debris

1. Place a standard gauze/lint dressing over the opening of a 50 ml plastic centrifuge tube, slightly depress the dressing in the middle.
2. Pour 10–20 ml of handling medium through the dressing. Discard the medium.
3. The cell suspension should be at $1–2 \times 10^7$/ml in handling medium. This is then carefully poured into the dressing. The cells which pass through the gauze/lint are collected in the centrifuge tube which is then centrifuged for 10 min at $200 \times g$ and the cells resuspended at an appropriate dilution.

2.5.2.4   Lymph Nodes

The lymph nodes are a good source of lymphocytes and, unlike the spleen, do not contain contaminating RBC if prepared carefully. The ratio of T-: B-cells in the normal lymph node is in the range of $2:1$ to $4:1$. The cervical, mesenteric and popliteal lymph nodes are the most commonly used because they are the most accessible. The popliteal lymph nodes are too cryptic in normal rodents for use but are often used after, e.g., a host-*versus*-graft reaction has been induced by the injection of allogeneic cells into the rear foot-pads; in such situations the nodes greatly increase in size. Ideally, if the cervical lymph nodes are required, the animal should be killed by anaesthetic overdose as cervical dislocation may damage them. The mesenteric lymph nodes are situated at the junction of the small and large intestines where they form a 'chain', they are distinguished from the surrounding fat and connective tissue by their darker colour and appearance as a chain of connected ovoids.

It is recommended that lymph nodes are handled in ice-cold medium as this causes adhering fat/connective tissue to turn white and thus the lymph nodes can be discerned and cleaned more easily. The cells may be dissociated from lymph nodes by crushing or teasing.

1. Apply minimal crushing pressure to lymph nodes held between two glass microscope slides to release cells, or
2. Crush lymph nodes in a minimal amount of handling medium in a 90 mm diameter *Petri* dish using a block of Perspex.
3. Increase the cell yield by subsequent gentle 'scraping' of the crushed lymph nodes, held by forceps, with a scalpel blade.
4. If a high cell yield is not required, trap lymph nodes in about 2 ml of handling medium in a 30 mm diameter *Petri* dish and gently tease apart using two 0.8 mm diameter hypodermic needles.
5. Aspirate the cell suspension into 10 ml conical centrifuge tubes and allow any debris to settle out.
6. Transfer the cell suspension to fresh tubes and wash the cells twice by centrifugation before finally resuspending them in handling medium.

2.5.2.5   *Peyer's Patches*

These are a rich source of B-cells (55–75 %). *Peyer's* patches are small, raised 'blisters' of a whitish colour found at intervals along the small intestine.

1. Kill the animal by a suitable humane method and place it on its back. Drench the abdomen with 70 % ethanol.
2. Make a long incision from the sternum to the groin and reflect the skin.

3. Using blunt-ended forceps gently pull the intestines from the body cavity (it is not necessary to dissect the intestines out as this increases the risk of contamination by the gut contents) and lay them out on a clean suface.

4. Isolate the small intestine, the *Peyer's* patches will be seen as described.

5. Holding the small intestine with blunt-ended forceps and using fine curved scissors cut the *Peyer's* patches from the gut wall. Transfer to a 60 mm diameter *Petri* dish containing 10 ml of handling medium (BSS + 2 % (v/v) calf serum). Rinse the tissues thoroughly to remove any adhering matter. Place the washed tissues in a fresh *Petri* dish containing 10 ml of handling medium.

6. The cells may be dispersed by (a) gentle 'scraping' of the *Peyer's* patches with a scalpel blade whilst securing the tissue with forceps or (b) enzymic digestion using collagenase which will result in a higher cell yield. Add collagenase (5 mg/ml in BSS) to the *Peyer's* patches in a test tube which is then capped and incubated at 37 °C for 20 min. Shake the tube periodically throughout the incubation period.

7. At the end of the incubation period aspirate the digested tissue into and out of a wide-bore *Pasteur* pipette in order to break the clumps of tissue. Leave to stand for a few moments in order to allow the debris to settle out.

8. Transfer the cell suspension, avoiding the debris, to a fresh centrifuge tube and wash twice in handling medium by centrifugation ($200 \times g$, 10 min).

9. Resuspend the cells to the desired concentration in handling medium.

2.5.2.6   Blood

The concentration of leucocytes is usually in the region of 5×10^6/ml, comprising approximately 60–70 % granulocytes, 25–30 % lymphocytes and 1–4 % monocytes. Blood is not often used as a source of rodent lymphocytes owing to the small volumes obtainable.

Obtain blood from (anaesthetized) rodents by cardiac puncture and collect into a tube containing heparin (10 U/ml) or sodium citrate. Fresh blood may be defibrinated, to remove platelets, by adding 1 glass bead (3 mm diameter) per ml of blood and mixing gently by end-over-end rotation for 10 min until a clot has formed. If blood has been collected in sodium citrate then it must be re-calcified before it can be defibrinated. The mononuclear cells may be isolated by density gradient centrifugation (c.f. 2.2.2). If, however, all peripheral white blood cells (lymphocytes, monocytes and granulocytes) are required, remove the RBC by ammonium chloride lysis (c.f. 2.5.2.3).

2.5.3   Preparation of Human Lymphoid Cells

Warning: All human tissues must be treated with caution as they are a potential source of HIV and hepatitis viruses. Cells from non-human primates are comparatively dangerous also. Safe handling procedures should be observed.

2.5.3.1 Tonsil

Tonsils are the most easily obtained human lymphoid organs. Because of the circumstances of their surgical removal, they may be microbially contaminated; aside from the hazard this involves, it may compromise the function of the cells. Handling and culture media should thus be supplemented with antibiotics (cf. 3.2).

1. Place the tonsil in a 60 mm diameter *Petri* dish containing cold handling medium (BSS + 2% calf serum), cut off fat and connective tissue.
2. Transfer the cleaned tonsil to a metal sieve held over a *Petri* dish containing fresh handling medium and roughly chop with scissors.
3. Use the rubber-ended plunger from a 5 ml syringe to push the tissue against the sieve. Wash 20 ml of handling medium through the sieve and collect the washings containing the cells in the *Petri* dish.
4. Transfer the cell suspension to fresh tubes and wash twice by centrifugation ($200 \times g$, 10 min). Resuspend the cells at a suitable concentration in handling medium. Remove contaminating RBC by ammonium chloride lysis (cf. 2.5.2.3) or density gradient centrifugation (cf. 2.2.2).

2.5.3.2 Blood

Blood should be collected and handled as described for rodents except, of course, venous blood is used as the source of human blood. It should be noted that defibrination of the blood will result in the loss of most of the B-cells.

Isolate lymphocytes from blood by density gradient centrifugation (cf. 2.2.2). If all leucocytes are required (granulocytes, monocytes and lymphocytes) then a buffy coat preparation can be prepared by simply centrifuging heparinized blood at $700 \times g$ for 5 min. The RBC form the bottom layer and the leucocytes form a white layer (buffy coat) on top. The yellow supernatant is the plasma which contains platelets. The buffy coats are carefully removed using a *Pasteur* pipette and the cells are washed by centrifugation in handling medium ($200 \times g$ for 10 min). Residual RBC may be removed by ammonium chloride lysis (cf. 2.5.2.3).

References

[1] *R.I. Mishell, R.W. Dutton,* Immunization of Dissociated Spleen Cell Cultures from Normal Mice, J. Exp. Med. 126 (1967) 423–442.
[2] *B.B. Mishell, S.M. Shiigi, C. Henry, E.L. Chan, J. North, R. Gallily, M. Slomich, K. Miller, J. Marbrook, D. Parks, A.H. Good,* Preparation of Mouse Cell Suspensions, in: *B.B. Mishell, S.M. Shiigi* (eds.), Selected Methods in Cellular Immunology, Freeman, San Francisco (1980) pp. 3–27.

2.6   Arthropod Tissues and Cells

Klaus-Peter Sieber

2.6.1   General Properties

Immunological methods have become crucial tools for elucidating the physiological nature and developmental role of endogenous and exogenous factors in biological systems. Immunochemical analysis in a wide range of studies in anatomy, biochemistry and molecular biology has increased logarithmically in the past 15 years. Although arthropods have provided excellent systems for *in-vitro* as well as *in-vivo* studies of biologically active factors, research in fields such as neurohormones has lagged behind the rapid advances in corresponding mammalian systems. One of the major difficulties is the scarcity of biological material, requiring the careful dissections of thousands of insect brains to elucidate the structure or function of a single factor. Another difficulty is the frequent need for time-consuming *in-vitro* bioassays to monitor bioactive fractions from purified material. The size and general nature of insects often dictate unique specialized cell and tissue preparation and cultivation techniques.

The search for alternative strategies in insect pest control as well as the possibility to utilize virus-infected insect cells as production sites of therapeutic and diagnostic agents have prompted scientists to deepen the understanding of neuroendocrinological and physiological processes in invertebrates as well as to improve insect cell culture technologies. New techniques have been established and older techniques modified in order to elucidate structural or functional properties of arthropod tissues and cells *in vitro*.

Research on arthropods, unlike that on vertebrates, deals with animal species with substantial differences in morphological as well as physiological properties due to their great evolutionary diversity. Rather than describe an isolated preparation technique of arthropod tissues, this section will focus on studies that include aspects of isolation and preparation of neural gland tissues and cells for biological *in-vitro* assays and immunohistochemistry because of common features of the nervous system within most arthropod species.

Often, the choice of dissection medium and incubation medium represents the only major difference from techniques applied in vertebrate science. The advantage of being able to induce and alter developmental processes which are rapid (ovarian development, ontogenesis) or unique (moulting, diapause) to arthropods, results in specific *in-vitro* experimental designs such as ovarian development *in vitro* or induction of physiological processes in which immunological tools are used. A schematic outline of a study is described here using tissues that contain bioactive factors (neural tissues) as well as tissues which act as target organs (glands).

The most obvious feature common to arthropods is their generally rigid exoskeleton. Therefore, growth involves completely different morphological features and processes (moulting, eclosion, imaginal discs), in which larval cells, except for nerve cells and malpighian tubules, are programmed to disintegrate. The cellular material is used for the construction of the adult, in which cell division (except in the gonads) does not occur: cells have already been determined and are competent to differentiate *in vitro*. The absence of blood vessels and the different organization of the nervous system become apparent once the specimen is dissected. Although arthropods do not seem to differ much from vertebrates with regard to their complement of hormones, neurotransmitters and neuropeptides (with highly conserved sequences), their neural structures and cells differ considerably from those of vertebrates. This makes uniquely identifiable neurones useful models for studies at the cellular level. Morphological and biochemical features of arthropod tissue and cells differ only in few aspects such as glycoprotein profile or lipid composition from vertebrate cells, facilitating purification procedures by use of preparation protocols already established for vertebrates. Because of inherent cytoarchitectural differences between invertebrates and vertebrates, descriptive classification derived from mammalian cell culture has limitations. Buffers and media are widely used for invertebrate cell culture that were originally designed for mammalian cells, although minimal and optimal nutritional requirements and culture parameters (pH, osmotic pressure) have to be evaluated and optimized for cells of various arthropod species.

2.6.2   Preparation of Tissues and Cells

2.6.2.1   General

The preparation of arthropod tissues for biochemical analysis is often performed by shock-freezing the whole animal in liquid nitrogen prior to grinding the tissues and extracting the molecules of interest. Specific procedures are available to ease the separation from other tissues: heads of mass-reared insects (mosquitoes, flies) can easily be separated from the body by shaking frozen adults in a chilled *Erlenmeyer* flask or polythene bag and by subsequent sieving detached heads through standard testing sieves. When working with larger specimens, a cork borer (5 mm) can be used to cut tissue portions containing the brain and the retrocerebral complex out of frozen heads. This material is homogenized in buffer or acetone and processed further by standard purification methods. Further purification methods of arthropod and mammalian tissues follow protocols which usually require specific buffers and solvents in which the molecule of interest is most stable and active; e.g., homogenization of tissues in electrophoresis sample buffer after injecting labelled tracers. Since purification protocols of insect tissues tend to make use of the various methods that have been developed for mammalian tissues and do not differ methodologically from isolation procedures of vertebrates [1], these procedures will not be dealt with here. An example is given below, describing the preparation of tissues for experiments in which bioactivity of factors is monitored in *in-vitro* experiments specific for arthropods.

2.6.2.2   Dissection

Insects are anaesthetized by placing them in crushed ice or by refrigerating them for 10–15 min. Pin them on wax in dissection dishes and cover the specimen with ice-cold PBS or another buffer of choice, cut open the cuticle and remove the tissue or organ under a dissecting microscope. Add protease inhibitors (cf. 2.6.5) to the dissection medium to prevent degradation of peptides to be analysed. Often, references for a certain preparation technique are already available (e. g., how to position the animal, the thorax or the head; which integument to cut or how to access glands). Pull the cuticle aside and pin to the wax exposing the tissues to be excised. When tissues (fat body) are difficult to dissect in certain species (e. g., mosquitoes) because of their fragility, perform the preparations with the organs still attached to other tissues (body wall) [2]. This ensures that the complete organ is removed and enables quantitative measurements to be made when protein content or synthesis rates are measured *in vitro*. Tissues should be washed free of adhering haemolymph in saline prior to incubations. Take care when dissecting tissues (nervous tissue, gut tissue), since practically all tissues are connected with an extensive and intricate network of tracheoles. Even trachea with small diameters are sturdy and a strong pull may easily rupture tissues.

2.6.2.3   Purification

As mentioned earlier, arthropod tissues are often prepared for immunological or biochemical analysis by freezing them in liquid nitrogen or by subjecting them to several freeze-thaw cycles. Previous purification methods [3] using whole insects, starting with homogenates in 7% (w/v) cold $HClO_4$ have been simplified with the introduction of liquid chromatography. Because of the size of the animals, the starting material often consists of highly impure preparations (whole animals) that often contain chitinaceous and sclerotinized rigid material. These homogenates can be agitated overnight at 4°C to increase the yield of soluble material from fragments [4] or heat-treated prior to centrifugation and filtration. Extensive purification protocols have been described which demonstrate the difficulty involved in isolating insect peptides. In isolating the peptide proctolin, a starting material of 125 kg cockroaches was necessary due to the minute amount of the peptide within the tissues [3]. Although using heads only from *Bombyx mori*, the starting material for a preparation of prothoracicotropic hormone (PTTH) consisted of 650000 heads (4.86 kg) that were extracted with 2% (w/v) NaCl, heat treated and precipitated (acetone, $(NH_4)_2SO_4$ or picric acid) prior to several chromatographic steps [5]. When tissue is easily accessible (ovaries) and the molecule to be purified is present in high amounts (vitellin), it is sufficient to excise the organs and solubilize ovarian proteins in NaCl, 0.15 mol/l. The proteins are then precipitated with ammonium sulphate solution (50% w/v) prior to dialysis and chromatographic purification steps (Sephacryl S-300, DEAE ion-exchange column and hydroxyapaptite column) for the production of specific antibodies.

Several commercial suppliers (*Boehringer Mannheim, Pharmacia, USB Biochemicals*) offer cocktails of protease inhibitors for stabilizing proteins during extraction steps, especially when neutral pH solvents are used (a much higher activity of enzymes is observed at non-acidic pH). High salt concentrations in buffers additionally decrease enzymatic activities.

Considerable degradation of peptides may occur in tissues during dissection. To prevent proteolysis, freeze tissues immediately in dry ice or liquid nitrogen. Purifications are simplified when using tissues with a high content of the bioactive peptide to be isolated. For example, for the purification of brain material containing PTTH, depending on the arthropod species and the developmental stage, either extirpated whole brains, glands or dissected cells containing PTTH-activity are used. (Brain tissues from day 0 pupae contain sufficient amounts of hormone to perform the *in-vitro* stimulation of glands with individual neurosecretory cells.) Rinse excised tissues in physiological solutions (i.e., lepidopteran *Ringer* solution) to remove contaminating haemolymph. If sites of synthesis or storage of bioactive factors are known, transfer the tissue to chilled medium CSM-2F [22] and dissect further. The osmolarity of CSM-2F medium prevents lysis of neurosecretory cells during dissection. For exact localization of bioactive factors, identifiable cells with known location can be separated from surrounding tissue with the aid of a stereo-microscope [24]. In an elegant study, *Flanagan* et al. [25] have shown that mAbs can be produced with immunogen that was obtained from only a few hundred somata of neurosecretory cells, thus eliminating the need for extensive purification of cell-specific proteins. Extraction of bioactive factors from homogenates of dissected tissues should be performed in solutions that fit the conditions of the bioassay. Best results are achieved with an extraction protocol using a chilled mixture of distilled water and insect medium (in a ratio of 2:1) or directly processed and diluted in insect medium (*Grace* [12]).

Heat treatment (100°C for 1–2 min) and subsequent centrifugation (10000 × g for 10 min) represents a 10-fold purification of PTTH and yields a greater amount of PTTH activity.

Extracts are usually concentrated by ultrafiltration or diafiltration and fractions are assayed for bioactivity for further analysis by chromatographic methods (gel filtration).

2.6.2.4   Cell Culture

Arthropod tissues (midguts, glands) can be dissociated enzymatically (0.1% w/v collagenase) shortly after dissection and used for *in-vitro* assays. They have been shown to incorporate label and synthesize hormones comparably to intact tissues [6]. Most studies with arthropod cell lines have been made with insect cell lines as substrates for insect-borne pathogens or for studies on the genetics, molecular biology and physiology of eukaryotic cells. They are increasingly used as host cells in baculovirus expression systems because of post-translational modifications that are absent from prokaryotic expression systems (nearly 200 insect cell lines have been developed in the 3 decades since the first insect cell lines were reported in 1962). In most cases it is not yet possible to isolate lines of specific cell types from given tissues, and, unlike mammalian cells, the identity of insect cell lines is somewhat unclear. In primary cultures, however, specific cells (nerve, muscle, fat body, tracheal or imaginal disc cells) can be identified. Significant variation can exist among cell lines derived from the same insect organ by the same method [7]. In the following, the establishment of a mosquito cell line is described.

Tissues for the establishment of larval or embryonic cell cultures are obtained from freshly hatched larvae or from crushed and homogenized embryos, respectively. Ovarian lines are derived from ovaries of adult females shortly after emergence. Of the available mosquito cell lines [8], *Aedes albopictus* is the best characterized. Prior to hatching, sterilize eggs briefly with acetone and by immersion in *White's* solution for 15 min, wash in sterile distilled water and allow to hatch under reduced pressure. Transfer freshly emerged (neonate) larvae to 1 ml of a solution of trypsin (0.25% w/v) in *Aedes* saline and mince it. Dilute the tissue suspension with an additional 5 ml trypsin solution and incubate at 37°C for 10 min. Mix the suspension gently with a *Pasteur* pipette, and centrifuge the cells at 200 × g. Wash the pellet in *Aedes* saline and adapt to *Eagles* MEM [9] supplemented with non-essential amino acids, glutamine and fetal bovine serum (5% v/v). Within 24 h most cells will attach to the culture flask plastic and can be subcultured [10]. Most insect cell lines are maintained under conditions different from those appropriate for mammalian cell lines, e.g., in temperature, pH and oxygen requirement described elsewhere (cf. 3.4).

2.6.2.5   Buffers and Media

Synthetic insect media initially used for organ culture were similar to the medium developed by *Grace* [12]. The composition of insect media was based on the ionic and osmotic analysis of final-stage larval insect haemolymph and its amino acid content with the Na/K ratio being the inverse of that necessary in mammalian media. Although the natural environment of arthropod cells is rather different from that of mammalian cells, insect cells can proliferate in a wide range of osmotic pressure and chloride levels (4–80 mmol/l) as well as with a different Na/K balance. Insect media are often more strongly buffered at a pH of around 6.2. Cell lines can be initiated in media specifically designed for the culture of arthropod cells (MM/VP12), containing salts, glucose, lactalbumin hydrolysate, bovine serum albumin (BSA), a vitamin mixture, inositol and choline [11]. Media have been increasingly used for the cultivation of arthropod cells, and they display greatly improved plating efficiencies, suitable for cloning [13]. Development of serum-free media for the propagation of insect cells is an important advance in cell culture technique [14–16], allowing large scale insect cell culture.

2.6.3   Assay Methods

2.6.3.1   Principle

A direct relationship between hormone and target tissue can be established and monitored in culture. In arthropods, the availability of high numbers of experimental animals allows the study of tissues at different stages of competence (readiness) as well as at different times after induction of developmental processes (bloodmeal, moulting). Target tissues, removed at defined developmental stages, are incubated *in vitro* in the presence of inducing factors, and their response to bioactive factors is quantified with biochemical or immunological methods. The presence of buffer salts or acids in bioactive fractions can interfere with most of the bioassays used to monitor the activity of molecules during purification. Volatile buffers (ammonium acetate, triethylammonium acetate) and volatile ion-pairing reagents (trifluoroacetic acid) allow fractions to be completely dried down (vacuum centrifuge) or lyophilized. Fractions from ion exchange columns have to be desalted (dialysis or reversed phase cartridge) because of their high concentrations of salts.

2.6.3.2   Quantitative Determination of *in vitro* Synthesized Vitellogenin

Excise tissue samples (fat body, thoracic muscles, midgut) under a dissecting microscope, wash in *Aedes aegypti* saline [11] and incubate with 100 µl silkmoth organ culture medium [17, 18]. Midguts (negative control tissue) should be washed free of their contents prior to incubation. Preparations of fat bodies remain connected to the epidermis of the abdomen and do not represent a culture of pure fat body cells. Control incubations in individual experimental systems have to demonstrate the non-interference of attached epidermal tissues in a bioassay.

Fat bodies, incubated *in vitro* can be used in a variety of studies.

Hormones, added to the incubation medium together with [³H]-phenylalanine, stimulate the fat body cells to synthesize radiolabelled vitellogenin (egg yolk protein) which can be precipitated and quantified with an antibody specific to vitellogenin [2]. Alternatively, aliquots of medium from incubated *Aedes aegypti* and *Drosophila melanogaster* are taken at defined time intervals for vitellogenin determination with

ELISA [19] for measuring the competence of fat body cells during development. With such studies it has been shown that the synthesis of vitellogenin in the fat bodies of as few as five individual *Drosophila* can produce vitellogenin well within the range of detectability.

2.6.3.3   Quantitative Determination of Prothoracicotropic Hormone (PTTH) *in vitro*

Excised prothoracicotropic glands from specific stages of pupae (inactive glands) or CO_2-anaesthetized larvae (more sensitive than pupal glands) should be dissected in lepidopteran saline [20], and maintained (washed) for up to 1 h in *Grace's* medium prior to use in bioassays. One of a pair of glands serves as the experimental gland and is incubated in medium containing samples to be measured for their bioactivity. The contralateral gland is incubated with medium alone and serves as control. The assay is performed in siliconized glass incubation dishes or in uncovered acrylic culture wells (*Linbro*) in 25 μl *Grace's* medium at a constant 26°C (water-bath, with shaking at 50 rpm).

Activation (A_r) is measured by induction of hormone synthesis (ecdysone) in a dose-dependent manner and released by the experimental gland over a time period of 2 h divided by the amount of hormone synthesized the control gland. A 10 μl aliquot of the incubation medium containing synthesized ecdysone is directly analysed in an ecdysone radioimmunoassay [21, 22].

Inhibition of bioactivity by antibodies present in the medium during the incubation period represents a modification of this assay. Adjustment of the pH from 6.2 (*Grace's* medium) to 6.8 with KOH enhances the binding of antibodies to PTTH.

The *in-vitro* bioassay is used to quantify PTTH-units. To determine the standard unit, the dose of brain extract from day 1 pupae (ED_{50}) is determined that half maximally activates the glands (A_{50}) *in vitro* (1 unit = 0.06 brain equivalents).

2.6.4   Preparation of Tissues for Immunocytochemistry

2.6.4.1   Insect Tissues

Dissection of nervous tissues or organs is performed in PBS, physiological saline, *Ringer* solution or insect medium. Vertebrate tissue usually requires fixation by transcardial perfusion for optimal tissue preservation at room temperature or body temperature of the experimental animal during perfusion. Tissues from arthropods are usually dissected on ice or as cold as possible and are fixed by immersion into cold fixative. Any surrounding sheath (neurolemma), inhibiting the fixative from penetrating the tissue should be removed since immunostaining without desheathing has been reported to be ineffective. When mild fixatives are used with desheathed whole ganglions or thick tissue preparations, post-fixation of sections on the glass slide is recommended.

When using complex tissues (central nervous system), the preparation is pinned in a Sylgard-coated dish [24].

A whole mount preparation of insect tissue allows for the convenient and rapid visualization of cell body location with respect to the positions of other cell bodies and in relation to the whole ganglion. It is used for visualizing immunoreactive factors in the soma and projections (axons) within the tissue. Fix tissues in *Bouin's* fixative for 2 h at 18°C and wash overnight at 4°C with PBS (0.1 mol/l) containing 0.1% (w/v) sodium azide (pH 7.4). After removing the connective tissue sheath from nervous tissues, permeabilize them in PBS containing 2% (v/v) Triton X-100 and store at 4°C. The immunochemical procedures for antibody incubations are generally conducted according to published procedures. (Immunofluorescent markers penetrate whole mount tissues better than the complex molecules in biotin-avidin detection systems.) When using milder fixatives (4% v/v phosphate-buffered paraformaldehyde), the sheath surrounding the tissues has to be removed prior to fixation. After applying antibodies, the tissues are cleared by dehydration through an alcohol series, mounted in methyl salicylate and analysed for distribution of immunoreactive material.

When prepararing arthropod tissues for sectioning, several aspects have to be considered. Chitinaceous structures might obstruct the cutting knife or rupture and deform sections. In contrast with sections of vertebrate tissues the loss of only few slices in serial sections might obscure the results since arthropod tissues (especially neural) may contain only a very limited number of cells (often only one or two cells) which are of interest. Since antigens might denature in paraffin sections when in contact with organic solvents, or when dehydrated through the alcohol series or by heat prior to immunostaining [26], it is recommended to use cryosections and a mild fixative (2% w/v paraformaldehyde and 0.4% w/v picric acid in phosphate buffer [0.1 mol/l, pH 7.4]) [27]. Triton X-100 facilitates the penetration of large biotin-avidin complexes in tissue section.

2.6.4.2   Crustacean Tissue (*Homarus americanus*)

To make a whole mount preparation dissect central ganglia with attached thoracic roots in cold lobster saline [27]. Fix tissues in 4% (w/v) paraformaldehyde in phosphate buffer (0.1 mol/l, pH 7.4) for 12 to 36 h. Rinse ganglia in several changes of phosphate buffer containing 0.3% (v/v) Triton X-100 and 0.1% (w/v) sodium azide for 6–8 h prior to incubation with primary antibody solution at 4°C. After incubation, rinse samples once in sodium carbonate buffer (4 mmol/l, pH 9.5) and mount samples in 80% (v/v) glycerol in carbonate buffer, 20 mmol/l, for viewing with an epifluorescent microscope.

2.6.5   Reagents and Solutions

Protocols for arthropod tissue preparation vary considerably depending on the species and the aim of the study. The list of buffers, saline and media given below covers those in common use.

- *Grace's* culture medium (*GIBCO,* Grand Island, NY)
  The medium resembles insect haemolymph and consists mainly of chemically pure amino acids, vitamins, organic acids and inorganic salts. Haemolymph, which was originally added, is now replaced by fetal bovine serum or bovine serum albumin.
- Medium CSM-2F [17] with osmolarity different from *Grace's* insect medium.
  Osmolarity of media can be measured by freezing-point depression (*Fiske* osmometer, G-62) and adjusted to 350 mOsmol/l by varying the sucrose concentration.
- Dissection buffers: PBS, *Aedes* saline [11], lepidopteran saline [20], *Ringer* solution
- Gel filtration: Phosphate buffer (0.05 mol/l NaH_2PO_4), (P-100 columns)
- Homogenization buffers (with protease inhibitors): Extraction protocols use a variety of buffers and depend on the tissue and the molecule to be purified. Some examples of extraction buffers are listed below.
  Various acidic solvents for purification of neuropeptides (i. e., 2 mol/l acetic acid)
  Tris-HCl buffer, 25 mmol/l (extraction of ovarian proteins)
  Tris-HCl buffer, 50 mmol/l, containing $CaCl_2$ (100 mmol/l, pH 7.9) for proteolytic enzymes
  Insect culture medium (*Grace's*)
  Ultrafiltration (*Amicon*) with distilled water on a YM-2 membrane (exclusion size $> M_r$ 1000)
- Inhibitors and their concentrations: (made up just before use, as PMSF is hydrolytically unstable. PMSF and pepstatin A are poorly soluble in water, they should be dissolved in acetic acid, which is then diluted in water.
  phenylthiourea (PTU, 0.01% w/v),
  phenylmethylsulphonyl fluoride (PMSF, 10^{-3}–10^{-4} mol/l)
  octyltrifluoropropanone (OTFP, 10^{-4} mol/l)
  pepstatin A
- Physiological saline (*Periplaneta*):
  NaCl, 140 mmol/l, KCl, 5 mmol/l, $CaCl_2$, 5 mmol/l, $NaHCO_3$, 4 mmol/l, $MgCl_2$,

1 mmol/l, trehalose, 5 mmol/l, sucrose, 100 mmol/l, HEPES or TES, 5 mmol/l, pH 7.2
- Crustacean Physiological saline (*Panulirus interruptus*):
  NaCl, 479 mmol/l, KCl, 12.8 mmol/l, CaCl$_2$, 13.7 mmol/l, Na$_2$SO$_4$, 3.9 mmol/l, MgSO$_4$, 10 mmol/l, Tris base 11 mmol/l [Tris (hydroxy-methyl)amino methane], maleic acid 4.8 mmol/l (pH 7.4–7.6)
- Crustacean Physiological saline (*Homarus americanus*):
  NaCl, 462 mmol/l, KCl, 16 mmol/l, CaCl$_2$, 26 mmol/l, MgCl$_2$, 8 mmol/l, glucose, 11.1 mmol/l, Tris base, 10 mmol/l, maleic acid, 10 mmol/l (pH 7.4)
- Lepidopteran saline (*Manduca sexta*), modified from [20]:
  KCl, 21 mmol/l, NaCl, 12 mmol/l, CaCl$_2$, 3 mmol/l, MgCl$_2$, 18 mmol/l, glucose, 170 mmol/l, piperazinediethanesulfonic acid, 5 mmol/l, KOH, 9 mmol/l (pH 6.6)
- Fixative: add paraformaldehyde to buffer, warm to 55°C and stir until solution has clear appearence (adding a few drops of NaOH). If necessary, titrate to pH 6.9–7.4. For fixing, paraformaldehyde is often used with physiological or hypotonic saline.
- PBS: Solution A: dissolve 1.4 g Na$_2$HPO$_4$ or 1.78 g Na$_2$HPO$_4$ · 2H$_2$O in 100 ml distilled water
  Solution B: dissolve 1.4 g NaH$_2$PO$_4$ · H$_2$O in 100 ml distilled water
  Mix 84.1 ml (solution A) and 15.9 ml (solution B),
  add 8.5 g NaCl and 900 ml distilled water for pH 6.9–7.4

References

[1] *K. J. Wilson*, Purification of Proteins/Peptides for Structural Studies, in: *A. S. Bhown* (ed.), Protein/Peptide Sequence Analysis: Current Methodologies, CRC Press, Boca Raton 1988, pp. 1–34.
[2] *T. R. Flanagan, H. H. Hagedorn*, Vitellogenin Synthesis in the Mosquito: the Role of Juvenile Hormone in the Development of Responsiveness to Ecdysone, Physiol. Entomol. *2*, 173–178 (1977).
[3] *B. E. Brown, A. N. Starratt*, Isolation of Proctolin, a Myotropic Peptide, from *Periplaneta americana*, J. Insect Physiol. *21*, 1879–1881 (1975).
[4] *D. Ben-Yakir, Y. K. Mumcuoglu*, Louse Antigens Recognized by Resistant Hosts: Immuno-blotting Studies, in: *D. Borovsky, A. Spielman* (eds.), Host Regulated Developmental Mechanisms in Vector Arthropods, Proc. 2nd Symp. 1989, Vero Beach, pp. 159–162.
[5] *H. Nagasawa, H. Kataoka, Y. Hori, A. Isogai, S. Tamura, A. Suzuki, F. Guo, X. Zhong, A. Mizoguchi, M. Fujishita, S. Y. Takahashi, E. Ohnishi, H. Ishizaki*, Isolation and Some Characterization of the Prothoracicotropic Hormone from *Bombyx mori*, Gen. Comp. Endocrinol. *53*, 143–152 (1984).
[6] *A.-S. Chiang, M. Gadot, C. Schal*, Changes in Number and Size of Corpus Allatum Cells of *Blattella germanica* During Oocyte Maturation, in: *A. B. Borkovec, E. P. Masler* (eds.), Insect Neurochemistry and Neurophysiology, The Humana Press Inc., Clifton, N.J. 1990, pp. 317–320.
[7] *R. H. Goodwin, G. H. Tompkins, P. McCawley*, Gypsy Moth Cell Lines Divergent in Viral Susceptibility. I. Culture and Identification, In Vitro *14*, 485–494 (1978).
[8] *T. J. Kurtti, U. G. Munderloh*, Mosquito Cell Culture, in: *K. Maramorosch* (ed.), Advances in Cell Culture, Vol. 3, Academic Press, New York 1984, pp. 259–301.

[9] *H. Eagle*, Amino Acid Metabolism in Mammalian Cell Cultures, Science *130*, 432–437 (1959).

[10] *K. R. P. Singh*, Cell Cultures Derived from Larvae of *Aedes albopictus* (Skuse) and *Aedes aegypti* (L.), Curr. Sci. *19*, 506–508 (1967).

[11] *M. G. R. Varma, M. Pudney*, The Growth and Serial Passage of Cell Lines from *Aedes aegypti* in Different Media, J. Med. Entomol. *6*, 432–439 (1969).

[12] *T. D. C. Grace*, Establishment of Four Strains of Cells from Insect Tissues Grown *in vitro*, Nature *195*, 788–789 (1962).

[13] *V. Deubel, J. P. Digoutte*, Morphogenesis of Yellow Fever Virus in *Aedes aegypti* Cultured Cells. 1. Isolation of Different Cellular Clones and the Study of Their Susceptibility to Infection with the Virus, Am. J. Trop. Med. Hyg. *30*, 1060–1070 (1981).

[14] *J. Mitsuhashi, R. H. Goodwin*, The Serum-free Culture of Insect Cells *in vitro*, in: *J. Mitsuhashi* (ed.), Invertebrate Cell System Applications, CRC Press, Boca Raton 1989, pp. 167–182.

[15] *D. Inlow, A. Shauger, B. Maiorella*, Insect Cell Culture and Baculovirus Propagation in Protein-free Medium, J. Tissue Cult. Methods *12*, 13–16 (1989).

[16] *X. Léry, G. Fédière*, A New Serum-free Medium for Lepidopteran Cell Culture, J. Invertebr. Pathol. *55*, 342–349 (1990).

[17] *E. Stevenson, G. R. Wyatt*, The Metabolism of Silkmoth Tissues. I. Incorporation of Leucine into Protein, Arch. Biochem. Biophys. *99*, 65–71 (1962).

[18] *H. H. Hagedorn, C. L. Judson*, Purification and Site of Synthesis of *Aedes aegypti* Yolk Proteins, J. Exp. Zool. *182*, 367–378 (1972).

[19] *M. Ma, K.-P. Sieber, J. Ballerino, S.-J. Wu*, ELISA and Monoclonal Antibodies, in: *L. I. Gilbert, T. A. Miller* (eds.), Immunological Techniques in Insect Biology, Springer Verlag, New York 1988, pp. 43–73.

[20] *R. D. Weevers*, A Lepidopteran Saline: Effects of Inorganic Cation Concentrations on Sensory, Reflex, and Motor Responses in a Herbivorous Insect, J. Exp. Biol. *44*, 163–175 (1966).

[21] *D. W. Borst, J. O'Connor*, Trace Analysis of Ecdysones by Gas-liquid Chromatography, Radioimmunoassay and Bioassay, Steroids *24*, 637–656 (1974).

[22] *J. T. Warren, L. I. Gilbert*, Radioimmunoassay: Ecdysteroids, in: *L. I. Gilbert, T. A. Miller* (eds.), Immunological Techniques in Insect Biology, Springer Verlag, New York 1988, pp. 181–214.

[23] *J. Mitsuhashi*, Tissue Culture of the Rise Stem Borer *Chilo suppressalis* Lepidoptera Pyralidae. II. Effects of Temperatures and Cold Storage on the Multiplication of the Cell Line from Larval Hemocytes Iridescent Virus, Appl. Entomol. Zool. *3*, 1–4 (1968).

[24] *N. Agui, N. A. Granger, L. A. Gilbert, W. E. Bollenbacher*, Cellular Localization of the Insect Prothoracicotropic Hormone: In vitro Assay of a Single Neurosecretory Cell, Proc. Natl. Acad. Sci. USA *76*, 5694–5698 (1979).

[25] *T. R. Flanagan, M. A. O'Brien, N. Agui, W. E. Bollenbacher*, Production of Antibodies to *Manduca sexta* Cerebral Neurosecretory Cells, Arch. Insect Biochem. Physiol. *12*, 219–229 (1989).

[26] *C. A. Bishop, M. O'Shea*, Neuropeptide Proctolin (H-Arg-Try-Leu-Pro-Thr-OH): Immunocytochemical Mapping of Neurons in the Central Nervous System of the Cockroach, J. Comp. Neurol. *207*, 223–238 (1982).

[27] *M. Otsuka, E. A. Kravitz, D. D. Potter*, Physiological and Chemical Architecture of a Lobster Ganglion with Particular Reference to Gamma-aminobutyrate and Glutamate, J. Neurophysiol. *30*, 725–752 (1967).

2.7   Plant Tissues and Cells

Hans-Willi Krell

2.7.1   General Properties of Plant Tissue

Immunological methods have given an enormous stimulus to the study of plant cell structure, to the identification and characterization of minor plant cell constituents, to the monitoring of secondary plant products, and to the detection of viruses. Moreover, in cases where large numbers of samples must be screened, immunological tests are particularly advantageous. In 1979 *Weiler and Zenk* claimed that more than 10000 samples could be tested on a visual basis in a day by an autoradiographic immunoassay [1].

The way in which the sample must be prepared is dictated by the problem to be solved. In general, immunological tests do not need much sample preparation, since antibodies can pick out the appropriate antigens in very complex biological matrices [2]. For example, many radioimmunoassays need only simple extraction procedures (e.g. using methanol) – with no further processing [1]. But if information is required about compartmentation of different plant organelles, these structures should be purified to avoid artificial results.

Plant tissues present some special problems in the isolation of enzymes and organelles. The reason is primarily the presence of a large variety, and frequently large quantities, of secondary products and of phenol oxidases. Moreover, in contrast to animal cells or bacteria, plant cells have two major properties which affect sample preparation. The first is the existence of a rigid, rather inflexible cell wall which separates the cells from each other [3]. Cell walls form the basic structural framework of the plant, defining the shape and size of plant cells and tissues [4]. They are usually classified as either primary or secondary, depending on their mechanical properties and chemical composition. Primary cell walls are composed of cellulose fibrils embedded in relatively large amounts of an amorphous mixture of polysaccharides and glycoproteins. In secondary cell walls, cellulose is relatively more abundant, and they contain significant amounts of lignins. Lignins are amorphous polymers from three basic components, namely p-cumarylalcohol, coniferylalcohol and sinapoylalcohol. They are responsible for high tensile and compressive strength, so extreme conditions are needed to break up certain kinds of plant tissues.

The second crucial property of plant cells is their possession of big vacuoles [5–7]. These are formed from different small vacuoles usally present in the young cell. Up to 90 % of the cell volume can be filled by the central vacuole. The aqueous solution of the vacuole contains inorganic ions, polyphosphates, a variety of organic compounds such as carboxylic and amino acids, phenols, quinones, tannins, flavones, sugars and alkaloids. Most of the secondary metabolites are stored in the vacuoles [8] as well as lytic enzymes such as proteinases, nucleases and phosphatases. In general, the vacuole is destroyed by disintegration methods if special precautions are not taken (cf. 2.7.4.8).

In plant tissues there is a large component of non-plasma material, mainly cell walls, and vacuolar soap and starch granules. For homogenization, it should be considered that in young spinach leaves more than 95 % of the fresh weight is water, minerals, fat and carbohydrates – only 3 % is extractable protein. Apple fruit contains only 0.3 % protein on a fresh weight basis, compared to nearly 20 % protein in beef liver [9].

The three-dimensional and temporal constituents [10] of the plant cell can change dramatically depending on its physiological state or period of development [11, 12]. A well-known example is the onset of secondary metabolite production in plant cells at the end of the stationary phase of culture [13]. In non-sterile growth conditions, such as are found with plants growing in the field, there are significant amounts of bacterial or fungal contamination. Plant tissues should therefore be thoroughly rinsed or peeled before disintegration.

2.7.2   Methods of Disintegration

The manner of disintegration has a profound effect on the yield and quality of the preparation. In tissues, cell-type or organ fractionation precedes disruption. In general, the way biological material is best broken up is a matter of trial and error. If possible, volumes should be kept small and the extract should be as concentrated as possible.

2.7.2.1   Disruption of Tissues and Cells

Cereals: To avoid bacterial contamination, wash leaves in tap water, rinse for 15 s in a solution of 0.1 % (w/v) sodium hypochlorite [1:50 dilution of household bleach] plus 0.05 % (v/v) nonionic detergent (e.g. Brij 58) in deionized water. Pat leaves dry and remove large ribs and veins.

Beans or seeds: They can be homogenized with a *Waring* blender. To avoid high temperatures the vessel should be cooled. Alternatively, surface sterilize seeds or beans by soaking 30 s in 0.1 % sodium hypochlorite and then rinse thoroughly with sterile deionized water. Swell seeds by soaking overnight at room temperature in sterile deionized water.

Ligninized material: Fibrous tissue should be ground to a fine powder after freezing in liquid nitrogen. For smaller amounts of ligninized plant material, a Microdismembrator (*Braun*, Melsungen, Germany) is very effective. Here, plant material frozen in liquid nitrogen is broken by metal balls. The powder can processed further by suspending in a suitable buffer (cf. 2.7.4.3). An alternative method for small-scale extracts is homogenization by grinding with acid-washed siliconized sand in a mortar and pestle [14].

Beside the methods described above, some others are also suitable. A very gentle means of preparation is enzymatic disruption with cell-wall hydrolases, as in the case of protoplast preparation (cf. 2.7.4.2). These hydrolases must be very highly purified.

Ultrasonic procedures [15] are in general not satisfactory with plant tissues and cultured plant cells. With plant cell cultures, a freeze-blast method has proved to be more effective [16]. The principle of the 'freeze-blast' method is to disintegrate cells by blowing a frozen cell suspension against a target panel in nitrogen gas at a high flow rate.

2.7.2.2 Media for Cell and Tissue Disintegration

To protect cell components, the media for disintegration should simulate the intracellular environment as much as possible and thereby protect the cell components from chemical or mechanical stress. Media normally contain a buffer, substances to maintain integrity, ions and chelates. The buffers used for homogenization of plant tissues typically include high concentrations of reducing agents and polyphenol inactivators, and of covalent protease inhibitors [for example cf. 17–19]. Many plant constituents, above all enzymes of the chloroplast stroma, require a reducing environment for activity. Typically, the preferred agents are dithioerythritol (DTT) at 2 to 5 mmol/l, or 2-mercaptoethanol at 14 mmol/l [19]. For isolation of chloroplasts, the more physiological compounds ascorbate [20] and reduced glutathione are preferred.

Specific requirements for ions in isolation media are largely empirical. However, low concentrations of Mg^{2+} (0.1 mmol/l) are important to stabilize the internal membranes. Usually, the pH should be maintained between 7 and 8. Preparation of isolates from tissues with big vacuoles requires buffers of high ionic strength. Furthermore, most plant tissues, especially seeds, are very rich in proteases. To preserve their structures, addition of protease inhibitors is sometimes useful [14, 21]. It must be ensured that none of the media components interferes with subsequent antigen-antibody interactions.

2.7.2.3 Post-treatment of Extracts

Homogenates can be cleared by centrifugation or by filtration through several layers of cheesecloth. In specialized cells of many species, the vacuoles contain alkaloids and polyphenolic compounds such as flavonoids or tannins [9]. These compounds can inhibit enzyme activity especially if polyphenol oxidase is present.

Protein determination is often used for a first characterization of the crude extracts. Many compounds present in crude extracts, however, inhibit classical protein determination techniques. For example, tannins react with the *Folin-Ciocalteu* reagent of the *Lowry* assay. The Coomassie Blue G-250 dye-binding assay [22] gives erroneous results in the presence of tannins bound to protein [23]. Also, spectroscopic determination in the 220- to 280-nm range is disturbed by high concentration of phenolics.

Phenolics and alkaloids can be removed from the crude plant extract by complexing with 1.5% (w/v) polyvinylpyrrolidone (PVP) or by gel filtration (e.g. on Sephadex G-50 or BioGel P-6DG). Phenol oxidase can be inhibited by a strongly reducing environment. Gel filtration (BioGel P-6DG or Sephadex G-50) is also very effective for removal of inhibitory compounds in extracts rich in tannins.

Polystyrene beads show great promise as agents for removing hydrophobic materials from plant extracts. Amberlite XAD has also been used to remove the detergents used in solubilizing membrane-bound enzymes or terpenoid compounds [24].

Precipitation with the synthetic polycation polyethyleneimine (PEI) is very effective for removing the bulk of nucleic acid and much of the phospholipid from extracts. This is especially useful for the preparation of extracts from dry material such as seeds or embryos, in which nucleic acids and lipids are concentrated [25].

2.7.3   Histological Methods

Immunocytochemical studies have become more important recently, especially for the study of transgenic plants [26], and can provide unique information [27] such as:

- Location of the precise cell or cells containing the defined macromolecule,
- Detection of changes in cellular distribution of the macromolecule during development,
- Identification of subcellular localization of the defined macromolecule,
- An indication at the ultrastructural level of the particular organelle synthesizing the defined macromolecule, or in which it may be sequestered in the cell.

Immunocytochemical methods are described in detail in chapter 5, but because of their differences from animal cells, there are particular considerations in applying such methods to plant cells.

Among the various labels for antibody, fluorochromes have proved to be particularly attractive for plant immunocytochemistry. It should be noted that tetramethylrhodamine isothiocyanate (TRITC) has often been used in preference to fluorescein isothiocyanate (FITC) because a high level of autofluorescence by some plant cells may mask the specific fluorochrome at the wavelength of FITC excitation. Plants rich in polyphenols, for example, show a very high autofluorescence between 400 and 500 nm which is the wavelength used in UV or blue-filter excitation systems for fluorescence microscopy. Non-tissue specific fluorescence may also result from aldehyde fixation, especially by glutaraldehyde or formaldehyde [28, 29].

In principle, pre- or post-embedding staining is possible. In the pre-embedding staining method (before fixation) the cells or tissues are directly exposed to the specific antibody. Few applications of this have been described because the antibody does not effectively penetrate the cells. Therefore post-embedding methods are used more widely because these enable direct access of the antibody to cellular antigens.

In plant tissues, antigen-antibody reactions can be disturbed by lectins. Some lectins may bind IgG. This kind of binding can be controlled by incorporating a monosaccharide inhibitor of lectin-binding in the antibody preparation. A variety of other plant glycoconjugates may also bind IgG, for example arabinogalactane proteins that are commonly present in the vascular tissues [30].

2.7.4   Preparation of Plant Cell Constituents

2.7.4.1   Cell Wall

Primary cell walls can be obtained readily from isolated plant tissues and from suspension cultures [31]. Usually the tissue is macerated and then cell walls are purified by extraction with water, salts, detergents and organic solvents, or by a combination of these [32, 33].

2.7.4.2   Protoplast

Protoplasts are isolated in large numbers after the enzymatic removal of the cell wall as pioneered by *Cocking* in 1960 [34]. Protoplasts are released by incubation of tissue pieces in a mixture of commercially available cell wall-degrading enzymes [35, 36, 37]. Incubation conditions depend strongly on the kind of tissue or cultured cells, conditions of plant growth and plant age [38]. The resulting protoplasts are separated by sieving the mixture through a mesh with 50–100 µm pores and are washed by low-speed centrifugation. Detailed procedures have been described [39, 40, 41].

2.7.4.3   Nuclei

Best results are achieved with plant tissues with thin cell walls and few lipid and starch granules [42]. Plant material is harvested and immediately frozen in liquid nitrogen, and can be stored at $-80\,°C$ for more than 1 year [43]. The cells are ground to a fine powder in liquid nitrogen and lysed in an iso-osmotic buffer containing the nonionic detergent Triton X100. After lysis, nuclei are collected by low-speed centrifugation and purified by centrifugation on a discontinuous Percoll gradient [43].

2.7.4.4   Plastids

The preferred way to purify intact chloroplasts is by Percoll density gradient centrifugation [44]. The density of chloroplasts of different tissues can vary with their developmental stage and species of origin. Healthy young plants are recommended; otherwise chloroplasts tend to be fragile and the yield of intact chloroplasts is poor [45, 46].

2.7.4.5   Mitochondria

To avoid damaging mitochondrial oxidative and phosphorylative capacities, leaf tissue should be homogenized for very short times in a blender [47]. Cotyledons or other parts of seedlings and fruits are chopped with razor blades and ground with a mortar and pestle. The main problem is to eliminate contaminating plastids, nuclear DNA, and cytoplasmic ribosomes. A key step in the mitochondrial isolation procedure is differential centrifugation to separate the bulk of nuclei, plastids, and cellular debris from the mitochondrial fraction which differs in particle size or density. Mitochondria may then be further separated from the remaining plastids and nuclear debris by gradient centrifugation (e.g. using sucrose or Percoll) [48].

2.7.4.6   Microbodies (Glyoxisomes, Peroxisomes)

Microbodies are respiratory subcellular orgenelles found in all eukaryotic plant and animal tissues. On the basis of the physiological and biochemical characteristics of isolated microbodies from different tissues, they are referred to as peroxisomes, from green photosynthetic tissues, or glyoxysomes, from germinating fatty seeds (e.g. castor bean) [49]. These organelles are very fragile, so gentle homogenization is recommended. To avoid damage by mechanical forces, osmotic shock or acid conditions, the tissue is chopped with razor blades and then gently ground, with a mortar and pestle, in a suitable buffered sucrose solution with protective reagents [50]. The homogenate is filtered through cheese cloth and cell debris removed by low-speed centrifugation. Microbodies can be enriched by isopycnic sucrose density gradient centrifugation and they generally band at a density between 1.24 and $1.26\,g/cm^3$ [49]. Alternatively, methods of differential centrifugation can be used [51].

2.7.4.7   *Golgi* Apparatus and Related Cell Components

Favoured tissues for the isolation of Golgi bodies are etiolated stems or non-green tissues [52]. After low-shear homogenization and filtration of the homogenate through cheese cloth, the dictyosomes are isolated by sucrose density gradient centrifugation. For the stabilization of the dictyosome stack, glutaraldehyde, 1–2 g/l, may be added to the freshly prepared homogenate [52].

2.7.4.8   Vacuoles

The vacuole of a plant cell has the functions both of a storage vesicle and also of a lysosome [53]. It can be a storage vesicle for inorganic ions, tricarboxylic acid [TCA] cycle intermediates, some alkaloids, sucrose and other sugars [7]. In addition, vacuoles may contain various hydrolases that include proteases.

The first generally accepted vacuole isolation method was published 1975 by *Wagner and Siegelmann* [54]. Mechanical forces can be avoided by first forming intermediate protoplasts. Phosphate buffer, 0.2 mol/l, pH 8.0, is used for a gentle osmotic rupture of the protoplasts, thereby releasing vacuoles that can then be recovered by centrifugation. The integrity of the vacuoles can be demonstrated by their ability to absorb vital neutral red dye from solution [6].

2.7.4.9   Plant Cell Membranes

Plant cells contain a system of intracellular membranes of varying complexity. The major aim in any purification procedure is to free the different cell membranes from cellular structures in a condition that preserves their natural composition and function. One of the consequences of tissue destruction is that enzymes (proteases, oxidases, etc.) that can modify membrane composition become activated. Here, working as quickly as possible at low temperatures and the addition of protease inhibitors is recommended. Membranes form aggregates in buffers. On the other hand, membranes can also dissociate from their binding sites. One gentle strategy involves the digestion of the cell wall and isolation of cell membranes or organelles from protoplasts [55, 56].

The endoplasmic reticulum (ER), isolated by sedimentation methods, can be contaminated heavily with other subcellular membranes [57]. Methods are available for the preparation of membrane fractions from cells grown in suspension cultures [58, 59].

The nuclear envelope may be obtained by subfractionation of a nuclear fraction after extraction of nucleoproteins in KCl, 2 mol/l, [60].

Tonoplasts are best prepared from isolated and purified vacuoles after osmotic lysis and sucrose density gradient centrifugation [61].

Plasmalemma is usally isolated by sucrose density gradient centrifugation of homogenates or plant cell protoplasts [62, 63, 64]. Membranes of the smooth or rough ER can be obtained from such homogenates if the extraction medium contains $MgCl_2$, 3 mmol/l, which preserves binding of ribosomes to the membranes without causing artificial aggregation of membranous structures. Fractions of the smooth and rough ER are subsequently separable when the homogenate is centrifuged into a density gradient [57].

References

[1]   E. W. Weiler, M. H. Zenk, Autoradiographic Immunoassays (ARIA), in: J. J. Langone, H. V. Vunakis (eds.), Methods in Enzymology, Vol. 73, Academic Press, New York 1981, pp. 394–406.

[2]   H. A. Kemp, M. R. A. Morgan, Use of Immunoassays in the Detection of Plant Cell Products, in: F. Constabel, I. K. Vasil (eds.), Cell Culture and Somatic Cell, Vol. 4, Academic Press, New York 1987, pp. 287–302.

[3]   A. Darvill, M. McNeil, P. Albertheim, D. P. Delmer, The Primary Cell Walls of Flowering Plants, in: P. K. Stumpf, E. E. Conn (eds.), The Biochemistry of Plants, Vol. 1, Academic Press, New York 1980, pp. 91–162.

[4]   R. D. Preston, The Physical Biology of Plant Cell Walls, Chapmann & Hall, London 1974.

[5]   Ph. Matile, The Lytic Compartment of Plant Cells, Cell Biology Monographs, Vol. 1, Springer-Verlag, Wien 1975.

[6]   F. Marty, D. Branton, R. A. Leigh, Plant Vacuoles, in: P. K. Stumpf, E. E. Conn (eds.), The Biochemistry of Plants, Vol. 1, Academic Press, New York 1980, pp. 625–658.

[7]   G. J. Wagner, Compartmentation in Plant Cells: The Role of the Vacuole, Recent Ad. Phytochem. 16, 1–45 (1982).

[8]   C. Werner, P. Matile, Accumulation of Coumaryl-glycosides in Vacuoles of Barley Mesophyll Protoplasts, J. Plant Physiol. 118, 237–249 (1985).

[9]   W. D. Loomis, Overcoming Problems of Phenolics and Quinones in the Isolation of Plant Enzymes and Organelles, in: S. Fleischer, L. Packer (eds.), Methods in Enzymology, Vol. 31, Academic Press, New York 1974, pp. 528–545.

[10] R. J. A. Budde, D. D. Randall, Light as a Signal Influencing the Phosphorylation Status of Plant Proteins, Plant. Physiol. 94, 1501–1504 (1990).

[11] J. Guern, J. P. Renaudin, S. C. Brown, The Compartmentation of Secondary Metabolites in Plant Cell Cultures, in: F. Constabel, I. K. Vasil (eds.), Cell Culture and Somatic Cell, Vol. 4, Academic Press, New York 1987, pp. 43–76.

[12] M. Wink, Physiology of the Accumulation of Secondary Metabolites with Special Reference to Alkaloids, in: F. Constabel, I. K. Vasil (eds.), Cell Culture and Somatic Cell, Vol. 4, Academic Press, New York 1987, pp. 17–42.

[13] M. Sakuta, A. Komamine, Cell Growth and Accumulation of Secondary Metabolites, in: F. Constabel, I. K. Vasil (eds.), Cell Culture and Somatic Cell, Vol. 4, Academic Press, New York 1987, pp. 97–114.

[14] P. Gegenheimer, Preparation of Extracts from Plants, in: M. P. Deutscher (ed.), Methods in Enzymology, Vol. 182, Academic Press, New York 1990, pp. 174–193.

[15] M. M. Smyk, Method of Sonication of Cell Suspensions, Bull Exp. Biol. Med. Engl. Transl. 84, 1669–1671 (1977).

[16] Y. Omori, M. Tsumura, T. Ichida, H. Nakajima, M. Ueda, F. Sato, Y. Yamada, A. Tanaka, Application of the Freeze-Blast Method to Disruption of Cultured Plant Cells, J. Ferment. Bioeng. 69, 132–134 (1990).

[17] L. Pick, J. Hurwitz, Purification of Wheat Germ RNA Ligase, J. Biol. Chem. 261, 6684–6693 (1986).

[18] *J. H. Wong, B. C. Yee, B. B. Buchanan*, A Novel Type of Phosphofructokinase from Plants, J. Biol. Chem. *262*, 3185–3191 (1987).

[19] *S. Heath-Pagliuso, D. C. Allyson, E. B. Kmiec*, Purification and Characterization of a Type-I Topoisomerase from Cultured Tobacco Cells, Plant Physiol. *94*, 599–606 (1990).

[20] *J. V. Anderson, J. L. Hess, B. I. Chevone*, Purification, Characterization, and Immunological Properties for Two Isoforms of Glutathion Reductase from Eastern White Pine Needles, Plant Physiol. *94*, 1402–1409 (1990).

[21] *C. H. Suelter*, A Practical Guide to Enzymology, Wiley, New York 1985.

[22] *M. M. Bradford*, A Rapid and Sensitive Method for the Quantification of Microgram Quantities of Protein Utilizing the Principle of Protein-Dye Binding, Anal. Biochem. *72*, 248–254 (1976).

[23] *R. L. Mattoo, M. Ishaq, M. Saleemuddin*, Protein Assay by Coomassie Brilliant Blue G-250-Binding Method is Unsuitable for Plant Tissues Rich in Phenols and Phenolase, Anal. Biochem. *163*, 376–384 (1987).

[24] *B. Croteau, A. J. Burbott, W. D. Loomis*, Enzymatic Cyclization of Neryl Pyrophosphate to α-Terpineol by Cell-free Extracts from Peppermint, Biochem. Biophys. Res. Commun. *50*, 1006–1012 (1973).

[25] *R. A. Bednar, J. R. Hadcock*, Purification and Characterization of Chalcone Isomerase from Soyabeans, J. Biol. Chem. *263*, 9582–9588 (1988).

[26] *R. A. J. Jefferson, T. A. Kavanagh, M. W. Bevan*, GUS Fusions: β-Glucuronidase as a Sensitive and Versatile Gene Fusion Marker in Higher Plants, EMBO J. *6*, 3901–3907 (1987).

[27] *R. B. Knox*, Methods for Locating and Identifying Antigens in Plant Tissues, in: *G. R. Bullock, P. Petrusz* (eds.), Techniques in Immunocytochemistry, Vol. 1, Academic Press, London 1982, pp. 205–238.

[28] *R. B. Knox*, Immunology and the Study of Plants, in: *J. J. Marchalonis, G. W. Warr* (eds.), Antibody as a Tool, John Wiley and Sons, Chichester 1982, pp. 293–346.

[29] *P. K. Nakane*, Ultrastructural Localization of Tissue Antigens with the Peroxidase-labelled Antibody Method, in: *E. Wisse, W. T. Daems, I. Molenaar, P. van Dujin* (eds.), Electron Microscopy and Cytochemistry, North-Holland Publishing Co., Amsterdam 1973, pp. 129–143.

[30] *A. E. Clarke, P. A. Gleeson, M. A. Jermyn, R. B. Knox*, Characterization and Localization of β-Lectins in Lower and Higher Plants, Aust. J. Plant Physiol. *5*, 707–722 (1978).

[31] *P. J. Harris*, Cell Walls, in: *J. L. Hall, A. C. Moore* (eds.), Isolation of Membranes and Organelles of Plant Cells, Academic Press, London 1983, pp. 25–53.

[32] *W. S. York, A. G. Darvill, M. McNeil, T. T. Stevenson, P. Albersheim*, Isolation and Characterization of Plant Cell Walls and Cell Wall Components, in: *A. Weissbach, H. Weissbach* (eds.), Methods for Plant Molecular Biology, Academic Press, San Diego 1988, pp. 3–40.

[33] *S. C. Fry*, Cell Wall-bound Proteins, in: *L. J. Rogers* (ed.), Methods in Plant Biochemistry, Vol. 5, Academic Press, London 1991, pp. 307–331.

[34] *E. C. A. Cocking*, A Method for Isolation of Plant Protoplasts and Vacuoles, Nature *187*, 927–963 (1960).

[35] *A. Ruesink*, Protoplasts of the Plant Cell, in: *S. P. Colowick, N. O. Kaplan* (eds.), Methods in Enzymology, Vol. 69, Academic Press, New York 1980, pp. 69–84.

[36] *D. N. Kuhn, P. K. Stumpf*, Preparation and Use of Protoplasts for Studies of Lipid Metabolism, in: *S. P. Colowick, N. O. Kaplan* (eds.), Methods in Enzymology, Vol. 72, Academic Press, New York 1981, pp. 774–783.

[37] *E. Galun*, Plant Protoplasts as Physiological Tools, Ann. Rev. Plant Physiol. *32*, 237–266 (1981).

[38] *T. R. Eriksson*, Protoplast Isolation and Culture, in: *L. C. Fowke, F. Constabel* (eds.), Plant Protoplasts, CFC Press, Boca Raton 1985, pp. 1–20.

[39] *E. U. Martinoia, U. Heck, A. Wiemken*, Vacuoles as Storage Compartments for Nitrate in Barley Leaves, Nature *289*, 292–294 (1981).

[40] *L. C. Fowke, F. Constable*, Plant Protoplasts, CRC Press, Boca Raton 1985.

[41] *I. Potrykus, R. D. Shillito,* Protoplasts: Isolation, Culture, Plant Regeneration, in: *A. Weissbach, H. Weissbach* (eds.), Methods for Plant Molecular Biology, Academic Press, San Diego 1988, pp. 335–383.

[42] *C. A. Price,* A Note on Isolation of Plant Nuclei, in: *E. Reid* (ed.), Methodological Surveys (B), Vol. 9, Plant Organelles, Ellis Horwood, Chichester 1979, pp. 200–206.

[43] *K. H. Cox, R. B. Goldberg,* Analysis of Plant Gene Expression, in: *C. H. Shaw* (ed.), Plant Molecular Biology, A Practical Approach, IRL Press, Oxford 1988, pp. 1–34.

[44] *J. J. Morgenthaler, M. P. F. Marsden, C. A. Price,* Factors Affecting the Separation of Photosynthetically Competent Chloroplasts in Gradients of Silica Soils, Arch. Biochem. Biophys. *168,* 289–301 (1975).

[45] *K. Keegstra, A. E. Yoursif,* Isolation and Characterization of Chloroplast Envelope Membranes, in: *A. Weissbach, H. Weissbach* (eds.), Methods for Plant Molecular Biology, Academic Press, San Diego 1988, pp. 173–182.

[46] *M. A. Schuler, R. E. Zielinski,* Methods in Plant Molecular Biology, Academic Press, San Diego 1989.

[47] *G. G. Laties,* Isolation of Mitochondria from Plant Material, in: *S. P. Colowick, N. O. Kaplan* (eds.), Methods in Enzymology, Vol. 31, Academic Press, New York 1974, pp. 589–600.

[48] *M. R. Hanson, M. L. Boeshore, P. E. McClean, M. A. O'Connell, H. T. Nivison,* The Isolation of Mitochondria and Mitochondrial DNA, in: *A. Weissbach, H. Weissbach* (eds.), Methods for Plant Molecular Biology, Academic Press, San Diego 1988, pp. 257–273.

[49] *N. E. Tolbert,* Microbodies-Peroxisomes and Glyoxysomes, in: *N. E. Tolbert* (ed.), The Biochemistry of Plants, Vol. 1, Academic Press, New York 1980, pp. 359–388.

[50] *E. L. Vigil, G. Wanner, R. R. Theimer,* Isolation of Plant Microbodies, in: *E. Reid* (ed.), Methodological Surveys (B), Vol. 9, Plant Organelles, Ellis Horwood, Chichester 1979, pp. 89–102.

[51] *H. Beevers, R. W. Breidenbach,* Glyoxisomes, in: *S. P. Colowick, N. O. Kaplan* (eds.), Methods in Enzymology, Vol. 31, Academic Press, New York 1974, pp. 565–571.

[52] *D. J. Morre, T. J. Buckhout,* Isolation of the *Golgi* Apparatus, in: *E. Reid* (ed.), Methodological Surveys (B), Vol. 9, Plant Organelles, Ellis Horwood, Chichester 1979, pp. 117–134.

[53] *T. W. Goodwin, E. I. Mercer,* Introduction of Plant Biochemistry, Pergamon, Oxford 1983.

[54] *G. J. Wagner, H. W. Siegelman,* Large-Scale Isolation of Intact Vacuoles and Isolation of Chloroplasts from Protoplasts of Mature Plant Tissue, Science *190,* 1298–1299 (1975).

[55] *P. J. Quinn, W. P. Williams,* Structure and Dynamics of Plant Membranes, in: *J. L. Haarwood, J. R. Bowyer* (eds.), Methods in Plant Biochemistry, Vol. 4, Academic Press, New York 1990, pp. 297–340.

[56] *T. K. Hodges, D. Mills,* Isolation of the Plasma Membrane, in: *A. Weissbach, H. Weissbach* (eds.), Methods for Plant Molecular Biology, Academic Press, San Diego 1988, pp. 41–54.

[57] *J. M. Lord, T. Kagawa, T. S. Moore, H. Beevers,* Endoplasmatic Reticulum as the Site of Lecithin Formation in Castor Bean Endosperm, J. Cell Biol. *57,* 659–667 (1973).

[58] *B. Gripsover, D. J. Morre, W. F. Boss,* Fractionation of Suspension Cultures of Wild Carrot and Kinetics of Membrane Labeling, Protoplasma *123,* 213–220 (1984).

[59] *D. J. Morre, A. O. Brightman, A. Stina, A. S. Sandelius,* Membrane Fractions from Plant Cells, in: *J. B. C. Findlay, W. H. Evans* (eds.), Biological Membranes, a Practical Approach, IRL Press, Oxford 1987, pp. 37–72.

[60] *W. W. Franke,* Zellkerne und Kernbestandteile, in: *G. Jacobi* (ed.), Biochemische Cytologie der Pflanzenzelle, Thieme Verlag, Stuttgart 1974, pp. 15–40.

[61] *R. A. Leigh, D. Branton, F. Marty,* Methods for the Isolation of Intact Vacuoles and Fragments of Tonoplasts, in: *E. Reid* (ed.), Methodological Surveys (B), Vol. 9, Plant Organelles, Ellis Horwood, Chichester 1979, pp. 69–80.

[62] *J. L. Hall, A. R. D. Taylor,* Isolation of the Plasma Membrane from Higher Plant Cells, in: *E. Reid* (ed.), Methodological Surveys (B), Vol. 9, Plant Organelles, Ellis Horwood, Chichester 1979, pp. 103–111.

[63] *D. S. Perlin, R. M. Spanswick,* Labeling and Isolation of Plasma Membranes Corn Leaf Protoplasts, Plant Physiol. *65,* 1053–1057 (1980).

[64] *P. H. Quail,* Plant Cell Fractionation, Annu. Rev. Plant Physiol. *30,* 425–484 (1979).

2.8   Prokaryotic Cells

Matthias C. C. Poetsch

Prokaryotic cells and their metabolites may serve as targets in methods of immunological analysis, for example, as whole cells, membranes, fractions of periplasm or cytoplasm, as well as providing macromolecules such as proteins, polysaccharides, lipids or nucleic acids. They are also sources of reagents for immunological analysis, e. g. streptavidin, enzymes such as β-galactosidase, or recombinant antibody-fragments.

Prokaryotic cells have certain advantages in immunological methods since their relatively short generation time provides reagents quickly and inexpensively. Bacterial growth proceeds by division into two identical daughter cells. Descendants of a single cell may be visualized as a single colony produced on an agar plate some hours later. After n divisions the number of cells in a colony corresponds to $N_0 \times 2^n$, where N_0 is the initial cell number. Therefore, a single cell of an organism with a typical generation time of 30 min would propagate on an agar plate to approximately 3×10^{15} cells within 24 h. Due to the exponential growth and the very short doubling times of many prokaryotes, very high yields of biomass may be obtained.

This section contains a general description for the preparation of prokaryotic cells with reference to the special requirements of the many different microorganisms that can be used in methods of immunological analysis. Further information on specific organisms should be drawn from the literature, e. g. [1].

In general, prokaryotic cells should be handled according to good standard microbiological practice.

2.8.1   Equipment

The equipment usually required in a microbiological laboratory is as below. Materials must tolerate the appropriate sterilization procedures.

In general, culture vessels are *Erlenmeyer* flasks, *Fernbach* flasks or other glass bottles, sealed with aluminium foil or cotton plugs. *Petri* dishes, covered cups and tubes may be of plastic or glass. Fermenters are made of glass or stainless steel. Tools for the preparation of media and propagation of the cultures are, for example, pipettes of glass or plastic, inoculation loops (platinium), *Drygalsky*-spatula, teflon-coated magnetic bars. Furthermore, a balance, pH-meter, magnetic stirrer, autoclave, laminar flow hood, gas burner, incubator and microscope are necessary. Centrifuge and sonicator (or *French* press, bead mill, etc.) are required for the harvest and disintegration of cells.

2.8.2   Sources of Microorganisms

Prokaryotic cells can be obtained from many sources: as isolates from natural habitats such as soil, air or water (particularly waste water), or as isolates from plants, animals or man. Characterize them in detail prior to further handling, in order to avoid the use of pathogenic strains without the required precautions including special containment. In general, the use of nonpathogenic strains is highly recommended. Kits are commercially available for the determination of the taxonomy of unidentified organisms. References to further methods for systematic characterization are given in [2]. National culture collections are sources of already classified microorganisms.

Recombinant bacteria have become highly important since methods of molecular engineering have enabled the expression of foreign proteins and antigens in them. Vast improvements in the development of new and more efficient expression systems are regularly reported, and are discussed in detail in a number of methods manuals among which that by *Sambrook* et al. (1989) is recommended [3].

2.8.3   Media

2.8.3.1   Composition

The basis for all media formulations is the elementary composition of the particular strain used. Optimal growth requires sufficient amounts of nutrients (macro-elements), substrates, trace elements (micro-elements), and supplements such as vitamins and growth factors. Further components may be added during growth (e. g., acid, alkali, anti-foam reagent, inducers, inhibitors, etc.). They are supplied as defined chemicals or as complex material derived from plant, animal or microbial sources.

For growth, prokaryotes usually require the following macro-elements: C, H, O, N, S, P, K, Ca, Mg. Furthermore, some micro-organisms need the addition of trace elements such as Mn, Mo, Zn, Co, Ni, V, B, Cl, Na, Se, Si, W, etc.; most of these may be present as contaminants of the macro-elements or in the water used to prepare the media. In addition, many organisms need very small amounts of supplements (0.005–0.15 mg/l). These are, for example, vitamins as part of coenzymes or prosthetic groups, or purines, pyrimidines and amino acids as compounds for synthesis of proteins and nucleic acids.

Genetically engineered organisms often require addition of amino acids or other metabolites for complementation of any auxotrophy they carry. Antibiotics are added according to need to select the strain desired among occasionally occurring revertants. The use of chemically defined or minimal media facilitates the preparation of cells for methods of, for example, immunological analysis by eliminating the necessity to remove medium proteins. Many non-fastidious organisms (e. g. *Escherichia coli* or *Pseudomonas sp.*) are able to grow up to their maximum specific growth rate (μ_{max}) in synthetic media composed of some of the elements listed above. In these cases, formulate media with respect to the specific requirements of the particular organisms.

Special media for most of the commonly used microorganisms are described by their commercial distributors. Therefore, the catalogues of culture collections, such as the American Type Culture Collection [4], German Collection of Microorganism and Cell Cultures [5], etc., are recommended as initial sources of information. More details on the nutritional requirements of particular organisms, e. g., their ability to use several sources of carbon for growth, are described in Bergey's Manual [2].

Several complete media are also available. These may be used following the manufacturers' instructions. Many are composed in part of complex raw materials such as extracts or hydrolysates from yeast, meat or plants. By products of industrial processes are also used because of low cost and high availability. These nutrients contain most of the elements listed above and supplements in sufficient amounts. Normally, however, their composition is not known in detail and differs slightly from batch to batch. Such media are usually enriched with glucose as substrate, and some macro- or micro-elements as required. When nutritional requirements are not known in detail, prokaryotes should be grown initially in a complex medium. The systematics of media design are given for example by *Fiechter* [6].

Media may contain either additives to control the pH at an optimum value with respect to the organisms' requirements. Achieve, this for instance, by adding $CaCO_3$, phosphate buffers or *Good* buffers [7]. Control foaming of the culture by adding a few drops of a chemical anti-foam emulsion (e. g. silicon oil, polyalcohols, etc.).

2.8.3.2   Preparation

Prepare all media by dissolving the ingredients in water with vigorous mixing. In order to prevent precipitation to insoluble complexes, add salts in chemically defined media with respect to their solubility constant. An example of the extreme care necessary to achieve an optimal preparation of a chemically defined medium is given by *Riesenberg* et al. [8]. They have developed a high density fermentation of recombinant *E. coli* with a dry-weight yield of cells up to 60 g/l. As a general rule the pH should be adjusted to the desired value before sterilization.

In order to minimize batch variation, the ingredients should be prepared as 10× or 100× stock solutions and stored at −20°C. Prepare the 1× basal medium, aliquot and sterilize it by autoclaving prior to use. Prepare glucose and sterilize separately and add prior to inoculation to prevent chemical modification by the *Maillard* reaction [9] during sterilization (see below).

2.8.3.3   Sterilization

In order to grow a pure culture of a desired prokaryote it is necessary to sterilize the media and equipment with which it will come in contact. Most potential microbial

contaminants are inactivated by autoclaving (20 min, 121°C, 101 kPa). Some ingredients such as starch, soya peptone and distiller's soluble extract, among others, may
form glutinous clots of undissolved material in spite of stirring during preparation. In
this case temperatures up to 135°C or an extension of sterilization time are needed.
Another method to deal with this problem is Tyndallization, which involves heating to
80°C followed by incubation at around 37°C until viable spores grow out; the procedure
is repeated twice thereafter. Sterilize thermolabile nutrients or supplements by passing
through 0.2 μm filters.

Sugars are partially decomposed when they are autoclaved in the presence of
inorganic salts and organic compounds [9]. Browning may occur as a result of the
Maillard reaction but as they are generally stable to autoclaving in pure solution, they
should be prepared separately and added to the medium after sterilization. Among
inorganic compounds, ammonium salts should be autoclaved at a pH less than 7,
otherwise ammonia is volatilized.

Other methods of sterilization include irradiation (e.g., by UV light), chemical
treatment (ethyleneoxide, formaldehyde, etc.) or dry heat (2 h, 160°C); these are
commonly used for glassware and equipment.

2.8.4   Culture

2.8.4.1   Propagation

The prerequisite for deposition in a cell bank is the preparation of a pure culture from
the isolate. Carry this out by growing cells on selective media and streaking on agar
plates to obtain single colonies. Repeat this cloning several times under different
conditions until the culture is homogeneous with respect to morphology of the
organisms and the colonies, and their physiological characteristics.

Prepare a standard inoculum by mixing a mid-logarithmic phase culture of the desired
prokaryote with an equal volume of sterile glycerol. Store aliquots frozen at −20 to
−196°C up to several years without any loss of viability. When required, the contents of a
vial should be thawed rapidly in a water-bath. Inocula may also be prepared by
concentration of cells by ultrafiltration under sterile conditions. Cultures may also be
stored as lyophilized stocks. Prepare these by drying cells from a mid-logarithmic phase
culture which has been mixed with an equal volume of freshly-prepared medium.

Check aliquots from the working cell bank routinely by thawing a sample and growing
a small culture as described below. Improvement of the strain is then focused on purity
of the culture, viability of the cells and physiological characteristics. Prepare inoculum
by rapidly thawing a vial from cell bank (above) in a water-bath at the desired
inoculation temperature. Inoculate pre-warmed medium with 0.3 to 10% of the culture
stock. When initiating from lyophilized stock, suspend cells in a sufficient amount of

medium or PBS and spread on a nutrient agar plate or dilute in 30–50 ml of medium in an *Erlenmeyer* flask. Grow to mid-logarithmic phase and use to inoculate further cultures.

Grow working cultures later on agar plates or slants and transfer to fresh medium every few days or weeks depending on the organism.

Propagate seed cultures, and preparations of cells up to an amount of 1 l, in *Erlenmeyer* flasks (without or with 1–4 indentations) on rotating shakers with agitation sufficient to meet the organisms' oxygen demand (usually 100–200 rpm). Fill culture flasks to 10–20% of their total volume to obtain optimal conditions for aeration of the culture. Aeration may also be achieved adequately in magnetically-stirred glass bottles up to a volume of 1–5 l.

Incubate cultures at temperatures from 15 to 80°C (and more) depending on the prokaryote to be grown. A temperature of 28–37°C is sufficient for most of the commonly used prokaryote.

Quality control of small cultures in shake flasks is restricted to two or three small samples taken from the culture. Generally there is no continuous measurement of growth but temperature and agitation are usually regulated. The cultures should be routinely checked for homogeneity using a microscope or by streaking on agar plates. The pH should be measured and the product determined before harvesting the cells. Biomass can be estimated by light scattering, determination of dry or wet weight, or counting under the microscope.

2.8.4.2 Harvest and Disruption of the Cells

Cells are sometimes required in as fresh a state as possible. Thus, handle at 4°C and with autoclaved solutions and equipment to prevent microbial contamination or artefactual results caused by proteases, etc. In general, recover cells by centrifugation at $5000–10000 \times g$ for 10–20 min. The g force required and the time of centrifugation will vary with the morphology of the cells or cell aggregates. It is important that supernatants are disposed of using proper techniques to kill any residual bacteria which may be pathogenic or potentially harmful genetically-engineered organisms.

Wash the pellet once or twice by centrifugation in Tris-HCl, 10 mmol/l, neutral pH, and then suspended in one-fiftieth of the original volume of wash buffer containing phenylmethylsulphonyl fluoride (PMSF), 2 mmol/l, to inhibit protease activity. Subsequent treatment of the cells will depend on the nature of the experiment. Freeze or resuspend again in special buffers or break for analysis of intracellular components.

Prokaryotic cells can be disrupted by chemical, physical and biological methods. Commonly, they are broken by sonication, with high presure, or in bead mills. Obtain crude extracts of the cells by centrifugation at $10000 \times g$ for 20 min at 4°C and withdraw the supernatant, which should be clarified by centrifugation a second time. The crude extracts of these pellets may then be treated for further analysis. Another method for the preparation of periplasmic proteins, for example, is osmotic shock lysis, which may provide proteins relatively free from contamination by cytoplasmic proteins.

References

[1] *B. Atkinson, F. Mavituna,* Biochemical Engineering And Biotechnology Handbook, The Nature Press, New York 1983.

[2] *J. G. Holt* (ed.), Bergey's Manual of Systematic Bacteriology, Williams & Wilkins, Baltimore 1984.

[3] *J. Sambrook, E. F. Fritsch, T. Maniatis,* Molecular Cloning: A Laboratory Manual, 2nd ed., Cold Spring Harbor Laboratory, New York 1989.

[4] American Type Culture Collection, Catalog of Bacteria and Bacteriophages, 17th edition, Rockville, Maryland, USA 1989.

[5] German Collection of Microorganisms and Cell Cultures, Catalog of Strains 1989, Fourth Edition Braunschweig 1989.

[6] *A. Fiechter,* Physical and Chemical Parameters of Microbial Growth, in: *A. Fiechter* (ed.), Adv. Biochem. Eng. Biotechnol. *30,* 7–60 (1984).

[7] *N. E. Good, G. D. Winget, W. Winter, T. N. Connolly, S. Izawa, R. M. M. Singh,* Hydrogen Ion Buffers, for Biological Research, Biochemistry *5,* 467–477 (1966).

[8] *D. Riesenberg, K. Menzel, V. Schulz, K. Schumann, G. Veith, G. Zuber, W. Knorre,* High Cell Density Fermentation of Recombinant *Escherichia coli* Expressing Human Interferon alpha 1, Appl. Microbiol. Biotechnol. *34,* 77–82 (1990).

[9] *D. Rewicki, M. Angrick,* Die Maillard Reaktion, Chemie in unserer Zeit *14,* 149–157 (1989).

3 Cell Culture

3.1   General Principles

Christopher B. Morris, Bryan J. Bolton and Jon M. Mowles

The origins of cell cultures go back to the start of the twentieth century, at a time when major advances in optical design through the development of compound lenses had allowed the evolution of the microscope to progress to a point where high resolution and magnification were possible. At about the same time attempts to elucidate the physiological role of tissues in higher animals had led to the discovery that simple salt solutions could maintain tissues in a "viable" condition for long periods of time.

Some of the earliest recorded experiments were undertaken with nerve tissue separated from a frog [1]. Outgrowth from fibres could be observed, which encouraged the idea that cell growth outside the body, i.e., *"in vitro"* was attainable. However, major obstacles had yet to be overcome. Microbial contamination, choice of a suitable vessel for cell growth and the formulation of culture medium that stimulated rather than merely maintained cells, were the prime areas of research during the following years. Today's high success rate with the many hundreds of different cell lines can be traced clearly through the joint development of aseptic techniques and cell culture media.

The following deals with the various requirements for setting up a successful cell culture laboratory and includes current thinking on the biosafety aspects of animal cell cultures.

3.1.1   Laboratory Design

Aseptic technique is the basis of success in all cell culture laboratories. The prevention of unintentional microbial and viral contamination is necessary at every stage of culture preparation and growth.

In early laboratory design the emphasis was on protecting the cell cultures, but not the operator. Lamina flow cabinets or rooms ensure a sterile air flow over the working area. This air can be directed either horizontally in a cabinet, or vertically as an "air curtain" in an aseptic cubicle, which means exposing the operator to air currents after they have passed over the cells being handled.

The term "sterile air", it should be explained, refers to air that has passed through a high-efficiency particulate air (HEPA) filter. This removes particles, including micro-organisms, down to 0.5 µm diameter.

Current cabinet design now also offers protection to the operator. There are four categories, or levels, of handling facility for microorganisms. These are designated according to the biohazard (potential pathogenicity) presented by the organism in question. The regulations applying to the United Kingdom are outlined in the publication, "Categorisation of Pathogens According to Hazard and Categories of Contaminent" [2]. There are small variations in terminology and interpretation in other countries' regulations controlling biohazardous organisms and their handling [3].

A working party on Safety in Biotechnology has been set up by the European Federation for Biotechnology to examine specific recommendations for working with animal cell cultures. A draft proposal has been issued in which safety precautions are outlined according to the origin of cell lines, such as established human diploid cell lines used in vaccine production (low risk), mammalian and non-haematogenous cell lines (medium risk) and human and primate blood and bone marrow-derived cell lines (high risk). The criteria for categorization are based on the cells' potential to carry pathogenic adventitious agents and, to this end, the guidelines for handling micro-organisms are followed [2, 3].

Ideally a cell culture laboratory should be purpose built, as for example in manufacturing and industrial laboratories. These comply with very strict requirements to ensure product integrity as well as operator protection. However, as most people have to convert existing facilities, what follows will take this into consideration, and is based on the guidelines from the U.K. and U.S.A. standards for containment (Biosafety) Level 2.

1. Rooms should be specifically designated for cell culture operations only and should be isolated from other areas, e. g. corridors, by doors or other suitable closures. Doors should be closed during all operations.
2. Access to the laboratory should be limited to essential personnel.
3. The laboratory should be easy to clean (all surfaces), with suitable bench surfaces which are impervious to water and resistant to acids, alkalis, solvents and disinfectants.
4. At least 24 m^3 should be allowed for each worker.
5. The laboratory should be mechanically ventilated to provide a negative pressure relative to adjacent rooms and areas, that is, air should flow into the laboratory. This can be achieved by venting the exhaust air from Class 2 cabinets, through ducting, to the external atmosphere. The air supply to the room(s) should preferably be HEPA filtered.
6. Class 2 cabinets and lamina flow cabinets (the latter for media and reagent preparation) must be located away from access doors, ventilation drafts and areas of regular personnel traffic.
7. The laboratory should contain a handwashing sink near the exit. Taps should be of a type that can be operated without touching by hand.
8. An autoclave should be readily accessible, either inside or in the vicinity of the laboratory.
9. If the laboratory has windows that open, they must be fitted with fly screens. However, the use of rooms with open windows is to be avoided if at all possible.

It is emphasized that these points only cover the most basic form of laboratory and that incubator rooms, cold rooms, and areas dedicated to media preparation and quality control require additional planning. Cell culture laboratories must never be located adjacent to areas where micro-organisms, or material containing micro-organisms, are handled. If media are to be prepared from powders, the room used for this must be ventilated under negative pressure relative to adjacent areas. Further information concerning these points can be found elsewhere [4].

If cell cultures are to be prepared for therapeutic or diagnostic use, a purpose-designed suite is essential. Here the emphasis is on protecting the product from extraneous contamination. Cell lines used in such processes have to satisfy rigorous quality control tests to ensure their safety for operators. In this case the cell culture laboratory is maintained at a positive air pressure relative to adjacent rooms. Such facilities have to be operated to Good Manufacturing Practice (GMP) standards [5, 6].

3.1.2   Equipment

In addition to the sterile air flow cabinets and autoclave mentioned above, a functional cell culture laboratory will require equipment [7] as described below.

3.1.2.1   Incubators

These should provide sufficient space to accommodate all possible needs. When choosing a model several points should be considered.

Temperature control must be very accurate, within $\pm 0.5°C$ or better. Most mammalian cells will grow between 33°C and 39°C. However, sensitive mutants or insect cell lines require lower temperatures, and some incubators are provided with refrigeration for this purpose. In general it is better to maintain incubators at a constant temperature and so it is preferable to have several with each dedicated to a particular set temperature. Circulated air is necessary to prevent temperature gradients within the incubator.

The incubator must be constructed of corrosion-resistant material such as stainless steel. Aluminium surfaces should be smooth or preferably polished for ease of cleaning. Note that the shelves and supports must be regularly cleaned and autoclaved, and the interior surfaces decontaminated, to prevent the build up of microbial contamination, especially moulds.

If CO_2 is required to buffer the culture medium an automatic CO_2 incubator is preferred, especially if open culture systems e. g. multi-well plates or *Petri* dishes are to be used. This type of incubator requires more maintenance than the dry type due to the need for a humidified atmosphere to provide accurate CO_2 control.

A constant supply of CO_2 is essential to prevent the loss of cultures, so the gas cylinders supplying the incubators must incorporate a dual circuit supply control system so that when one set of cylinders becomes empty there is an automatic switch over to another set.

If CO_2 incubators are not available, a supply of 5% CO_2/95% air will be needed to gas culture flasks individually. The gas supply line should be fitted with an in-line 0.2 μm filter designed for use with gas mixtures. Flasks can then be gassed through sterile plugged plastic or glass pipettes to ensure sterility.

3.1.2.2   Microscope

Regular, in many cases daily, examination of cultures requires an inverted phase contrast microscope. Essential design features include, ease of use, and a sturdy stage suitable for examination of a variety of culture vessels from *Petri* dishes to large flasks. If roller bottles are to be examined a long-focus objective lens is required. A useful addition is an attachment tube for a camera. This will enable photographs to be taken.

3.1.2.3   Other Items

These include items routinely required to maintain and manipulate cell cultures in the laboratory.

Water-bath for thawing frozen ampoules and warming media. This must be cleaned at least once a week, using only purified water (distilled or cartridge purified) with a suitable disinfectant to inhibit growth of microorganisms.

Haemocytometer which is a glass cell-counting chamber used to estimate both the total and viable cells in a population. The Improved *Neubauer* type is most suitable for animal cells. A vital stain, e. g. Trypan Blue, is used to measure viable cells. A full description of this method is given in 2.1.1.2.

Culture flasks and pipettes. Many laboratories use pre-sterilised plastic culture-ware rather than glass, to reduce the need for special glassware washing facilities. However, should it be necessary to use glassware, the correct types of cleaning agents, suitable for cell culture, must be used. Rinsing with tap water must be followed by extensive rinsing with purified water to ensure that no residue remains on the glass. Automatic washing machines therefore provide the best solution to this problem. Note that cell lines are extremely sensitive to ionic and non-ionic detergents.

Pipetting aids. Mouth pipetting is strictly forbidden. Many mechanical aids to pipetting are available. Routine subculture requires the use of 1 ml – 25 ml pipettes, and can be best achieved by using an automatic pipetting aid comprising a small electric pump which controls pressure through vacuum lines attached to a special handle designed to hold the pipettes. Button controls allow repetitive pipetting to be accurately controlled with one hand. For smaller quantities, various negative, or air, displacement micropipettes are available.

Germicidal solutions. These are best made available in spray or squeeze bottles as solutions suitable for surface decontamination of flow cabinets and bench tops. Traditionally 70% ethanol in distilled water has been used. Alternatively, formalin- and propanol-based solutions are more efficient because they avoid the problem of fixing protein residues, as in serum, on surfaces where alcohol is used. A 2% v/v solution of Tegodor *(Goldschmidt Ltd.)* can be used for both surface decontamination and for immersion of discarded pipettes.

Programmable freezer. As it is impractical to maintain most cell lines indefinitely in culture, a system for freezing cells it necessary [8].

To achieve the maximum viability, freeze cells slowly at a rate between 1°C and 3°C/min. This can be most accurately achieved with a controlled rate, programmable freezer *(Planer Products, Savant Instruments)*. In practice resuscitated cells have similar viability to those in culture at the time of freezing. Since this type of freezer is expensive an alternative is to use insulated containers specially designed for use with −80°C freezers *(Nalgene, Biocell)*. These have been designed to achieve a cooling rate of 1°C/min. However, this method of freezing cannot compensate for the heat released during the phase transition from liquid to solid which is the most critical point of freezing. Therefore, for truly reproducible results a programmable freezer is necessary. Methods of cryopreservation are described in 3.2.4.

Nitrogen storage vessels. Frozen cells must be stored at −130°C or below to maintain their viability. Electrical freezers can now achieve this temperature, but they are expensive to purchase and operate. Liquid nitrogen vessels offer several advantages over electrical freezers. They operate down to −196°C, are inexpensive to run, do not generate heat and are available in a wide range of sizes *(Statebourne, MVE, Taylor-Wharton, L'Air Liquide, Cryomed)*.

It must be stressed that full protective clothing (full face mask, insulated gloves and splash proof coat) must be worn at all times when handling liquid nitrogen, otherwise severe frostbite can result. It is also advisable to install an oxygen monitor, as oxygen levels below 16% may cause drowsiness and fainting. As a safeguard against rapid loss of nitrogen, e.g. through vacuum failure, an alarm system should be fitted to the vessel(s). Systems are now available which can be linked to the telephone network, providing autodialling to selected numbers when a fault occurs.

3.1.3   Good Laboratory Practice

The essential requirements of Good Laboratory Practice (GLP) involve adherence to strict protocols or Standard Operating Procedures (SOP) which are all based on a sound common sense approach to avoiding problems. These fundamental points can be translated to the laboratory environment by producing instruction protocols.

Each procedure undertaken should be written in a concise instructional manner, with all formulation and equipment requirements included. Preparation of media, sterility tests, handling of different cell lines, disposal of liquid and solid waste, and handling of radioisotopes are a few examples. The simplest approach to providing sufficient protocols is to itemize the sequence of events in the laboratory from start to finish over each day. In this way it will be possible to separate the various functions and operations taking place. Some of the items that will need addressing are described below.

Quality Control of Media. This includes testing of components for their ability to support cell growth, for example, serum batch testing and checks for contamination by bacteria, fungi and mycoplasma.

Handling of Cell Lines. This includes safety categories according to the risk factor to operators, such as cell lines carrying category 2 and 3 micro-organisms, subculture routines for adherent and suspension lines and bulking up procedures.

Quality Control of Cell Lines. This involves testing for microorganisms and mycoplasma, cell characterization, for example by isoenzyme analysis, and viability checks of cryopreserved stocks.

General Laboratory Procedures. These include general safety aspects and accident reporting, laboratory clothing, personal hygiene, disposal of non-toxic, toxic and radioactive waste.

Equipment. SOPs for equipment include setting-up and operating procedures, maintenance and standardization records.

Documentation. This involves staff training records, equipment testing, safety requirement forms, storage records, e. g. batch numbers and expiry dates of reagents, locations of cryopreserved cell lines.

An approach to GLP is to document each procedure according to local statutory regulations such as the Control of Substances Hazardous to Health Regulations (COSHH) issued by the Health and Safety Executive, that became a legal requirement in the United Kingdom in October 1989. In this way a protocol with the incorporated appropriate safety procedures can be produced for each laboratory operation.

Industrial laboratories have to perform their functions to the highest standards set by the regulatory body for that country. A fully descriptive Standard Operating Procedure (SOP) must be written for every aspect of operation. A SOP must provide sufficient information for any trained member of personnel to be able to perform the task from the written instructions. All SOPs are essentially derived from basic protocols and so any laboratory wishing to upgrade its operating standards can use these as the basis for a SOP. Useful background reading on the approach needed to comply with regulatory standards can be found in [9, 10].

References

[1] *R. G. Harrison,* Observations on the Living Developing Nerve Fiber, Proc. Soc. Exp. Biol. Med. *4,* 140–143 (1907).

[2] Advisory Committee on Dangerous Pathogens, Categorisation of pathogens according to hazard and categories of containment, HMSO publications, London (1990).

[3] U.S. Department of Health and Human Services (Public Health Service), Biosafety in Microbiological and Biomedical Laboratories, U.S. Government Printing Office, Washington 1988.

[4] *W. Scheirer,* Laboratory Management of Animal Cell Culture Processes, Trends in Biotechnol. *5,* 261–265 (1987).

[5] *J. R. Sharp* (Ed.), Guide to Good Pharmaceutical Manufacturing Practice, HMSO Publications, London 1983.

[6] Food and Drug Administration, General Biological Production Standards; Cell Lines Used for Manufacturing Biological Products, U.S. Federal Register 51, No. 237, 44451–44454, 1986.

[7] *A. Doyle, C. B. Morris,* Maintenance of Animal Cells, in: *B. E. Kirsop, A. Doyle* (eds.), Maintenance of Microorganisms, Academic Press, London 1991, pp. 234–236.

[8] *A. Doyle, C. B. Morris, W. J. Armitage,* Cryopreservation of Animal Cells, in: *A. Mizrahi* (ed.), Advances in Biotechnological Processes, Vol. 7, A. R. Liss, New York 1988, pp. 1–17.

[9] FDA, Points to Consider in the Characterisation of Cell Lines Used to Produce Biologicals from FDA Congressional Consumer and International Affairs Staff, Rockville, Maryland 1987.

[10] Draft Outline on, Requirements for the Production and Quality Control of Monoclonal Antibodies of Murine Origin Intended for Use in Man; from Commission of the European Communities III/859/86-ENN (1986).

3.2   Long-term Cultures and Cell Lines

Bryan J. Bolton, Christopher B. Morris and Jon M. Mowles

3.2.1   Types of Cell Lines

The following sub-sections consist of broad definitions of different categories of cell lines. More detailed descriptions of culture techniques for different types of cell lines are given elsewhere [1] and in this volume.

Primary cell cultures. These are cultures isolated directly from animal tissue. They are prepared by disaggregation techniques involving manual and/or enzymatic digestion. The enzyme usually used is trypsin (EC 3.4.21.4) but others include collagenase (EC 3.4.24.8), elastase (EC 3.4.21.36), hyaluronidase (EC 4.2.2.1), DNaseI (EC 3.1.21.1), pronase* (EC 3.4.24.4), dispase** or various combinations of these. Embryonic tissue yields more viable cells and tends to proliferate more rapidly than adult tissue.

Finite cell lines. Finite cell lines are usually derived from a primary cell culture and have a defined number of population doublings before senescence occurs. The number of doublings can be as high as 70 with human diploid cell lines, e. g. MRC-5. However, with many adult or differentiated cell types the number of doublings is extremely limited.

Transformed cell lines. There are many types of transformation which result in a continuous cell line. Transformation can be spontaneous, as following a "crisis" phase in a cell line during which all growth apparently ceases, and then a population of cells forming a continuous line appears. These usually have the general characteristics of reduced cell size, increased tumourigenicity and variable karyology. Transformed cell lines may also be derived directly from tumour tissue or be established *in vitro* by viruses such as SV40 and EBV or by DNA fragments derived from a transforming virus using vector systems. It is also possible to generate transformed cell lines using chemical carcinogens such as tetradecanoyl phrobol-13-acetate (TPA).

Although transformed cell lines have the advantage of growing continually it is very difficult to generate transformed cell lines with highly differentiated characteristics. In long-term culture there is continuous selection for cells with the highest growth rates and these generally demonstrate the least functional differentiation.

---

 * non-specific protease from *Streptomyces griseus*
** neutral protease

Hybridomas. Hybridomas that secrete monoclonal antibodies are produced after fusion of antibody-secreting B-cells from an immunized patient or an animal with a malignant myeloma cell line capable of indefinite growth *in vitro*. They may be unstable and difficult to maintain, since as they can loose whole chromosomes. This may prevent the cells from producing the antibody which was of first interest. T-cell hybridomas can be produced by analogous methods. Detailed protocols and further discussions can be found in 3.3, in Volume 2, section 4.3 and elsewhere [1].

3.2.2   Media

Many articles and books have been written on this subject, however certain principles and guidelines can be outlined here as a means of introduction to the topic. The principle of cell-culture media is to mimic the physiological conditions the cells would normally be under within tissues and organs. Media generally have a near neutral pH and contain serum, balanced salt solutions, glucose, salts, vitamins, amino acids and other growth factors [1].

3.2.2.1   Types, Choice and Preparation

There are no hard and fast rules on which media to use for different types of cell lines. There are many defined media available commercially; the more common ones in use include *Eagle's* minimum essential medium (MEM); *Dulbecco's* MEM; *Ham's* F10 und F12, RPMI 1640, Medium 199, *Fischer's* and *Waymouth's* MB 752/1. Although defined, they are usually supplemented with 5–20% serum which is usually fetal bovine in origin. If a cell line has been obtained from a culture collection (e. g. ECACC, ATCC) then the required medium and growth conditions will be recommended. If this is not so, one approach is to start with a rich medium such as *Ham's* F12: *Dulbecco's* MEM (1:1) supplemented with 20% fetal bovine serum and then gradually reduce the serum concentration and manipulate the concentration of the other constituents such as amino acids and the various salts. Often other growth factors and hormones are added which in the case of hybridomas may include 2-mercaptoethanol (50 µmol/l), sodium pyruvate (1 mmol/l) or insulin (5 µg/l). Other important growth factors include fibroblast and epidermal growth factors, and hydrocortisone.

Defined media are available commercially in either powder form for preparation and sterilization in the laboratory, or in liquid form in 1× to 10× concentration. Powdered media have the advantage of being cheaper, although the preparation is time-consuming and labour-intensive. If ready-to-use liquid media are used, serum and L-glutamine have to be added prior to use, therefore requiring a programme of microbiological quality control (cf. 3.2.5).

The choice of serum is an important consideration, particularly for hybridomas which tend to be fastidious in their requirements. Therefore, test different batches of serum for their ability to maintain the cell lines to be cultured. A further consideration in the purchase of serum is the country of origin, since foot and mouth disease and other viruses are endemic in certain regions of the world. The use of serum from any country of origin other than Zone I (U.S.A., Canada, U.K. and New Zealand) may lead to difficulty in importing cell lines to the U.S.A., for example.

3.2.2.2 Serum-free Media

It is often desirable to culture cell lines in media without serum. Serum free medium has many advantages including
a) the constitution of the medium for a particular cell line is defined, standardized and therefore reproducible;
b) the need for extensive testing of new batches of serum is not required;
c) downstream processing of cell culture products is simpler due to the lower protein content; and
d) since serum may be contaminated with viruses it is necessary to demonstrate to regulatory authorities the absence of such viruses from the final product. This should not be necessary with serum-free media.

Serum contributes a major part of the costs of cell culture media. However, the use of serum-free media will not necessarily significantly reduce this cost due to the high cost at present of serum-free media. In addition, the time necessarily spent in adapting the line to grow in serum-free media must also be taken into account.

3.2.3 Subculture and Maintenance

Maintain cell cultures at their optimum condition by keeping them in the log phase of growth. The doubling time for animal cells is generally between 24 and 48 hours. Prolonged periods in the stationary growth phase often result in cell lines losing their plating efficiency and their overall quality and healthiness will decline.

There are two general methods of subculture dependent on whether the cell line grows attached or in suspension, and protocols for both are given below. Cell lines are supplied either as growing cultures or cryopreserved. Details for starting from a frozen culture are given in 3.2.4.2.

3.2.3.1   Attached Cell Lines

Examine cells under an inverted microscope ($\times$ 100 magnification) and if cells are confluent then sub-culture them as follows:

1. Discard spent culture medium and gently pour or pipette PBS to the same volume of the original culture medium. Gently swirl the PBS to wash the cells. Discard the PBS and repeat.
2. Add trypsin-EDTA solution (1–2 ml/25 cm^2) and gently swirl to ensure all the surface is covered. Pour off most of the solution leaving just sufficient to wet the cells. Incubate at 37°C until the cells start to detach from the surface of the flask. This usually takes 2–10 min. If cells are slow to detach, the flask can gently be knocked or shaken to loosen the cells.
3. If the cells are to be cryopreserved see 3.2.4.2, otherwise proceed as follows. Resuspend cells in cell culture medium and add to pre-prepared tissue culture flasks at 37°C (or other appropriate incubation temperature) with the required volume of culture medium, e. g. 5–7 ml for a 25 cm^2, 20–30 ml for a 75 cm^2 and 50–100 ml for a 175 cm^2 flask. Gas with a 5% CO_2/95% air mixture, where required.
4. Prior to adding the cells to the flasks, perform a viable cell count (cf. 2.1.1.2) to determine the correct split ratio. A cell count is not always necessary once the split ratio of a cell line is known. The size of culture flask to use depends entirely upon the number of cells required, since saturation densities for adherent cell lines range from about 10^5 cells/cm^2 to 3 to 4×10^5 cells/cm^2 when multilayers are formed.

3.2.3.2   Suspension Cell Lines

As for attached cell lines, examine cultures microscopically for signs of cell deterioration. The colour of the medium can also be used as an indicator of cell density, red-orange is normal whereas yellow indicates that the culture has become acidic and is at risk of going into stationary phase and decline. However, some cell lines, e. g., EBV-transformed lymphoblastoid lines, prefer acidic conditions. Typical growing densities for suspension cell lines fall between 10^5 and 10^6 cells/ml, but some lines may be able to withstand higher dilutions or may reach higher densities. Subculture suspension lines as follows:

1. If a viable count is to be carried out, mix well without shaking too vigorously and sample for counting (cf. 3.2.3.3, and 2.1.1.1).
2. Decant cells into a centrifuge tube and spin for 5 min at 80–100 $\times$ g. Resuspend the cell pellet in freshly prepared flasks at 2–5 $\times$ 10^5 cells/ml, gas with 5% CO_2/95% air mixture and incubate at 37°C.
3. It may not always be necessary to centrifuge the cells or replenish the whole medium. Stand the flasks upright for a few h at 37°C to allow the cells to settle, decant

medium, and resuspend cells in fresh pre-warmed medium to the required volume. This is often the method of choice for hybridomas and lymphoblastoid cell lines.

3.2.3.3   Cell Counting

It is important, both during subculture and cyropreservation procedure to know the percentage of viable cells in a cell culture. The simplest method for doing this uses a vital strain such as trypan blue, and a haemocytometer (improved *Neubauer* type), as described in 2.1.1. A normal healthy culture should be more than 90% viable. A viability less than this would indicate that either the cells are being exposed to sub-optimal growth conditions or that they have exhausted their nutrient supply.

3.2.4   Cryopreservation

The reason for preserving cell lines is to ensure adequate supplies for future use. Continual maintenance of cell cultures is not only impractical but may permit or induce genetic drift or deviation from the parent material.

The concept of preparing cell stocks can be best understood by outlining the principles of cell banking used in industry. The genealogy of a cell line is very important if it is to be used in a manufacturing process, as is its species and tissue of origin, age and exposure risk to contamination from other cell lines and extraneous agents. Hence cell banks are prepared as shown in Figure 1.

The age of a cell line is measured in population doublings, that is the number of times it has replicated in culture. As this can only be measured by taking regular cell counts, most laboratories only estimate a cell's age by the number of times it has been subcultured.

The approach illustrated to cell stock preparation ensures that supplies are checked for authenticity and contamination at each stage (cf. 3.2.5 and 3.2.6) and that reproducibility is ensured by returning to the Working Bank after a fixed number of population doublings subcultures. The token freeze is maintained as a back-up in the event of problems with the Master and Working Banks.

3.2.4.1   Equipment and Materials

The essential requirements for the cryopreservation of cells are as follows.

1. Sterile plastic ampoules of 1.2–1.8 ml capacity *(Nunc, Corning, Costar)*.
2. Ampoule racks *(Nunc)*.
3. Indelible marking pens suitable for low temperatures.
4. Sterile pipettes and centrifuge tubes.
5. Improved *Neubauer* haemocytomers.
6. 0.4% v/v Trypan Blue in PBS.

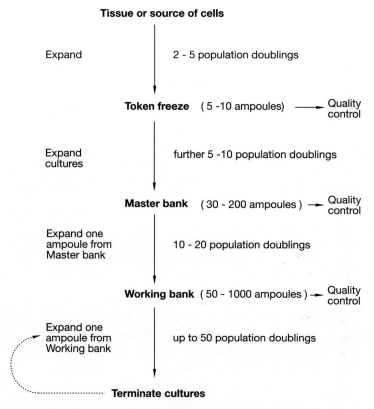

Fig. 1. Cell bank preparation. Generalised outline of a cell procedure for establishing master and working stocks. The basic principles involved are establishing cell banks with a lineage as close to the original source as possible, and generating working banks from a master bank ampoule, after quality control checks have been completed. Cultures derived from the working bank are terminated after a prescribed number of subcultures or population doublings and then restarted from a new working bank ampoule. This procedure ensures that a regular supply of reproducible cultures is maintained.

7. Freezing mixture, such as growth medium containing 25% serum or whole serum with sterile 7–10% (v/v) cryoprotectant. The cryoprotectant most widely used is dimethyl sulphoxide (DMSO). Alternatively glycerol can be used and may be preferable for some cell lines, e.g., mouse T-cells. DMSO should be of the highest grade and must be filtered, but only with filters specifically designed for this purpose, e.g., *Nalgene,* Cat. No. 01952020. Glycerol can be sterilized by autoclaving.

   A recommended freeze medium is whole serum, (e.g. fetal bovine) to which 7–10% v/v cryoprotectant is added. Alternatively the same percentage of cryoprotectant can be added to growth medium, in which the serum level has been raised to 25%. The freeze medium should always be freshly prepared because DMSO denatures serum and increases the pH of hydrogen carbonate-based medium.

8. A programmable freezer *(Planer)* or two-stage freezer.
9. Liquid nitrogen storage vessel *(Statebourne, MVE, Taylor-Wharton, l'Air Liquide).*
10. Protective face mask, gloves and apron for handling liquid nitrogen.
11. Inventory record plan of the cell storage system.
12. Record book for freeze runs, to record details of cell lines, quantity of cells frozen, numbers of ampoules and locations.

3.2.4.2   Method

This method is based on the use of plastic screw-top ampoules ("cryotubes") and either a programmable freezer or two-stage freezer.

1. Freeze only healthy cultures, i.e., those in log-phase growth.
2. Perform a viable cell count (cf. 3.2.3.3). The viability must be greater than 80%, and preferably 95–100%.
3. Prepare sufficient cells, by centrifugation, to fill ampoules with at least 4×10^6 cells each (maximum 1×10^7). If cells have been trypsinized to remove them from flasks, neutralise the trypsin by adding medium containing an equal volume of serum, before centrifugation.
4. Prepare sufficient freezing medium to fill ampoules with 1 ml each.
5. Resuspend the cells in the freezing medium and dispense in 1 ml aliquots into pre-marked ampoules. Each ampoule should be labelled with cell designation, passage number and date of freezing.
6. Freeze ampoules at a rate between -1 to $-5°C/min$ until at least $-60°C$. After this point the rate can be increased to $-10°C/min$. When using a programmable freezer, set the start temperature of the run at the same temperature as the ampoules. For ampoules prepared at ambient temperature, start at $+15°C$ to $+25°C$; for ampoules prepared in pre-cooled medium start at $+4°C$ to $+10°C$.

When first freezing a new cell line a rate of $-2°C/min$ is recommended until $-60°C$ is reached. If this is successful a faster rate, i.e. $-3°C/min$ can be tried.

The two stage freezer allows ampoules to be placed at a pre-determined depth in the gas-phase of a *Dewar* flask containing liquid nitrogen. After a period of 10–20 min, the ampoules are plunged into the nitrogen.

7. Immediately after freezing, transfer ampoules to a nitrogen storage vessel.

8. Test at least one ampoule from each cell type for viability and sterility. During all stages of handling ampoules that have been stored in nitrogen (gas or liquid), full face and hand protection must be worn.

   To avoid the explosion risk which is greatest during defrosting, unscrew the ampoule top about 1/4 turn, after removing from nitrogen storage, to release pressure. Leave at room temperature for 1–2 min and re-tighten the top.

   Rapidly thaw the ampoule(s) in a water bath at the cells' normal growing temperature, i.e. 25°C for amphibian, 37°C for mammalian cells. To ensure water does not enter the ampoules, float them in a piece of thin polystyrene or foam so that they are not submerged above the neck of the screw-top.

9. Wipe thawed ampoules with ethanol before opening. Transfer the contents either directly into prepared culture flasks or into a 15 ml centrifuge tube. Add 1 ml medium dropwise to the tube, followed by a faster addition of 8 ml medium. If a viable cell count is to be performed, remove 0.2–0.5 ml and centrifuge the remainder at low speed, i.e. $70–80 \times g$ for 3–5 min. Then inoculate the pellet into flasks. Centrifugation is normally only used if it is essential to remove the cryoprotectant.

10. Start new cultures at between 30%–50% of their final (maximum) cell density, to allow rapid conditioning of the medium. The cultures should be monitored for growth and sterility in the absence of all antibiotics.

Keep accurate records of all frozen banks to include their source of origin, freeze medium, date of freezing, quality control results and storage location. As well as written records, computer software for storage documentation is readily available (Cardbox Plus from *Business Simulations Ltd* or dBase 4 from *Ashton-Tate*). Further information on the cryopreservation of animal cells can be found in the article by *Doyle* et al. [2].

3.2.5   Microbiological Quality Control

Microbiological quality control is an essential part of routine cell culture: it should not be neglected. It is concerned with the testing of culture media and cell lines for a variety of microorganisms, including bacteria, fungi, yeasts and mycoplasma.

3.2.5.1   Testing for Bacteria and Fungi

If cell lines are cultured in antibiotic-free media, contamination by bacteria or fungi is easily observed by an increase in turbidity of the medium or a change in pH. A problem may arise with cell lines routinely cultured in antibiotic-containing media since the antibiotics may reduce the level of contamination present thereby making it more difficult to detect. Reagents added during the preparation of all culture media, e. g. fetal calf serum, contribute to the risk of contamination, therefore it is good practice to set up quality control checks on culture medium prior to its use. The two methods generally used for the detection of bacteria and fungi involve isolation or direct observation using *Gram's* stain.

Detection by isolation. Two types of isolation media should be used. Those suggested by the *U.S. Code of Federal Regulations* [3] and the *European Pharmacopoeia* [4] are (a) fluid thioglycollate medium for the detection of aerobic and anaerobic forms, and (b) soybean-casein digest (tryptone soya broth) for the detection of aerobes, facultative anaerobes and fungi.

Inoculate test material into each of two *Universal* containers (15 ml) of the above media. One broth of each pair is incubated at 35°C and the other at 25°C. If bacteria are present the broths usually become turbid very quickly, i. e. within 1–2 days, although incubation may require as long as two weeks. Positive controls should be used, e. g. *Bacillus subtilis* as the aerobe and *Clostridium sporogenes* as the anaerobe. Type strains are available from the *National Collection of Type Cultures* [5] and the *American Type Culture Collection* [6].

Detection by *Gram's* stain. Sediment the test material by centrifugation at a minimum of $1000 \times g$ for 15 min. Decant supernatant leaving as small a volume as possible to resuspend the pellet which may not be visible to the naked eye. Add the sample to a labelled slide using a sterile inoculating loop and allow to dry. Heat fix and stain using standard procedures [7]. This method has the advantages of speed and of detecting fastidious bacteria and fungi which may be difficult to culture [8].

3.2.5.2   Testing for Mycoplasma

Mycoplasma infection of cell cultures was first observed by *Robinson* et al. in 1956 [9] and the incidence since then of mycoplasma infected cell cultures has been found to vary from laboratory to laboratory. It is very important to use mycoplasma-free cell lines as they can: affect the growth rate of cells [10]; induce morphology changes [11]; cause chromosome aberrations [12]; influence amino acid and nucleic acid metabolism [13, 14] and induce cell transformation [15]. Of equal importance, Regulatory Bodies insist that cell cultures used for the production of reagents for diagnostic kits or therapeutic agents are free from mycoplasma infection [3, 4].

Various methods exist for the detection of mycoplasma [for reviews cf. 16, 17]. The two methods which are used routinely in the quality control laboratory at *ECACC* and are recommended by the FDA [18] are the *Hoechst* stain method and microbiological culture. Common to all detection methods is the requirement for cells to be grown in antibiotic-free and cryoprotectant-free media for a minimum of two passages so as to avoid the masking of infection. Also, with the exception of the *Hoechst* stain method, cultures should not receive a medium renewal within 3 days of testing.

Hoechst 33258 DNA stain method

The fluorochrome dye *Hoechst* 33258 binds specifically to DNA causing fluorescence when viewed under UV light. A fluorescence microscope equipped for epi-fluorescence with a 340–380 nm excitation filter and 430 nm emission filter is required. In view of fundamental requirement for mycoplasma-free cell lines in tissue culture a detailed outline of this technique is provided.

1. Harvest adherent cells by the usual subculture method and resuspend in the original culture medium at approximately 5×10^5 ml. Test suspension cells directly at a similar concentration. The number of cells used should be sufficient to produce a semi-confluent spread at the time of staining. Add approximately 2–3 ml of test cells to each of two 22 mm sterile coverslips in 35 mm diameter tissue culture dishes. Incubate overnight at 37°C in a humidified atmosphere of 5% CO_2 and 95% air. Test one sample at 24 h, and examine the other after 72 h.
2. Before fixing, examine the cells on an inverted microscope ($\times$ 10 objective) for evidence of microbial contamination.
3. Add 2 ml *Carnoy's* fixative (methanol:glacial acetic acid, 3:1 v/v) dropwise from the edge of the culture dish and leave for 3 min. Take care not to sweep unattached cells to one side of the dish. Pour the fixative into a waste bottle and immediately add another 2 ml of fixative. Leave for a further 3 min.
4. Dry the coverslip in air on the inverted tissue culture dish lid for 30 min. Wearing gloves, add 2 ml freshly prepared *Hoechst* 33258 stain (0.05 mg/l in distilled water) and leave for 5 min. Shield the coverslip from light at this point. Decant the stain to a waste bottle. Note that the stain is toxic and must be disposed of correctly.
5. Add one drop of mountant to a glass slide and mount the coverslip, cell side down.
6. Examine under ultraviolet fluorescence with a $\times$100 oil immersion objective.

Uncontaminated cells show only brightly fluorescing cell nuclei, whereas mycoplasma-infected cultures contain small cocci or filaments which may or may not cytadsorb to the cells (Fig. 2).

For reasons of standardization the assay may be performed using a monolayer culture as an indicator onto which is inoculated a test sample. This method also has the advantage of being able to screen serum, cell culture supernatants and other reagents

a)

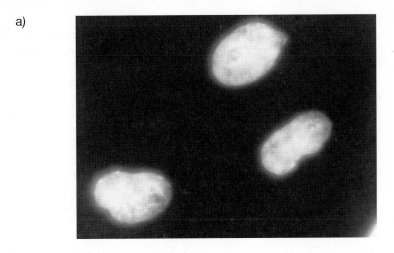

b)

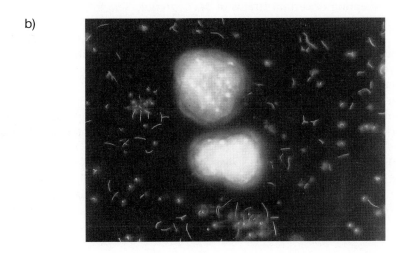

Fig. 2. Cell preparations stained with *Hoechst* 33258 DNA stain and viewed with a 100× oil immersion objective using a fluorescence microscope.
a) mycoplasma – negative cell line
b) mycoplasma – positive cell line

which do not contain cells. Inoculate indicator cells, which should have a high cytoplasm/nucleus ratio, e. g. Vero cells, to tissue culture dishes containing coverslips 12–24 h prior to inoculation of test sample. As with test cells, inoculate indicator cells at a concentration at which a semi-confluent monolayer is formed at the time of observation.

Some preparations may show extracellular fluorescence caused by disintegrating nuclei which are usually not of a uniform size and are too large to be mycoplasma. Contaminating bacteria or fungi will also stain if present, but will appear much larger and brighter than mycoplasma. Compare with positive and negative slides.

The main advantages of this method are the speed (less than 1 day) at which results are obtained, and that the non-cultivatable *M. hyorhinis* strains can be detected. However, the sensitivity of this method is not as good as the culture method (below). It is generally considered that *circa* 10^4 mycoplasmas are required to produce a clear positive result.

Microbiological culture

Most mycoplasma cell culture contaminants will grow on standardised agar and broth media with the exception of certain strains of *M. hyorhinis*. The following is a brief outline of the method given in more detail elsewhere [19].

1. Harvest adherent cells using a sterile swab, and resuspend in the culture medium in which they were growing to a concentration of approximately 5×10^5 cells/ml. Test suspension cells direct at the same concentration.
2. Inoculate an agar plate with 0.1 ml of the test sample.
3. Inoculate 2 ml broth with 0.2 ml of the test sample.
4. Incubate the test plate under anaerobic conditions *(Gaspak)* at 36°C for 21 days and the test broth aerobically at 36°C.
5. Subculture the test broth (0.1 ml) onto agar plates at approximately 7 and 14 days postinoculation and incubate anaerobically at 36°C.
6. Examine all agar plates after 7, 14, and 21 days incubation using an inverted microscope (×40 or ×100 objective) for detection of mycoplasma colonies (Figure 3).

Both agar and broth media should be checked prior to use for their ability to grow species of mycoplasma known to contaminate cell lines, e. g. *A. laidlawii, M. arginini, M. fermentans, M. hominis, M. hyorhinis,* and *M. orale.* Type strains are available from the National Collection of Type Cultures [5] or the American Type Culture Collection [6]. For further discussion on interpretation of results see [19].

Other methods of detection. Regulatory requirements may limit the methods of detection to those given above. However, for those laboratories which have no necessity to follow these, other methods of detection, available in kits, may prove useful.

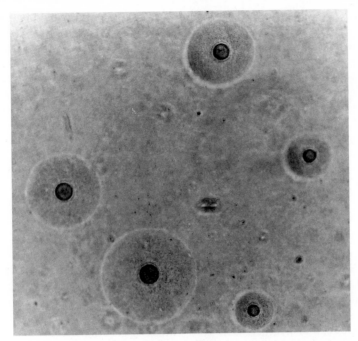

Fig. 3. Mycoplasma colonies on agar viewed with an inverted microscope (×40 objective).

One such method is Gen-Probe [20] which requires no cultural procedure and gives same-day results. The protocol requires incubation of a ^{3}H-labelled DNA probe with either cell culture supernatant or the cells themselves. Hydroxyapatite is utilized to separate bound from unbound probe prior to scintillation counting. The DNA probe used is homologous to mycoplasma rRNA, which hybridizes with different species of mycoplasma, but not with mammalian cellular or mitochondrial r-RNAs. The disadvantage of this method is that it is expensive.

Another commercially available indirect method is the Myco-Tect [21] system which requires co-cultivation of cells to be tested with 6-methylpurine deoxyriboside. For a comparison of this method with others see [17].

Finally, a mycoplasma detection kit is available from *Boehringer Mannheim* [22] which involves an enzyme-immunoassay. This kit is currently being evaluated in the *ECACC* quality control laboratory but has disadvantages in terms of sensitivity and specificity (only four species being detectable).

3.2.5.3   Elimination of Mycoplasma

Cell cultures contaminated with mycoplasmas should ideally be discarded. There are, however, occasions when this is not possible due to the non-availability of mycoplasma-free cell stocks. Although no one method of mycoplasma elimination is universally successful, the most efficient and easy to use is the addition of antibiotics to cell culture media. The most effective antibiotics to date are ciprofloxacin (Cyproxin – *Bayer, Sigma*) [23] and Mycoplasma Removal Agent (*ICN-Flow*). As with all antibiotics, anti-mycoplasma agents should not be persistently added to cell cultures because of the risk of inducing resistance.

3.2.6   Authenticity of Cell Lines

Cell line authentication is an essential requirement in good cell culture technique. It is important that authentication is undertaken to show culture purity from the point of view of cell species verification as well as of microbial contamination [24].

The occurence of cross-contamination within cell cultures is often underestimated and is illustrated by the presence of *HeLa* markers in many cell lines [25, 26]. There are many ways this can be avoided such as by obtaining certified cell lines from *bona fide* culture collections such as the *ECACC* [27] or *ATCC* [6] and by good laboratory practices (Section 3.1.3). At *ECACC*, species verification is performed by isoenzyme analysis on master cell stocks and DNA fingerprinting for individual identification. Cytogenetic analysis is not performed on a routine basis, but is used to fulfil regulatory requirements when necessary. The following outlines the general principles involved.

3.2.6.1   Isoenzyme Analysis

This is a quick and simple method for determining the species of a cell line. Isoenzymes are polymorphic variants which have different electrophoretic mobility [28]. A simplified method, The Authentikit System [29] *(Innovative Chemistry Inc.)* is available. The basic kit offers seven different enzymes and the choice reflects the need to identify the supposed species against known species. In most cases a good initial test enzyme is lactate dehydrogenase, as it can give up to five distinct bands which in themselves may provide sufficient information to distinguish certain species. By using several enzymes, a composite picture analogous to fingerprinting is built up of the species of origin. Isoenzyme analysis can detect mixtures from two species provided the level of the contaminant cell line is at least 20%.

Although karyotyping (see below) can be used for species verification, isoenzyme analysis is the method of choice because of its speed and simplicity of interpretation.

3.2.6.2   Cytogenetic Analysis

Cytogenetic analysis is used to establish the normal karyology of species and cell lines, and for identifying changes in them, e. g. verification of cross-contamination of cell lines, quality control of cell lines used to produce biologicals and changes associated with transformation or long-term culture. In comparison to isoenzyme analysis it is a more complicated technique and requires the operator to have more training and experience.

There are many different techniques described for staining and banding chromosomes; these include *Giemsa* (G) banding, Quinacrine (Q) banding and G-11 banding. The most common and useful type of banding used is G-banding.

With trypsin and *Giemsa* stain, banding patterns (G-bands) are obtained on the chromosomes which are characteristic of each chromosome pair [30].

Quinacrine banding (Q-banding) uses quinacrine to produce fluorescent bands within chromosomes which mostly correspond to G-bands. The technique is particularly useful for looking at the Y chromosome in man which is more distinctive when this method is used.

G-1 banding may be used when examining human/rodent hybrids. By using *Giemsa* stain at pH 11 instead of the usual pH 6.8 differential staining of species occurs.

Detailed protocols and discussion of these techniques are available [31, 32].

3.2.6.3   DNA Fingerprinting

The discovery of variable regions within genes and the resulting development of DNA fingerprinting by *Jeffreys* in 1985 enabled the specific identification of human individuals [33]. It was soon realised that this technique could be applied to the analysis of a wide range of species, and it is now widely used in animal cell technology. By use of the multi-locus probes 33.6 and 33.15, a specific fingerprint of a cell line can be generated based on the visualization of repetitive DNA sequences.

The method can be used for the quality control of cell banks, e. g. to demonstrate genetic stability between master and working cell banks (Figures 1, 4) [34]. It is also possible to detect cross-contamination with other cell lines of the same or different species down to approximately 5% contamination compared with 20% with isoenzyme analysis.

The procedures involve complete digestion of extracted cell line genomic DNA with the restriction enzyme HinfI followed by separation using agarose gel electrophoresis. After depurination, the DNA is blotted onto a nylon membrane and hybridized with *Jeffreys'* probes 33.6 or 33.15. The membranes are then exposed to X-ray film producing the characteristic fingerprint shown in Figure 4. The probe 33.15 is the more informative of the two probes in most cases. Both probes are available commercially from *Cambridge Research Biochemicals* [35]. Exact conditions for use of the probes are provided by the manufacturers and other protocol details are published [36, 37].

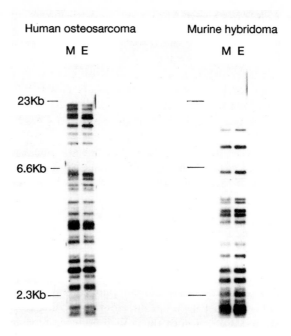

Fig. 4. DNA Fingerprints of two cell lines of master (M) and extended (E) cell banks. The illustrated fingerprints show Southern blots of cell line DNA digested with the Hinf I restriction enzyme and probed with ^{32}P labelled multilocus probe 33.6 [33] (photograph courtesy of G. Stacey, ECACC)

References

[1] R. I. Freshney, Culture of Animal Cells – A Manual of Basic Technique, Alan R. Liss, New York 1987, pp. 99–128.
[2] A. Doyle, C. B. Morris, W. J. Armitage, Cryopreservation of Animal Cells, in: A. Mizrahi (ed.), Advances in Biotechnological Processes, Vol. 7. A. R. Liss, New York 1988, pp. 1–17.
[3] Detection of Mycoplasma Contamination. Office of the Federal Register National Archives and Records Administration, Washington, 113–128, 379.
[4] European Pharmacopoeia, Biological Tests, 2nd Ed., Part 1, Mycoplasmas, Maisonneuve, Sainte-Ruffine 1980, pp. V.2.1.3.
[5] National Collection of Type Cultures, Central Public Health Laboratory, 61 Colindale Avenue, Colindale, London NW9 5HT.
[6] American Type Culture Collection, 12301 Parklawn Drive, Rockville, Maryland 20852, USA.
[7] Cowan and Steel's Manual for Identification of Medical Bacteria, Cambridge University Press, Cambridge 1979, pp. 163.
[8] J. M. Mowles, A. Doyle, M. J. Kearns, Y. Cerisier, Isolation of an Unusual Fastidious Contaminant Bacterium from an Adherent Cell Line Using a Novel Technique, in: R. E. Spier, J. B. Griffiths, J. Stephenson, P. J. Crooy, (eds.), Advances in Animal Cell Biology and Technology for Bioprocesses, Butterworths, Sevenoaks 1988, Section 3: pp. 111–113.

[9] *L. B. Robinson, R. B. Wichelhausen, B. Roizman*, Contamination of Human Cell Cultures by Pleuropneumenia-like Organisms, Science *124*, 1147–1148 (1956).

[10] *G. J. McGarrity, D. Phillips, A. Vaidya*, Mycoplasmal Infection of Lymphocyte Cultures: Infection with *M. salivarium*, In Vitro *16*, 346–356 (1980).

[11] *M. Butler, R. H. Leach*, A Mycoplasma that Reduces Acidity and Cytopathic Effect in Tissue Culture, J. Gen. Microbiol. *34*, 285–294 (1964).

[12] *P. Aula, W. W. Nichols*, The Cytogenetic Effects of Mycoplasma in Human Leucocyte Cultures, J. Cell. Physiol. *70*, 281–290 (1967).

[13] *E. J. Stanbridge, L. Hayflick, F. T. Perkins*, Modification of Amino Acid Concentrations Induced by Mycoplasmas in Cell Culture Medium, Nature *232*, 242–244 (1971).

[14] *E. M. Levine, L. Thomas, D. McGregor, L. V. Hayflick, H. Eagle*, Altered Nucleic Acid Metabolism in Human Cell Cultures Infected with Mycoplasma, Proc. Natl. Acad. Sci. U.S.A. *60*, 583–589 (1968).

[15] *I. MacPherson, W. Russel*, Transformations in Hamster Cells Mediated by Mycoplasmas, Nature *210*, 1343–1345 (1966).

[16] *J. J. Hessling, S. E. Miller, N. L. Levy*, A Direct Comparison of Procedures for the Detection of Mycoplasma in Tissue Culture, J. Immunol. Methods *38*, 3151–3324 (1980).

[17] *J. McGarrity, H. Kotani, D. Carson*, Comparative Studies to Determine the Efficiency of 6-methylpurine Deoxyribose to Detect Cell Culture Mycoplasmas, In Vitro Cell. Dev. Biol. *22*, 310–304 (1986).

[18] Points to Consider in the Characterisation of Cell Lines used to Produce Biologicals, November 18th, 1987. Issued by Director, Office of Biologicals Research and Review, Department of Health and Human Sciences, Food and Drug Administration, Bethesda MD 20205, U.S.A.

[19] *J. M. Mowles*, Mycoplasma Detection, in: *J. W. Pollard, J. M. Walker* (eds.), Methods in Molecular Biology, Vol. 5, Animal Cell Culture, The Humana Press, Clifton 1990, pp. 65–74.

[20] Gen-Probe Inc. 9620 Chesapeake Drive, San Diego, California 92123, U.S.A.

[21] Myco-Tect, Bethesda Research Laboratories Inc., Gaithersburg, Maryland 20877, U.S.A.

[22] Boehringer-Mannheim Biochemica, Mycoplasma Detection Kit, Bell Lane, Lewes, East Sussex, BN7 1LG.

[23] *J. M. Mowles*, The Use of Ciprofloxacin for the Elimination of Mycoplasma from Naturally Infected Cell Lines, Cytotechnology *1*, 355–358 (1988).

[24] *J. M. Mowles, A. Doyle*, Cell Culture Standards – Time for a Rethink?, Cytotechnology *3*, 107–108 (1990).

[25] *W. A. Nelson-Rees, D. W. Daniels, R. R. Flandermeyer*, Cross Contamination of Cells in Culture, Science *212*, 446–452 (1981).

[26] *B. Hukku*, Cell Culture Quality Control by Rapid Isoenzymatic Characterisation, In Vitro *19*, 16–24 (1983).

[27] European Collection of Animal Cell Cultures, PHLS Centre for Applied Microbiology & Research, Porton Down, Salibury, SP4 OJG.

[28] *S. J. O'Brien, J. E. Shannon, M. H. Gail*, A Molecular Approach to the Identification and Individualisation of Human and Animal Cells in Culture: Isozyme and Allozyme Genetic Signatures, In Vitro *16*, 119–135 (1981).

[29] Authentikit Innovative Chemistry Inc., PO Box 90, Marshfield, MA 02050, U.S.A.

[30] *M. Seabright*, A Rapid Banding Technique for Human Chromosomes, Lancet *2*, 971–972 (1971).

[31] *D. E. Rooney, B. H. Czepulkowski*, Human Cytogenetics, IRL Press, Oxford 1986.

[32] *H. Macgregor, J. Varley*, Working with Animal Chromosomes, 2nd Edition, Wiley, Chichester 1988.

[33] *A. J. Jeffreys, V. Wilson, S. L. Thein*, Individual Specific Fingerprints of Human DNA, Nature *316*, 76–79 (1985).

[34] *T. Burke, G. Dold, A. J. Jeffreys, R. Wolff* (eds.), in: DNA Fingerprinting Approaches and Applications, Birkhäuser Verlag, Basel 1991, pp. 361–370.

[35] Cambridge Research Biochemicals Ltd., Gadbrook Park, Northwich, Cheshire CW9 7RA.

[36] *L. J. Kirby*, DNA Fingerprinting, Macmillan Publishers, Basingstoke 1990.

[37] *G. N. Stacey, B. J. Bolton, A. Doyle*, The Quality Control of Cell Banks Using DNA Fingerprinting, in: *T. Burke, G. Dolt, A. J. Jeffreys, R. Wolff* (eds.), DNA Fingerprinting: Approaches and Applications, Birkhäuser Verlag, Basel 1991, pp. 361–370.

3.3   Lymphocyte Clones

Robyn E. O'Hehir, Brigitte A. Askonas and Jonathan R. Lamb

The extensive heterogeneity of specificity and function inherent in the T-lymphocyte pool has long been appreciated and has provided the scientific rationale for the isolation of single populations of immunocompetent cells. However, the technical advances needed to produce clones of T-cells were hampered by an incomplete knowledge of the physiology of T-cells. It had been assumed that T-cell antigen receptors would have identical functional and structural characteristics to those of B cells, in that they would display the property of binding directly to native antigen in free form, and would be secreted into the supernatants of cultured cells. It is now well-recognized that the activation of both CD4+ and CD8+ T-lymphocytes and the subsequent induction of an immune response is dependent on the formation of molecular interactions between the T-cell antigen receptor and peptide fragments of antigen in association with gene products of the major histocompatibility complex (MHC) [reviewed in 1–5]. This characteristic of T-cell antigen recognition provided a molecular explanation for the failure to isolate T-cells using free native soluble antigen.

As the different biological signals and receptors required for T-cell activation and proliferation began to be identified as antigen non-specific lymphokines, the technical constraints on the expansion of monoclonal populations of T-cells were eased. Two major sets of experimental results eventually facilitated the cloning of T-cells. From the demonstration that the interaction between T-cells and antigen is MHC-dependent, it became apparent that for T-cell activation, proliferation and target cell recognition, a source of histocompatible antigen presenting cells would be necessary. Secondly, *Morgan, Ruscetti & Gallo* [6] reported in 1976 that the addition of tissue culture medium conditioned with mitogen-stimulated human peripheral blood lymphocytes resulted in the *in vitro* proliferation of lymphoblasts that were of T-cell origin. The antigen-nonspecific growth factor in the conditioned medium was identified as IL-2 [7] and allowed the expansion of antigen-specific murine and human cytotoxic [8, 9] and helper [10–16] T-cells subsequently.

The manipulation of the IL-2-dependence of activated T-cells is, however, not the only method for the generation of T-cell clones and the alternative techniques that include hybridization [e.g. 17] and viral transformation [18, 19] are mentioned.

This chapter describes methods for the selection and maintenance of human CD4+ and CD8+ antigen-specific T-cell lines and clones as well as the important functional assays that are required. Obviously, the basic methods vary with different antigen systems and individual laboratories use their own modifications. Therefore, the representative recipes can be developed to suit specific requirements.

3.3.1   Lymphocyte Cultures

Incubate cultures under maximal humidification, with an atmosphere of 5–6 % CO_2 in air at 37 °C. For non-copper-lined incubators, add copper sulphate to the water trays to minimize fungal contamination.

3.3.1.1   Media

Commonly used tissue culture media include RPMI-1640, *Dulbecco's* modified *Eagle's* medium (DMEM) and *Iscove's* modified *Dulbecco's* medium (IMDM). Powdered preparations or liquid media are obtainable. With powdered media, use only high quality, endotoxin-free distilled water. Buffering, such as with sodium hydrogen carbonate and/or HEPES, facilitates equilibration to pH 7.4 at 5 % CO_2. Antibiotic supplementation (penicillin, 10^5 I.U./l, and streptomycin, 100 mg/l, or gentamicin, 50 mg/l) is usual. Routine use of antimycoplasma agents is not recommended but Antimycoplasma Removal Agent (*Flow*) or Ciproflaxacin (*Bayer*) are useful if mild contamination is identified. Routinely, commercially prepared RPMI-1640 with sodium bicarbonate, 2 g/l, supplemented with L-glutamine 2 mM/l, penicillin, and streptomycin (as above) are used for all lymphocyte cultures.

Serum supplementation is needed: fetal calf serum or normal human serum (preferably AB) are suitable. The more readily available A+ serum is also suitable. Batch screening is mandatory. Standard proliferation assays should be performed against a common recall antigen, such as BCG or tetanus, in medium containing serum at 5, 10, or 20 % with a requirement for good positive responses and low background proliferation. Sera should be heat inactivated at 56 °C for 30 min and then may be stored at −70 °C for extended periods. Optimal concentration for cultures should be determined for each batch but is usually 5–10 %. A variety of commercial serum replacements are now available and may be useful for some cultures.

Short term tissue culture in IMDM or *Yssel's* medium allows replacement of serum by soybean lipids (20 mg/l), bovine serum albumin (500 mg/l) and iron-saturated transferrin (5 mg/l) [20] (all obtainable from *Boehringer Mannheim GmbH, Mannheim*). Serum-free preparations prove less reliable for long-term cultures.

Routinely, media for human T cell culture are supplemented with human AB or A serum, for EBV-transformed B cell lines and murine L cell cultures with FCS.

3.3.1.2   Lymphocyte Preparation

Density centrifugation

Isolate peripheral blood mononuclear cells (PBMC) from heparinized (preservative-free, 5 U/ml; *Paines and Byrne Ltd., Greenford, U.K.*) peripheral venous blood. Mix one volume of whole blood with an equal volume of medium and layer over 1 volume Ficoll Hypaque (density 1.077) or equivalent lymphocyte separation medium. Harvest mononuclear cells from the plasma density gradient interface by centrifugation at 1200 $\times$ g for 20 min at room temperature, and wash twice (800 $\times$ g for 15 min then 400 $\times$ g for 10 min). If large numbers of PBMC are present, add 1 % additive-free heparin to the first wash. As T-cells represent 75 % of PBMC, further purification is usually not required prior to culture.

Cryopreservation and thawing

For storage, resuspend cells at the required concentration in complete medium. Add chilled 15 % solution of DMSO in FCS dropwise to an equal volume of cell suspension, mixing throughout, at 4 °C. Add 1 ml aliquots of the final cell suspension to sterile cryovials and freeze slowly in a rate-controlled freezer or a polystyrene box which is sealed and placed at −70 °C overnight. Vials may then be transferred to liquid nitrogen storage (−180 °C); cf. 3.2.4 for full details.

Remove frozen vials of cells from −180 °C storage and rapidly thaw over 1–2 min in a 37 °C water-bath. Add the cell suspension to a Universal bottle and add dropwise 1 ml of complete medium with continuous mixing. Add a further 20 ml of medium to dilute the DMSO. Recover the cells by centrifugation at 300 $\times$ g for 10 min. Resuspend the pellet to the required concentration in complete medium for culture.

3.3.2   CD4+ T-Cell Growth *in vitro*

CD4+ T-cells produce a large number of lymphokines after stimulation with antigen in association with MHC class II molecules. While the regulation of their secretion is not yet fully understood, it has been observed that in the mouse there are definite subsets of CD4+ T-cells (TH1 and TH2) which vary in the secretion of several of the lymphokines [21]. In the human, such subsets are not so clearly defined but differential lymphokine secretion has been observed [22]. Different experimental approaches have resulted in inconsistent results with human CD4+ T-cells. A lack of kinetic studies and the failure to correlate mRNA levels with their soluble products has been misleading.

In general, CD4+ T-cells proliferate on antigenic stimulation and provide a helper/inducer function for B-cells and in the amplification of CD8+ T-cells. With long-term culture, however, not all CD4+ T-cell clones maintain their stable expression of lymphokines [23] as growth in IL-2 may inhibit IL-2 production by the clones. In addition, most CD4+ T-cell clones acquire cytolytic capacity [24]; particularly in the presence of adjuvant, CD4+ T-cells may become lytic *in vivo* [25]. Culture and characterization of CD4+ T-cells must therefore be done with consideration of their various properties.

3.3.2.1 T-Cell Proliferative Assays

Polyclonal responses

Culture PBMC (5×10^4/well) with antigen over a dose range in 96-well round bottom microtitre plates. Determine optimal conditions for culture by incubating over a concentration range for various periods of time. Pulse cultures with $0.5–1 \mu Ci$ tritiated methyl thymidine ([^{3}H]-TdR, 28 Ci/mmol specific activity; *Amersham*) for 6–16 h before harvesting on to glass-fibre filters. Proliferation is measured by liquid scintillation spectroscopy using a β counter. Express results as the mean counts per minute (cpm) of (3–6) replicate cultures.

T-cell lines and clones

Culture T cells from oligoclonal and monoclonal T-cell populations (10^4/well) with antigen in 96-well round bottom microtitre plates in the presence of accessory (antigen presenting) cells (2.5×10^4 irradiated PBMC/well or 1×10^4 irradiated EBV-transformed B-cells/well). After incubation for 48 h (soluble antigen) or 72 h (particulate antigen), pulse and harvest cultures as above. If mitomycin-C treated murine L cells are used as accessory cells (2×10^4/well), use 96-well flat bottom microtitre plates with increased T-cell numbers (2×10^4/well). Background counts may be minimized by pulsing the accessory cells overnight with antigen prior to the addition of T-cells.

Accessory cells for antigen presentation

T-cell activation and the subsequent induction of an immune response is dependent on molecular interactions between the specific T-cell antigen receptor, MHC molecules on the surface of the accessory cell and peptidic fragments of foreign antigen. Therefore, for the establishment and maintenance of long term T-cell cultures, a source of antigen and histocompatible antigen presenting cells or feeders is necessary.

Cell division is not required for functional accessory activity and should be prevented to avoid contamination of T-cell populations. Treat cells by either irradiation (a γ-emitting source such as ^{60}Co or ^{137}Cs or any X-ray source), or mitomycin-C treatment.

PBMC

Optimal antigen presentation is provided by fresh or cryopreserved histocompatible PBMC (autologous or allogeneic; 0.5–1.0 × 10^6/ml). T-cell depletion of PBMC is not necessary. Ideally, fresh autologous irradiated PBMC (2500–3000 rad) should be used, but buffy coats provide a good PBMC supply for cryopreservation.

Epstein-Barr virus (EBV)-transformed B-cells

Transformed B-cell lines are useful feeders in short term assays [26, 27], but long term cultures are poorly supported when transformed cells are the sole accessory cells. Relative radioresistance of transformed B-cells necessitates radiation doses of 5–6000 rad.

Human B-cells may be transformed using EBV obtained from the cell line B95.8 which is derived from cotton-topped marmoset PBMC infected with EBV obtained from a cell line derived from a patient with infectious mononucleosis [28]. Grow the cells to confluence, harvest the culture supernatant and pass through a 0.45 μ filter. Infect B-cells by resuspending up to 10^7 PBMC, washed in serum-free complete medium, in 1 ml B95.8 culture supernatant for 1 h at 37 °C with gentle agitation. Pellet the cells, remove the supernatant and culture the cells. Obtain immortalized EBV-infected B-cell lines from infected cells seeded at 5 × 10^5 cells/ml, in complete medium containing 10 % FCS, in 24-well plates. T-cell lysis is promoted by the addition of Cyclosporin A (Sandoz; 10 mg/l) for the first 2–3 weeks of culture. Alternatively, PHA may be used to remove T-cell populations. Feed cultures bi-weekly and replace half the medium without disturbing the cell layer. By use of an inverted microscope, foci of proliferating transformed B cells are usually identifiable after 1–2 weeks although many lines may take as long as 6 weeks. As the transformed cells approach confluence (10^6 cells/ml) dilute them to 10^5 cells/ml.

Transfected murine fibroblasts (L-cells)

Murine fibroblasts have no endogenous MHC class II molecules and, therefore, the use of L-cells expressing the products of transfected human MHC class II genes as accessory cells allows the MHC class II products to be studied in isolation. Prepare L-cells in serum-free complete medium by treatment with mitomycin-C (50 mg/l for 45 min at 37 °C), wash four times in complete medium plus serum, and then use in assays [29] Wash thoroughly to avoid contamination of T-cell cultures.

3.3.2.2   T-Cell Hybridization

Adaptations of technology designed originally for the propagation of B-cell hybridomas have fused normal T-cells and AKR thymoma BW 5147 [e.g. 17, 30] to establish monoclonal T-cells. Although effective for the generation of murine CD4$^+$ T-cell hybridomas, results with human T-cell populations have been disappointing. Normal PBMC activated *in vitro* with antigen or mitogen have been fused to human T lymphoblastoid cells by means of polyethylene glycol and stable lines cloned by limiting dilution [31, 32]. The T-cell lymphoma *Jurkat* line has been fused to antigen specific IL-2-dependent T-cell lines to obtain functional antigen specific human T-cell hybrids [33]. However, attempts to develop IL-2-dependent antigen-specific cytotoxic T-cell hybridomas have been less successful. Complications associated with human hybridoma technology are chromosomal loss with phenotypic and functional changes.

3.3.2.3   Viral Transformation

Human T-lymphocytes have been successfully transformed by co-cultivation with neoplastic T-cell lines secreting the RNA retrovirus, human T-cell leukaemia/lymphoma virus (HTLV-I), that is tropic for CD4 T cells [19, 34]. Problems with dysregulation, however, have induced changes in activation requirements, B-cell help and lymphokine production [35], thus minimizing the usefulness of this approach also for the study of normal T-cell physiology.

3.3.2.4   Sources of IL-2

T-cell growth factor or interleukin 2 is required to maintain T-cells in long-term culture [6, 7]. Human and gibbon IL-2 are able to support human T-cells.

MLA-144

This gibbon cell line constitutively secretes IL-2 which may be recovered from cell culture ($1–2 \times 10^6$/ml) supernatants. Mycoplasma contamination of the cell line, however, is frequent and should be vigilantly avoided.

Lectin-stimulated human T-cells

Culture PBMC at 10^6/ml in complete medium with normal human serum and PHA 0.1 mg/l (or Con A 5 mg/l) for 48 h. Harvest the IL-2-containing supernatant and store at

−20 °C. Commercial preparations, such as Lymphocult-T Lectin Free (*Biotest Folex*, FRG) are highly effective. Optimal concentration for supplementation should be determined but is usually 5–20 %.

Recombinant IL-2

Gene cloning in bacteria [36] has allowed the production of recombinant human IL-2, which is now commercially available from several sources. Problems of lectin and mycoplasma contamination are avoided but lack of glycosylation may decrease stability and low levels of bacterial products may be present. Concentrations of approximately 5 µg/l are usually optimal.

Assay for IL-2

IL-2-dependent cell lines such as HT2 [37] or CTLl [7] may be used in a bioassay for IL-2 production. Serially dilute test supernatants and culture with cells (5×10^3/well) in 96-well round bottom microtitre plates at a volume of 200 µl/well. Pulse plates with [3H]-TdR after 24 h and harvest 6 h later. Read IL-2 concentrations off a standard curve generated by using recombinant IL-2 of known concentration.

In addition to this functional assay, immunoassays of lymphokines other than IL-2 have been introduced recently (e.g. γ-interferon, IL-4, IL-5) and more specific tests are currently under development. This has been discussed by *deVries* et al. [22, 38], which interested investigators should consult.

3.3.3   Cloning Techniques for Human CD4+ T-Cells

3.3.3.1   Primary Cultures

Peripheral blood mononuclear cells (PBMC)

Prepare PBMC at 2.5×10^5 cells/ml in complete medium +5 % A+ serum, and stimulate with antigen extract. The concentration of antigen required to produce optimal stimulation, assayed by the incorporation of [^{3}H]TdR should be determined beforehand using standard proliferation assay kinetic studies. After mixing, plate 200 µl aliquots of the cell suspensions into 96-well round bottom tissue culture plates and incubate for 6–8 days (as selected from proliferative assay kinetic studies). Alternatively, prepare a bulk culture by incubating $1–1.5 \times 10^6$ PBMC in complete medium +5% A+ serum with optimal antigen concentration in volumes of 2 ml in a 24-well tissue culture plate.

Tissue sites (antigen unknown)

Skin punch biopsy. Culture tissue fragments for 10–14 days in 2 ml complete medium +5% A+ serum in a 24-well plate in the presence of 10% IL-2 to expand *in vivo* activated T-cells. Release of T-cells is facilitated by teasing with sterile needles. After 4 days, if T-cell expansion is slow, activate cells with insolubilized anti-CD3 antibody (OKT3; 12 mg/l) and 10% IL-2 which stimulates through the TCR. Expansion with IL-2 may then be continued.

Synovial fluid. Isolate mononuclear cells from heparinized aspirated synovial fluid using the same method as for the preparation of PBMC. Expand the *in vivo* activated T cells in 2 ml complete medium +5% A+ serum in 24-well megatitre plate in the presence of 10% IL-2 for 10–14 days. Anti-CD3 activation may also be used, if necessary.

3.3.3.2   Established T-Cell Lines

After primary culture under the optimal conditions, antigen concentration and duration of culture, recover the T blast cells by density centrifugation over Ficoll-Paque for 20 min at $1200 \times g$. Dilute blast-enriched cell suspensions at the interface to 1×10^5/ml of complete medium +5% A+ serum supplemented with autologous PBMC X-irradiated (2500 rad) 5×10^5/ml as antigen presenting cells, optimal concentration of antigen and 10% IL-2. Aliquot cultures in 10 ml volumes in 25 ml tissue culture flasks or 2 ml volumes in 24-well plates and incubate in humidified chambers at 37 °C in 5% CO_2 in air.

If limited autologous or allogeneic PBMC are available for use as accessory cells, a combination of pooled, irradiated, allogeneic PBMC (10^6/ml; 2500–3000 rad), autologous or histocompatible, irradiated, EBV-transformed B-cell line cells (10^5/ml; 6000 rad) and PHA-P (0.5 mg/l) may be used. If the antigen is known, an optimal concentration of antigen should also be added. Supplementary IL-2 (10% Lymphocult-T) should be added after 4 days with further splitting as required. Freeze seed vials when T-cells are resting, at least 10–14 days after the last addition of PHA.

3.3.3.3   Limiting Dilution Isolation of T-Cell Clones

Autologous or allogeneic accessory cells

Cloning from a long term T-cell line

The antigen-specific T-cell lines may be used to isolate antigen-specific T-cell clones. Recover T blasts by density centrifugation, wash and then resuspend in complete medium +5% A+ serum. Plate by limiting dilution in microtest-II trays with 0.3 blasts/well, 10^4 accessory cells and optimal antigen concentration in the presence of IL-2 10% v/v with a total volume of 20 µl/well. Incubate cultures for 6 days after which the growing clones can be identified using an inverted microscope: transfer them to fresh medium (200 µl) containing 10% IL-2, accessory cells (10^5/well) and antigen in 96-well flat bottom plates. After 7 additional days of culture, transfer the clones to 24-well plates containing the same concentration of IL-2, accessory cells and antigen each in a total volume of 2 ml.

Cloning from a Primary Culture

After 7 days primary culture, harvest cells by density centrifugation. Dilute blast-enriched suspensions to 15 blasts/ml of complete medium +5% A+ serum containing 10% IL-2, 5×10^5 accessory cells/ml and antigen, and add to microtest-II trays in 20 µl aliquots as detailed above.

Autologous or histocompatible allogeneic EBV-transformed B-cells combined with non-histocompatible allogeneic PBMC

If insufficient autologous or histocompatible accessory cells are available an alternative feeding suspension may be used. This should contain autologous or histocompatible EBV transformed B cells (6000 rad; 10^5/ml), a pool of 2 or more non-histocompatible, allogeneic PBMC (2500 rad; 10^6/ml), optimal antigen concentration and 0.5 µg/ml PHA. The feeding mixture of non-histocompatible cells in the presence of PHA induces a vigorous mixed lymphocyte reaction with release of a cocktail of cytokines to drive T-cell growth [*H. Spits*, personal communication, 39]. Supplement with fresh medium and 10% IL-2 after 4–5 days. This method is also suitable for cloning from tissue sites where the antigen is unknown; for example, synovial compartment T-cells. Clone, using this accessory cell mixture, in microtest-II trays (20 µl/well) or 96-well round or flat bottom plates (200 µl/well). Clones generated in this way should not be used for assays until at least 10–14 days after the last stimulation with PHA, by which time cells should be in resting phase. Background proliferation counts should be less than 1000 cpm at this stage.

Semi-solid agar

After 7 days primary culture, suspend T-cell blasts with accessory cells (10^5–10^6/ml) and antigen in soft agar (0.2–0.5 % in culture medium at 45 °C) and plate onto a pre-formed feeder layer of 0.5 % agar in tissue culture medium. IL-2 is added at this stage in some protocols. Colonies of cell growth appear near the surface of the agar after an interval of 4–7 days [10]. With a fine glass capillary tube, transfer growing colonies to liquid culture in 200 µl of feeding suspension containing antigen, accessory cells and IL-2 for expansion. The probability of clonality using this method is decreased and once colonies of potential interest have been established, multiple recloning at high plating efficiency is essential to secure clonality. This method has been successfully used by a few groups [10, 14].

3.3.4   CD8+ Cytotoxic T-Cell Growth *in vitro*

3.3.4.1   Background

CD8+ and class I MHC-restricted T-cells differ in their induction requirements when compared to CD4+ T-cells [40]. The latter are able to respond to infectious agents, most purified proteins or appropriate peptide epitopes. CD8+ T-cells on the other hand are best primed by infection of the cell donor, rather than by purified proteins. In a secondary response, CTL can be stimulated by infected APC, or specific peptides and only rarely by soluble proteins. Low primary anti-viral CTL responses have been induced *in vivo* by presentation with peptide-pulsed dendritic cells *in vitro* [41] or with adjuvant [e.g. 42] or peptides with fatty acid tails [43]. In exceptional cases purified proteins (e.g. influenza nucleoprotein [44], or APC loaded with high concentrations of foreign protein by osmotic shock [45], have been shown to prime low levels of CTL *in vivo* or to stimulate secondary responses *in vitro*. Alloreactive CTL are selected by allogeneic cells but not by purified alloantigens.

In recent years *Townsend* et al [46] demonstrated that recognition by class I restricted CTL of virus infected cells can be defined by protein fragments, i.e. short peptides derived from the viral components, and these vary with different MHC restriction molecules [reviewed in 5]. If the peptide epitope for a given virus-specific CTL response has been defined, it is possible to stimulate CTL with that particular peptide. In general, infection of a donor generates circulating memory CTL that are not cytotoxic *per se;* these need to be restimulated with antigen *in vitro* to generate cytotoxic activity. However, in certain acute infections, particularly in AIDS, fresh PBL do show strong virus-specific and class I MHC-restricted cytolytic activity [e.g. 47]. Presumably this can be attributed to continuous antigenic stimulation by infected circulating monocytes and dendritic cells. The first virus-specific and class I MHC-restricted human CTL were reported by *McMichael* and associates [48] and then *Biddison* et al. [49] in the influenza system; this system mainly will be used to illustrate the principles of the techniques used to generate and assay cytotoxic T-cells in humans. It must be noted that every virus or other infective agent behaves differently in tissue tropism, infectivity, and so on; therefore, the techniques to select CTL will vary and will have to be adapted for each pathogen. For details, refer to papers dealing with the different systems.

3.3.4.2   The Generation of CTL and Their Culture

Isolate human PBMC on Ficoll-Paque as described above; incubate responder white blood cells at 1.5×10^6/ml in RPMI-1640 medium for 1–2 h with antigen in an upright 50 ml plastic tissue culture bottle (8 ml total volume). Include FCS, specifically chosen for this type of culture, at 10 % v/v, although in many instances autologous serum is preferable.

For stimulation with influenza virus, incubate the cells with 5–10 HAU of virus; do this in the absence of serum to prevent infectivity, and add serum after 1–2 h incubation at 37 °C. With many infective agents with high virulence or a tropism for the T-cells themselves, it is necessary to stimulate with autologous APC that are infected and washed or pulsed with peptide. Stimulator cells are generally autologous PBMC, (preferably after activation with PHA) or irradiated EBV-transformed B-cell lines (BCL) at 1/10 or 1/20 the number of responder T-cells [50].

With human PBMC (although the donor will have been exposed to the infection), the first *in vitro* antigen stimulation often results in very low antigen-specific cytotoxicity. However, CTL lines with strong reactivity can be selected by re-stimulating several times with APC (infected or peptide pulsed and then washed as detailed above). Feed cultures with 1/2 the medium every 3–4 days and re-stimulate with antigen every 8–12 days. After the second stimulation add a source of IL-2 (5–10 U of rIL-2 or Lymphocult T at 5–10 %, v/v).

3.3.5   Cloning Techniques for CD8+ Cytotoxic T-Cells

In mouse systems extensive work has been published with cloned CD8+ CTL to study the repertoire of CTL for components of viruses or parasites and to define the role of

CTL effector function in infections *in vivo* by transferring CTL clones into infected hosts in animal models. Detailed methods have been described in many publications relating to influenza [9, 51, 52], respiratory syncytial virus [53], malaria [54] and LCMV [55, 56] amongst others. There are fewer publications dealing with human CD8+ virus-specific T-cell clones although alloreactive clones are more easily obtained [16]. In general, the methods used are similar to those developed for murine cells. In early attempts to clone human CTL, overgrowth by CD4+ cells was often observed. In such cases, it is preferable to select positively for CD8+ T-cells with magnetic beads or to remove CD4+ cells with antibody and complement. Cloning can be done by limiting dilution using re-stimulated cultures [57, 58] – if the peptide epitope has been defined the best selection for the desired clones is to re-stimulate with peptide-pulsed, autologous irradiated APC or BCL, although infected stimulator cells can be used. Then distribute activated T-cells in various numbers (e.g. 50, 10, 3 and 1/well) into 96-well plastic microtitre plates in the presence of 10^4–10^5 antigen-pulsed APC and rIL-2 or Lymphocult T in a total volume of about 150 μl. Every few days feed the wells with RPMI 1640 +10 % FCS medium containing a source of IL-2. Once the cells grow, transfer to 24-well *Costar* plates and re-stimulate with antigen-pulsed APC (responder : stimulator cell ratio of 1:1) and feed with IL-2 as detailed for the CTL lines.

3.3.5.1 Target Cells for Cytotoxicity Assay

Target cells need to be labelled wth $Na_2^{51}CrO_4$ and loaded with antigen, either by infection with the agent under test, or by pulsing with peptides to be tested or the appropriate peptide if the epitope has been defined. Tumour cells sharing class I MHC HLA molecules with the T-cells, either by expressing these molecules constitutively or following transfection, are suitable. For the assays with human cells, autologous EBV-transformed BCL are most widely utilized, but mouse cell lines transfected with shared HLA class I MHC molecules are also useful [e.g. 50, 58]. If neither of these is available, then PHA-activated autologous PBMC can serve as target cells though they are less efficiently lysed by CTL.

Wash the target cells, label with ^{51}Cr (100 μc/1–3 $\times$ 10^6 cells) for 1 h at 37 °C in 0.1–0.2 ml serum-free medium, wash and then infect with about 1000 HAU influenza virus (in a very small volume of serum-free medium; 0.1–0.2 ml) for 1–2 h at 37 °C. With some viruses the radiolabelling and infection can be done at the same time. Then wash the cells 3 times in full medium (RPMI 1640 +10 % FCS), incubate for 4 h at 37 °C (for adequate expression of viral proteins) wash 3 times in RPMI 1640, resuspend in 1 ml RPMI 1640 +10 % FCS and count viable cells.

Alternatively, pulse target cells with peptide after the ^{51}Cr labelling by incubating for 1 h at 37 °C in RPMI +10 % FCS with an excess of peptide, generally about 10^{-6} mol/l, depending on the affinity or sensitivity of the peptide, wash 3 times and dilute to 2 $\times$ 10^5 cells/ml to be dispensed for the assay (see below). Another way of titrating out the peptide concentration required for CTL recognition and target cells lysis is to add peptide to the assay at various concentrations ranging from 10^{-5} to 10^{-12} mol/l and to leave the peptide in the wells during the assay period.

Since purified proteins cannot be used for target cell formation, recombinant vaccinia viruses encoding individual proteins of pathogens have been most useful to determine which proteins are recognized by the CTL [50]. Infect the target cells with 10–20 pfu of virus/cell, incubate for 1–2 h at 37 °C, extensively wash in full medium and incubate at 37 °C for 4 h for the expression of virally encoded proteins before CTL-mediated lysis is determined.

3.3.5.2   Cytotoxicity Assay

Suspend the CTL and ^{51}Cr-labelled target cells separately in RPMI 1640 +10 % FCS. Add target cells to 96-well round bottom microwell plates in a volume of 50 or 100 µl (usually 1–2 × 10^4 cells/well). Distribute the killer cells in different numbers at least in duplicate, and in triplicate if possible, to achieve killer : target ratios varying from 50:1 to 1:1. For cell lines or clones the lower K : T ratios are sufficient. It is essential to have 8–10 wells with the target cells alone. Use 4 of these to obtain the total radioactivity of the target cells seeded out in each well and 4–6 to determine the spontaneous ^{51}Cr release into the supernatant during the incubation (control release). The final volume in every well has to be the same (i.e. 200 µl) during the incubation, except for the wells destined to give the total radioactivity of the target cells which remain at 100 µl; at the end of the incubation time, treat these with 100 µl of 5 % Triton X 100. Centrifuge the plates lightly (30 s at 500 rpm) and incubate at 37 °C for 3–5 h depending on the particular system under test and the level of cytotoxicity. After incubation centrifuge the plates (5 min at 1000 rpm) and withdraw 100 µl of the supernatant into small tubes to count the released radioactivity in a gamma counter. The % specific target lysis is calculated as follows:

$$\frac{\text{cpm experimental sample} - \text{cpm control release}}{\text{cpm of total target cells} - \text{cpm control release}} \times 100$$

For smaller assays, 20 µl of supernatant can be removed onto filter papers which are dried and counted in scintillation fluid on a flat bed gamma/beta counter [59].

Not all cell types are equally susceptible to CTL-mediated lysis and normal cells generally show a lower lysis plateau than established tumour cell lines.

3.3.6   Applications of T-Cell Clones

Undoubtedly, knowledge of the natural history of the many different T-cell populations is incomplete. Nevertheless, the considerable advances in our understanding of the physiological mechanisms regulating T-cell differentiation and function owe much to the technological developments that facilitated the isolation and expansion of monoclonal populations of antigen-specific T-cells [60]. In general, the technical approaches for generating T-cell clones are based on the observation that T-cell activation depends on the recognition of antigen in association with self MHC gene products [1, 2]. It is, perhaps, a lack of information on the molecular basis of antigen recognition and signalling requirements that has hindered the ability to isolate certain regulatory T-cells with inhibitory function.

The application of T-cell clones has allowed investigations of a wide range of immunological problems that were not possible with unfractionated lymphocyte populations. These concerned the recognition pattern and repertoire of T-cell subpopulations as well as their functional properties [61]. Antigen-induced lymphokine production can be examined *in vitro* while functional assays to define protective or deleterious effects in infection *in vivo* clearly require animal models. In many instances cloned antigen-specific CD8+ T-cells transferred into infected hosts have accelerated clearance of intracellular pathogens or showed protective effects in infections such as influenza [51, 52], lymphocytic choriomeningitis virus [55], mouse cytomegalovirus [57], malaria [54] and herpes virus [62]. On the other hand CD4+ T-cells, as well as CD8+ T-cells, may enhance immunopathology and exacerbate disease if the infective agent localizes in important tissues or areas where tissue damage is particularly deleterious – this can be observed for example with CD8+ T-cells specific for respiratory syncytial virus where infection spreads to the fine air passages [53], or with virus-specific CD8+ CTL after intracerebral LCMV infection or widespread LCMV infection in neonatally infected hosts [55], or myelin basic protein specific CD4+ T-cells causing damage in the CNS [63]. In addition, T-cell clones have helped to define CD4+ T-cell subpopulations that can produce different lymphokines [21] important in regulating the Ig subclass of the antibody formed by B-cells [64]. Thus, in leishmania the IL-4 producing T helper cells are deleterious while the IL-2 and IFN-γ secretors limit the infection [65, 66].

Studies with T-cell clones have also brought great progress in understanding of the requirements for the interaction between peptides and MHC molecules respectively. Experimental approaches have included exon shuffling of the heavy chains of class I MHC, mutations in specific regions or residues of the MHC molecule, particularly residues in the helical walls or the floor of the antigen binding groove formed by the $\alpha1$ and $\alpha2$ domains of the heavy chain [e.g. 67]. Such experiments are defining the MHC residues critical for the binding of peptides in different haplotypes and for different peptide epitopes. It was through T-cell cloning that, contrary to expectation, it was found that CD8+ CTL in many viral infections predominantly react to peptide fragments derived from internal viral proteins rather than from the glycoproteins expressed at the cell surface at high levels [5]. Similarly, it has been possible to map critical residues in T cell determinants based on the ability of peptides synthesized with amino acid substitutions to stimulate T cell clones [68, 69].

In addition to the fine detail of specificity that the analysis of monoclonal T-cell populations allows, it has been suggested that examination of panels of T-cell clones, despite the obvious limitation in numbers, reflects the antigen specificity of the T-cell repertoire as a whole. However, it is likely that multiple antigen re-stimulations *in vitro* will select for dominant clones with high precursor frequency in the donor cells or with TCR expressing very high avidities or affinities for certain peptide-MHC complexes. With T-cell antigen receptors of defined antigen and restriction specificity isolated from T-cell clones it has been possible to examine repertoire selection by introducing these TCR as transgenes into host mice [70, 71]. Manipulation of the thymic environment by variation of the MHC haplotype and exposure to specific antigen have provided information on mechanims of positive and negative selection in the thymus. The introduction of TCR αβ transgenes derived from CD4+ or CD8+ T-cell clones has confirmed the importance of these accessory molecules in repertoire selection [72].

The isolation of T-cell antigen receptors followed the ability to precipitate heterodimeric molecules of 92 kD molecular weight with antibody uniquely reactive with the immunizing population of cloned T-cells [73]. Further immunoprecipitation studies with anti-receptor antibodies demonstrated that CD3 is part of the T-cell receptor complex. For certain T-cell clones, co-modulation of CD4 and Ti-CD3 with anti-clonotypic antibodies suggests that CD4 may physically form part of the antigen recognition structure [74]. From biochemical studies, including these, the preliminary protein structure of T-cell antigen receptors was established [75]. Although clonotypic antibodies were first raised against IL-2-dependent T-cell clones, the inability to generate antigen-specific T-cell hybridomas has hindered the analysis of receptor structure using conventional biochemical techniques. However, by constructing DNA subtraction libraries between T- and B-cells, genes for the TCR-β chain were isolated and cloned [76]. Molecular probes reactive with constant regions of the murine genes have facilitated the isolation of the equivalent molecules in human T-cells [77]. Subsequently, with cloning of the α, β, γ and δ chains the genetic organization of the TCR genes has been explored in detail [78].

In addition to their application in the isolation of TCR structure, monoclonal T-cell populations have contributed to the analysis of signal transduction under conditions that induce activation or anergy respectively [79].

The primary information on T-cell-derived cytokines is based on the investigation of supernatants of activated T-cell clones to influence the differentiation, growth or biological function of different cell lineages. Immunization using lymphokines purified biochemically has raised antibodies reactive with a variety of lymphokines and facilitated the cloning and expression of the appropriate genes. These recombinant lymphokines may then be used in binding studies for the identification of receptors. Thus, from the biological activity originally identified in the supernatants of mono-clonal cells, the role of cloned lymphokines and their receptors in T-cell signalling may be explored.

In this discussion, the major contributions that cloned T-cells have made to our understanding of T-cell biology are outlined. As more T-cell populations are isolated at the clonal level, differences in T-cell structure and the interaction of signals regulating the growth and functions of T-cells and their role in the homeostasis of the host will be resolved. The value of this knowledge is in the manipulation of T-cells in the prevention and control of disease.

References

[1] *R. M. Zinkernagel, P. C. Doherty,* MHC-restricted Cytotoxic T Cells: Studies on the Biological Role of Polymorphic Major Transplantation Antigens Determining T Cell Restriction – Specificity, Function and Responsiveness. Adv. Immunol. *27,* 51–177 (1979).

[2] *E. M. Shevach, A. S. Rosenthal,* Function of Macrophages in Antigen Recognition by Guinea Pig T Lymphocytes. II Role of the Macrophage in the Regulation of Genetic Control of the Immune Response, J. Exp. Med. *138,* 1213–1229 (1973).

[3] *P. M. Allen, B. P. Babbitt, E. R. Unanue,* T Cell Recognition of Lysozyme: the Biochemical Basis of Presentation, Immunol. Rev. *98,* 171–187 (1987).

[4] *R. H. Schwartz,* T Lymphocyte Recognition of Antigen in Association with Gene Products of the Major Histocompatibility Complex, Annu. Rev. Immunol. *3,* 237–261 (1985).

[5] *A. Townsend, H. Bodmer,* Antigen Recognition by Class I Restricted T Lymphocytes, Annu. Rev. Immunol. *7,* 601–624 (1989).

[6] *D. A. Morgan, F. W. Ruscetti, R. C. Gallo,* Selective in vitro Growth of T Lymphocytes from Normal Human Bone Marrow, Science *193,* 1007–1008 (1976).

[7] *S. Gillis, K. A. Smith,* Long Term Culture of Tumour Specific Cytotoxic T Cells, Nature *268,* 154–156 (1977).

[8] *H. Von Boehmer, H. Hengartner, M. Nabholtz, W. Lernhardt, M. H. Schreier, W. Haas,* Fine Specificity of a Continuously Growing Killer-cell Clone Specific for HY Antigen, Eur. J. Immunol. *9,* 592–597 (1979).

[9] *Y. L. Lin, B. A. Askonas,* Biological Properties of an Influenza A Virus-specific Killer T Cell Clone. Inhibition of Virus Replication in vivo and Induction of Delayed Type Hypersensitivity Reactions, J. Exp. Med. *154,* 225–234 (1981).

[10] *C. G. Fathman, H. Hengartner,* Clones of Alloreactive T Cells, Nature *272,* 617–618 (1978).

[11] *M. Nabholtz, H. D. Engers, D. Collaro, M. North,* Cloned T Cell Lines with Specific Cytolytic Activity, Curr. Top. Microbiol. Immunol. *81,* 176–187 (1978).

[12] *F. H. Bach, H. Inouye, J. A. Hank, B. J. Alter,* Human T Lymphocyte Clones Reactive in Primed Lymphocyte Typing in Cytotoxicity, Nature *281,* 307–310 (1979).

[13] *M. H. Schreier, T. Tees,* Clonal Induction of Helper T Cells. Conversion of Specific Signals to Non-specific Signals, Int. Arch. Allergy Appl. Immunol. *61,* 227–237 (1980).

[14] *B. Sredni, D. Yolkman, R. H. Schwartz, A. S. Fauci,* Antigen Specific Human T Cell Clones: Development of Clones Requiring HLA-DR Compatible Presenting Cells for Stimulation in the Presence of Antigen, Proc. Natl. Acad. Sci. U.S.A. *78,* 1858–1862 (1981).

[15] *J. R. Lamb, D. D. Eckels, P. Lake, A. H. Johnson, R. J. Hartzman, J. N. Woody,* Antigen Specific Human T Lymphocyte Clones; Induction, Antigen Specificity and MHC Restriction of Influenza Virus Immune Clones. J. Immunol. *128,* 233–238 (1982).

[16] *H. Spits, J. Borst, C. Terhorst, J. E. de Vries,* The Role of T Cell Differentiation Markers in Antigen Specific and Lectin Dependent Cellular Cytotoxicity Mediated by T8+ and T4+ Human Cytotoxic T Cell Clones Directed at Class I and Class II MHC Antigens, J. Immunol. *129,* 1563–1569 (1982).

[17] *J. W. Kappler, B. Skidmore, J. White, P. Marrack,* Antigen-inducible, H-2 Restricted, Interleukin-2 Producing T Cell Hybridomas. Lack of Independent Antigen and H-2 Recognition, J. Exp. Med. *153,* 1198–1214 (1981).

[18] *O. J. Finn, J. Boniver, H. S. Kaplan,* Induction, Establishment in vitro and Characterisation of Functional, Antigen-specific, Carrier Primed Murine T Cell Lymphomas, Proc. Natl. Acad. Sci. U.S.A. *76,* 4033–4037 (1979).

[19] *M. Popovic, G. Lange-Wantzin, P. S. Sarin, D. Mann, R. C. Gallo,* Transformation of Human Umbilical Cord Blood T Cells by Human T Cell Leukaemia/Lymphoma Virus, Proc. Natl. Acad. Sci. U.S.A *80,* 5402–5406 (1983).

[20] *N. N. Iscove, M. Melchers,* Complete Replacement of Serum by Albumin, Transferrin and Soybean Lipid in Cultures of Lipopolysaccharide-reactive B Lymphocytes, J. Exp. Med. *147,* 23–933 (1978).

[21] *T. R. Mosmann, R. L. Coffman*, TH1 and TH2 Cells: Different Patterns of Lymphokine Secretion Lead to Different Functional Properties, Annu. Rev. Immunol. *7*, 145–173 (1989).

[22] *J. E. DeVries, L. P., de Waal, R. Malefyt, H.Yssel, M. G. Roncarolo, H. Spits*, Do Human T_H1 and T_H2 CD4+ Clones Exist? Res. Immunol. *142*, 59–63 (1991).

[23] *P. M.Taylor, F. Esquitel, B. A. Askonas*, Murine CD4+ T Cell Clones Vary in Function in vitro and in Influenza Infections in vivo. Internat. Immunol. *2*, 323–328 (1990).

[24] *B. Fleischer*, Acquisition of Specific Cytotoxic Activity by Human T4 Lymphocytes in Culture, Nature *308*, 365–367 (1984).

[25] *J. P. Tite, S. M. Russell, G. Dougan, D. O'Callaghan, I. Jones, G. Brownlee, F. Y. Liew*, Antiviral Immunity Induced by Recombinant Nucleoprotein of Influenza A Virus. I. Characteristics and Cross-reactivity of T Cell Responses, J. Immunol. *141*, 3980–3987 (1988).

[26] *D. McKean, A. Infante, A. Nilson, M. Kimoto, C. G. Fathman, E. Walker, N. Warner*, Major Histocompatibility Complex-restricted Antigen Presentation to Antigen-reactive T Cells by B Lymphocyte Tumour Cells, J. Exp. Med. *154*, 1419–1431 (1981).

[27] *M. J. H. Ratcliffe, M. H. Julius, K.-J. Kim*, Heterogeneity in the Response of T Cells to Antigens Presented by B Lymphoma Cells, Cell. Immunol. *88*, 49–60 (1984).

[28] *G. Miller, M. Lipman*, Release of Infectious Epstein-Barr Virus by Transformed Marmoset Leukocytes, Proc. Natl. Acad. Sci. U.S.A. *69*, 383–387 (1973).

[29] *R. N. Germain, B. Malissen*, Analysis of the Expression and Function of Class II Major Histocompatibility Complex-encoded Molecules by DNA-mediated Gene Transfer, Annu. Rev. Immunol. *4*, 281–316 (1986).

[30] *M. Nabholz, M. Cianfriglia, O. Acuto, A. Conzelmann, W. Haas, H. von Boehmer, H. R. MacDonald, H. Pohlit, J. P. Johnson*, Cytolytically Active Murine T Cell Hybrids, Nature *287*, 437–440 (1980).

[31] *M. Okada, N. Yoshimura, T. Kaieda, Y. Yamamura, T. Kishimoto*, Establishment and Characterisation of Human T Hybrid Cells Secreting Immunoregulatory Molecules, Proc. Natl. Acad. Sci. U.S.A. *78*, 7717–7721 (1981).

[32] *J. L. Butler, A. Muraguchi, H. C. Lane, A. S. Fauci*, Development of a Human T-T Cell Hybridoma Secreting B Cell Growth Factor, J. Exp. Med. *157*, 60–67 (1983).

[33] *E. C. De Freitas, S. Vella, A. Linnenbach, C. Zimijewski, H. Koprowski, C. M. Croce*, Antigen-specific Human T Cell Hybrids with Helper Activity, Proc. Natl. Acad. Sci. U.S.A. *79*, 6646–6650 (1982).

[34] *M. Popovic, N. Flomenberg, D. J.Volkman, D. Mann, A. S. Fauci, B. Dupont, R. C. Gallo*, Alteration of T Cell Functions by Infection with HTLV-I or HTLV-II, Science *226*, 459–462 (1984).

[35] *D. J.Volkman, M. Popovic, R. C. Gallo, A. S. Fauci*, Human T Cell Leukaemia/Lymphoma Virus-infected Antigen Specific T Cell Clones: Indiscriminant Helper Function and Lymphokine Production, J. Immunol. *134*, 4237–4243 (1985).

[36] *T. Taniguchi, H. Matsui, T. Fujita, C. Takaoka, N. Kashima, R. Yoshimoto, J. Hamuro*, Structure and Expression of a Cloned cDNA for Human Interleukin-2, Nature *302*, 305–310 (1983).

[37] *J. Watson*, Continuous Proliferation of Murine Antigen-specific Helper T Lymphocytes in Culture, J. Exp. Med. *150*, 1510–1519 (1979).

[38] *R. E. O'Hehir, H. Yssel, S. Verma, J. E. de Vries, H. Spits, J. R. Lamb*, Clonal Analysis of Differential Lymphokine Production in Peptide and Superantigen Induced T Cell Anergy, Internat. Immunol. *3*, 819–826 (1991).

[39] *W. C. A. Van Schooten, T. H. M. Ottenhof, P. R. Klatser, J. Thole, R. R. P. De Vries, A. H. J. Kolk*, T Cell Epitopes on the 36 K and 65 K *Mycobacterium leprae* Antigens Defined by Human T Cell Clones, Eur. J. Immunol. *18*, 849–854 (1988).

[40] *L. A. Morrison, A. E. Lukacher,V. L. Braciale, D. Fan, T. J. Braciale*, Differences in Antigen Presentation to MHC Class I and Class II Restricted Influenza Virus-specific Cytolytic T Lymphocyte T Cell Clones, J. Exp. Med. *163*, 903–921 (1986).

[41] *S. E. Macatonia, P. M.Taylor, S. C. Knight, B. A. Askonas*, Primary Stimulation by Dendritic Cells Induces Anti-viral Proliferative and Cytotoxic T Cell Responses in vitro, J. Exp. Med. *169*, 1255–1264 (1989).

[42] *W. M. Kast, A. M. Bronkhorst, L. P. DeWaal, C. J. M. Melief*, Cooperation between Cytotoxic and Helper T Lymphocytes in Protection against Lethal *Sendai* Virus Infection. Protection by T Cells Is MHC Restricted and MHC-regulated, a Model for MHC Disease Associations, J. Exp. Med. *164*, 723–738 (1986).

[43] *K. Deres, H. Schild, K. H. Wiesmuller, G. Jung, H. G. Ramensee*, In vivo Priming of Virus Specific Cytotoxic T Lymphocytes with Synthetic Lipopeptide Vaccine, Nature *342*, 561–564 (1989).

[44] *D. C. Wraith, B. A. Askonas*, Induction of Influenza A Virus Cross-reactive Cytotoxic T Cells by a Nucleoprotein/Haemagglutinin Preparation, J. Gen. Virol. *66*, 1327–1331 (1985).

[45] *M. W. Moore, F. R. Carbone, M. J. Bevan*, Introduction of Soluble Protein into the Class I Pathway of Antigen Processing and Presentation, Cell *54*, 777–785 (1988).

[46] *A. R. M. Townsend, J. Rothbard, F. M. Gotch, G. Bahadur, D. Wraith, A. J. McMichael*, The Epitopes of Influenza Nucleoprotein Recognised by Cytotoxic T Lymphocytes Can Be Defined with Short Synthetic Peptides, Cell *44*, 959–968 (1986).

[47] *B. D. Walker, S. Chakraharti, B. Moss, T. J. Paradis, T. Flynn, A. G. Durno, R. S. Blumberg, J. C. Kaplan, M. S. Hirsch, R. T. Schooley*, HIV-specific Cytotoxic T Lymphocytes in Seropositive Individuals, Nature *328*, 345–348 (1987).

[48] *A. J. McMichael, B. A. Askonas*, Influenza Virus Specific Cytotoxic T Cells in Man: Induction and Properties of the Cytotoxic T Cell, Eur. J. Immunol. *8*, 705–711 (1978).

[49] *W. E. Biddison, M. S. Krangel, J. L. Strominger, F. E. Ward, G. M. Hearer, S. Shaw*, Virus Immune Cytotoxic T Cells recognise Structural Differences between Serologically Indistinguishable HLA-A2 Molecules, Hum. Immunol. *3*, 225–232 (1980).

[50] *F. M. Gotch, A. J. McMichael, G. L. Smith, B. Moss*, Identification of the Virus Molecules Recognised by Influenza Specific Human Cytotoxic T Lymphocytes, J. Exp. Med. *165*, 408–414 (1987).

[51] *C. D. Mackenzie, P. M. Taylor, B. A. Askonas*, Rapid Recovery of Lung Histology Correlates with Clearance of Influenza Virus by Specific CD8+ Cytotoxic T Cells, Immunology *67*, 375–382 (1989).

[52] *E. Lukacher, V. L. Braciale, T. J. Braciale*, In Vivo Effector Function of Influenza Virus Specific Cytotoxic T Lymphocyte Clones is Highly Specific, J. Exp. Med. *160*, 1560–1565 (1984).

[53] *M. J. Cannon, P. J. M. Openshaw, B. A. Askonas*, Cytotoxic T Cells Clear Virus but Augment Lung Pathology in Mice Infected with Respiratory Syncytial Virus, J. Exp. Med. *168*, 1163–1168 (1988).

[54] *P. Romero, J. L. Maryanski, G. Corradin, R. S. Nussenzweig, V. Nussenzweig, F. Zavala*, Cloned Cytotoxic T Cells Recognise an Epitope in the Circumsporozoite Protein and Protect against Malaria, Nature *341*, 323–326 (1989).

[55] *J. A. Byrne, M. B. A. Oldstone*, Biology of Cloned Cytotoxic T Lymphocytes Specific for LCMV, J. Immunol. *136*, 698–704 (1986).

[56] *J. Baenziger, H. Hengartner, R. M. Zinkernagel, G. A. Cole*, Induction and Prevention of Immunopathological Disease by Cloned Cytotoxic T Cell Lines Specific for Lymphocytic Choriomeningitis Virus, Eur. J. Immunol. *16*, 387–393 (1986).

[57] *F. M. Gotch, D. F. Nixon, N. Alp, A. J. McMichael, L. K. Borysiewicz*, High Frequency of Memory and Effector Gag Specific Cytotoxic T Cells in HIV Seropositive Individuals, Internat. Immunol. *2*, 707–712 (1990).

[58] *H. Bodmer, F. Gotch, A. J. McMichael*, Class I Cross Restricted T Cells Reveal Low Responder Alleles due to Processing of Viral Antigen, Nature *337*, 653–655 (1989).

[59] *C. G. Potter, F. Gotch, G. T. Warner, Y. Oestrup*, Lymphocyte Proliferation and Cytotoxic Assays Using Flat Bed Scintillation Counting, J. Immunol. Methods *105*, 171–177 (1987).

[60] *C. G. Fathman, F. W. Fitch*, Isolation, Characterisation and Utilisation of T Lymphocyte Clones, Academic Press, New York 1982.

[61] *R. E. O'Hehir, R. Garman, J. Greenstein, J. R. Lamb*, The Specificity and Regulation of T-cell Responsiveness to Allergens, Annu. Rev. Immunol. *9*, 67–95 (1991).

[62] *A. A. Nash, A. Jayasuriya, J. Phelan, S. P. Cobbold, H. Waldmann, T. Prospero,* Different Roles of L3T4 and Lyt 2+ T Cell Subsets in the Control of an Acute Herpes Simplex Virus Infection of the Skin and Nervous System, J. Gen. Virol. *68,* 825–833 (1987).

[63] *B. Engelhardt, T. Diamantolscin, H. Weckerle,* Immunotherapy of Experimental Autoimmune Encephalomyelitis: Differential Effect of Anti-IL-2 Receptor Antibody Therapy on Actively Induced and T-line Mediated EAE of the Lewis Rat, J. Autoimmunity *2,* 61–73 (1989).

[64] *R. L. Coffman, J. Carty,* A T Cell Activity that Enhances Polyclonal IgE Production and Its Inhibition by Interferon-gamma, J. Immunol. *136,* 949–954 (1986).

[65] *F. Y. Liew,* Functional Heterogeneity of CD4+ T Cells in Leishmaniasis, Immunol. Today *10,* 40–45 (1989).

[66] *I. Muller, T. Pedrazzini, J. P. Farrell, J. Louis,* T Cell Responses and Immunity to Experimental Infection with Leishmania Major, Annu. Rev. Immunol. *7,* 561–579 (1989).

[67] *A. J. McMichael, B. A. Askonas, J. Frelinger,* Processing and Presentation of Viral Antigens with Class I MHC Molecules, in: *J. McCluskey* (ed.), Antigen Processing and Recognition, C.R.C. Press, Boca Raton, Florida 1991, pp. 85–107.

[68] *J. B. Rothbard, R. I. Lechler, K. Howland, V. Bal, D. D. Eckels, R. P. Sekaly, E. O. Long, W. R. Taylor, J. R. Lamb,* Structural Model of HLA-DR1 Restricted T Cell Antigen Recognition, Cell *52,* 515–523 (1988).

[69] *J. B. Rothard, R. M. Pemberton, H. C. Bodmer, B. A. Askonas, W. R. Taylor,* Identification of Residues Necessary for Clonally Specific Recognition of a Cytotoxic T-cell Determinant, EMBO J. *8,* 2321–2328 (1989).

[70] *C. Benoist, D. Mattis,* Positive Selection of the T Cell Repertoire: Where and When Does It Occur, Cell *58,* 1027–1033 (1989).

[71] *H. von Boehmer, P. Kisielow,* Self-nonself Discrimination by T Cells, Science *248,* 1369–1373 (1990).

[72] *P. Kisielow, H. Teh, H. Bluthman, H. von Boehmer,* Positive Selection of Antigen-specific T Cells in Thymus by Restricting MHC Molecules, Nature *335,* 730–733 (1988).

[73] *S. C. Meuer, O. Acuto, R. E. Hussey, J. C. Hodgdon, K. A. Fitzgerald, S. R. Schlossman, E. L. Reinherz,* Evidence for T Cell Associated 90 kD Heterodimer as the T Cell Antigen Receptor, Nature *303,* 808–811 (1983).

[74] *K. Saizawa, J. Rojo, C. A. Janeway,* Physical Association of CD4 and the CD3: αβ T Cell Receptor, Nature *328,* 260–263 (1987).

[75] *P. Marrack, J. Kappler,* The Antigen-specific, Major-histocompatibility Complex-restricted Receptor on T Cells, Annu. Rev. Immunol. *38,* 1–30 (1986).

[76] *S. M. Hedrick, E. A. Nielsen, J. Kavaler, D. J. Cohen, M. M. Davis,* Sequence Relationships Between Putative T Cell Receptor Polypeptides and Immunoglobulins, Nature *308,* 153–158 (1984).

[77] *Y. Yanagi, Y. Yoshikai, K. Leggett, S. P. Clark, I. Aleksander, T. W. Mak,* A Human T Cell Specific cDNA Clone Encodes a Protein Having Extensive Homology to Immunoglobulin Chains, Nature *308,* 145–149 (1984).

[78] *D. H. Roulet,* The Structure Function and Molecular Genetics of the γδ T Cell Receptor, Annu. Rev. Immunol. *7,* 175–209 (1989).

[79] *R. H. Schwartz,* A Cell Culture Model for T Lymphocyte Clonal Anergy, Science *248,* 1349–56 (1990).

3.4   Arthropod Cells

Klaus-Peter Sieber

Efforts to understand the metabolism of insect cells have received greater attention with the introduction of new technologies in viral expression vector systems, important for large scale commercial applications in medicine and agriculture. The increased significance of arthropod cell culture (primarily insect cell culture) is reflected by its application in the production of proteins as diagnostics, vaccines, therapeutics or reagents of medical, pharmaceutical and veterinary importance [1] as well as by its commercial use to develop pathogens for insect pests in bioreactors. Earlier attempts to culture arthropod cells as prototypes for studies on the physiology, molecular biology or genetics of eukaryotic cells were laborious and difficult, due to the lack of defined media and culture conditions.

3.4.1   Setting up Arthropod Cell Cultures

3.4.1.1   Starting Material

Arthropod cell lines usually originate from primary explants of embryonic tissue or from tissues of young larvae or pupae. Although cells from tissue and organs of older larvae or adults have been cultured in primary cell cultures, these attempts have had little success in dipterans. Cells from imaginal discs proliferate *in vitro* at rates comparable to growth *in vivo* [2], however, they do not grow in standard media but in a complex, serum-free medium [3]. The source of most insect cell lines, as well as tick cell lines [4, 5], has been a complex organ (ovaries) or the whole embryo. Several approaches can be selected. Some examples are given here for the preparation of embryonic cell cultures.

1. Cut embryos into 2 or 3 fragments and subject to enzymatic treatment, e. g., trypsin (0.1–0.25%, w/v), collagenase (0.2%, w/v), hyaluronidase (0.25%, w/v), pronase (0.1%, w/v) or chitinase (0.25%, w/v) in *Rinaldini's* salt solution (RSS) [6] and culture in glass flasks with medium.
2. Mechanically dissociate embryonic cells and dispense in medium with 15% FBS, which can be enriched with a 10% (w/v) extract of *Drosophila* pupae [7–10]. Subculture cells every 3 to 7 days, when they cover approximately 60% of the culture

flask surface or feed twice a week (replacing 80% of the spent medium with an equal volume of fresh medium).

3. Mechanically mince embryos from 0 day old (4–20 h) dechorionated eggs in balanced saline solution [11] in a high speed mechanical stirrer. Suspend cell clumps and fragmented organs in M3 medium. At high densities transfer supernatants to new culture flasks and subsequently split into subcultures [12].

Most lepidopteran cell lines that are currently used in virus expression vector work are derived from adult ovarian tissues (*Trichoplusia ni*, [9]) or pupal ovarian tissues (*Mamestra brassica* [44], *Spodoptera frugiperda*, [13]) and subcloned (SF-9 cells, ATCC CRL 1711). Of unclear origin, but most likely from pupal ovarian cells, are several *Bombyx mori* sub cell lines which are used as host cells in nuclear polyhedrosis virus (NPV) work [14].

3.4.1.2   Primary Cell Culture

Embryonic tissues

Dissociated, rapidly proliferating tissues (embryonic or young larvae/pupae) of heterogenous origin (whole embryo or complex organs, e. g., ovaries and testes) contain cells of unknown identity. Although lines of specific cell types from a given tissue cannot be obtained, larval or embryonic tissues represent acceptable sources for the establishment of cell lines. Most identifiable cells of the larva are competent to complete their differentiation *in vitro* [2] and are programmed to reach their final differentiated state in the absence of signals from adjacent cells. Within 6 h after plating the cell homogenates of postgastrulation embryos, differentiating and aggregating myocytes can be distinguished between small clusters of primary fat body cells which subsequently enlarge due to accumulating fat. Muscle cells tend to aggregate but do not proliferate. Myoblasts can be separated from other cells within the primary culture and used for differentiation studies by adding EGTA (as a chelating agent) to the medium. Neuroblasts (from blastoderm cells) are also detectable early on in the primary culture, subsequently forming a net of axons over the culture dish surface and clusters of ganglion cells. Cells identifiable on the basis of their morphology or physiology (nerve, muscle, trachea, macrophages) usually disappear by the 2nd or 3rd week of culture.

Insect hormones, although not necessary for the initiation or maintenance of established cell lines, have been shown to stimulate cell division and differentiation and to induce cuticle synthesis (β-ecdysone) in primary cell culture [15]. Cell lines from cell types, distinguishable in primary cultures (epithelial-like, fibroblast-like cells, vesicles or round cells), will be successful only several weeks after starting the primary culture [19] and can take as long as several months [16]. Mostly epitheloid cells remain in stable lines after subcloning [17], although the morphology of the cells can vary with culture condition, medium composition and passage number. When embryonic tissues from most dipteran species are cultured, multicellular single-layered vesicles (epithelial-like cells forming a sphere) can form [10, 18], which sometimes display a cuticle-like membrane [15]. Vesicles can be dissociated mechanically and subcultured. Cell lines established this way will adhere to the plastic surface [19]; others have been reported to grow continuously in vesicles [20]. Although these vesicles seem to be imaginal disc tissue [21], their origin is not defined.

Adult tissue

Cells from most organs of adult arthropods are differentiated and do not proliferate, although they can be held in short term culture in various media. Adult ovaries have been successfully used as a source to establish continuous cell lines [22]. Originating from minced adult ovaries [9], a continuous cell line (TN-368) is commonly used for replication of *Autographa californica* nuclear polyhedrosis virus (AcMNPV), which grows well in cell monolayers.

3.4.1.3   Cell Lines

Stable cell lines from more than 70 insect species [23] and 7 species of Acari (Ixodidae) [24] have been cultured to date. Although insect cell lines are not substrate-dependent, they can be maintained as monolayer cultures on a variety of surfaces and substrates or grown in suspension. The degree of attachment is not only dependent on culture conditions but also varies on different surfaces [25]. *Spodoptera frugiperda* (SF 9) cells are anchorage-independent and grow well both in suspension in stirred 50 to 250 ml spinner flasks and as monolayer cultures in tissue culture flasks. Since arthropod cells do not adhere to plastic as tightly as many vertebrate cells, they can be recovered by pipetting or by using a rubber "policeman" and do not require trypsinization. Lag-phases of cellular growth after subcloning, or cellular death after harvesting cells that grow as attached monolayers, can be avoided by using dispase, a neutral protease [26]. If cells of a suspension culture aggregate, as found in the cell line TN-368 or with some dipteran cells, determination of cell number is facilitated by counting nuclei with a haemocytometer after suspending cells in PBS containing NP-40 (0.1%, w/v).

New cell lines should be characterized routinely before releasing them to other laboratories. Cross-contamination and misidentification of cell lines is detected by enzyme isoelectric focusing [27] and isoenzyme analysis [28, 29] with commercially available kits. Karyotyping (chromosomal analysis) [30, 31], a widely used method, is of limited use for distinguishing among cell lines from lepidopteran species [32]; however, it can be applied to distinguish between dipteran and lepidopteran cells [33]. When used in combination, sufficient markers should be available to characterize the cell line of interest.

3.4.1.4   Media

The early media for organ culture were based on the known composition of the haemolymph of the silkworm *Bombyx mori* [14, 34], or of particular invertebrate species, and used for culture of insect cell lines. Today, most basal insect media are modifications of the original media and supply basic nutrients (salts, sugars, amino acids, organic acids, vitamins and trace elements), and differ only in the relative amounts of these factors. Three basic formulations are most commonly used for lepidopteran cell lines. These are *Grace's* Antheraea medium [14], IPL-41 [35] and TC 100 [36]. These media, as well as *Schneider's* M3 medium [37] and other dipteran media [38], commonly used for culturing *Drosophila* cells, contain peptones or lactalbumin hydrolysate (LH) as substitutes for known peptides and proteins of insect haemolymph, and yeastolate (YE, a source for nucleotides and B-vitamins) or inosine [39]. Originally designed for cultures of cells of leafhopper embryonic, nymphal and adult stages, the most widely used medium for mosquito cells is M&M medium [40]. In addition, mosquito cell lines were reported to be isolated with greatly improved plating efficiencies in *Leibovitz's* L-15, a vertebrate cell culture medium [20]. Cells maintained on undefined media can be gradually shifted to defined media at times of subculturing.

Different from mammalian media, which generally use a CO_2-bicarbonate buffer system, insect media have a pH of approximately 6.2 with Na-phosphate as buffer. The pH of dipteran culture media is usually between 6.8 and 7.0, although pH values of dipteran haemolymph can vary between 6.3 and 7.7, depending on the stages within development. Invertebrate media lack phenol red, commonly used in mammalian media, therefore most insect media are clear or yellow.

Arthropod media are commonly supplemented with 10% (v/v) heat inactivated (56°C for 30 min) fetal bovine serum (FBS), however, concentrations can range between 20% [41] and 0.5% [42, 43]. Serum provides additional nutrients and protects cells from hydrodynamic stress in suspension culture. The concentration of FBS can be reduced with time and the cells can be adapted gradually to grow in serum-free media. Reduction of serum in the medium may be necessary to promote adhesion of *Mamestra brassicae* cells on the surface of culture vessels [44]. The recent development of serum-free media facilitates low-cost propagation of lepidopteran cells [42, 44, 45], with low protein content and containing cholesterol, cod liver oil fatty acid methyl esters, Tween 80, alpha tocopherol acetate and Pluronic F-68 (*BASF*) [46] as an emulsifying agent. These supplements are commercially available, and protocols for their preparation are available [46]. Cells may take 2–3 months to adapt from a complete medium to a serum-free medium and they may exhibit longer lag periods on subculture compared to those grown in a complete medium [47].

Omitting antibiotic-antimycotic supplements from the medium may facilitate the identification of contaminated cultures, since routine use of these supplements may mask contaminants.

3.4.1.5   Cell Culture of *Spodoptera frugiperdis* Cells (SF9-cells)

Since this cell line grows well in both suspension and monolayer cultures (other cell lines may vary in characteristics from this example), stock cultures are maintained in monolayer culture (higher viability and growth rate) and used to seed suspension cultures when needed. The cells are grown at 28°C in a humidified incubator with a population doubling rate of 18–24 h and subcultured twice a week at 80%–90% confluency.

Subculturing monolayer cultures

Under the inverted microscope, healthy cells have a rounded appearence, without granules. If cultures are too dense, cells tend to float (lack of contact inhibition). Contaminations (bacteria and fungus) should be visible at this point as cloudiness of medium (not to be confused with occasionally amorphous precipitated serum proteins). Lysed cells and changed morphology of cells point to viral contamination. Cultures with suspected contamination should not be opened but discarded in autoclave bags.

1. Pipette cells gently off the surface of the culture flask (SF9 cells do not need trypsinization or EDTA for detachment).
2. Determine cell viability of the culture in a small aliquot by adding 1/10 of the volume of trypan blue solution and analyse on a haemocytometer (cf. 2.1) (approximately > 98% of cells should be viable).
3. Seed a 25 cm^2 tissue culture flask with 2×10^6 cells (in approximately 5 ml), or a 75 cm^2 flask with 5×10^6 cells (in approximately 10 ml). Within 3 to 4 days, the cultures will be confluent (1–2×10^7 cells/25 cm^2). One day after subculturing the flasks should be examined for contamination.

Suspension cultures

Cells are cultured in glass bottles with a magnetic stir bar (in 500 ml medium bottles on magnetic stirrer plate or in hanging-bar spinner/microcarrier spinner flasks) or alternatively agitated on a shaking platform.

1. Inoculate vessels with 2–4×10^5 cells/ml and incubate in flasks which are stirred at 60–100 rpm. They will reach a density of 10^6 cells/ml within 3–4 days (incubated at 28°C), and can now be used for monolayer cultures (i.e. for plaque assays). Subculture by transferring 1/10 to 1/3 of the culture to a new flask containing fresh medium.
2. Wash spinner flasks with distilled water and autoclave (without bleach or disinfectants in flasks) for reuse.

3.4.1.6   Cloning Methods

In order to overcome the heterogeneity of cells in continuous lines (cells from organs or from hundreds of embryos) cloning may be necessary or desirable to maximize yield of expression, to increase susceptibility to viral infection or to isolate biochemical variants.

1. Dilute the cells to a concentration of one cell/ml and transfer aliquots to wells of a 96-well microtiter plate (cloning by limiting dilution). This is the most common method [48, 49]. By use of an inverted microscope, mark the presence of single cells in individual wells, and transfer viable, growing clones to larger flasks in (usually) 2–3 weeks.
2. Alternatively, single cells can be picked from a cell line by the capillary tube method [50] or with a micromanipulator and propagated.
3. Isolated colonies can be produced in soft agar (0.33% agar in medium) in sealed dishes with a base layer of 1–2% (w/v) agar in medium with heart infusion broth or in medium alone [51].

Insect cells grow very poorly when inoculated at low densities or as single cells. Conditioned medium (medium from fast growing cultures, which has been centrifuged and sterilized) usually improves the colony-forming efficiency.

3.4.1.7   Culture Parameters

Although arthropod cells tolerate a wide range of temperatures, the optimal temperature for the growth of cell cultures (population doubling time and adaptation to change in medium composition) has been found to be 28°C for most cell lines [52]. A CO_2 supply to the incubator is not required, so cultures are maintained in ambient atmosphere. The osmotic pressure in insect media is not critical and can vary more than in mammalian tissue culture media (290–300 mOsm/l). Some arthropod cells can be shifted from 290 to 400 mOsm/l with little effect other than the requirement of adaptation [52]. The high oxygen requirement and the high fragility (shear sensitivity) of insect cells, especially when virus infected, may become a problem in scale up suspension cultures in stirred vessels (fermentors) and sparging is required [53] (cf. 3.6). Cells are better able to withstand hydrodynamic stress in the presence of Pluronic F-68 [46].

3.4.2   Applications

The importance of arthropods as vectors of viral and protozoan pathogens as well as the search for alternatives to insecticides provides an increasing rationale for experiments with arthropod cell culture.

3.4.2.1   Arthropod-transmitted Virus

Arbovirus (arthropod-borne virus, i.e., encephalitis, yellow fever virus, *Dengue*) can be grown in dipteran and tick cell lines, and culture is rarely accompanied by cytopathic effects (CPE). Isolation and characterization of arboviruses as well as epidemiological studies have been facilitated greatly by using continuous arthropod cell lines.

3.4.2.2   Studies on Differentiation and Genetics

In the past 20 years, research studying development and differentiation has increasingly used insect cell cultures, especially because of the wealth of information on the genetics and the large numbers of mutants available in the *Drosophila* system. Besides the biochemistry and genetics of dipteran cells in culture [55], *Drosophila* cells have also been used as tools for studying more general problems, i.e. heat shock proteins. When cells *in vitro* are moved from their usual culture temperature of 25°C to 37°C, a complete change in the pattern of transcription, translation and processing occurs, thus providing a system to study the functional organization of a group of genes.

3.4.2.3   Gene Expression in Transfected Insect Cells

Stable *Drosophila* cell lines (*Schneider 2*) have been established that produce and secrete high levels of foreign gene products (e.g. envelope proteins from different HIV-isolates [56]). It is clear that, with the development of the baculovirus expression vector system [57], invertebrate cell culture represents a very important technology to produce a rapidly increasing number of proteins [1]. The presence on the viral DNA of a very strong promoter preceding the polyhedrin gene, which can be replaced by other genes, results in the synthesis of large amounts of the desired protein in the baculovirus expression system. Foreign proteins, expressed in insect cells are enzymatically, antigenically, immunologically and functionally similar to their authentic counterparts. Unlike in many prokaryotic expression systems, proteins are folded correctly when expressed in insect cells with baculovirus vectors. Like higher eukaryotic cell systems, they possess the necessary enzymes for post-translational modifications involving recognition and cleavage of signal peptides and secretion of the protein in its soluble form into the medium. Vaccines and subunit vaccines, as well as therapeutics, are available through the expression of high amounts of viral proteins. These developments have contributed to the popularity of the expression in insect cells.

References

[1] V. A. Luckow, M. D. Summers, Trends in the Development of Baculovirus Expression Vectors, Bio/Technology 6, 47–55 (1988).

[2] G. Shields, A. Dübendorfer, J. H. Sang, Differentiation in vitro of Larval Cell Types from Early Embryonic Cells of Drosophila melanogaster, J. Embryol. Exp. Morphol. 33, 159–175 (1975).

[3] K. T. Davis, A. Shearn, In vitro Growth of Imaginal Discs from Drosophila melanogaster, Science 169, 438–440 (1977).

[4] U. K. M. Bhat, C. E. Yunker, Establishment and Characterization of a Diploid Cell Line from the Tick Dermacentor parumapertus Neumann, (Acarina: Ixodidae), J. Parasitol. 63, 1092–1098 (1977).

[5] C. E. Yunker, J. Cory, H. Meibos, Continuous Cell Lines from Embryonic Tissues of Ticks, In Vitro 17, 139–142 (1981).

[6] L. M. A. Rinaldini, A Quantitative Method for Growing Animal Cells in vitro, Nature 173, 1134–1136 (1954).

[7] T. J. Kurtti, U. G. Munderloh, Mosquito Cell Culture, in: K. Maramorosch (ed.), Advances in Cell Culture, Vol. 3, Academic Press, New York 1984, pp. 259–302.

[8] G. Echalier, A. Ohanessian, Isolation in in vitro Cultures of Diploid Cell Lines of Drosophila melanogaster, C. R. Acad. Sci. Paris 268, 1771–1773 (1969).

[9] W. F. Hink, Established Insect Cell Line from the Cabbage Looper, Trichoplusia ni, Nature 226, 466–467 (1970).

[10] I. Schneider, Cell Lines Derived from Late Embryonic Stages of Drosophila melanogaster, J. Embryol. Exp. Morphol. 27, 353–356 (1972).

[11] L. N. Chan, W. Gehring, Determination of Blastoderm Cells in Drosophila melanogaster, Proc. Natl. Acad. Sci. USA 68, 2217–2221 (1971).

[12] U. Regenass, H. P. Bernhard, Rudimentary Mutants of Drosophila melanogaster, Wilhelm Roux Arch. Dev. Biol. 187, 167–177 (1979).

[13] K. L. Vaughn, R. H. Goodwin, G. J. Tompkins, P. McCawley, The Establishment of Two Cell Lines from the Insect Spodoptera frugiperda (Lepidoptera: Noctuidae), In Vitro 13, 213–217 (1977).

[14] T. D. C. Grace, Establishment of Four Strains of Cells from Insect Tissues Grown in vitro, Nature 195, 788–789 (1962).

[15] M. P. Kambysellis, I. Schneider, In Vitro Development of Insect Cells. III. Effects of Ecdysone on Neonatal Larval Cells, Dev. Biol. 44, 198–203 (1975).

[16] S. Kitamura, Establishment of Cell Line from Culex Mosquito, Kobe J. Med. Sci. 16, 41–46 (1970).

[17] U. K. M. Bhat, K. R. P. Singh, Studies on the Characterization of Cells in Aedes albopictus Cell Cultures, Indian J. Exp. Biol. 9, 153–160 (1971).

[18] U. K. M. Bhat, K. R. P. Singh, Structure and Development of Vesicles in Larval Tissue Culture of Aedes aegypti (L.), J. Med. Entomol. 6, 71–76 (1969).

[19] R. B. Tesh, Establishment of Two Cell Lines from the Mosquito Toxorhynchites amboinensis (Diptera: Culicidae) and Their Susceptibility to Infection with Arboviruses, J. Med. Entomol. 17, 338–343 (1980).

[20] U. G. Munderloh, T. J. Kurtti, K. Maramorosch, Anopheles stephensi and Toxorhynchites amboinensis: Aseptic Rearing of Mosquito Larvae on Cultured Cells, J. Parasitol. 68, 1085–1091 (1982).

[21] A. Dübendorfer, G. Shields, J. H. Sang, Development and Differentiation in vitro of Drosophila melanogaster Imaginal Disc Cells from Dissociated Early Embryos, J. Embryol. Exp. Morphol. 33, 487–498 (1975).

[22] S. H. Hsu, S. Y. Li, J. H. Cross, A Cell Line Derived from Ovarian Tissue of Culex tritaeniorhynchus Summorosus Dyar, J. Med. Entomol. 9, 86–91 (1972).

[23] W. F. Hink, D. R. Bezanson, Invertebrate Cell Culture Media and Cell Lines, in: E. Kurstak (ed.), Techniques in the Life Sciences, Vol. C1, Techniques in Setting Up and Maintenance of Tissue and Cell Cultures, Elsevier Scientific, New York 1985, pp. C111/1–C111/30.

[24] *T. J. Kurtti, U. G. Munderloh,* Tick Cell Culture: Characteristics, Growth Requirements and Applications to Parasitology, in: *K. Maramorosch, J. Mitsuhashi* (eds.), Invertebrate Cell Culture Applications, Academic Press, New York 1982, pp. 195–232.

[25] *R. H. Goodwin,* Growth of Insect Cells in Serum-free Media, in: *E. Kurstak* (ed.), Techniques in the Life Sciences, Vol. C1, Cell Biology Techniques in Setting Up and Maintenance of Tissue and Cell Cultures, Elsevier Scientific, New York 1985, pp. C109/1–C109/28.

[26] *P. L. Roberts,* The Use of Proteolytic Enzymes for Harvesting Insect Cell Lines which Support Nuclear Polyhedrosis Virus Replication, FEMS Microbiol. Lett. *29,* 189–191 (1985).

[27] *A. H. McIntosh, C. M. Ignoffo,* Replication and Infectivity of the Single-embedded Nuclear Polyhedrosis Virus, *Baculovirus heliothis,* in Homologous Cell Lines, J. Invertebr. Pathol. *37,* 258–264 (1981).

[28] *W. J. Tabachnick, D. L. Knudson,* Characterization of Invertebrate Cell Lines, II. Isozyme Analyses Employing Starch Gel Electrophoresis, In Vitro *16,* 392–398 (1980).

[29] *D. E. Lynn, E. M. Dougherty, J. T. McClintock, M. Loeb,* Development of Cell Lines from Various Tissues of Lepidoptera, in: *Y. Kuroda, E. Kurstak, K. Maramorosch* (eds.), Invertebrate and Fish Tissue Culture, Springer Verlag, Berlin 1988, pp. 239–242.

[30] *M. Pudney, M. G. R. Varma, Anopheles stephensi* var. mysorensis: Establishment of a Larval Cell Line (Mos. 43), Exp. Parasitol. *29,* 7–12 (1971).

[31] *D. E. Lynn, A. Stoppleworth,* Established Cell Lines from the Beetle, *Diabrotica undecimpunctata* (Coleoptera: Chrysomelidae), In Vitro *20,* 365–368 (1984).

[32] *I. Schneider,* Characteristics of Insect Cells, in: *P. F. Kruse Jr., M. K. Patterson Jr.* (eds.), Tissue Culture Methods and Applications, Karyology of Cells in Culture, Academic Press, New York 1973, pp. 788–790.

[33] *B. H. Sweet, J. S. McHale,* Characterization of Cell Lines Derived from *Culiseta inornata* and *Aedes vexans* Mosquitoes, Exp. Cell. Res. *61,* 51–63 (1970).

[34] *S. S. Wyatt,* Culture *in vitro* of Tissue from the Silkworm, *Bombyx mori* L., J. Gen. Physiol. *39,* 841–857 (1956).

[35] *S. A. Weiss, J. L. Vaughn,* Cell Culture Methods for Large-scale Propagations of Baculoviruses, in: *R. R. Granados, B. A. Federici* (eds.), The Biology of Baculoviruses, Vol. 2, CRC Press, Boca Raton 1986, pp. 63–87.

[36] *G. R. Gardiner, H. Stockdale,* Two Tissue-culture Media for Production of Lepidopteran Cells and Nuclear Polyhedrosisis Viruses, J. Invertebr. Pathol. *25,* 363–370 (1975).

[37] *S. Lindquist, S. Sonoedo, T. Cox, K. Slusser,* Instant Medium for *Drosophila* Tissue Culture Cells, Drosophila Inf. Serv. *58,* 163–164 (1982).

[38] *J. H. Sang, Drosophila* Cells and Cell Lines, in: *K. Maramorosch* (ed.), Advances in Cell Culture, Vol. 1, CRC Press, Boca Raton 1981, pp. 125–182.

[39] *T. Marunouchi, T. Miyake,* Substitution of Inosine for Yeastolate in the Culture Medium for *Drosophila* Cells, In Vitro *14,* 1010–1014 (1978).

[40] *M. Mitsuhashi, K. Maramorosch,* Leafhopper Tissue Culture: Embryonic, Nymphal and Imaginal Tissues from Aseptic Insects, Contrib. Boyce Thompson Inst. *22,* 435 (1964).

[41] *A. H. McIntosh, C. M. Ignoffo,* Characterization of Five Cell Lines Established from Species of Heliothis, Appl. Entomol. Zool. *18,* 262–269 (1983).

[42] *W. F. Hink,* A Serum-free Medium for the Culture of Insect Cells and Production of Recombinant Proteins, In Vitro Cell. Dev. Biol. *27,* 397–401 (1991).

[43] *D. M. DiSorbo, W. G. Whitford, S. A. Weiss,* Accessory Reagents to Enhance Quantitation of Baculovirus Expression in Serum-free Invertebrate Cell Culture, Focus *13,* 16–18 BRL (1991).

[44] *L. A. King, S. G. Mann, A. M. Lawrie, S. H. Mulshaw,* Replication of Wild-type and Recombinant *Autographa californica* Nuclear Polyhedrosis Virus in a Cell Line Derived from *Mamestra brassicae,* Virus Res. *19,* 93–104 (1991).

[45] *X. Léry, G. Fédière,* A New Serum-free Medium for Lepidopteran Cell Culture, J. Invertebr. Pathol. *55,* 342–349 (1990).

[46] *D. Inlow, A. Shauger, B. Maiorella,* Insect Cell Culture and Baculovirus Propagation in Protein-free Medium, J. Tissue Cult. Methods *12,* 13–16 (1989).

[47] *M. Mitsuhashi, R. H. Goodwin,* The Serum-free Culture of Insect Cells *in vitro,* in: *J. Mitsuhashi* (ed.), Invertebrate Cell System Applications, CRC Press, Boca Raton 1989, pp. 167–182.

[48] *B. G. Corsaro, M. J. Fraser,* Characterization of Cloned Populations of the *Heliothis zea* Cell Line IPLB-HZ 1075, In Vitro Cell. Dev. Biol. *23,* 855–862 (1987).

[49] *V. Deubel, J. P. Digoutte,* Morphogenesis of a Yellow Fever Virus in *Aedes aegypti* Cultured Cells, I. Isolation of Different Cellular Clones and the Study of Their Susceptibility to Infection with the Virus, Am. J. Trop. Med. Hyg. *30,* 1060–1070 (1981).

[50] *E. C. Suitor Jr., L. L. Chang, H. A. Liu,* Establishment and Characterization of a Clone from Grace's *in vitro* Cultured Mosquito *Aedes aegypti* (L.) Cells, Exp. Cell Res. *44,* 572–578 (1966).

[51] *A. H. McIntosh, C. Rechtoris,* Insect Cells: Colony Formation and Cloning in Agar Medium, In Vitro *10,* 1–5 (1974).

[52] *N. Sarver, V. Stollar,* Sindbis Virus-induced Cytopatic Effect of *Aedes albopictus* (Singh) Cells, Virology *80,* 390–400 (1977).

[53] *W. F. Hink, E. M. Strauss,* Semi-continuous Culture of the TN-368 Cell Line in Fermentors with Virus Production in Harvested Cells, in: *E. Kurstak, K. Maramorosch, A. Dübendorfer* (eds.), Invertebrate Systems in Vitro, Elsevier, Amsterdam 1980, pp. 27–33.

[54] *V. Stollar,* Togaviruses in Cultured Arthropod Cells, in: *R. W. Schlesinger* (ed.), The Togaviruses, Academic Press, New York 1980, pp. 583–621.

[55] *A. M. Fallon, V. Stollar,* The Biochemistry and Genetics of Mosquito Cells in Culture, in: *K. Maramorosch* (ed.), Advances in Cell Culture, Vol. 5, Academic Press, New York 1984, pp. 97–137.

[56] *J. S. Culp, H. Johansen, B. Hellmig, J. Beck, T. J. Matthews, A. Delers, M. Rosenberg,* Regulated Expression Allows High Level Production and Secretion of HIV-1 gp120 Envelope Glycoprotein in *Drosophila* Schneider Cells, Bio/Technology *9,* 173–177 (1991).

[57] *G. E. Smith, M. J. Fraser, M. D. Summers,* Molecular Engineering of the *Autographa californica* Nuclear Polyhedrosis Virus Genome: Deletion Mutations within the Polyhedrin Gene, J. Virol. *46,* 584–593 (1983).

3.5   Plant Cells

Hans-Willi Krell

Plant tissue cultures are aseptic *in vitro* cultures of any plant part in a nutrient medium.

During the last century *Scheiden* (1838) and *Schwann* (1839) recognized that cells are the basic functional units of living organisms, but it was not until 1939 that *Nobecourt, Gautheret and White* demonstrated that plant cells can live outside the tissue in a totipotent manner [1]. These authors published independently that infinite growth of non-differentiated cells – the so-called callus – is possible. A single cell can sustain an independent metabolism and can regenerate to a whole plant without any loss of genetic information [2].

Working with cultures of plant tissue has some important advantages over the use of intact plants.

- In tissue culture, cells can be maintained under controlled and constant conditions, free of micro-organisms.
- Cell cultures can be used for the production of secondary metabolites [3].
- Plant cell cultures can be used in biotransformation.
- Plant cells are ideal material for the study of cell metabolism.
- Cells can be used as a source of intermediate metabolites which are difficult to obtain from the whole plant. This is very useful in studying the degradation of xenobiotics or for the elucidation of metabolic pathways.
- In culture, the spectrum of metabolites can differ quantitatively and qualitatively from intact plants; therefore, new metabolites with interesting physiological or pharmacological actions can be found.
- Tissue cultures are used for mass propagation of genetically uniform, economically important crops or ornamental plants.
- By manipulation of single cells, mutants with desired properties (e.g. salt resistance) can be selected.

3.5.1 Setting Up Plant Tissue Cultures

Several very useful methodological and practically – oriented text books have been published on this general area [4, 5, 6].

3.5.1.1 Plant Material

Today almost any tissue can be used to start a culture [7]. First of all, the original tissue must be aseptic [8], and there are two principal ways to achieve this:

1. Cells are derived from plants grown under conditions free of micro-organisms. This is rather simply achieved if seeds can be surface-sterilized (e.g. with 96 % ethanol).
2. Cells from plants grown under greenhouse conditions, are directly separated from the original tissue. In this case, the small tissue pieces must be surface-sterilized in a way that does not damage the inner cells.

Beside nutrient medium and physiological growth factors, the nature of the original plant material will influence growth and development of the *in-vitro* culture [9]. The important factors are genotype, age of the plant, tissue or organ, its physiological state, the original location of the explant within the plant, the method of inoculation, preparation and nurse effects.

3.5.1.2   Induction of a Callus Culture

The cultures are initiated by planting a section of sterile plant tissue on a nutrient medium solidified by agar. It is important for success that the explant is in the right biological state and, generally speaking, young tissues are the most suitable.

Within several weeks a callus may be produced. This is a mass of unorganized cells as produced in a wound response. The callus mass is subcultured by transferring small pieces with a sterile scalpel to fresh agar medium. The pieces transferred should not be too small, as further growth may be inhibited.

3.5.1.3   Suspension Cultures

To establish a suspension culture, a small piece of callus is transferred to a vessel with liquid medium. A relatively large initial inoculum is advantageous. The vessel is placed on a shaker (30–150 rpm), and the shear forces generated will wash cells from the callus and ensure optimal aeration. At the first subculture to fresh medium only the finer or smallest aggregates of cells should be transferred with a pipette. For each cell line there is a characteristic minimum inoculum size below which the culture will not grow. Growth rate and effective dispersion of the culture will depend very much on the plant species. For example, soya cell suspension cultures produce very small aggregates, in contrast to wheat cell suspensions.

The advantages of cell suspension cultures are that large amounts of material may be obtained rapidly, that homogenesus cell populations can be harvested and that growth or metabolism of homogeneous cultures can be examined [10].

3.5.1.4   Haploid Cell Cultures

Cultures of cells with a gametic chromosome number (original chromosome number is reduced by half) may be prepared by a number of means, each of which relies upon abnormal embryo development. Haploid cultures are especially important for the production of homozygous plants by chromosome doubling with the help of, for example, colchicine.

The production of haploid cells *in vitro* can be improved by many different techniques including gynogenensis, androgenesis, chemical treatment or irradiation with X-rays [9]. Androgenesis has become the most important of these [11]. Anthers containing pollen are removed from the plant and placed on a culture medium designed to permit the survival and development of microspores. The optimum requirements for each species are different, and have been described in detail [12].

3.5.1.5   Media

The basic nutritional requirements of cultured plant cells are very similiar to those of whole plants [13]. Nutrient media [6] generally consist of

– macroelements (inorganic salts)
– microelements or trace elements (inorganic salts)
– carbon sources
– organic supplements (vitamins, amino acids),
– phytohormones (growth regulators).

The media often contain chelated iron in the form of ferrous-EDTA, so the availability of iron at pH values up to 8.0 and throughout the growth cycle of the cultures is guaranteed. Usually several inorganic salts and vitamins can be combined to minimize the number of stock solutions that must be prepared.

Without exception, cultured plant cells can use glucose or sucrose equally well. Plant cell culture media are therefore rich in substrates which make growth of fungi or bacteria possible. However, the addition of antimicrobial compounds to the medium can result in complications and phytotoxicity to the explants [14].

Media very useful for cells of many different plant cells, tissues, and organs were first described for tobacco [15, 16], or soybean [17]. The *Murashige & Skoog* (MS) [15], *Gamborg* (B5) [17] and *Schenk & Hildebrand* (SH) [18] media are among those most commonly used. They differ significantly with respect to their nitrogen and phosphorus contents (Table 1).

In the absence of a formulation for a specific medium from the literature, MS, SH or *Gamborg's* B5 standard medium is used, sometimes with variations in the concentrations of the plant growth regulators auxin and cytokinin.

For the best reproducibility, fully defined media should be used if possible. However, some plant cell cultures grow better in the presence of complex supplements such as coconut milk or casein hydrolysate. In such cases large batches should be prepared to avoid variation.

For semi-solid media, agar, 6–10 g/l is added. Before autoclaving the pH should be adjusted to between 5.5 and 6.0. It will drop slightly as a result of the production of sugar acids during autoclaving. Moreover, sucrose can break down into fructose and glucose. As mentioned, autoclaving at too high a temperature can caramelize sugars which may become toxic as a result. Therefore, sterilization procedures should be as short as possible. Normally 121 °C for 20 min is sufficient, so that saccharose in still intact. To avoid precipitation, iron salts should be sterilized separately.

Table 1. Macro-salt content of the most important media (in mg/l) [9]:

Components	Gamborg et al. B5 [17]	Schenk & Hildebrandt [18]	Murashige & Skoog [19]
KNO_3	2 500	2 500	1 900
$NaNO_3$	–	–	–
$Ca(NO_3)_2 \cdot 4H_2O$	–	–	–
NH_4NO_3	–	–	1 650
$(NH_4)_2SO_4$	134	–	–
$NH_4H_2PO_4$	–	300	–
$NaH_2PO_4 \cdot H_2O$	150	–	–
KH_2PO_4	–	–	170
KCl	–	–	–
$CaCl_2 \cdot 2H_2O$	150	200	440
$MgSO_4 \cdot 7H_2O$	250	400	370

Ion contents of the most important media (in mmol/l)

N-total	26.756	27.336	60.017
NH_4^+	2.028	2.608	20.612
NO_3^-	24.728	24.728	39.405
$H_2PO_4^-$	1.087	2.608	1.249
K^+	25.815	24.728	20.042
Ca^{2+}	1.163	1.360	2.993
Mg^{2+}	1.014	1.623	1.501
SO_4^{2-}	2.028	1.623	1.501
Na^+	–	–	–
Cl^-	2.325	2.721	5.986
Total	60.188	61.999	93.289

Micro-salt content of the most important media (in mg/l)

$FeCl_3 \cdot 6H_2O$	–	–	–
$FeSO_4 \cdot 7H_2O$	27.8	15	27.8
$MnSO_4 \cdot 4H_2O$	13.2	13.2	22.3
$ZnSO_4 \cdot 7H_2O$	2.0	1.0	8.6
H_3BO_3	3.0	5.0	6.2
KI	0.75	1.0	0.83
$CuSO_4 \cdot 5H_2O$	0.025	0.2	0.025
$Na_2MoO_4 \cdot 2H_2O$	0.25	0.1	0.25
$CoCl_2 \cdot 6H_2O$	0.025	0.1	0.025
$NiCl_2 \cdot 6H_2O$	–	–	–
$AlCl_3$	–	–	–
Na_2EDTA	37.3	20	37.3

3.5.2   Applications

3.5.2.1   Somaclonal Variation

Genetic variation and mutation occur naturally during cultivation of a plant cells in tissue culture. Culture-associated variability has been called "somaclonal variation", defined as the variation among plants derived from any form of cell culture [19]. Somaclonal variation is particularly valuable in plants which naturally show little variation, and its exploitation permits the selection of numerous types of biochemical and agronomic mutants at the cellular level [20]. The list of agriculturally useful mutant plants selected *in vitro* is growing rapidly [21].

3.5.2.2   Protoplast Fusion

Isolated plant protoplasts are 'naked' cells that have had their cell walls removed either by mechanical action or by enzymatic digestion [22]. The only barrier between the cytoplasm and the external environment becomes the plasma membrane. As a consequence, spontaneous fusion can occur. To speed up the fusion rate, polyethylene glycol (PEG), first described for this purpose in 1974, may be used as a fusogen [23]. The correct amount of PEG to be used must be established experimentally in each system. Over-addition will cause massive agglutination of the protoplasts whereas addition of too little will cause the protoplasts to adhere but not fuse.

3.5.2.3   Transformed (transgenetic) Plants

Combining methods of recombinant DNA and protoplast technologies with classical plant breeding techniques has revolutionized plant improvement. Plant cell transformation can be achieved either by introduction of naked DNA directly into plant cell protoplasts or by using a vector. Such gene vectors include *Agrobacterium* Ti-plasmids, plant DNA viruses, and plant RNA viruses [24].

3.5.2.4   Plant Regeneration

Various cells, tissues and organs from many plant species can be manipulated to regenerate whole plants [25]. This is a very important process, and without it protoplast hybridization, growth and differentiation studies, generation of genetic variant plants, commercial cloning or disease-elimination through meristem culture would be useless [26].

3.5.2.5   Production of Secondary Metabolites

The production of secondary metabolites by plant cell cultures *in vitro* has for a long time been considered a promising alternative to using intact plants for the same purpose. Over 30 cell culture systems are known to be better producers of defined secondary metabolites than their respective parent plants [27]. Plant cells have now been cultured in a wide range of bioreactors in volumes from 21 to 75.0001 [28–32]. However, very few processes have yet reached a commercial application such as in the production of shikonin, a plant pigment derived from *Lithospermum erythrorhizon*, by Mitsui Petrochemical Industries Ltd. [33].

In general, secondary metabolite production is very closely correlated with the growth and morphological differentiation of cells [34]. Metabolites are generally produced at the beginning of the stationary growth phase. Several procedures have been described for the selection of high producing cell lines [35, 36].

References

[1] *R. J. Gautheret,* History of Plant Tissue and Cell Culture: A Personal Account, in: *I. K. Vasil* (ed.), Cell Cultures and Somatic Cell Genetics of Plants, Vol. 2, Academic Press, Orlando 1985, pp. 1–59.

[2] *M. G. K. Jones, A. Karp,* Plant Tissue Culture Technology and Crop Improvement, in: *A. Mizrahi, A. L. van Wezel* (eds.), Advances in Biotechnological Processes, Vol. 5, Alan R. Liss Inc., New York 1985, pp. 91–122.

[3] *O. Sahai, M. Knuth,* Commercializing Plant Tissue Culture Processes: Economics, Problems and Prospects, Biotechn. Prog. *1,* 1–9 (1985).

[4] *I. K. Vasil* (ed.), Cell Culture and Somatic Cell Genetics of Plants, Academic Press, Orlando 1984

[5] *L. R. Wetter, F. Constabel* (eds.), Plant Tissue Culture Methods, National Research Council of Canada, NRCC 19876, Saskatoon 1982.

[6] *R. A. Dixon,* Plant Cell Culture, IRL Press, Oxford 1985.

[7] *O. L. Gamborg,* Callus and Cell Culture, in: *L. R. Wetter, F. Constabel* (eds.), Plant Tissue Culture Methods, National Research Council of Canada, NRCC 19876, Saskatoon 1982, pp. 1–9.

[8] *C. Leifert, W. M. Waites,* Contaminants of Plant Tissue Cultures, Newsletter International Association for Plant Tissue Culture *60,* 2–13 (1990).

[9] *R. L. M. Pierik,* In Vitro Culture of Higher Plants, Martinus Niyhoff Publishers, Dordrecht 1987.

[10] *P. J. King,* Induction and Maintenance of Cell Suspension Cultures, in: *I. K. Vasil* (ed.), Cell Culture and Somatic Cell Genetics of Plants, Academic Press, Orlando 1984, pp. 130–138.

[11] *B. Foroughi-Wehr, G. Wenzel,* Androgenetic Haploid Production, Newsletter International Association for Plant Tissue Culture *58,* 11–18 (1989).

[12] *J. M. Dunwell,* Haploid Cell Culture, in: *R. A. Dixon* (ed.), Plant Cell Culture, IRL Press, Oxford 1985, pp. 21–36.

[13] *O. L. Gamborg*, Plant Cell Cultures: Nutrition and Media, in: *I. K. Vasil* (ed.), Cell Culture and Somatic Cell Genetics of Plants, Vol. 1, Academic Press, Orlando 1984, pp. 18–26.

[14] *R. H. Smith*, Establishment of Calli and Suspension Cultures, in: *A. Weissbach, H. Weissbach* (eds.), Methods for Plant Molecular Biology, Academic Press, San Diego 1988, pp. 343–353.

[15] *T. Murashige, F. Skoog*, A Revised Medium for Rapid Growth and Bioassays with Tobacco Cultures, Physiol. Plant. *15*, 473–479 (1962).

[16] *E. M. Linsmaier, F. Skoog*, Organic Growth Factor Requirements of Tobacco Tissue Culture, Physiol. Plant *18*, 100–127 (1965).

[17] *O. L. Gamborg, R. A. Miller, K. Ojima*, Nutrient Requirements of Suspension Cultures of Soybean Root Cells, Exp. Cell Res. *50*, 151–158 (1968).

[18] *R. U. Schenk, A. C. Hildebrandt*, Medium and Techniques for Induction and Growth of Monocotyledonous and Dicotyledonous Plant Cell Cultures, Can. J. Bot. *50*, 199–204 (1972).

[19] *W. R. Scowcroft*, Somaclonal Variation: The Myth of Clonal Uniformity, in: *B. Hohn, E. S. Dennis* (eds.), Plant Gene Research: Basic Knowledge and Application, Genetic Flux in Plants, Springer, New York 1985, pp. 217–245.

[20] *D. A. Evans, W. R. Sharp*, Somaclonal Variation and its Application in Plant Breeding, Newsletter International Association for Plant Tissue Culture *54*, 2–10 (1988).

[21] *B. T. Reisch*, Genetic Instability in Plant Cell Cultures: Utilization in Plant Breeding and Genetic Studies, in: *M. S. S. Pais, F. Mavituna, J. M. Novais* (eds.), NATO ASI Series, Vol. 18, Springer, Berlin 1988, pp. 87–95.

[22] *T. Bengochea, J. H. Dodds*, Plant Protoplasts, Chapman and Hall, London 1986.

[23] *K. N. Kao, M. R. Michayluk*, A Method for High Frequency Intergeneric Fusion of Plant Protoplasts, Planta *115*, 355–367 (1974).

[24] *F. Mavituna*, Introduction to Plant Biotechnology, in: *M. S. S. Pais, F. Mavituna, J. N. Novais*, NATO ASI Series, Vol. 18, Springer, Berlin 1988, pp. 1–14.

[25] *B. Tisserat*, Embryogenesis, Organogenesis and Plant Regeneration, in: *R. A. Dixon* (ed.), Plant Cell Culture, IRL Press, Oxford 1985, pp. 79–105.

[26] *B. Tisserat, E. B. Esan, T. Murashige*, Somatic Embryogenesis in Angiosperms, Hortic. Rev. *1*, 1–76 (1977).

[27] *M. Wink*, Physiology of the Accumulation of Secondary Metabolites with Special Reference to Alkaloids, in: *F. Constabel, I. K. Vasil* (eds.), Cell Cultures and Somatic Cell Genetics of Plants, Vol. 4, Academic Press, San Diego 1988, pp. 17–42.

[28] *M. W. Fowler*, Large-Scale Cultures of Cells in Suspension, in: *I. K. Vasil* (ed.), Cell Culture and Somatic Cell Genetics of Plants, Academic Press, Orlando 1984, pp. 167–174.

[29] *M. W. Fowler, A. H. Scragg*, Natural Products from Higher Plants and Plant Cell Cultures, in: *M. S. S. Pais, F. Mavituna, J. M. Novais* (eds.), Plant Cell Biotechnology, Springer Verlag, Heidelberg 1988, pp. 165–177.

[30] *M. Luckner*, Secondary Metabolism in Microorganisms, Plants, and Animals, Gustav Fischer Verlag, Jena 1990.

[31] *E. Rittershaus, J. Ulrich, K. Westphal*, Large-Scale Production of Plant Cell Cultures, Newsletter International Association for Plant Tissue Culture *61*, 2–10 (1990).

[32] *K. Westphal*, Large Scale Production of New Biologically Active Compounds in Plant Cell Cultures, Abstracts VIIth Int. Congress on Plant Tissue and Cell Culture, Amsterdam 1990, p. 326.

[33] *H. Deno, C. Suga, T. Morimoto, Y. Fujita*, Production of Shikonin Derivatives by Cell Suspension Cultures of *Lithospermum erythrorhizon*, Plant Cell Rep. *6*, 197–199 (1987).

[34] *M. Sakatu, A. Komamine*, Cell Growth and Accumulation of Secondary Metabolites, in: *F. Constabel, I. K. Vasil* (eds.), Cell Cultures and Somatic Cell Genetics of Plants, Vol. 4, Academic Press, San Diego 1988, pp. 97–114.

[35] *J. M. Widholm*, Selection of Mutants Which Accumulate Desirable Secondary Compounds, in: *F. Constabel, I. K. Vasil* (eds.), Cell Cultures and Somatic Cell Genetics of Plants, Vol. 4, Academic Press, San Diego 1988, pp. 125–137.

[36] *U. Eilert*, Elicitation: Methodology and Aspects of Application, in: *F. Constabel, I. K. Vasil* (eds.), Cell Cultures and Somatic Cell Genetics of Plants, Vol. 4, Academic Press, San Diego 1988, pp. 153–196.

3.6   Prokaryotic Cells

Matthias C. C. Poetsch

Monod [1] was the first to demonstrate that the kinetics of growth in bacterial systems obeyed the *Michaelis-Menten* equation for enzymatic substrate conversion to product. He presented experimental data which fitted exactly the mathematical relationship for enzyme kinetics in non-inhibited systems, *Monod's* equation is described as follows

$$\mu = \mu_{max} \frac{S}{K_S + S} \;.$$

The specific growth rate μ of an organism depends on the concentration of the growth-limiting substrate (S) in the medium. K_S is the *Monod* saturation constant, numerically equal to the substrate concentration at which $\mu = 1/2 \, \mu_{max}$. Its maximum value, which expresses the unrestricted function of an entire set of active enzymes, can be achieved only under the condition of excess medium components and it depends critically on the constancy of physical parameters (dicussed below). Under certain conditions, deviations from μ_{max} indicate that the regulatory situation has diverged from unrestricted growth or metabolic functioning. This is normally due to the presence of inhibitors, unusual substrates or undefined limitations of nutrients [2].

During the growth of prokaryotic cells in batch cultures (e. g. shaking flasks) the environment will change continuously. Therefore, growth rate may be lowered, for example by a decrease in pH to suboptimal levels, although substrate has not yet become limiting. To counteract these changes in physicochemical parameters, long term cultures are carried out in fermenters that are equipped with controlling devices to maintain constant conditions. The greater volume of fermenters compared with conventional flask cultures enables samples to be taken during the course of the culture in which intracellular products within the biomass may be checked or analysed.

This section introduces basic principles of prokaryotic cell culture. Advanced methods of fermentation technology, fermenter instrumentation and control have been described in detail by, for example, *Pirt* [3] and *Wang* et al. [4] which are recommended for further reading.

3.6.1   Bioreactors

Fermenters are closed culture vessels fitted with a gas inlet and agitator. They have additional features for maintaining optimal growth conditions, monitoring the physiological state and growth kinetics, and controlling the process. A standard bioreactor is illustrated in Fig. 1.

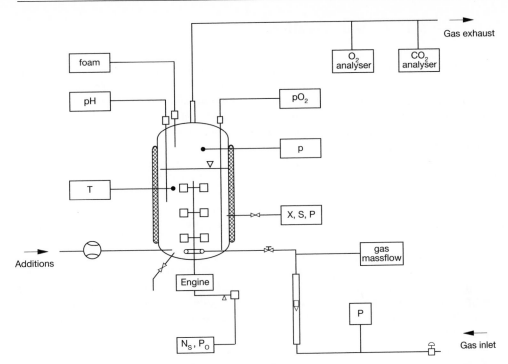

Fig. 1. Standard bioreactor instrumentation scheme in which the boxes represent measurement and input of the values into automatic control systems: negative logarithm of hydrogen ion concentration (pH), pressure (p), temperature (T), dissolved oxygen (pO_2), concentrations of biomass (X), substrate (S) and product (P) in the culture, concentration of O_2 and CO_2 in the gas exhaust (O_2- and CO_2-analyser), speed number of the stirrer (N_S), external power for the agitator (P_0), and gas mass flow and pressure (p) in the gas inlet.

The construction is usually of high grade stainless steel to prevent corrosion or leakage of toxic metal salts into the growth medium. Furthermore, all surfaces or modules that come in contact with wet heat during sterilization need to be resistant to the procedure. A perfect reactor system maintains high mass transfer and short mixing times, it prevents concentration gradients and any effects of flotation or sedimentation, wall growth or overflow of foam, while ensuring sterile operating conditions.

Although many attempts have been made to develop new mixing systems, it is surprising that the fermenters commonly used for industrial production are closely related to the stirred tank reactor (STR) described below. *Schügerl* [5], in his comprehensive review, lists and evaluates the various systems for mixing and agitation. Only the group of air-lift reactors, as reviewed by *Schügerl* [5, 6] and *Sittig* [7], represent a real alternative to the STR. It should be noted that a valid comparision of various agitation and aeration systems can only be made with data from bioprocesses that use identical strains and media.

Provision must be made in the fermenter for the addition of the culture inoculum, supplementary media requirements and other components (e. g. inducers) under sterile conditions.

3.6.1.1   Mixing and Aeration

The mixing process has several functions. It is required for uniform temperature throughout the reactor and for accurate pH control. Mixing also has to provide optimal supplies of nutrients and gas (i. e. oxygen). Most industrial fermentations applied to the large scale cultivation of microbes are aerobic processes, although the supply of dissolved oxygen to the fermentation broth is a fundamental problem. Oxygen is quite insoluble in aqueous solutions (ca. 6.6–8.1 mg/l water at 25–40°C and 101 kPa). The maximum oxygen absorption rate has been found to be limited to about 15 mmol/l per h in a roller bottle [8], and about 50 mmol/l per h in 500 ml *Erlenmeyer* flasks containing 50 ml medium [9]. In small cultures up to a volume of 1 l it is possible to achieve cell densities of 1–2 g/l dry wt before oxygen becomes limiting. In general, in modern fermentation equipment, a transfer of oxygen around 200 mmol/l per h is achieved at an operation rate of 1 v/v per min and 500 cm/s tip speed.

In large scale culture, and at high cell density, the oxygen demand may be satisfied by vigorous aeration and/or increased presure (101–150 kPa). In the classical STR the agitation and aeration system may consist of a 3–4 stage flat blade turbine (FBT) with *Rushton* impellers combined with several baffles, and a gas sparger at the bottom of the vessel. Typical dimensions of the elements of this system are described, for example, by *Finn* [10].

3.6.1.2   Temperature and pH Control

Heat exchange is achieved by passing steam or cooling water through the vessel jacket and/or coils inside the vessel. First of all the vessel containing the medium is heated to 121°C for 20 min to sterilize it. The temperature is then adjusted to the optimum for the growth of the particular prokaryote. During growth of the culture, metabolic heat can be countered by cooling and thermostatic regulation. Finally, the culture is cooled rapidly in order to stop all metabolic processes during harvest of the cells and further preparation of the products.

While the prokaryotes are growing, the pH of the surrounding medium changes due to the metabolism of the cells. Usually, the pH is monitored in the fermentation broth on-line with a pH probe *in situ*. To maintain a fixed pH, acid and alkali from sterile reservoirs are added, which may be connected to the reactor by flexible tubings. Avoid the use of $CaCO_3$ in vessels with a bottom drive to prevent damage to the mechanical seals.

3.6.1.3   Foam Control

Foaming as a result of agitation and aeration of the growing culture can be detected by means of a simple probe placed above the medium in the headspace of a fermenter.

When the foam touches the probe it completes an electrical circuit and this activates a mechanical foam-breaker or a pump connected to a supply of an anti-foaming reagent. The amount of anti-foam added throughout the entire fermentation run should not exceed more than 1% of final volume to prevent any impairment during downstream processing.

3.6.1.4   Sterilization

One of the main problems in long term cultivation is maintaining a pure culture. Sterilize the entire fermenter and ancillary equipment *in situ* with steam prior to inoculation. In addition, sterilize by filtration the gas supplied during the fermentation and the exhaust gas. This is not only a safety requirement with respect to the prevention of contamination of the pure culture and the products therein, but it also prevents the release of organisms into the environment. No mechanical breaks should occur anywhere in the fermenter system that will allow the entry of micro-organisms. At the point where the agitator shaft enters the vessel, sterility is maintained by double mechanical seals, which are lubricated with condensed steam. Furthermore, storage tanks for acid, alkali, anti-foam emulsion, substrate and other additives have to be filled and connected to the vessel under sterile conditions.

3.6.2   Characteristics of the Culture Procedure

3.6.2.1   Media

The composition of culture media will depend on the organism, the desired growth and yield of products, and the energy requirements of the organism during the process [2]. Estimates of the yield can be made from the elementary composition of the biomass. The requirements of different micro-organisms and the preparation of appropriate media have been described (cf. 2.8.3).

3.6.2.2   From Colony to Large Scale Culture

The size of the inoculum for prokaryotes is generally a mid- or end- log phase culture of the order of 0.3–10% of the total end-volume of the fermentation medium. If it is smaller, or the concentration of the cells in the inoculum is low, the lag phase of the inoculated culture may be prolonged before growth commences. Therefore, the inoculum for a large scale fermentation is usually prepared stepwise, beginning in shaking flasks followed by preculturing in fermenters with a three- to ten-fold increase in volume. Because the operating conditions are different on each scale, there is a need for further process development by scaling up, especially with regard to the parameters for the conditions of mixing and aeration.

A possible strategy for scale up could involve, for example, attaining constancy in the volumetric oxygen transfer rate, impeller tip speed, volumetric power input and equal mixing times [4].

3.6.2.3   Monitoring and Control of Fermentation

In fermenters, several on-line parameters are monitored, and automatic control systems maintain a constant environment (above). On the other hand, physical and chemical parameters can be monitored by suitable sensors or off-line readings, in order to obtain additional information on the physiological state of the cells. They can be measured directly or by "gateway" sensors: for example, the pH control coupled with differential and integral monitoring of base addition can give the rate of acid product formation. The estimation of the biomass, if it is not carried out by light scattering or determination of metabolites within the cells in off-line samples, can be calculated from the rate of CO_2 evolution measured by the analysis of exhaust gas. Metabolites can also be measured on-line in the supernatant and in crude extracts of the cells by use of autoanalysers [11]. For an introduction to fermentation instrumentation, control and computer applications consult, for example, *Wang* et al. [4].

3.6.2.4   Kinetics of Growth in Batch Culture

For batch fermentations, sterilize the bioreactor and fill with sterile medium before inoculation. The organism is allowed to grow such that, during the course of the process, nutrients will be consumed; add acid or alkali and an anti-foam agent as necessary (manually or automatically). Air or other gases are supplied continuously usually by sparging; excess gases and the exhaust gases are then given up from the liquid phase. On completion, harvest the biomass and/or supernatant. Prepare the bioreactor for the next run.

In a batch culture the specific growth rate (μ) changes through about six phases. In the lag phase, inoculated cells rest and attain physicochemical equilibration with the environment ($\mu \approx 0$). During the following period the cells start an accelerated growing phase with an increasing μ. When the maximum specific growth rate is achieved the culture will grow at μ_{max} in the logarithmic phase until growth becomes limited. Then μ will fall in a decline phase which leads to a steady state in a stationary phase in which cell growth and lysis are in equilibrium ($\mu \approx 0$). Finally, lysis of cells will predominate in the so called death phase ($\mu < 0$).

When it is desired to obtain primary metabolic products which normally reach their maximum concentrations during the logarithmic phase, harvest the culture in the late logarythmic phase. If, in contrast, the product is a secondary metabolite, its accumulation will occur late in the growth cycle or stationary phase and thus harvest it much later and at the optimal product concentration.

There are different types of fed batch culture in which a single substrate or the full medium may be added once or repeatedly by pulsation. Alternatively, medium may be added continuously and depending on the physiological state of the culture (e.g., a set-point is given by pH or pO_2). This can influence biochemical pathways and the intracellular metabolic control. The type of feeding will depend on the kind of product sought, the kinetics of its formation and whether a soluble protein or an inclusion body is desired.

3.6.2.5   Kinetics of Growth in Continuous Culture

In continuous fermentation, raw materials are supplied to the bioreactor at a rate volumetrically equal to that at which product and spent medium are withdrawn.

As summarized by *Pimrose* [12], for unicellular microbes growing exponentially in a nutrient medium, the rate of change of cell number (n) with time (t) is proportional to the number of cells, that is

$$\frac{dn}{dt} = \mu n$$

where the specific growth rate (μ) is the constant of proportionality. Eventually, if some nutrient becomes limiting, μ will decrease proportionally to the consumption of the nutrient. In practice therefore, in continuous cultures fresh nutrients are added constantly to the medium and an equal volume of culture is removed concurrently, so that the total volume of the culture remains the same throughout culture.

In *turbidostats* the turbidity of the culture is monitored constantly and when it exceeds a pre-set value the culture will be diluted by the addition of fresh medium and the removal of an equal volume by an overflow mechanism.

In *chemostats* all nutrients except one are maintained in excess. Thus the concentration of the limiting substrate determines cell density. If fresh medium is added to a chemostat at a rate F and the volume of medium is V, then the rate of loss of organisms from the fermenter is given by:

$$-\frac{dn}{dt} = \frac{F}{V} n = Dn$$

The ratio F/V is known as the dilution rate (D). At the steady state, dn/dt should be zero, in which case $\mu = D$. Clearly, if D is allowed to exceed μ, cells will be lost from the culture faster than they can grow and washout will occur.

In a chemostat culture cells propagate at submaximal rates except when the value of D approaches that of μ. The nutrients which can be used to limit growth include sources of carbon, nitrogen, phosphorus, sulphur or metal ions. Different limiting nutrients effect cell physiology in different ways. Consequently, the chemostat culture is an appropriate tool for quantitative and qualitative research. It can also be used to study the competition of prokaryotes for growth-limiting substrates and for the selection of mutants or strains with a better K_m for the corresponding enzyme related to the substrate. In a turbidostat culture, however, cells grow at the maximum rate possible within the selected medium chosen.

Two advantages of continuous culture compared to batch culture are that the growth rate of the cells can be maintained at a value that is optimal for product formation, and that the environment surrounding the cells remains constant.

3.6.2.6   Harvest of Cells

When the fermentation process is completed, recover the desired product which may be located in or as part of the biomass, or as a metabolite present in the supernatant. Downstream processing can be started by cooling the culture within the bioreactor, or by pumping the culture over a heat exchanger. Sediment the biomass by centrifugation. The clarified supernatant will contain metabolites and (extracellular) enzymes. Many methods are available for their recovery, including ion-exchange chromatography, precipitation and solvent extraction. If the desired product is contained within the cells, disrupt the cells. Among several methods, high pressure homogenization or disruption in a high speed bead mill is usually suitable for large scale preparations.

References

[1] *J. Monod*, Recherche sur la Croissance des Cultures Bacteriennes, Herman, Paris 1940.
[2] *A. Fiechter*, Physical and Chemical Parameters of Microbial Growth, in: *A. Fiechter* (ed.), Adv. Biochem. Eng. Biotechnol. *30*, 7–60 (1984).
[3] *S. J. Pirt*, Principles of Microbe and Cell Cultivation, Blackwell Scientific Publications, Oxford 1975.
[4] *D. I. C. Wang, C. L. Cooney, A. L. Demain, P. Dunnill, A. E. Humphrey, M. D. Lilley*, Fermentation and Enzyme Technology, John Wiley & Sons, New York 1979.
[5] *K. Schügerl*, Neue Bioreaktoren für Aerobe Prozesse, Chem. Ing. Tech. *52*, 951–965 (1980).
[6] *K. Schügerl*, Verwendung von Blasensäulen als Bioreaktoren, in: *R. L. Lafferty* (ed.), Rothenburger Symposium 1978, Fermentationstechnik, Gutenberg, Melsungen 1978.
[7] *W. Sittig*, Biochemische Reaktionen, Fortschr. Verfahrenstech. *15*, 354–369 (1977).
[8] *B. M. Hall*, Performance of Roller Agitators for Cultivation of Microorganisms, Appl. Microbiol. *8*, 378–382 (1960).

[9] *D. Freedmann*, The Shaker in Bioengineering, Process Biochem. *4*, 35–40 (1969).

[10] *R. K. Finn*, Agitation – Aeration in the Laboratory and in Industry, Bacteriol. Rev. *18*, 254–274 (1954).

[11] *N. Ahlmann, A. Niehoff, U. Rinas, T. Scheper, K. Schügerl*, Continuous On-line Monitoring of Intracellular Enzyme Activity, in: *H. Chmiel, W. P. Hammen, J. E. Bailey* (eds.), Biochemical Engineering, Fischer, Stuttgart, New York 1987.

[12] *M. B. Pimrose*, Modern Biotechnology, Scientific Publications Heidelberg 1987.

4 Cell Fractionation and Purification

4.1   General

Norman A. Staines

The study of cells requires in many cases that they are used as pure populations or that components or organelles are purified from them for study. Accordingly, many sections of this book are devoted to the isolation and culture of some of the many different types of cells that are the important objects of investigation.

Cell separation methods are designed to yield pure or relatively pure populations of cells of defined phenotype. Such methods exploit the fact that cells differ in their size, density, charge or adherence characteristics. One special approach to the physical separation of cells utilises the exquisite specificity of antibodies against cell surface antigens to isolate cells of particular phenotypes. This is dealt with in section 4.2 which covers methods that either involve adherence of cells to an antibody-coated matrix or use preparative flow cytometry that itself can identify cells according to their antibody-defined phenotype, size and granularity. Further discussion of analytical flow cytometric methods will be found in 5.11.

Without recourse to antibody-based methods, the two cardinal ways in which cells can be separated and purified depend upon simple adherence methods, described in 4.2, or upon centrifugation methods (cf. 2.2 and 4.3). These methods are relatively cheap to use, but it is important to remember that their successful application in purifying cells will depend upon the availability of ways of assessing cell purity according to the physical or morphological properties of the cells.

There are special problems involved in working with cells from living donors, especially humans. For this reason, tissue biopsy material is centrally important as it can be obtained in amounts that satisfy both ethical standards and scientific imperatives. In section 4.3 biopsy methods are discussed and the ways in which biopsied tissue can be fractionated into its component parts are dealt with in detail. The fractionation methods are relevant to animal and human tissue material recovered *post mortem*, and not just to small samples from living donors. Other aspects of tissue disintegration and fractionation have been considered in section 2.2 of Volume 2 of this series.

4.2   Differential Adherence and Antibody-based Methods

Deborah J. Bevan

4.2.1   Methods Employing Cell Adherence to a Solid Matrix

Various materials and surfaces have been used as matrices for the removal of adherent cells from a variety of populations. They include glass beads, nylon wool, plastic and cross-linked dextrans. *Shortman* et al. [1] and *Elliot* et al. [2] have utilized glass beads in column chromatography in order to remove adherent cells from heterogeneous suspensions. The adhering cells may subsequently be recovered from the column by the addition of EDTA to the Mg^{2+}- and Ca^{2+}-deficient washing buffer. Nylon wool columns, as devised by *Julius* et al. [3], form a substrate to which macrophages and B-cells adhere allowing T-cells to pass through the column. Sequential adherence, to remove and/or to enrich macrophages and/or dendritic cells, by allowing cells to adhere to plastic *Petri* dishes within prescribed time periods is described by *Klinkert* et al. [4] and *Van Voorhis* [5]. Species differences occur with regard to the adherence properties of cells, as is demonstrated by dendritic cells: rat dendritic cells are not adherent whereas those of human and mouse origin show transient adherence.

The distinction between "physical" and "active" adherence has been made by *Shortman* et al. [1]. The active adherence of cells is temperature-dependent, appears to correlate with the phagocytic activity of the cells and requires calcium and magnesium ions (Ca^{2+}, Mg^{2+}), whereas physical adherence is temperature-independent and is enhanced by a lack of serum in the handling medium. It is important to be aware that monocyte adherence provides a regulatory signal resulting in the induction of high levels of expression of the TNFα and CSF-1 genes [6]. Therefore, monocytes harvested by means of adherence methods will not be typical of a "resting" population.

Note: The fetal calf serum (FCS) used in these methods is heat-inactivated (56 °C, 30 min). Room temperature is assumed to be 22 °C.

4.2.1.1   Glass Bead Column Filtration for Removal of Adherent Cells

1. Acid wash (HCl, 1 mol/l) glass beads of approximately 300 μm diameter followed by 6 washes in distilled water and subsequent siliconizing using dichlorodimethylsilane. Wash again with several changes of distilled water and dry. If a sterile separation is required the beads may be autoclaved.
2. Plug a 30 ml syringe with a siliconized glass wool plug and attach a 3-way tap and 21 gauge needle to the syringe.
3. Turn the tap off and add 15 ml saline (0.9% w/v NaCl) to the syringe. Resuspend the glass beads in saline and, using a *Pasteur* pipette, introduce the beads below the liquid's surface up to the 30 ml mark. To assist the beads in settling allow the saline to flow through the column slowly (1 drop/s).
4. Wash the column with 60 ml HBSS without bicarbonate, seal and equilibrate at 37 °C.
5. Run 30 ml warm HBSS containing 10–20% (v/v) FCS into the column and stop the flow when the medium is just above the beads.
6. Resuspend the cells in HBSS/20% FCS to a concentration of 5×10^7/ml. Add 4 ml cell suspension to the top, and allow it to enter the column. Rinse the cells into the column with a further 4 ml of medium.
7. Elute the non-adherent cells with 30 ml warm medium, collect and centrifuge the cells (200 x*g*, 10 min) and resuspend in fresh medium.
   Note: The cells should take approximately 10 min to be eluted from the column. If necessary, adjust the flow rate to achieve this.
8. Recover the adherent cells by elution with Ca^{2+}- and Mg^{2+}-free HBSS containing 5% FCS using either of the following. (a) Wash with 2 column volumes of medium by reverse flow pumping; or (b) seal the column, gently invert and allow the beads to settle, then flush cells out of the column by the addition of further medium. Pellet cells by centrifugation and resuspend in fresh medium.

4.2.1.2   Gel Filtration for Removal of Adherent Cells

Sephadex G-10 (*Pharmacia*) may be used to remove monocytes from cell preparations [7, 8].

1. Add 10 g Sephadex G-10 to 100 ml saline, gently swirl and allow the beads to swell for 3 h at room temperature or overnight at 4 °C. Decant and discard any fine particles which do not sediment; add fresh saline; gently mix and allow the gel to settle. Decant any remaining fines. If necessary, the Sephadex may be autoclaved at this stage.
2. Weigh out about 1.5 g each of 300 μm and 500–600 μm diameter glass beads (keep separate) and prepare as detailed in 4.2.1.1. The beads may then be autoclaved if desired.

3. To prepare a 15 ml column take a 20 ml plastic syringe, remove the plunger and attach a 3-way tap. Pour the larger beads into the column followed by the smaller beads, close the tap and add 4 ml HBSS-5% FCS (medium) to the column.
4. Remove sufficient saline from the Sephadex suspension so that a thick slurry is formed (about 75% settled gel content).
5. Pour the Sephadex slurry down the column's inside wall until it reaches the top of the column. Open the tap and allow the medium to run out of the column which assists the bedding-down of the Sephadex. Continue topping-up the column with a total volume of 40 ml fresh medium, ensuring that the column does not dry out. Close the tap.
6. Add 1×10^8 cells in 4 ml medium to the column, open the tap and allow the cells to enter the gel bed. Wash out the non-adherent cells with 30 ml medium.

4.2.1.3   Affinity Chromatography

Attachment of ligands to a matrix, for example, lectins or protein A conjugated to agarose beads, can be used to provide a more specific column adherence method for cell selection. *Schlossman & Hudson* [9] were amongst the first to utilize affinity chromatography for cell depletion. They conjugated anti-Fab antibodies to Sephadex and used this matrix to deplete cell suspensions of B-cells. Cells may be incubated with specific mAbs prior to adherence to a protein A-Sepharose column; lectins such as *Helix pomatia* lectin or wheat germ lectin conjugated to agarose will bind specific subsets of lymphocytes. Lymphocytes bound to lectin-conjugated columns may be released by competition with the appropriate free sugar [10]. These methods will not be detailed here: a good source of information is the *Pharmacia/LKB* booklets on cell chromatography.

4.2.1.4   Nylon Wool Adherence

Julius et al. [3] and *Greaves & Brown* [11], working with mouse and human cells respectively, were able to demonstrate that cell suspensions could be depleted of macrophages and B-cells by passage over nylon wool. Excellent purifications for T-cells may be obtained with this method (98–99% T-cells).

1. Place the nylon wool (*Travenol,* 3 denier) in boiling distilled water for 10 min, allow it to cool, rinse in 6 changes of distilled water and dry in a dust-free environment.
2. Gently tease apart 0.6 g of the dry nylon wool and pack it into a 10 ml syringe up to the 6 ml mark.
3. Rinse column with 25 ml BSS followed by 25 ml BSS containing 5% FCS (medium). Fill the column with fresh medium, seal and incubate at 37 °C for 30 min.

4. Wash the column with 25 ml warm (37 °C) medium, add the cells (maximum 1×10^8) in 2 ml medium and allow them to enter the column. Add 0.5 ml medium to the top of column and seal. Incubate for 30 min at 37 °C.
5. Attach a 3-way tap and 21 gauge needle to the column. Elute the non-adherent cells with 25 ml warm medium. Adjust the flow rate to approximately 1 drop/s.
6. The adherent cells may be forcibly eluted from the column by the addition of cold normal saline followed by insertion and depression of the plunger. However, it is recommended not to use this method for macrophage or B-cell enrichment as the viability of the recovered cells is very low.

4.2.1.5   Sequential Adherence for Purification/Removal of Monocytes and Dendritic Cells

Macrophages and dendritic cells (DCs) have both been shown to act as antigen-presenting cells. Of the two cell types, dendritic cells are the more potent accessory cells [4, 5]. Isolation of DCs has been hampered by their rarity and also by lack of unique cell surface markers. This has necessitated lengthy purification procedures based on physical criteria. DCs from lymphoid tissue may be more suitable for functional studies than those obtained from blood since peripheral DCs may undergo further differentiation [12].

Macrophages may be separated from DCs by differential adherence [13] and also by removing Fc receptor-positive (FcR+) cells (macrophages are FcR+, DCs are not) by EA rosetting. DCs of human and mouse origin are transiently adherent and may be isolated from heterogeneous populations by overnight adherence. Unfortunately, rat DCs do not adhere at all [14]; therefore, a different approach is required in order to isolate these cells.

Isolation of dendritic cells of mouse or human origin

1. Resuspend 5×10^7 peripheral blood mononuclear cells (PBMC) in 25 ml RPMI 1640-5% FCS. Add to a 100 mm plastic *Petri* dish and incubate for 1 h at 37 °C in 5% CO_2 in air.
2. Remove the non-adherent cells (mainly T- and B-cells) with 4 rinses of medium. Add fresh medium to the plate and incubate for a further 16 h at 37 °C.
3. Remove non-adherent cells (rich in DCs) with 4 rinses of medium. Recover adherent monocytes by adding PBS containing EDTA 10 mmol/l buffered to pH 7.2 to the plate and incubating for 20 min at room temperature followed by swirling of the plate.
4. Remove residual monocytes from the DC-rich fraction by re-adhering the cells for 1 h at 37 °C.

5. Remove any remaining T-, B- or FcR$^+$-cells by simultaneous rosetting with E (for human T-cells) and EA (anti-immunoglobulin conjugated SRBC and anti-CD3 conjugated SRBC) (mouse or human B-cells).

Isolation of rat dendritic cells

1. Add 5×10^7 mononuclear cells in 25 ml of medium to a 100 mm plastic *Petri* dish and incubate for 1 h at 37 °C.
2. Remove non-adherent cells (T-, B- and DCs) with 4 rinses of the plate.
3. The non-adherent fraction may be depleted of T-, B- and FcR$^+$-cells by panning and/or rosetting (cf. 4.2.2.2, 4.2.2.3). Use EA and SRBC conjugated with anti-immunoglobulin and anti-CD3 antibodies for simultaneous rosetting. Alternatively, coat plates with anti-rat immunoglobulin (whole molecule) or anti-mouse immunoglobulin for direct and indirect panning respectively.

Various authors have used density gradient separation on BSA. Percoll or metrizamide as an initial purification step (cf. 2.2). The low density fraction has been shown to be enriched for DCs [14–16]. This procedure may be used in conjunction with the above methods.

4.2.2   Cell Separation Methods Utilizing Antibodies

Cell separation techniques based on the use of defined antibodies (usually monoclonal) that bind to specific cell surface structures may be seen to be superior in fractionating complex cell mixtures to those techniques, such as density gradient centrifugation, which utilize the physical attributes of cells. Indeed, the physical methods of cell separation are often used as a preliminary purification step. The great advantage of the antibody-based techniques is their exquisite specificity. Cytotoxic antibodies and complement may be used to ablate particular cell types which share a specific antigen. Alternatively, the antibody is attached or coated onto a solid matrix, which may be a cell, a paramagnetic bead or a plastic surface, and the specifically adhering cells may be harvested or discarded (positive or negative selection, respectively).

Immunologically-based techniques are dependent on the specificity and activity of the primary antibody or protein used. Care must be taken in the selection of a suitable antibody particularly with regard to its possible cross-reactions.

4.2.2.1   Complement-mediated Cytolysis

The ablation of subpopulations of cells expressing a specific antigen by the relevant antibody is necessarily restricted to those antibodies which are capable of fixing complement. Mouse mAbs of the IgG_1 isotype do not do this, for example. This method of negative selection may be either a one- or two-step procedure.

Batches of complement should be tested for their inherent toxicity (natural antibodies) against cells. If a low-toxicity batch cannot be found, pre-screened batches may be purchased or pre-absorption of the serum with cells may be carried out. Rabbit serum has been found to be preferable as a source of complement with autologous systems such as HLA typing [17], rather than guinea-pig serum. However, some mAbs appear to work more efficiently with guinea-pig serum. If fresh serum is to be the source of complement it should be used within 30 min of harvesting or, alternatively, it may be stored frozen at -70 °C but should not be refrozen after thawing.

A "cocktail" of cytotoxic antibodies may be used in this method providing that they do not compete for the same epitope(s).

One-step method

Mg^{2+} and Ca^{2+} must be present in the medium.

1. Add 2 ml antibody at appropriate dilution in BSS (previously titrated) to 5×10^7 pelleted cells. Add complement at a suitable concentration (usually at 10 to 20% final concentration). Mix and incubate for 1 h at 37 °C in a shaking water-bath.
2. Wash the cells twice in BSS-2% FCS; resuspend the cells and layer onto a Ficoll-Hypaque density gradient. Centrifuge for 15 min at $1000 \times g$.
3. Harvest the viable cells from the interface and wash twice in BSS-FCS.

Two-step method

Based on the method of *Hercend* et al. [18].

1. Add 1 ml of antibody at appropriate dilution in BSS to 5×10^7 pelleted cells. Mix and incubate for 30 min at 4 °C.
2. Wash the cells twice in BSS and resuspend to 2 ml in complement diluted in BSS. Incubate for 1 h at 37 °C in a shaking water-bath.
3. Continue as for the one-step method from (2).

Note: If "capping" of the antibody is seen to be a problem the two-step method should be used.

4.2.2.2   Panning

This may be either a direct or indirect method.

Mononuclear cells pre-incubated with mAb are added to a *Petri* dish coated with affinity-purified anti-mouse IgG.

Alternatively, for B-cell depletion, add cells directly to a dish coated with polyclonal anti-Ig which is specific for the species from which the cells are derived. Following incubation, the non-adherent (negative) cells are recovered by gentle washing of the plate whilst the adherent (positive) cells are released by one of several means. In order to ensure that FcR^+-cells do not bind to the Fc portion of the antibody coated onto the plate, a $F(ab')_2$ fragment preparation of the anti-Ig antibodies should be used. However, the binding of $F(ab')_2$ fragments to the dish is slightly less efficient than that of the whole immunoglobulin molecule [19]. Excessive concentrations of the polyclonal antibody used for coating the plate should not be used as it causes adherent cells to become very tightly bound so that they cannot be released by competition and/or vigorous pipetting [20].

Method

Based on methods of *Engleman* [21] and *Wysocki* [19] illustrated in Figure 1.

1. Dilute the affinity-purified rabbit or goat anti-mouse IgG $F(ab')_2$ to a concentration of 10 µg/ml, either in PBS or in Tris, 0.05 mol/l, pH 9.5. Add 10 ml of the antibody solution to a bacteriological-grade *Petri* dish (100 mm diameter) and incubate for 1 h at room temperature or overnight at 4 °C.
2. Wash the dish 3 times with PBS followed by a final rinse of PBS containing 1% FCS. (The coated dishes, with all liquid removed, may be stored at -20 °C for subsequent use. Rinse twice with PBS after thawing.)
3. For indirect binding: resuspend 10^8 cells to 4 ml in PBS 1% FCS (handling medium) containing 80–100 µg mAb and incubate for 30 min at 4 °C. Wash the cells 3 times and resuspend the cells in 4 ml handling medium.
4. Add a maximum of 10^8 cells (untreated or pre-incubated with mAb) to the dish and incubate for 1 h at 4 °C. Gently swirl the cells around the dish several times during the incubation. Ensure that the dish is level.
5. Decant the non-adherent cells and gently rinse the plates 4 times with handling medium in order to recover any residual non-adherent cells.
6. Remove adherent cells. Either (a) add 5 ml handling medium containing 25% mouse serum (after direct panning of mouse B cells or indirect panning of other species cells) to the plate and incubate for 30 min at room temperature followed by vigorous pipetting or (b) substitute PBS containing 0.02% EDTA.

Inspect the dish on an inverted microscope to ensure that the adherent cells have been recovered.

1.

Fluid

Petri dish

4.

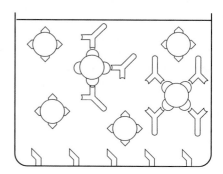

2.

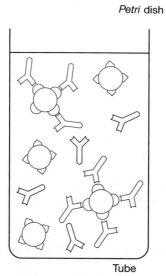

Tube

5.

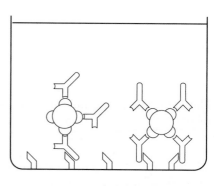

3.

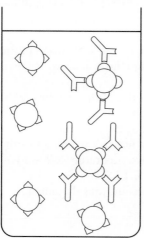

6.

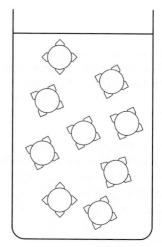

If a cell preparation containing a high proportion of macrophages is to be used the macrophages should be removed by plastic adherence prior to panning, in order to ensure that the antibody-coated dish is not overloaded.

4.2.2.3   Rosetting Methods Utilizing Erythrocytes

The basis of this method is the binding of antibody-coated "spheres" (i. e., erythrocytes or paramagnetic beads) to specific target antigens on cells to form rosettes and to enable the subsequent isolation of the rosetted cells from the non-rosetted cells by density gradient centrifugation.

Direct or indirect rosetting methods may be used.

The basis of direct rosetting is the binding of erythrocytes, with or without bound antibody, to specific targets on cells (usually of other species). This type of rosetting may occur in four ways:

1. The utilization of the inherent ability of some erythrocytes to form spontaneous rosettes with other species' leucocytes: for example, human T-cells [22] and certain mouse macrophages [23] will bind to untreated SRBC.
2. Antibody directed against the erythrocytes themselves is allowed to bind to the erythrocytes (usually sheep or ox), thereby forming erythrocyte-antibody complexes (EA) on which the Fc portion of the antibody is available for binding Fc receptor-positive cells [24].
3. EAC (erythrocyte-antibody-complement complexes) rosetting involves the addition of complement components to EA complexes thereby forming a target for complement receptor-positive (CR$^+$) cells [11, 25].
4. The binding of mAbs directed against specific nucleated cell surface determinants to erythrocytes by chemical coupling methods [26].

Direct erythrocyte (E) rosetting of human T-cells

Sheep erythrocytes (SRBC) are able to form spontaneous rosettes with human peripheral T-cells, *via* the CD2 antigen on the T-cells [22, 27, 28]. However, these rosettes are unstable at 37 °C and the majority readily dissociate. Therefore, the SRBC

◄ **Fig. 1.** Schematic diagram of the basic principle of panning.
  1. Coat *Petri* dish with goat anti-mouse IgG F(ab')$_2$.
  2. Pre-incubate the cell suspension with mAb to a specific cell surface antigen in test tube.
  3. Remove excess mAb by centrifugal washing of the cells.
  4. Add the cells to the coated *Petri* dish.
  5. Remove non adherent cells by gentle rinsing of the dish.
  6. Collect and wash non-adherent cells and resuspend.

are pre-treated with 2-aminoethyl*iso*thiouronium bromide hydrobromide (AET) or neuraminidase in order to stabilize the rosettes. If pre-treatment of the SRBC is not possible, it is essential first to incubate the SRBC and lymphocytes for 5 min at 37 °C and then to carry out all rosetting procedures (including density gradient separation) at 4 °C.

Neuraminidase pre-treatment of SRBC

Based on the protocols of *Bentwich* et al. [29] and *Han & Minowada* [30].

1. Wash SRBC (up to two weeks old, stored in *Alsever's* solution at 4 °C) twice in RPMI 1640 by centrifugation and resuspend to 5% (v/v).
2. Add 0.02 U of *Vibrio cholerae* neuraminidase (EC 3.2.1.18) per ml of SRBC suspension and incubate for 45 min at 37 °C, followed by 3 washes in RPMI 1640.

AET pre-treatment of SRBC

Based on the protocols of *Pellegrino* et al. [31] and *Saxon* et al. [32].

1. Mix SRBC suspension and AET, 0.14 mol/l, pH 8.0 in a 1:4 ratio and incubate for 20 min at 37 °C with stirring.
2. Wash SRBC 4 times in PBS by centrifugation then resuspend in RPMI 1640 containing a small amount of serum. The cells may be kept for up to 5 days if stored at 4 °C.

Method

Fig. 2 shows typical E rosettes of peripheral blood T-cells prior to density gradient separation.

1. Isolate lymphocytes from anticoagulated venous blood as described in 2.2. Adjust their concentration to about 5×10^6/ml.
2. Wash the pre-treated SRBC in BSS by centrifugation, $400 \times g$ for 10 min. Adjust to 2% (v/v) in BSS.
3. Mix equal volumes of the lymphocyte and SRBC suspensions and incubate at 37 °C for 5 min.
4. Centrifuge at $200 \times g$ for 10 min and incubate for 1 h at 4 °C.
5. Gently resuspend the cells and layer onto Ficoll-Hypaque (specific gravity 1.077) and centrifuge for 20 min at $400 \times g$.
6. Aspirate the non-rosetting mononuclear cells at the interface (E−) and wash 3 times with PBS (0.15 mol/l). Resuspend the cells at the required concentration in BSS.
7. To recover the rosetted (E+) cells, resuspend the cell pellet, which contains the E+ and free SRBC, and wash and follow with tris-ammonium chloride lysis (0.87% tris-buffered NH_4Cl) of the SRBC. Wash T-cells twice in PBS and resuspend in BSS.

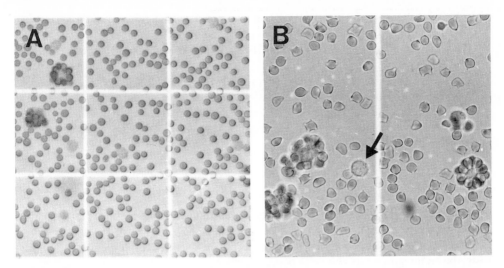

Fig. 2. Direct E rosetting of human T-cells. (A) Low-power magnification. Within the field are two rosettes. (B) High-power magnification. Within the field one unrosetted leucocyte (arrowed) may also be seen.

EA rosetting

Developed from the method of *Parish* [24].

   This method is used to remove Fc receptor-positive cells (FcR$^+$). SRBC are coated with a sub-agglutinating dose of hyperimmune (IgG) rabbit anti-SRBC serum. These sensitized SRBC are then used to rosette out FcR$^+$ cells.

Method

It is necessary to titrate the heat-inactivated (56 °C, 30 min) anti-SRBC serum to ascertain a suitable non-agglutinating dilution as follows.

1. Wash the SRBC 3 times in normal saline (400 × g, 10 min).
2. Aliquot 20 µl volumes of packed SRBC into several tubes, add 1 ml per tube of a range of antibody dilutions (in BSS), mix and incubate for 30 min at room temperature with mixing.
3. Wash the SRBC twice in BSS, resuspend the cells to 400 µl in BSS (5% v/v EA).
4. Check microscopically for agglutination of the SRBC, ascertain the non-agglutinating dilution range of the antibody.
5. Test the non-agglutinating dilutions of antibody for their ability to form rosettes with FcR$^+$ cells. The dilution of antibody for preparation of EA should be that which gives the greatest number of rosettes at the highest dilution.

6. Add 0.4 ml sensitized SRBC (EA) at 5% (v/v) to 0.4 ml of mononuclear cell suspension at 1.5 to 2×10^7/ml in BSS.
7. Mix the cells prior to pelleting by centrifugation ($200 \times g$, 10 min). Incubate for 30 min at 4 °C.
8. Resuspend the cell pellet gently, layer onto a density gradient and proceed as described for recovery of E rosettes, above. If, instead of human mononuclear cells, those of mouse or rat origin are used, the Ficoll-Hypaque density of the gradients used for separating the rosetted cells from the non-rosetted cells should be 1.083 or 1.095 respectively.

EAC rosetting

Complement receptor-positive cells may be separated using this method [11]. Sensitize SRBC with rabbit anti-SRBC (IgM) at a dilution not able to form EA rosettes with FcR^+ cells, and further incubate with fresh serum (source of complement components) from the same species as the cells being separated.

Chemical coupling of antibody to SRBC

Antibodies or other proteins may be coupled to SRBC by means of chromic chloride [26, 33, 34]. The treated SRBC are then incubated with the mixed leucocyte population where they bind to those cells which have the relevant surface antigen, forming rosettes which may be separated from unrosetted cells by density gradient centrifugation or by careful and rapid centrifugation alone. In the case of those cells separated on a density gradient, the rosetted cells (antigen +ve) will be found in the pellet along with dead cells, debris and the excess SRBC. The unrosetted leucocytes (antigen −ve) will remain at the interface. Centrifugation without density gradient medium will result in the rosetted cells and excess SRBC being pelleted whilst unrosetted leucocytes remain in the supernatant.

Purity levels of 95–99% may be achieved; the yields may be increased by resuspending the cell pellet and re-rosetting. If the antigen-positive cells (rosetted cells) are required for further use or analysis the SRBC attached to them may be lysed. However, it should be noted that the target antigen on the leucocyte used for the rosetting will remain "masked" by the attached antibody; overnight culture at 37 °C should result in the shedding and resynthesis of the antigen. It is recommended that erythrocytes from species capable of forming spontaneous rosettes with leucocytes from other species are not used for indirect rosetting. For example, ox red blood cells (ORBC) should be substituted for SRBC if human lymphocyte subsets are to be rosetted.

Preparation of coupling reagent (chromic chloride)

Use solution of chromic chloride for the antibody coupling. Best results will be achieved if the solution is "aged".

1. Dissolve 0.5 g chromic chloride ($CrCl_3.6H_2O$) in 500 ml 0.9% sodium chloride solution at room temperature to give a concentration of 1 g/l.
2. Adjust the pH to 5.0 by the addition of NaOH, 1 mol/l.
3. Readjust the pH back to 5.0 every few days over a 3-week period, after which the pH will remain stable. The solution may be kept for at least one year at room temperature.

Coupling of antibody to SRBC

Note: Phosphate buffers must not be used in the preparation and conjugation of antibody to SRBC – the phosphate prevents the coupling.

1. Wash the SRBC 4 times in saline, after the final wash do not resuspend the cells.
2. Add 0.5 to 1 ml of antibody at 1 mg/ml in saline to 0.5 ml packed SRBC and 9 ml saline. Add 0.5 ml chromic chloride solution dropwise with mixing. Incubate for 5 min at room temperature.
3. Wash the SRBC 3 times in PBS (to stop the reaction) by centrifugation, $400 \times g$ for 8 min, and resuspend finally to 5% (v/v) in BSS containing 0.5% BSA.

Direct rosetting

If mAbs directed against specific cell determinants are coupled to SRBC (chromic chloride method) direct rosetting of the target cells may be carried out. The method for E rosetting of T-cells is used, substituting the mAb-coated SRBC for the uncoated SRBC (described above).

Indirect rosetting

Indirect rosetting involves the conjugation of a "capture" reagent to the erythrocytes; these are then mixed with the heterogeneous cell suspension which has been pre-incubated with a cell-specific mAb (usually mouse). The "capture" reagent may be a polyclonal anti-mouse immunoglobulin, protein A [35, 36] or, if biotinylated mAbs are to be used, avidin [37]. Use the chromic chloride method above to couple protein A or avidin to SRBC substituting 1 ml protein A at 2 mg/ml in saline or 0.4 ml avidin (0.5 mg/ml in saline) for antibody.

Method

1. Incubate the mononuclear cell suspension with an appropriate dilution of mAb for 30 min at 4 °C in BSS.
2. Wash the cells twice in BSS containing 2% FCS and resuspend to 5×10^6/ml.

3. Add an equal volume of 5% (v/v) SRBC coated with the relevant "capture" reagent to the cell suspension. Mix and pellet the cells by centrifugation ($400 \times g$, 10 min). Incubate for 30 min at 4 °C.
4. Gently resuspend the cells and layer onto a density gradient. Separate the rosetted and unrosetted cells as described previously.

4.2.2.4   Immunomagnetic Rosetting Methods

Magnetic material is attached to specific cell types using defined mAbs bound to paramagnetic microbeads (direct rosetting). Alternatively, a polyclonal secondary antibody, attached to the magnetic beads, is incubated with a cell suspension pre-incubated with a specific mAb (indirect rosetting) followed by the application of a magnetic field in order to immobilize the rosetted cells.

Ugelstad [38] developed M-450 paramagnetic microsperes which are polystyrene beads with maghaemite dispersed throughout. Antibodies can be covalently coupled to them *via* the hydroxyl groups on the beads' surface. These beads are available from *Dynal Ltd* and the methods described are based on their use. Paramagnetic beads and various pre-coated beads are also available from other suppliers. Pre-activated beads may be purchased and other antibodies coated onto these beads in the laboratory. Once the beads have been attached to the target cells they are separated out by the application of a magnetic field which is generated by a strong permanent magnet. Suitable magnets include samarium/cobalt and neodymium/iron/boron and are available in various holders or stands.

Immunomagnetic rosetting is a quick and efficient method for specific cell depletion and/or enrichment. However, if used for enrichment of cell populations, the paramagnetic beads attached to the selected cells preclude many subsequent experiments owing to (1) their size (4.5 µm) and (2) the masking of the cell surface antigen used for the initial cell selection. These problems may be overcome by using very small beads (approximately 20 nm, MACS system *Becton Dickinson Ltd*) which do not alter the size and granularity profiles of the cells when analysed by flow cytofluorography. These microbeads are magnetically relatively weak: therefore, they can only be used in conjunction with extremely strong (and relatively expensive) magnets which are capable of generating high field gradients [39, 40]. Alternatively, the beads may be detached by overnight culture at 37 °C, or an anti-mouse Fab reagent may be added to directly-rosetted cells in order competitively to remove the mAb from the cell surface.

Direct immunomagnetic rosetting

Fig. 3 demonstrates the binding of magnetic beads to cells.

1. Prepare the cell suspension as described in the relevant part of section 2; resuspend the cells to 5×10^6/ml in PBS containing 2% FCS, maintain the suspension at 4 °C.

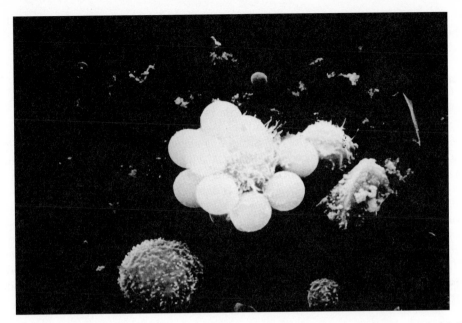

Fig. 3. Scanning electron micrograph of a *Burkitt's* lymphoma cell rosetted by magnetic M-450 beads *(Dynal Ltd.)*. Magnification × 15000. This photograph is published courtesy of *Dynal AS* (Norway), original work by *S. Funderud, G. Kvalheim, A. Reith* (DnR LMK).

2. Wash the mAb-coated magnetic beads by resuspending the required number of beads in 5 ml of cold PBS containing 1% FCS or 0.1% BSA in a test-tube (preferably glass). Apply the strong magnet to the side of the tube and wait for 2 min. Keeping the magnet in position, aspirate and discard the supernatant. Repeat.
3. Add the cell suspension to the magnetic beads and mix gently by rolling and/or rotating at 4 °C for 30 min.
4. Separate the rosetted cells by applying the magnet to the side of the tube. After 2 min remove the supernatant (containing the unrosetted cells) and add 10 ml fresh PBS/BSA to the rosetted cells in the tube.
5. Remove the magnet and gently mix the rosetted cells by inversion. Wash several times in the same manner.

The number of beads required will vary according to the nature of the separation required and with the numbers and ratio of the target cell in the population to be fractionated. The following may be applied as a guide. For positive selection (recovery of cells from beads) use a bead:cell ratio of 3:1; thus to recover 10^7 cells use 3×10^7 beads. For negative selection (removal of cells on beads) use a ratio of 10:1. To achieve a final contamination of less than 1%, use a ratio of up to 40:1, or two sequential depletions with a ratio of 10:1 beads:cells.

These ratios are applicable to clean starting cell populations devoid of debris and erythrocytes. Increase the ratio further if whole blood, for example, is used. These ratios apply to M-450 Dynabeads: adjust ratios as appropriate for beads of other types.

Detachment of beads from directly-rosetted cells

Either (1) culture the rosetted cells overnight in RPMI 1640 and 2% FCS at 37 °C, 5% CO_2.

Or (2) detach the beads by use of a competing reagent, polyclonal anti-mouse IgFab. If a commercial preparation is used, *(Dynal Ltd.)* the reagent will be ready for use since unwanted cross-reactions to species immunoglobulin have been removed. Titrate anti-Fab antibodies from other sources to determine their suitability, and remove cross-reactive antibody by absorption or affinity chromatography. The anti-Fab reagent binds to the bead-bound mAb dissociating it from the relevant cell surface antigen without damaging or activating the cell. This method is suitable for cells isolated *via* the direct rosetting method only. If used for cells isolated by the indirect method problems will occur as the anti-mouse Fab will probably cross-react with the secondary antibody bound to the magnetic bead, causing detachment of the bead and secondary antibody but possibly leaving some of the mAb attached to the cell.

Method

Titrate the anti-Fab reagent against each mAb to ascertain the amount required to effect complete detachment. Fig. 4 depicts the results obtained from an immunomagnetic depletion/enrichment experiment followed by detachment of the magnetic beads from the rosetted cells.

1. Resuspend 10^6–10^7 positively selected cells in 100 µl RPMI 1640 + Hepes + 2% FCS.
2. Add the required amount of anti-Fab reagent to the cell suspension and incubate for 1 h at room temperature with gentle mixing (not end-over-end).
3. Remove the detached beads by placing within a magnetic field for 2 min, aspirate and retain the supernatant whilst the tube remains within the magnetic field.
4. To obtain maximal cell recovery add 1 ml of medium to the detached beads, mix gently and re-apply the magnetic field. Aspirate remaining trapped cells.
5. Wash the cells 3 times by centrifugation, and resuspend the cells in fresh medium.

Indirect immunomagnetic rosetting

Cells are pre-incubated with the chosen mAb before the addition of paramagnetic beads coated with an anti-mouse antibody. A magnetic field is then applied to select out the rosetted cells.

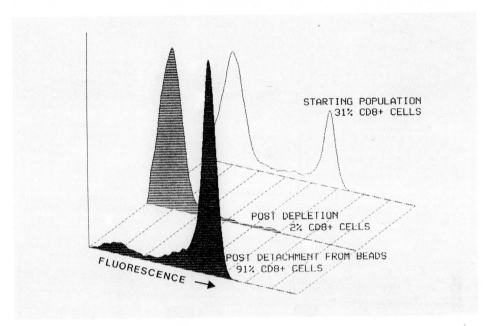

Fig. 4. Immunomagnetic depletion/enrichment of CD8⁺-cells from human PBL with subsequent detachment of cells from the paramagnetic beads by competition. Human PBL were depleted of CD8⁺-cells by direct immunomagnetic rosetting using an anti-CD8 mAb directly bound to the paramagnetic beads. The rosetted cells were subsequently detached from the beads. Samples were stained using a phycoerythrin-conjugated anti-CD8 mAb, followed by analysis using a *Becton-Dickinson* FACSTAR.

The log fluorescence intensity is plotted on the horizontal axis of the 3-D histogram. The data show that of the 31% CD8⁺-cells in the starting population only 2% remain in the post-depletion sample. Of the cells recovered from the beads, 91% were CD8⁺; the remaining 9% of cells (CD8⁻) may either be cells which have lost the CD8 antigen during the detachment process or cells which have non-specifically adhered to the beads.

1. Incubate cells with mAb for 30 min at 4 °C.
2. Wash the cells 3 times by centrifugation (200 x*g*, 10 min) using a balanced salt solution containing 1% FCS to remove excess mAb.
3. Resuspend and wash the required number of anti-mouse IgG coated beads. Add to the cell suspension. Incubate with gentle mixing at 4 °C for 10 min if positive selection of cells is required or for 30 min for negative selection.

Magnetic cell sorting (using high-gradient magnetic separation)

Fig. 5 demonstrates the basic principle of magnetic cell sorting.

The cells are specifically labelled with biotinylated mAbs to which micro superparamagnetic beads are coupled ("MACS" system; *Becton Dickinson Ltd.*) *via* an avidin

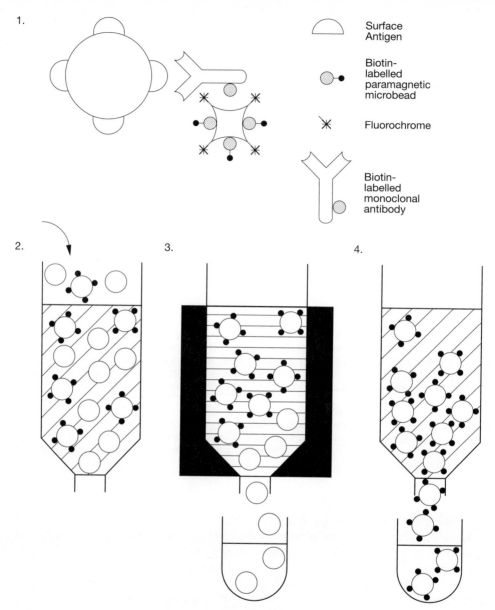

Fig. 5. Positive/negative cell selection using the magnetic cell sorting method.
1. Label a subpopulation of cells specifically with paramagnetic beads *via* an avidin-biotin bridge.
2. Add the cell mixture, containing the labelled cells, to the separation column which contains a magnetizable matrix.
3. Apply a strong magnetic field to the column; the "magnetically"-labelled cells are retained whilst unlabelled cells are eluted.
4. Remove the magnetic field and recover the labelled cells.

bridge. The avidin molecule may be linked to a fluorochrome to allow identification of positive cells in a flow cytometer or by fluorescence microscopy. The cell suspension containing the magnetically stained cells is put through a separation column which contains magnetizable steel wool. The column is placed within an extremely strong magnetic field ($\times 1000$ stronger than most other systems) and the labelled cells are retained within the column whilst the unlabelled cells pass through. The "magnetic" cell fraction is subsequently eluted by removing the magnetic field and flushing the column with medium.

The "MACS" system utilizes micro-beads (50–100 nm) which do not alter the light scattering parameters of stained cells; therefore, the positively selected cells may be further analysed, with fluorochrome-labelled mAbs against other cell surface antigens, by flow cytometry or fluorescence microscopy. The beads are also bio-degradable in culture. A detailed description of this method has been published by *Miltenyi* et al. [41].

4.2.2.5   Preparative Flow Cytometry

Cell sorting by flow cytometry, although a highly discriminating and multiparameter cell separation method [42, 43], is limited not only by the amount of time required to separate rare cells, but also by the cost of the instrument and the expertise required to use it.

The principles behind the operation of flow cytometers are described in detail in 5.11. Follow details there for the labelling of cells with fluorochromated antibodies. Note that the alignment of the system is as critical for efficient and accurate sorting as it is for analytical purposes. Cells may be sorted according to up to four parameters: forward scatter (size), side scatter (granularity) and one or two fluorescent parameters. Two populations may be recovered simultaneously if desired.

Preparation for sterile sorting

If the sorted cells are to be subsequently cultured sort in a sterile manner.

1. Connect a 0.22 μm filter to the fluid supply line.
2. Flush the tubing with a 1% (w/v) solution of sodium hypochlorite (or 70% alcohol) followed by sterile distilled water and finally sterile PBS.
3. Clean the sorting chamber and door and also the collection tube holder with 70% alcohol.
4. Add 0.5 ml sterile PBS containing 5–10% FCS and antibiotics to the collecting tubes and swirl around to coat the inside of the tubes. Prepare several tubes, store at 4 °C.
5. Ensure that the starting cell population is sterile.

Method

Fig. 6 illustrates window settings on a population of cells and the resulting populations obtained by sorting.

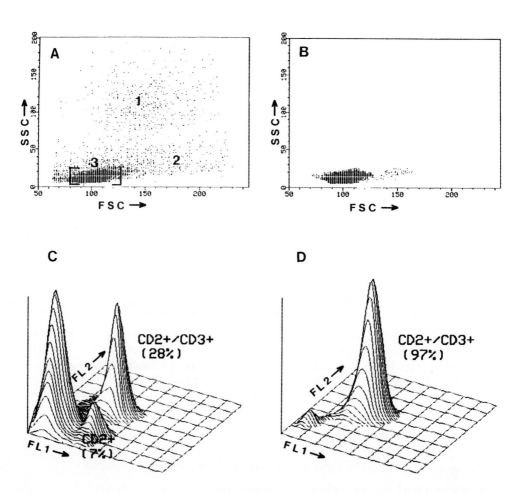

Fig. 6. Cell sorting. Two sorting gates were set on a population of spleen cells. The cells were sorted from one gate (FSC/SSC) through to the next (FL1/FL2). (A) Shows a dot plot of size (FSC) versus granularity (SSC) of the starting population of spleen cells. Three different populations of cells are shown (1 = granulocytes; 2 = lymphoblasts/macrophages; 3 = lymphocytes). The first sorting gate is set around the lymphocytes excluding the other cell types. (B) A dot plot of the sorted population showing that 99% of the sorted cells fell within the lymphocyte gate. (C) A 3-D plot of 2 fluorescence parameters. The spleen starting population was stained with anti CD2-FITC (FL1) and anti CD3-PE (FL2). The majority of CD2$^+$-cells are also CD3$^+$ (T-cells) whilst a subpopulation are CD3 (NK cells). The second sorting gate is set around the CD2$^+$/CD3$^+$ double positive cells. (D) A 3-D plot of the sorted population showing that 97% of the cells are CD2$^+$/CD3$^+$.

1. Analyse the population of cells and identify which populations are to be sorted.
2. Set the sorting windows ("gates" through which only the desired cells will pass) either manually *via* the electronic console or by using the computer data-management program and transferring the defined windows to the electronic console. Windows are often set on a dot plot (Fig. 6). Care should be taken if two populations are being sorted simultaneously that the windows set for each population do not overlap. Activate the sorting windows. The identified populations, when being sorted, will be sent either to the right or left collecting tubes.
3. Initiate oscillation of the nozzle which emits the fluid stream containing the cells. This will cause the fluid stream containing the analysed cells to break up into droplets. These will become electrically charged (positive and negative), as determined by the sort windows, and as they pass through the electric field formed between two metal "deflection" plates, −ve droplets will be deflected towards the +ve plate and *vice versa*, forming two side-streams of gated cells whilst the ungated cells remain in the central stream.
4. Collect the gated cells into the prepared tubes maintained at 4 °C. The collection tubes are pre-coated with medium so that the collected cells do not stick to the tube walls. Keep them at 4 °C by placing the tubes in an ice-bath or by circulating chilled water around the collection chamber to ensure the cells remain in good condition because a sort can last for several hours. Change the collection tubes regularly in case of tube blockages, side-stream shifts, etc., altering the alignment and hence possibly affecting the sorted populations.

   If a rare cell population is to be sorted, the side-stream containing these cells will probably not be visible as very few droplets will be deflected. In these cases it is sometimes helpful to also sort another more common cell type within the population at the same time, as the side-stream for this population will be visible. Light sources for viewing the fluid streams should not be used when sorting rare cells as the light will have a drying effect on the droplets.
5. Wash the sorted cells by centrifuging twice in fresh medium containing FCS and antibiotics.
6. Resuspend the cells in tissue culture medium.

References

[1] *K. Shortman, N. Williams, H. Jackson, P. Russell, P. Byrt, E. Diener,* The Separation of Different Cell Classes from Lymphoid Organs, J. Cell. Biol. *48,* 1566–1579 (1971).
[2] *L. H. Elliot, T. L. Roszman,* Suppressor Cell Regulation of the Spontaneously Induced *in vitro* Secondary Antibody Response, Cell. Immunol. *40,* 46–57 (1978).
[3] *M. H. Julius, E. Simpson, L. A. Herzenberg,* A Rapid Method for the Isolation of Functional Thymus-derived Murine Lymphocytes, Eur. J. Immunol. *3,* 645–649 (1973).
[4] *W. E. F. Klinkert, J. H. LaBadie, W. E. Bowers,* Accessory and Stimulating Properties of Dendritic Cells and Macrophages Isolated from Various Rat Tissues, J. Exp. Med. *156,* 1–19 (1982).
[5] *W. C. Van Voohis, L. S. Hair, R. M. Steinman, G. Kaplan,* Human Dendritic Cells. Enrichment and Characterization from Peripheral Blood, J. Exp. Med. *155,* 1172–1187 (1982).

[6] *S. Haskill, C. Johnson, D. Eierman, S. Becker, K. Warren,* Adherence Induces Selective mRNA Expression of Monocyte Mediators and Proto-oncogenes, J. Immunol. *140,* 1690–1694 (1988).

[7] *I. A. Ly, R. I. Mishell,* Separation of Mouse Spleen Cells by Passage through Columns of Sephadex G-10, J. Immunol. Methods 5, 239–247 (1974).

[8] *C. M. Alonso, R. R. Bernabe, E. Moreno, F. D. De Espada,* Depletion of Monocytes from Human Peripheral Blood Leucocytes by Passage through Sephadex G-10 Columns, J. Immunol. Methods *22,* 361–368 (1978).

[9] *S. F. Schlossman, L. Hudson,* Specific Purification of Lymphocyte Populations on a Digestible Immunoabsorbent, J. Immunol. *110,* 313–315 (1973).

[10] *U. Hellstrom, M. L. Dillner, S. Hammarstrom, P. Perlman,* Fractionation of Human T Lymphocytes on Wheat Germ Agglutinin-sepharose, Scand. J. Immunol. 5, 45–54 (1976).

[11] *M. F. Greaves, G. Brown,* Purification of Human T and B Lymphocytes, J. Immunol. *112,* 420–423 (1974).

[12] *P. D. King, D. R. Katz,* Mechanisms of Dendritic Cell Function, Immunol. Today *11,* 206–211 (1990).

[13] *R. M. Steinman, G. Kaplan, M. D. Witmer, Z. A. Cohn,* Identification of a Novel Cell Type in Peripheral Lymphoid Organs of Mice, J. Exp. Med. *149,* 1–16 (1979).

[14] *W. E. F. Klinkert, J. H. LaBadie, J. P. O'Brien, C. F. Beyer, W. E. Bowers,* Rat Dendritic Cells Function as Accessory Cells and Control the Production of a Soluble Factor Required for Mitogenic Responses of T Lymphocytes, Proc. Natl. Acad. Sci. U.S.A. *77,* 5414–5418 (1980).

[15] *D. Landry, M. Lafontaine, M. Cossette, H. Barthelemy, C. Chartrand, S. Montplaisir, M. Pelletier,* Human Thymic Dendritic Cells. Characterization, Isolation and Functional Assays, Immunology *65,* 135–142 (1988).

[16] *S. C. Knight, J. Mertin, A. Stackpoole, J. Clark,* Induction of Immune Responses *in vivo* with Small Numbers of Veiled (Dendritic) Cells, Proc. Natl. Acad. Sci. U.S.A. *80,* 6032–6035 (1983).

[17] *P. I. Terasaki, J. D. McClelland,* Microdroplet Assay of Human Serum Cytotoxins, Nature *204,* 998–1000 (1964).

[18] *T. Hercend, S. Meuer, E. L. Reinherz, S. F. Schlossman, J. Ritz,* Generation of a Cloned NK Cell Line Derived from the "Null Cell" Fraction of Human Peripheral Blood, J. Immunol. *129,* 1299–1305 (1982).

[19] *L. J. Wysocki, V. L. Sato,* "Panning" for Lymphocytes. A Method for Cell Selection, Proc. Natl. Acad. Sci. U.S.A. *75,* 2844–2848 (1978).

[20] *M. G. Mage, L. L. McHugh, T. L. Rothstein,* Mouse Lymphocytes with and without Surface Immunoglobulin: Preparative Scale Separation in Polystyrene Tissue Culture Dishes Coated with Specifically Purified Anti-Immunoglobulin, J. Immunol. Methods *15,* 47–56 (1977).

[21] *E. G. Englemann, C. J. Benike, F. C. Grumet, R. L. Evans,* Activation of Human T Lymphocyte Subsets: Helper and Suppressor/Cytotoxic T Cells Recognize and Respond to Distinct Histocompatibility Antigens, J. Immunol. *127,* 2124–2129 (1981).

[22] *M. Jondal, G. Holm, H. Wigzell,* Surface Markers on Human T and B Lymphocytes, J. Exp. Med. *136,* 207–215 (1972).

[23] *P. R. Crocker, S. Gordon,* Mouse Macrophage Hemagglutinin (Sheep Erythrocyte Receptor) with Specificity for Sialylated Glycoconjugates Characterized by a Monoclonal Antibody, J. Exp. Med. *169,* 1333–1346 (1989).

[24] *C. R. Parish, J. A. Hayward,* The Lymphocyte Surface. II. Separation of Fc Receptor, C'3 Receptor and Surface Immunoglobulin-bearing Lymphocytes, Proc. R. Soc. Edinburgh Sect. B: Biol. *187,* 47–63 (1974).

[25] *C. Bianco, R. Patrick, V. Nussenzweig,* A Population of Lymphocytes Bearing a Membrane Receptor for Antigen-antibody-complement Complexes, J. Exp. Med. *132,* 702–720 (1970).

[26] *C. R. Parish, I. F. C. McKenzie,* A Sensitive Rosetting Method for Detecting Subpopulations of Lymphocytes which React with Alloantisera, J. Immunol. Methods *20,* 173–183 (1978).

[27] W. H. Lay, N. F. Mendes, C. Bianco, V. Nussenzweig, Binding of Sheep Red Blood Cells to a Large Population of Human Lymphocytes, Nature 230, 531–532 (1971).

[28] J. Wybran, M. C. Carr, H. H. Fudenberg, The Human Rosette-forming Cell as a Marker of a Population of Thymus-derived Cells, J. Clin. Invest. 51, 2537–2543 (1972).

[29] Z. Bentwich, S. D. Douglas, E. Skutelsky, H. G. Kunkel, Sheep Red Cell Binding to Human Lymphocytes Treated with Neuraminidase; Enhancement of T Cell Binding and Identification of a Subpopulation of B Cells, J. Exp. Med. 137, 1532–1537 (1973).

[30] T. Han, J. Minowada, Enhanced E- and EAC-rosette Formation by Neuraminidase, J. Immunol. Methods 12, 252–260 (1976).

[31] M. A. Pellegrino, S. Ferrone, M. P. Dierich, R. A. Reisfeld, Enhancement of Sheep Red Blood Cell Human Lymphocyte Rosette Formation by the Sulfhydryl Compound 2-Amino Ethylisothiouronium Bromide, Clin. Immunol. Immunopathol. 3, 324–333 (1975).

[32] A. Saxon, J. Feldhaus, R. A. Robins, Single Step Separation of Human T and B Cells Using AET Treated SRBC Rosettes, J. Immunol. Methods 12, 285–288 (1976).

[33] E. R. Gold, H. H. Fudenberg, Chromic Chloride: a Coupling Reagent for Passive Hemagglutination Reactions, J. Immunol. 9, 859–863 (1967).

[34] K. C. Anderson, J. D. Griffin, M. P. Bates, B. C. Slaughenhoupt, S. F. Schlossman, L. M. Nadler, Isolation and Characterisation of Human B Lymphocyte Enriched Populations. I. Purification of B Cells by Immune Rosette Depletion, J. Immunol. Methods 61, 283–292 (1983).

[35] A. Forsgren, J. Sjoquist, "Protein A" from S. Aureus, J. Immunol. 97, 822–827 (1966).

[36] V. Ghetie, K. Nilsson, J. Sjoquist, Detection and Quantitation of IgG on the Surface of Human Lymphoid Cells by Rosette Formation with Protein A-coated Sheep Red Blood Cells, Scand. J. Immunol. 3, 397–403 (1974).

[37] D. Levitt, R. Danen, Separation of Lymphocyte Subpopulations Using Biotin-avidin Erythrocyte Rosettes, J. Immunol. Methods 89, 207–211 (1986).

[38] J. Ugelstad, T. Ellingsen, A. Berge, M. B. Steen, K. Nustad, New Developments in Production and Application of Monosized Polymers Particles, Proc. ACS Div. Polymeric Materials 54, 521–525 (1986).

[39] C. S. Owen, E. Moore, High Gradient Magnetic Separation of Rosette-forming Cells, Cell Biophys. 3, 141–153 (1981).

[40] H. Abts, M. Emmerich, S. Miltenyi, A. Radbruch, H. Tesch, CD20 Positive Human B Lymphocytes Separated with the Magnetic Cell Sorter (MACS) can be Induced to Proliferation and Antibody Secretion in vitro, J. Immunol. Methods 125, 19–28 (1989).

[41] S. Miltenyi, W. Muller, W. Weichel, A. Radbruch, High Gradient Magnetic Cell Separation with MACS, Cytometry 11, 231–238 (1990).

[42] M. R. Loken, L. A. Herzenberg, Analysis of Cell Populations with a Fluorescence-activated Cell Sorter, Ann. N. Y. Acad. Sci. 254, 163–171 (1975).

[43] M. R. Loken, A. M. Stall, Flow Cytometry as an Analytical and Preparative Tool in Immunology, J. Immunol. Methods 50, R85–R112 (1982).

4.3   Biopsy-based Methods

Timothy J. Peters

4.3.1   Principles

The analysis of tissue biopsies by morphological, immunological or biochemical techniques, although well established in clinical diagnosis, is of increasing interest in experimental physiological and pathological studies [1, 2]. Investigation of biopsy-sized tissue fragments allows detailed studies of small structures, e.g., endocrine and nervous tissues or multiple sequential studies of larger organs, e.g., liver, kidney and muscle. Use of small tissue samples for such studies will also reduce the number of animals needed for studies, particularly in costly long-term toxicity studies.

4.3.1.1   Sample Variability

It should be noted, however, that there are potential problems in biopsy studies of experimental animals which have long been recognized in diagnostic pathology laboratories. Analysis of small tissue samples inevitably means that the analytical variation of the assay methods used is increased but, more importantly, the problem of sampling errors and tissue variability arises. Even for a relatively large and homogenous organ such as the liver, biopsy samples may show variations, particularly if needle biopsy samples are used. An example of tissue variability in the liver is the difference in fibrous tissue elements at the liver edge as compared to the central region of the liver. This observation is well known to diagnostic pathologists, but may be misleading to experimentalists.

Sample variation is even more marked in organs showing regional organization such as the kidney organized into a cortex and medulla. Similarly, muscle studies often fail to take account of predominant fibre types in a particular muscle. Thus, in man most muscles are mixed Type I and Type II fibres, whereas in the rat certain muscles may show a marked predominance of a particular fibre type. For example, the *plantaris* is predominantly composed of anaerobic glycolytic Type II fibres and those of the *soleus* are principally the aerobic glycolytic Type I fibres. In addition, because of the different mechanical functions of the various muscle groups, e.g., axial, proximal and distal muscle, the responses to physiological and pathological process are likely to differ markedly. Similarly, differences in the response of left-, right- and inter-ventricular cardiac muscle to systemic or pulmonary circulatory changes may be striking. Selective biopsies will heighten the differences compared to whole organ analyses and this will have critical importance in interpreting the results. Multiple biopsies, wherever possible, will reduce these variations.

4.3.1.2   Sample Collection

The procedures necessary for the biopsy may cause marked functional and even morphological changes. The use of general anaesthetics, preoperative fasting, restraining of the animals, etc., may have effects which may mask the variable under investigation. Again, a well known example from clinical studies concerns biopsy of human liver. Surgical biopsies are commonly collected from the liver edge by oversewing the margins of a small segment so that the tissue sample can be collected without excessive haemorrhage. As well as having an increased collagen content compared with the bulk of the liver, such biopsies commonly show increased numbers of leucocytes as an early response to tissue ischaemia and thus misleading conclusions may ensue from the histological appearance.

Following tissue sampling, either by open or by closed biopsy procedures, subsequent processing will depend on the intended analysis. For morphological studies, both at the light and electron microscopic level, aldehyde fixatives are commonly employed. For special studies and particularly for histochemical studies, alternative fixatives are available. For the highest morphological resolution, use of *in-vivo* perfusion fixation is recommended, particularly for rapidly autolysed tissues such as those of the gastro-intestinal tract. Histochemical light microscopical and cytochemical electron microscopical studies of biopsy specimens are usually undertaken on fixed tissue samples, but it must be recognized that the fixation procedure usually inhibits enzyme activities by over 95 % and thus the activity displayed may well not be representative of the enzyme distribution in the intact tissue. Most of the enzymes studied by this approach are hydrolases and less than one tenth of the total number of known enzymes can currently be studied by histochemical and cytochemical methods. The use of frozen section procedures, although associated with inferior ultrastructural preservation, allow more enzymes to be studied with minimal inactivation of enzyme activities. Similar considerations also apply to immunocytochemical techniques (cf 5.1 and 5.6).

4.3.1.3   Tissue Preservation

Preservation of tissue samples for subsequent biochemical analysis, particularly for compartmental analysis, offers particular challenges. Where assay of stable components, e.g., ions, trace elements, simple metabolites, is required, storage in the frozen state is usually quite satisfactory. However, it must be remembered that the reference unit, e.g., wet weight, non-collagenous protein or DNA, will be affected by storage. Bacterial and fungal degradation and dehydration may occur at $-20\,°C$. Similarly, cold-labile enzymes will be rapidly inactivated by cold storage. The use of preservation media ranging from 0.25 mol/l sucrose or 50 % (v/v) glycerol solutions to complex mixtures and the use of controlled freezing and defrosting regimens are particularly valuable in maintaining membrane integrity [3]. It should be noted that unbuffered preservation media will be acidic (as low as pH 4.0) and this may contribute to analyte degradation, including enzyme inactivation.

It is also clear that preservation of tissue constituents is superior if the biopsy fragment is maintained intact in a small volume of buffered isotonic medium, e.g., 0.25 mol/l sucrose containing 10 mmol/l TRIS-HCl buffer, pH 7.4, than if it is stored as an homogenate. Although some of the more fragile organelles, such as lysosomes and peroxisomes, are disrupted by a single freeze-thaw cycle, other organelles including mitochondria, *Golgi,* endoplasmic reticulum and nuclei, retain a remarkable degree of integrity when stored frozen. Thus it is still possible to isolate reasonably intact mitochondria from frozen tissue, for example, as a starting point for purification of their constituents. However, more sophisticated functions, such as *Krebs* cycle activities and oxidative phosphorylation, are largely lost in the process of freeze-thawing tissue specimens.

The addition of certain reagents may improve tissue preservation. Thus the addition of mmol/l concentrations of their substrates may reduce inactivation of some enzymes [4]. For example, routine addition of 0.1 % (v/v) hydrogen peroxide, a substrate for the peroxidatic activity of catalase, will considerably reduce the loss of catalase activity on storage. The addition of 0.1–1 mmol/l EDTA will prevent heavy metal inhibition of certain enzyme activities, 1–10 mmol/l mercaptoethanol oxidation of critical thiols and a cocktail of protease inhibitors will considerably reduce acid (catheptic) and neutral proleolytic degradation.

4.3.2   Cell Isolation Procedures

For several reasons, methods have been developed for the isolation of cells from tissue samples and whole organs. The general strategy is a two-step procedure involving release of the constituent cells and separation and isolation of specific cell populations. For the release of cells, methods for the dissolution of the extracellular matrix and specific cell-cell junctional complexes are used.

Hyaluronidase has been used with some success to degrade the extracellular matrix, thereby releasing cell constituents. However, most enzyme preparations used successfully have been impure and it is likely that contaminating hydrolases, most notably proteases, were important for the hyaluronidase effect. More recently, collagenase (EC 3.4.24), either alone or in combination with hyaluronidase (EC 3.2.1.35), has been successfully used to isolate constituent cells from a variety of tissues. Again, impure (protease-contaminated) collagenases are superior to highly purified collagenase preparations. The enzymic dissolution methods work most successfully when used *via* vascular perfusion and thus are most frequently employed in experimental animal studies, although they may be applied to excised organs including human tissues. An alternative strategy which may also be used in combination with enzymic digestion is the use of Ca^{2+} chelators, most usually EDTA, EGTA or phosphate buffers; these latter methods appear to be less damaging to the cell surface proteins. The isolated cells can be fractionated by a variety of techniques described elsewhere in this series and, if of interest, subjected to subcellular fractionation techniques to isolate, identify and characterize the individual organelles.

4.3.3 Subcellular Fractionation Techniques

Detailed description of equipment and procedures are provided in several monographs and key references [4–8]. This discussion will be confined to general principles, key strategies and tactical issues.

4.3.3.1 Homogenization Assessments

This is the key but often most empirical step in the cell disruption procedure [6]. The principal aim is to breach the cell membrane, releasing the intracellular organelles with minimal damage; that is, a selective disruption of the plasma membrane. A variety of homogenizers and tissue disrupters are available and selection of the most appropriate and optimal conditions is generally by a trial and error approach. Monitoring of the degree of disruption is usually performed by sequential phase-microscopic observation of the homogenate during repeated disruption; e.g., after every 5 passes of the homogenizer. A more quantitative approach can be sequential measurement of the percentage sedimentability of an appropriate organelle, e.g., mitochondria or lysosomes, as reflected by a specific marker enzyme in the low-speed ($250–1000 \times g$) pellet. After minimal disruption, up to 70 % of the enzyme will be recovered in the low-speed pellet. Further cellular disruption is continued until at least 70 % of the marker enzyme is recovered in the supernatant. However, it is likely that further homogenization will lead to damage to the released organelles. This can be minimized by removing the supernatant after partial cellular disruption and, after adding fresh medium, by repeating the homogenization step: this is usually repeated three times [4].

In parallel with quantitative monitoring of tissue disruption, it is usual in establishing an optimal fractionation procedure to assess integrity of the released organelles.

Lysosomes are a particularly suitable organelle for this role. They are readily released from disrupted cells, they are not adsorbed to other intracellular structures such as nuclei or myofibrils, they are relatively fragile and thus maintenance of their integrity is encouraging with respect to other organelles, and their marker enzymes are relatively stable and are easily assayed. Organelle stability can be assessed quantitatively by measuring sedimentability (usually $10,000–15,000 \times g$ for 10–30 min) or more simply by assaying latent enzyme activity. This technique is based on the observation that intact organelles are impermeable to enzyme substrates and, when incubated with the substrate of an intra-organelle marker enzyme, will show no cleavage of the substrate. However, disruption of the organelle by a detergent will allow the enzyme to be exposed to the substrate. The result is usually expressed as the percentage latent activity of the marker enzyme. The value obtained approximates to, but is usually slightly lower than, the percentage sedimentability of the same marker enzyme. A ratio of latent to sedimentable activity of lysosomal marker enzymes in the homogenate or post-nuclear supernatant of greater than 70 % is considered satisfactory [4].

4.3.3.2   Homogenization Procedures

The most commonly used homogenization procedures involve the tube and pestle approach either manually *(Dounce)* or mechanically *(Potter)* driven [8]. Avoidance of local heating of the homogenate is important in preventing organelle damage and is generally achieved by ice-cooling and slow disruption rates. It is often forgotten that the major variable that is usually poorly controlled in the disruption process are the shear forces in the vertical movement of the pestle in the tube. The clearance and accuracy of the pestle and tube diameters are clearly important but are readily definable. The rate of rotation of the pestle and the number of passes, usually detailed in the description of the method, are much less critical than the rate of passage of the pestle through the homogenate. This latter is rarely noted in publications. It is thus important for the experimenter to determine the optimal procedure for maximal cell disruption with minimal organelle damage for the particular study. This should be verified for each tissue, both normal and, if appropriate, pathological, that is the subject of such a study. It is important that each experimenter should confirm that optimal conditions are being used since it is common to find that disrupting shear forces vary from operator to operator. It is also wise to restandardize conditions if a new homogenizer is used.

Homogenization of isolated cell suspensions poses particular difficulties as the clearance and shear forces generated in the usual homogenizers are insufficient to disrupt cells in suspension. Vigorous homogenization sufficient to disrupt the cells frequently causes extensive organelle damage. Improved disruption can be achieved if the cells are pelleted in the homogenizer tube itself and disrupted in a small volume of medium (i.e., aggregating the cells as tissue). Alternative approaches are to use a hypotonic homogenization medium which causes cells to swell, rendering them more fragile and thus facilitating cellular disruption. Restoration of isotonicity should be made as soon as possible after completing the homogenization to avoid organelle damage. Addition of small concentrations of detergents (e.g. 0.01–0.1 mg/ml digitonin) to the homogenization medium may facilitate disruption of the cell membrane but the likelihood of organelle damage is high. An alternative approach has been to use more vigorous disruption procedures. The use of pressure cells in which the cell suspension is equilibrated with high-pressure nitrogen, followed by rapid release of the pressure so that microbubbles of dissolved gas are released very rapidly within the cells thus disrupting them, has many advocates. This procedure is useful if membranous components are required but more fragile organelles such as lysosomes are liable to damage by this approach.

Having disrupted the cell to produce what should correctly be called a heterogenate, the next step is the separation/isolation of the cell organelles. There are two fundamentally different approaches to the localization of constituents, components and function to organelles. These are: (i) does a particular organelle contain that constituent, etc?, and (ii) what, without prejudice, is the subcellular location of the constituent? These two approaches are specifically and respectively called (i) preparative and (ii) analytical subcellular fractionation [9].

4.3.3.3 Principles of Analytical and Preparative Techniques

Analytical subcellular fractionation does not aim to isolate individual organelles to a high purity. Using a variety of methods based on differences in the biophysical or biochemical properties of the individual organelles, they are separated (resolved) from each other. The organelles are identified in the separated fractions mainly by assay of their marker enzymes (Table 1). Analytical subcellular fractionation is quantitative, in that all the organelles in the tissue sample are accounted for. This is particularly important in the study of diseased tissue where alterations in the properties of certain organelles may occur. By use of the analytical approach, changes in the physical properties of the organelles can be detected and this information can be used to indicate organelle pathology.

Preparative subcellular fractionation aims to isolate specific organelles to a high degree of purity. Much of our current knowledge of cell biology and biochemistry has been obtained by this approach. It employs large amounts of starting material and uses several different fractionation techniques, successively, to isolate the organelles, often with little regard to yield or quantitative recoveries. Morphological methods are frequently used to assess organelle purity. Clearly, this approach has only very limited application to tissue biopsy samples which are usually only available in milligram quantities.

Table 1. Marker Enzymes for Principal Subcellular Organelles

Organelle	Marker	
Plasma Membrane	5-Nucleotidase	(EC 3.1.3.5)
	Na$^+$, K$^+$ ATPase	(EC 3.6.1.3)
	Adenylate Cyclase	
Brush Border (intestine)	γ-Glutamyltransferase	(EC 2.3.2.2)
	Alkaline phosphatase	(EC 3.1.3.1)
	Sucrase	(EC 3.2.1.26)
Golgi apparatus	Galactosyl transferase	(EC 2.4.13.8)
	Sialyl transferase	(EC 2.4.99.1)
Endoplasmic Reticulum	Cytochrome P450	
	Ribosomal RNA	
Mitochondria	Succinate dehydrogenase	(EC 3.2.1.30)
	Glutamate dehydrogenase	(EC 1.4.1.3)
	Cytochrome Oxidase	(EC 1.9.3.1)
	Monoamine Oxidase	(EC 1.4.3.4)
Peroxisomes	Catalase	(EC 1.11.1.6)
	D Amino-acid Oxidase	(EC 1.4.3.3)
Lysosomes	N Acetyl-β-glucosaminidase	(EC 3.2.1.20)
	Acid Phosphatase	(EC 3.1.3.2)
Cytosol	Lactate dehydrogenase	(EC 1.1.1.27)
	Glucose 6 phosphate dehydrogenase	(EC 1.1.1.49)
Nuclei	DNA	

4.3.3.4   Centrifugation Methods

Centrifugation techniques rely on differences in organelle density or size (sedimentation coefficient) to effect a separation [9]. Separations based on density differences in organelles involve layering the tissue homogenate or extract in isotonic medium (usually sucrose) onto a linear density gradient and centrifugation for prolonged periods until the organelles reach their equilibrium densities. This is a useful technique, since the individual organelles usually have a narrow density range and are readily resolved from one another; furthermore, providing that equilibrium densities are achieved, the exact centrifugation conditions are not critical. Sucrose is the most commonly used medium but sugar polymers, e.g. Ficoll, glycogen, Stractan, have also been used. These high molecular weight polymers are of particular value if the organelles are damaged by hypertonic solutions. A relatively recent addition to this range of polymers has been the introduction of Percoll. Percoll forms a self-generating gradient and is also particularly suitable for separating cells. Colloidal silica had previously been used as a density gradient medium but its use had largely been abandoned because of its cytotoxicity: coating the particles with polyvinylpyrrolidone overcame the problem.

In order to overcome many of the disadvantages of these high molecular weight polymers, iodinated organic compounds have been introduced. These are of high density and low viscosity, with low toxicity and relatively low osmotic activity. Again, these compounds (e.g. metrizamide) have been frequently used for subcellular fractionation of tissue organelles [10]. Separations of a broad range of organelles in a single tissue sample have been disappointing but the use of iodinated media in the isolation of specific organelles has been useful as part of a multi-step procedure.

Apart from the introduction of new media, there have been other innovations designed to overcome the problems of density gradient centrifugation. One of the disadvantages mentioned above has been that prolonged centrifugation times are necessary to reach equilibrium densities, particularly with the highly viscous media. Two approaches have been used to overcome this problem. Firstly, the introduction of very high speed centrifuges capable of generating over $500,000 \times g$ has considerably shortened centrifugation times. However, an unexpected problem with high speed centrifugation has been organelle disruption due to the high hydrostatic pressure generated in the swinging bucket rotors. This particularly affects mitochondria, but other organelles are also affected [11]. The hydrostatic pressure appears to disrupt the inner mitochondrial membrane. This renders it permeable to sucrose so that the equilibrium density increases. The phenomenon can be minimized by centrifugation at higher temperatures and slower speeds, by the use of protective agents or use of zonal rather than swinging-bucket rotors [12, 13].

The second and more useful approach to shortening the centrifugation time needed to achieve equilibrium density is to reduce the pathlength of organelles in the gradient. This can be achieved with the small volume automatic zonal centrifuge designed by *Beaufay* [14]. This rotor, which is unfortunately not commercially available, has a smaller chamber, peripherally placed in the rotor. It allows organelles to be separated more rapidly (five fold) than with conventional swing-out rotors. In many ways the recently-introduced vertical pocket re-orientating rotor combines the advantages of the *Beaufay* rotor with ability to process several samples simultaneously. In addition, these rotors are commercially available for most ultracentrifuges [15].

Rate zonal and differential centrifugation separate organelles on the basis of differences in their sedimentation coefficients. Zonal centrifugation is performed in either swinging-bucket or zonal rotors. The latter are generally of larger volume and thus are more suitable for preparative fractionation. Zonal rotors minimize wall effects and avoid the disturbance of the separated zones which occurs during stopping the rotor prior to collection of the fractions. However, they are more expensive, and require complex ancillary equipment including pumps, gradient-making devices and various monitors. Differential pelleting (centrifugation) is a form of separation based on differences in the sedimentation coefficients of the organelles. It was the earliest form of centrifugation technique to be developed and applied to organelle isolation, and still has many applications. It yields limited numbers of fractions, simplifying analysis. Moreover, the composition of the principal fractions for several tissues, particularly liver, are well defined. Differential centrifugation has the particular advantage that throughout the procedure the organelles are exposed only to isotonic isolation media.

4.3.3.5   Affinity Chromatography

This method of organelle separation relies on the presence of certain proteins or glycoproteins on the exposed surface of the organelle. Immobilized antibodies to organelle surface proteins, or lectins attached to inert column materials, should provide selective isolation of the particular organelles. Problems due to steric hindrance of the ligands, accessibility to organelle constituents and difficulties of eluting the organelles without disrupting them, has so far meant that these potentially elegant techniques have not been fully exploited in the separation or isolation of subcellular organelles. The technique also relies on the formation of vesicles of a consistent "sidedness", e.g., from plasma membrane and endoplasmic reticulum. A consistent sidedness implies that the vesicles must always form in such a way that a particular surface is accessible to the binding agent.

4.3.3.6   Gel Permeation Chromatography

In view of the value of this technique in the separation of many different molecules of biological interest, it is surprising that separation of subcellular organelles by this approach has been attempted to a limited extent only. Polysaccharides including Sepharose 6B and Sepharose 1000M have been used to fractionate microsomal components [16]. In particular, they have been used to separate adsorbed cytosolic proteins from the membraneous components. Their exclusion volume is too small to resolve adequately larger subcellular organelles.

Chromatography on controlled-porosity glass beads has been used to a limited extent in the purification of vesicles, including synaptosomal vesicles [17] and fragments of intestinal brush border vesicles [18]. Separation is largely on the basis of apparent molecular volume but hydrophobic and ionic interactions may play a role. It is likely that, if suitable matrices can be developed, chromatographic methods for the separation and isolation of intracellular organelles will be of increasing value.

4.3.3.7   Phasepartition Chromatography

Phasepartition, particularly with immiscible organic phases, has been used for the separation of molecules of biological interest for many years. The introduction, by *Albertsson* and colleagues [19], of two-phase systems of dextran and polyethylene glycol polymers has enabled this approach to be used for the isolation of biological macromolecules, subcellular organelles, viruses and bacteria, and even intact cells [20]. Mixtures of dextran and polyethylene glycol above their critical concentrations yield an upper, polyethylene glycol-rich phase and a lower, dextran-rich phase. Various ions, in particular phosphate, distribute unequally between the two phases and thus there is a charge- and ionic-gradient between the two phases. Many different phase mixtures can be employed, including substituted dextrans and polyethylene glycol derivatives, enhancing ionic and hydrophobic interactions between the two phases. The attachment of ligands to one or other of the phase constituents can further be used to enhance the separation and some remarkably effective isolation techniques have been reported [21].

Phase separations are very sensitive to alterations in the polymer composition and there are often marked variations in organelle separations using different batches of reagents. Careful standardization of the mixtures, particularly the dextran, is important.

4.3.3.8 Electrophoretic Methods

Separation of subcellular organelles by electrophoretic techniques, like chromatographic procedures, has been limited by problems with support matrices. However, the introduction of carrier-free electrophoresis has overcome these problems and useful separations of intact cells, organelles, bacteria and viruses have been obtained [22]. At present the equipment is costly and is not yet suitable for processing small amounts of tissue.

4.3.4 Enzyme Analysis of Biopsies and Fractions

The approach adopted in, what is in fact a biochemical approach to tissue pathology, is to assay selected marker enzymes for individual organelles [2]. Where possible, marker enzymes solely confined to a particular organelle are assayed [23]. However, limitations due to low activities or insensitive assays may necessitate the use of markers that are less than ideal. The most appropriate markers differ, in some cases, from one tissue to another, particularly for plasma membrane domains. Table 1 lists the principal marker enzymes used in biopsy studies, where only milligram quantities of samples are available. Detailed procedures are given in the appropriate references, but the assays rely on radiometric or fluorimetric techniques [1, 2]. Hydrolases are readily determined with 4-methylumbelliferyl or coumarin derivatives. Dehydrogenases can be assayed at high sensitivity with the methods of *Lowry* [24], and radiometric assays are available for most other analyses.

Analysis of tissue samples for representative organelle marker enzymes entails many assays, particularly if the sample has been subjected to subcellular fractionation. Clearly, automated analysis should prove particularly valuable. Unfortunately, automated methods for most of the radioassays are not yet available and the complete requirements for fully automated assay of tissue samples and sucrose density gradient fractions by fluorimetric techniques are not met by commercially available instruments. The specific requirements are that the tissue homogenates are kept at 4 °C during sampling and that minimal amounts of material are used for duplicate assays. Analysis of gradient fractions which many contain up to 60 % (w/w) sucrose or other media also poses a problem for many automatic analysers because of their high viscosity. We have coupled the *Pye-Unican* AURA analyser to a *Perkin Elmer* 1000M spectrofluorimeter and a *Hewlett Packard* desk top calculator to provide automatic enzyme analysis of density gradient fractions. Most hydrolases, dehydrogenases and oxidases can be readily assayed. Excellent linear enzyme kinetics are obtained, even in the presence of high sucrose concentrations and there is very close agreement between enzyme distribution determined manually and with the automatic enzyme analyser [25].

References

[1] *T. J. Peters*, Investigation of Tissue Organelles by a Combination of Analytical Subcellular Fractionation and Enzymic Microanalysis: A New Approach to Pathology, J. Clin. Path. *34*, 1–12 (1981).

[2] *T. J. Peters*, Application of Analytical Subcellular Fractionation Techniques and Tissue Enzymic Analysis to the Study of Human Pathology, Clin. Sci. Mol. Med. *53*, 505–511 (1977).

[3] *J. Farrant*, General Observations on Cell Preservation. In: M. J. Ashwood-Smith and J. Farrant (eds.), Low Temperature Preservation in Medicine and Biology, Pitman Medical Tunbridge Wells, Kent 1980, 1–18.

[4] *T. J. Peters, C. A. Seymor*, Analytical Subcellular Fractionation of Needle Biopsy Specimens from Human Liver, Biochem. J. *174*, 435–446 (1978).

[5] *D. Rickwood*, Centrifugation: A Practical Approach, IRL Press, Oxford 1984, pp. 352.

[6] *C. De Duve, H. Beaufay*, A Short History of Tissue Fractionation, J. Cell. Biol. *91*, 293–295 (1981).

[7] *T. J. Peters*, Subcellular Fractionation and Enzymatic Analysis of Tissue Biopsy Specimens. In: H. U. Bergmeyer (ed.), Methods in Enzymatic Analysis, 3rd edition. Verlag Chemie, Weinheim 1983, pp. 49–66.

[8] *W. H. Evans*, Preparation and Characterization of Mammalian Plasma Membranes, North Holland, Amsterdam 1978, pp. 266.

[9] *C. De Duve*, Tissue Fractionation Past and Present, J. Cell. Biol. *50*, 20–55D (1971).

[10] *D. Rickwood*, Biological Separations in Iodinated Density Gradient Media, Information Retrieval Ltd, London 1976.

[11] *M. Collot, S. Wattiaux-De Coninck, R. Wattiaux*, Deterioration of Rat Liver Mitochondria during Isopyonic Centrifugation in an Isoosmotic Medium, Eur. J. Biochem. *51*, 603–608 (1975).

[12] *S. Wattiaux-De Coninck, M. F. Ronveaux-Dupal, F. Dubois, R. Wattiaux*, Effect of Temperature on the Behaviour of Rat Liver Mitochondria during Centrifugation in a Sucrose Gradient, Eur. J. Biochem. *39*, 93–99 (1973).

[13] *S. Wattiaux-De Coninck, F. Dubois, R. Wattiaux*, Effect of Imipramine on the Behaviour of Rat Liver Mitochondria during Centrifugation in a Sucrose Gradient, Eur. J. Biochem. *48*, 407–416 (1974)

[14] *H. Beaufay*, La centrifugation en gradient de densité (Thèse d'Agrégation de l'Enseignement Supérieur Université Catholique de Louvain, Louvain, Belgium). Ceuterick S.A., Louvain, Belgium 1966, pp. 132.

[15] *D. Rickwood*, An Assessment of Vertical Rotors, Anal. Biochem. *122*, 33–40 (1982).

[16] *J. A. Higgins, J. E. Mazurkiewicz,* A Rapid Method for the Separation of Free and Membrane-bound Polysomes of Rat Liver by Gel Filtration on Columns of Sepharose 4B, Prep. Biochem. *10,* 317–330 (1980).

[17] *A. Nagy, R. R. Baker, S. J. Morris, V. P. Whittaker,* The Preparation and Characterisation of Synaptic Vesicles of High Purity, Brain Res. *109,* 285–309 (1976).

[18] *K. Ohsawa, A. Kano, T. Hoshi,* Purification of Intestinal Brush Border Membrane Vesicles by the Use of Controlled Pore Glass-Bead Column, Life Sci. *24,* 669–678 (1979).

[19] *P. A. Albertsson,* Partition of Cell Particles and Macromolecules, Wiley-Interscience, New York 1971.

[20] *D. Fisher,* The Separation of Cells and Organelles by Partitioning in Two-Polymer Aqueous Phases, Biochem. J. *196,* 1–10 (1981).

[21] *P. A. Albertsson, B. Andersson, C. Larsson, H. E. Akerlund,* Phase Partition – A Method for Purification and Analysis of Cell Organelles and Membrane Vesicles, Methods Biochem. Anal. *28,* 115–150 (1982).

[22] *S. Menashi, H. Weintraub, N. Crawford,* Characterisation of Human Platelet Surface and Intracellular Membranes Isolated by Free-Flow Electrophoresis, J. Biol. Chem. *256,* 4095–4101 (1981).

[23] *D. J. Moore, G. B. Cline, R. Coleman, W. H. Evans, H. Glaumann, D. R. Headon, E. Reid, G. Siebert, C. C. Widenell,* Markers of Membraneous Cell Components, Eur. J. Cell. Biol. *20,* 195–199 (1979).

[24] *O. H. Lowry, J. V. Pasionean,* A Flexible System of Enzymatic Analysis, Academic Press, New York 1972.

[25] *T. Shah, D. Heywood-Waddington, G. D. Smith, T. J. Peters,* Automated Enzymic, Protein and DNA Microanalysis of Tissue Biopsy Samples and Subcellular Fractions, Clin. Chim. Acta *138,* 125–132 (1984).

5 Methods of Phenotype Analysis

5.1 General Features of Immunocytochemistry

Susan Van Noorden

The characteristic properties of differentiated cells can be investigated by morphological and functional studies. The gross nature of a tissue such as, for example, bone, muscle or nerve, and its relationship with neighbouring tissues are the subject of anatomical study. Microscopical investigation with histological stains will show whether the tissue is normal or diseased. Biochemical methods can analyse and quantify the chemical constituents of the tissue, some of which can be localized at a cellular or subcellular level by histochemical reactions, and are essential in functional studies when they are used to measure the amount of a product secreted by living cells *in vitro* or by organs or glands *in vivo*.

The exquisitely matched interactions between antigens and antibodies have been exploited in many different ways to provide means of studying tissue constituents and cell function. These interactions are employed in immunocytochemistry in the microscopical demonstration of the make-up of normal and diseased cells and tissues in a more specific way than conventional histochemistry allows.

5.1.1 Principles

A distinction might be made between immunohistochemistry at the tissue level to define the tissue type, e. g. muscle or epithelium, and immunocytochemistry at the cellular or sub-cellular levels to identify, for instance, the hormone in intracellular secretory granules of an endocrine cell, or growth-factor receptors on a cell surface membrane. However, there is no real difference in principle since many identifiable Ags may be present in cells or in the extracellular matrix and all are tissue constituents. The term immunocytochemistry will therefore be used throughout.

5.1.2   Choice of Reagents

Immunocytochemistry is the identification and localization of antigenic substances in cells and tissues by application of labelled Abs, the label being designed to produce a microscopically visible product at the site of the Ag-Ab reaction. The technique is histochemical in that the reaction has a known chemical basis, and it complements immunological assays of tissue extracts which can identify the Ag and measure the total amount of it in an extract using the same or similar Abs, but which cannot pinpoint its cellular localization. Although immunocytochemistry is less sensitive than radioimmunoassay in that it cannot detect such small concentrations of Ag, if the Ag is confined to a few cells only, immunocytochemical methods will have a greater chance of detecting it in those cells than an assay of an extract in which the Ag will be greatly diluted.

Any substance that can be used to raise an Ab can be identified by immunocytochemistry, provided that it can be immobilized in the tissue substrate with its antigenic sites exposed. However, the greater the purity of the original Ag, the greater are the chances of producing a monospecific Ab which will provide accurate localization. Synthesized, rather than purified extracted immunogens, may therefore be preferable. Affinity-purification can improve the specificity of polyclonal Abs, but may only be possible with Abs of relatively low affinity. Monoclonal Abs can be selected with absolute monospecificity, whether produced from pure or heterogeneous immunogens.

Immunocytochemistry demands Abs of high affinity that are unlikely to be detached from their binding sites by the extensive washing processes essential to the technique. Polyclonal antisera must contain a high titre of Ab so that they can be diluted greatly to remove unwanted serum components. Monoclonal Abs are not subject to this constraint, unless they are in the form of ascites fluid which unavoidably contains contaminants from the host species, and the degree to which they can be diluted is therefore less important, except from the point of view of cost. The most useful Abs for immunocytochemistry are of the IgG class because their small size allows efficient penetration of the tissue sample and, if necessary, even smaller Fab fractions can be produced. However, IgM molecules may have advantages when a high ratio of label to Ag is required.

Although immunocytochemistry provides the only truly morphological assessment of tissue Ag content, the principle of identification of Ab bound to Ag is the same as in other types of immunoassay.

5.1.3   Methodology

In order to identify an Ag *in situ,* an Ab, raised in a species immunologically different from that carrying the Ag, is applied to the substrate, which may be a tissue section or cell preparation, or a membrane in a blotting method. After reaction the unbound Ab is washed off the substrate and the bound Ab is revealed, either by a pre-attached (conjugated) label or, itself acting as an Ag, by further labelled Abs and other reagents applied in sequence. Labels used in light microscopical immunocytochemistry include fluorescent dyes, enzymes, colloidal gold, radioactive elements and biotin or haptens serving as bridges for other, labelled molecules. The label may be visible microscopically (e.g. fluorescent dyes) or may require further treatment (e.g., enzyme-catalysed reactions to produce a visible reaction product, silver intensification of colloidal gold, or autoradiographic exposure of a radiolabel).

Dyes were first attached to Abs in 1934 [1] but the intensity of colour was too low to be seen in the microscope. A fluorescent label, fluorescein isocyanate, was introduced by *Coons* and colleagues in the early nineteen forties [2], and the principle of immuno-cytochemistry was established [3]. The fluorescence of fluorescein under near ultraviolet light is a bright apple green, easily distinguishable from tissue autofluorescence which tends towards a blue colour. Several other fluorescent compounds, emitting green, red or blue light, may be used to label Abs but fluorescein, in the form of fluorescein isothiocyanate (FITC) which is easier to conjugate to Abs [4], remains one of the most widely used labels.

At first, immunostaining relied on a one-step direct method in which the fluorescent label was conjugated to the primary Ab. However, a two-step, indirect method was found to be more efficient [3]. In this, the primary Ab was unlabelled and was detected by a second layer consisting of a fluorescein-labelled Ab raised against the immuno-globulin of the species providing the primary Ab. The amount of label localized at the site of the primary Ag-Ab reaction is thereby increased and the primary Ab can be diluted further than in a direct method, giving reduced background staining.

In order to overcome the problems associated with fluorescence (fading, and the need for a specialized microscope) enzymes were introduced as labels [5], the first and still the most widely used being horseradish peroxidase, POD (EC 1.11.1.7). The enzyme itself is not visible but its presence is revealed at the end of the immunocytochemical procedure by adding a soluble substrate (hydrogen peroxide when POD is the enzyme concerned) and a chromogenic electron donor, thus producing an insoluble coloured product to identify the tissue Ag site.

The qualities that make an enzyme suitable as a label are a chemical structure suitable for conjugation to an Ab, and the ability to react with a soluble substrate to produce an insoluble, intensely coloured end-product that is deposited at the site of reaction and does not diffuse away from it.

The advantages of enzyme labels over fluorescent labels are that permanent preparations may be made when the reaction product is insoluble, the resulting stain can be seen in an ordinary light microscope, and the stained structures are visible in the context of the tissue substrate which may be counterstained with suitable histological techniques to provide more information.

There are some disadvantages: enzyme-conjugated Abs are less suitable than fluorescent Abs in the direct method because the conjugation process lessens the immunoreactivity of the Ab and the reactivity of the enzyme. However, indirect and three-layer methods with their amplified labelling are suitable (cf. 5.4) and improvement of the conjugation method by incorporation of an intermediate step [6] allows more of the enzyme activity to be retained and raises the detectability of the reaction to the level of the fluorescent Ab methods. A development step is necessary after the immunoreaction which prolongs the process and introduces yet more variables. Endogenous enzyme may present a problem, but confusion with the applied enzyme-linked immunoreagents can be prevented by prior blocking of the endogenous reaction.

Immunocytochemistry became accessible to all through the use of enzyme labels; by the nineteen seventies it was part of the armament of diagnostic and research laboratories in most branches of biomedical science, with reagents being supplied by an increasing number of commercial companies. Four enzymes are now in common use as labels in immunocytochemistry. The differently coloured end-products of their reactions makes then highly adaptable for multiple labelling techniques (cf. 5.4.6). One of the most popular chromogens for the peroxidase reaction, providing a dark brown, insoluble end-product, is 3,3'-diaminobenzidine (DAB) [7]. An additional advantage of this product is that it can react with osmium tetroxide, reducing it to osmium black which is electron-dense. Thus immunoperoxidase methods can be used for Ag identification at the electron-microscopical level.

Building on the foundations of the method, *Sternberger* [8] developed an even more sensitive three-layer technique, the unlabelled Ab-enzyme method, in which the primary and secondary Abs were both unlabelled. The site of reaction was marked by a third layer, a stable, cyclic peroxidase anti-peroxidase complex (PAP). The method (cf. 5.4.3) provided an intense and very clean reaction. Enzymes other than POD have now been used to make similar third layer complexes.

The only other novel concept introduced was the incorporation of a non-immunological and very stable bond, that between a vitamin, biotin, and a glycoprotein, avidin [9–11]. Various methods of combining these molecules with labels, with each other and with Abs have been devised (e. g. avidin-biotin methods, 5.4.3.2) resulting in a labelling intensity that may be considerably higher than for the PAP method. Although there are some inherent problems, they can be overcome and the method has been widely adopted.

All other modifications of these immunocytochemical techniques have been concerned with the search for new labels with different properties, for ever greater sensitivity and detectability, for reduction of nonspecific reactions and for better Ag preservation and availability. The reader is referred to several publications [12–14] for a more extensive review of the theory, practice and applications of immunocytochemistry than can be given here.

5.1.4   Applicability

Immunocytochemical techniques have had an enormous impact in all fields of biomedical science that require accurate localization of defined substances in tissues, whether plant or animal. The provisions are that the substance can be made immunogenic enough to provoke an Ab in another species, preferably immunologically removed from the one in which the Ag is to be identified, and that it can be immobilized at its tissue site by fixation while retaining the availability and antigenicity of its Ab-binding sites. Even living cells can be used, for example in analytical and preparative flow cytometry (cf. 5.11 and 4.2.2) by fluorescent Ab binding (cf. also 5.2.7), but usually cells and tissues must be frozen or chemically fixed at some stage in the method. Any of the techniques discussed above can be used for any preparation, but many factors will determine which is the most suitable, such as the nature of the tissue, the nature of the Ag and whether immunocytochemistry is to be combined with other techniques.

The combination of immunocytochemistry with other methods of morphological analysis increases its range even further. Thus receptor sites can be identified by immunolabelling of the bound ligand, while the messenger RNA for a cell product can be identified by *in situ* hybridization in the same preparation as the immunolabelled product itself. If the hybridization probe carries a non-radioactive label, e. g., biotin or digoxygenin, an immunocytochemical reaction using Ab to the label can be used to reveal the hybridization reaction. As an example, tracer molecules transported along nerve axons in a retrograde direction from the nerve terminal can be used to identify the neuronal origin of the nerve and can be seen simultaneously with immunostains able to identify the neurochemical produced by the neurone. Tissue enzyme histochemistry can be combined with immunocytochemistry for other cell products.

5.1.5   Limitations

In common with other methods of phenotype analysis, immunocytochemistry can only demonstrate what is in the cell at the moment of localization. The dynamics of production or output can only be inferred from alteration of experimental conditions or artificial functional studies such as the reverse haemolytic plaque assay. Measurement of the amounts of immunocytochemically-identified substances in cells is still limited to comparative rather than absolute quantities (cf. 5.4.7 and 5.8).

Of course, as with enzyme histochemistry, mere localization of a cell product does not imply that the product is biologically active, but only that the antigenic groups are available to the applied Ab.

Tissue preparation techniques (cf. 5.2) may alter the antigenicity of substances so that their reaction with Abs is impaired. Another limit to the use of the method is set by the concentration of the substance at the tissue site which, at some point, must be below the detection range. Both these problems can be overcome to some extent by compromising between mild fixation and good morphology, and by choosing amplified and enhanced immunocytochemical methods.

Numerous factors affect the achievement of an intense, clean and specific immuno-cytochemical reaction. The most common problem is unwanted background staining, although false negative staining and specific but unwanted cross-reactions of Abs with Ags other than the desired one also take place. In practice, simple remedies such as further dilution of the Abs, raising the ionic content of the buffers by adding NaCl to 0.5 mol/l, and blocking unwanted reactions with normal serum usually suffice. Some problems and solutions are outlined in 5.6 and a detailed discussion will be found in [14].

References

[1] *J. Marrac*, Nature of Antibodies. Nature *133*, 292–293 (1934).
[2] *A. H. Coons, H. J. Creech, R. N. Jones*, Immunological Properties of an Antibody Containing a Fluorescent Group, Proc. Soc. Exp. Biol. Med. *47*, 200–202 (1941).
[3] *A. H. Coons, E. H. Leduc, J. M. Connolly*, Studies on Antibody Production, I. A Method for the Histochemical Demonstration of Specific Antibody and Its Application to a Study of the Hyperimmune Rabbit, J. Exp. Med. *102*, 49–60 (1955).
[4] *J. L. Riggs, R. J. Seiwald, J. H. Burckhalter, C. M. Downs, T. Metcalf,* Isothiocyanate Compounds as Fluorescent Labeling Agents for Immune Serum, Am. J. Pathol. *34*, 1081–1097 (1958).
[5] *P. K. Nakane, G. B. Pierce, Jr.*, Enzyme-Labeled Antibodies: Preparation and Application for the Localization of Antigen, J. Histochem. Cytochem. *14*, 929–931 (1966).
[6] *S. Avrameas*, Coupling of Enzymes to Proteins with Glutaraldehyde. Use of the Conjugates for the Detection of Antigens and Antibodies, Immunochemistry 6, 43–52 (1969).
[7] *R. C. Graham, M. J. Karnovsky*, The Early Stages of Absorption of Injected Horseradish Peroxidase in the Proximal Tubules of Mouse Kidney. Ultrastructural Cytochemistry by a New Technique, J. Histochem. Cytochem. *14*, 291–302 (1966).
[8] *L. A. Sternberger, P. H. Hardy, Jr., J. J. Cuculis, H. G. Meyer*, The Unlabeled Antibody-Enzyme Method of Immunohistochemistry. Preparation and Properties of Soluble Antigen-Antibody Complex (Horseradish Peroxidase – Antihorseradish Peroxidase) and Its Use in Identification of Spirochetes, J. Histochem. Cytochem. *18*, 315–333 (1970).
[9] *M. H. Heggenes, J. F. Ash*, Use of the Avidin-Biotin Complex for the Localization of Actin and Myosin with Fluorescence Microscopy, J. Cell Biol. *73*, 783–788 (1977).
[10] *J. L. Guesdon, T. Ternynck, S. Avrameas*, The Use of Avidin-Biotin Interaction in Immunoenzymatic Techniques. J. Histochem. Cytochem. *27*, 1131–1139 (1979).
[11] *S. M. Hsu, L. Raine, H. Fanger*, Use of Avidin-Biotin-Peroxidase Complex (ABC) in Immunoperoxidase Techniques: a Comparison between ABC and Unlabeled Antibody (PAP) Procedures. J. Histochem. Cytochem. *29*, 577–580 (1981).
[12] *L. A. Sternberger*, Immunocytochemistry, 3rd edition, John Wiley and Sons, New York 1986.
[13] *J. M. Polak, S. Van Noorden* (eds.), Immunocytochemistry, Modern Methods and Applications, 2nd edition, John Wright & Sons, Bristol 1986.
[14] *L.-I. Larsson*, Immunocytochemistry: Theory and Practice. C. R. C. Press, Boca Raton 1988.

5.2   Preparation of Specimens for Immuno-cytochemistry

Susan Van Noorden

Immunocytochemical methods can only be successful if the Ag-Ab reaction site can be accurately localized in the tissue substrate. Both the Ag and the tissue structure must therefore be preserved. Unfortunately, the two conditions are sometimes incompatible since adequate tissue preservation can destroy some Ags. However, a compromise is usually reached.

5.2.1   Purpose of Fixation

The chemical preservation of tissue is known as fixation. Its purpose is to prevent autolysis, the breakdown of tissue by endogenous enzymes, and to render the tissue components insoluble, including the Ags under investigation. For study by transmitted-light microscopy thin (2–6 μm) sections or monolayers of cell preparations are required. Fixation stabilizes the structure of tissue proteins so that they withstand further processing through solvents and impregnation of the tissue in paraffin wax, resin or other hard medium for sectioning. For preservation of Ags or structures that may be affected by processing, tissues can be frozen after fixation instead of being processed and immunocytochemistry carried out on frozen sections.

Alternative procedures include snap-freezing fresh tissue to immobilize its constituents, then cutting sections from the frozen block and fixing them before immuno-staining. Whole cell preparations can be fixed in suspension or as monolayers on slides or coverslips. Live cells can be immunostained before fixation if this is necessary to demonstrate a particular Ag.

5.2.1.1   Action of Fixatives

Precipitant: alcohols and acetone are examples of fixatives which precipitate carbohydrates and coagulate proteins. Mixtures such as *Carnoy's* fixative and Methacarn are also used. They fix rapidly but penetrate tissue poorly, and are used for fixing small blocks, sections from fresh frozen material, cells in monolayer culture or cytocentrifuge preparations. A similar type of fixation is achieved by air-drying which denatures proteins.

Cross-linking: tissue blocks are usually fixed in solutions of aldehydes such as formaldehyde or, mainly for electron microscopy, glutaraldehyde. These penetrate well and fix tissue proteins by forming methylene bridges between their basic amino acids. The structure of the tissue is excellently preserved by aldehyde fixatives but a disadvantage for immunocytochemistry is that strong cross-linking can change the antigenic sites and prevent an immunoreaction. For some Ags this can be reversed by protease digestion (cf. 5.5.2) or by washing.

Formaldehyde mixtures: many patent additions have been made to formaldehyde in efforts to create the perfect fixative, i.e., rapid penetration, no swelling or shrinkage, precipitation as well as cross-linking. Among the most popular are picric acid (a precipitant) in *Bouin's* fluid and in *Zamboni's (Stefanini's)* fixative [1] which is similar but phosphate-buffered. Most small peptides are well preserved for immunocytochemistry by these fixatives. Glycoproteins are particularly suited by a mixture of periodate and lysine with formaldehyde [2]: it is believed that the periodate oxidizes the carbohydrate groups to aldehydes which are then cross-linked with lysine and further preserved by formaldehyde. The addition of dichromate preserves lipids also and has been recommended for immunocytochemistry of lymphoid cell surface Ags [3].

Alternatives to formaldehyde: milder cross-linking fixatives such as diethyl pyrocarbonate or *para*benzoquinone have been suggested; in particular, for small soluble peptides [4]. They can be used, as can *para*formaldehyde, in vapour form to fix freeze-dried tissue blocks, thus combining the advantages of snap-freezing with cross-linking. Freeze-dried, vapour-fixed tissue is used less than formerly because of the development of Abs that react well with formalin-fixed Ags.

5.2.2   Processing for Paraffin Sections of Pre-fixed Material

Adopt a fixation and processing regime according to the type of tissue and Ag to be studied. A standard fixation and processing schedule for routine diagnostic histopathology is given here. Cf. 5.2.9 for composition of fixatives.

5.2.2.1   Fixation

Immerse small blocks of freshly obtained tissue (not more than 5 mm thick) in a formaldehyde fixative (see above) for 6–24 h or perfuse a terminally anaesthetized experimental animal with fixative, dissect out the tissues of interest and immerse them in the same fixative until the full time has elapsed.

Perfusion ensures that the fixative reaches the tissues rapidly through the circulatory system, avoiding the danger that the centre of a tissue block may become autolysed before a diffusing fixative reaches it. The volume of fixative in which a block is immersed must be at least ten times greater than the volume of the block itself to allow adequate exchange of fluids.

5.2.2.2   Washing

Wash out the fixative before processing by immersing blocks in running water or several changes of buffer for some hours to reverse some of the effects of over-fixation (too much cross-linking). If fixation time is not more than 24 h, this is not usually necessary.

5.2.2.3   Dehydrating and Embedding in Paraffin

Do this "by hand" with tissues in screw-top jars and agitate from time to time or continuously on a shaker or roller: an automatic processor is more convenient. The water in the tissue is gradually replaced by alcohol, the alcohol by a solvent and the solvent by wax.

1. Take the tissues through a graded series of alcohols (70%, 90%, 2× 100%) then two changes of an alcohol-miscible solvent such as xylene or chloroform (or a less toxic alternative such as Histoclear (*National Diagnostics,* Hull, UK) and two changes of molten (56 °C melting point) paraffin wax, for at least 1 h in each step.
2. Embed the tissue block in a mould in fresh molten paraffin wax, with the surface to be cut facing down.
3. Solidify the wax on a cold plate and remove the block.

Paraffin sections: section cutting is a skill acquired by experience helped by practical instruction. Most Ags will be preserved indefinitely in paraffin sections if fixation has been adequate.

1. Cut sections 2–4 μm thick on a microtome and float them out on a water bath at 40 °C.
2. When they are flattened and wrinkle-free, pick them up on clean uncoated slides or slides coated with a tissue adhesive such as *poly*-L-lysine [5] (cf. 5.2.10).
3. Dry them well at 25–37 °C (several hours to overnight) and store them at room temperature. Do not bake sections onto slides (e.g. on a hot-plate at more than 50 °C) as this may damage some Ags.

Removing paraffin from sections: before immunostaining, de-wax sections in solvent (two changes) and bring them to water through graded alcohols (100% × 2, 90%, 70%, 2 min in each).

Removing mercury pigment: if mercuric salts were included in the fixative the resultant precipitate in the tissue sections, visible in the microscope as black crystals, can be removed without harm to tissue Ags at this stage or even after development of an enzyme label.

Immerse the preparations for 5 min in *Lugol's* iodine (1% w/v iodine in 2% potassium iodide w/v in water), then bleach the yellow colour produced by this treatment by immersion in 2.5% w/v sodium thiosulphate in water for 1 min.

5.2.2.4   Processing to Epoxy Resin

If the greater resolution provided by very thin sections is required, prepare tissue blocks in various resins which are harder than wax and produce less shrinkage. Any fixative is suitable, but if sections from the same block are to be taken to the electron microscope some kind of aldehyde fixative is essential. Because of the viscous nature of resins, penetration of the tissue may be inadequate and it is only possible to use blocks of less than 3 mm thickness. After dehydration in alcohol or acetone, mixtures of the resin and the final dehydration medium are followed by impregnation with the resin and then the resin with the required accelerator prior to embedding and polymerization (cf. 5.7 for details). The epoxy resins, Araldite® and Epon®, are suitable for light microscopical immunocytochemistry, as they can be removed easily from the sections (see below).

Some acrylic resins can also be used. Lowicryl K4M®, useful for processing and embedding at low temperatures, does not need to be removed from the sections. LR White®, another acrylic resin with no known solvent for the polymerized form, is sometimes suitable for light microscopical immunocytochemistry, but glycol methacrylate, much used in histology, is unfortunately not yet routinely usable because of its specialized tissue fixation and processing requirements [6].

Epoxy resin sections: Again, cutting such sections is a skilled procedure. Sections may be stored indefinitely.

1. Cut sections of 0.5–1 μm using an ultramicrotome and a glass knife.
2. Pick them up dry or float them on water or 10% acetone in a trough attached to the knife, depending on the resin.
3. Transfer the sections to a drop of water or 10% acetone on a *poly*-L-lysine-coated slide.
4. Allow the fluid to evaporate on a warm surface (37–40 °C) and dry the preparations thoroughly at 25–37 °C for several hours.

Resin removal with saturated alcoholic sodium hydroxide [7]

1. Make a saturated solution by adding solid sodium hydroxide pellets to absolute alcohol.
2. Shake at intervals for a week. The solution is ready when it is pale yellow to dark brown and remains effective for several months.
3. Remove the resin from epoxy resin sections by soaking in alcoholic sodium hydroxide for 10–20 min.
4. Rinse in several changes of 100% alcohol, check microscopically (with a lowered condenser) that the resin has dissolved and bring to water through graded alcohols.

5.2.2.5   Uses of Paraffin or Resin Sections

Provided that the Ags of interest are preserved, these provide the most convenient way of studying their distribution. Storage of blocks and sections is easy. Large areas of tissue can be sampled in paraffin blocks, although this is not true of resin blocks where sampling error could be a problem. The tissue structure is well preserved, providing good localization, and thin sections give good resolution. Many Ags can be stained in the same piece of tissue, using serial sections for comparison of results, which should be reproducible over a long period as deterioration in the block or sections is minimal. Immunocytochemical methods can be used that will combine easily with other morphological methods such as *in situ* hybridization. Archive material can be used, and even sections which have previously been histologically stained can be de-stained and re-used for immunocytochemistry. Routine histopathological diagnosis, to which immunocytochemistry has become indispensable, relies on the use of paraffin sections. Sections from resin blocks, if suitably fixed, can be used to compare light microscopical and electron microscopical immunolabelling.

5.2.3   Preparation of Frozen Fixed Tissue Blocks

Wash out excess fixative for several hours at 4 °C in several changes of buffer containing a cryoprotectant such as sucrose (12–15% w/v).

To store for several weeks, keep tissues in buffer with sucrose at 4 °C with a preservative such as sodium azide (0.1–1% w/v).

1. Cut the tissue into blocks not more than 5 mm thick.
2. Blot gently and arrange the block on a drop of adhesive such as OCT compound on a cork mat or moistened wad of filter-paper, with the surface to be cut uppermost.

3. Lable the cork in advance by writing on the underside with a ball-point pen.
4. Have ready a beaker containing the inert gas, arcton (Freon), which has been previously solidified by cooling in liquid nitrogen. An alternative, free from fluorinated hydrocarbons, is *iso*-pentane. (These substances are good conductors of heat and allow very rapid freezing, preventing the formation of ice crystals which disrupt the structure of the tissue.)
5. Allow the solidified freezing medium to melt at room temperature until there is some liquid and some solid in the beaker, to achieve the lowest possible temperature in the liquid state.
6. Immerse the mounted block rapidly and completely in the freezing medium for a few seconds until it is frozen.
7. Place block in a cryostat for sectioning or store it in liquid nitrogen or a freezer, preferably at a temperature lower than $-40\,°C$, until it is used.

Tissue blocks can also be made by placing them in a mould made from aluminium foil wrapped round a suitable template then detached from it. This method has the advantage of producing a block of tissue surrounded by OCT in a regular shape which is easier to section.

1. Place the tissue in the mould with the cutting surface down.
2. Fill the mould with OCT compound and place a labelled cork mat on top, in contact with the OCT.
3. After freezing, remove the foil.
4. For long-term storage, use liquid nitrogen or a $-70\,°C$ freezer, keep the block in a sealed container excluding air as much as possible to prevent the tissue drying out. Once frozen, tissue blocks must not be allowed to thaw.

5.2.3.1   Sections of Frozen Fixed Tissue Blocks

1. Cut the block in a cryostat (a microtome kept in a cold chamber at about $-20\,°C$).
2. Pick up the sections, from 4–20 µm thickness, according to need, from the surface of the knife on slides coated with *poly*-L-lysine (cf. 5.2.10) or chrome-gelatine and allow them to dry at room temperature for at least 1 h.
3. Store at $4\,°C$.

5.2.3.2   Semithin or Ultrathin Frozen Fixed Tissue Sections

It is possible to cut sections at 0.5–1 µm if they are needed for greater resolution, and even thinner for electron microscopy. However, a specialized microtome cooled by liquid nitrogen is required [8].

5.2.3.3   Uses of Pre-fixed Frozen Sections

Frozen fixed material provides the advantages of good tissue preservation without the damage that might be done to some Ags, such as lipid-associated substances, by processing through solvents and embedding media. The thicker sections that are available from a cryostat (15–20 μm) are much better than thin sections, for example, for examining the irregular course of nerves that have been stained by immunofluorescence, and confocal microscopy has recently enhanced this application by its ability to focus on successive planes through the thickness of a section (cf. 5.10).

Immunocytochemistry on pre-fixed frozen sections can be used in combination with other methods requiring such preparations.. They can also been used for selection of an immunocytochemically reactive area of a block for further processing for electron microscopy, or sections or parts of sections may be directly embedded for electron microscopy after DAB-identified immunoperoxidase staining. Some *in situ* hybridization studies on mRNA require fixed frozen tissue and benefit from combined immunocytochemistry.

5.2.4   Unembedded, Unfrozen Pre-fixed Material

5.2.4.1   Vibratome® Sections

Cut fixed tissue blocks without freezing on a specialized microtome with a vibrating blade. Sections are necessarily thick (50–100 μm) and are usually immunostained "free floating" in the various solutions so that reagents can penetrate them from both sides.

5.2.4.2   Whole-Mount Material

Any thick tissue preparations that are carried from one reagent to the next without being mounted on a slide until the reaction is ready for microscopy are known as whole-mount preparations. Examples are thick Vibratome or frozen sections, microdissected layers of the gut wall or structures such as diaphragm or iris membranes which are subsequently stretched onto slides. Special procedures are necessary for immunostaining these preparations (cf. 5.5.2).

5.2.4.3   Uses of Vibratome and Whole-Mount Preparations

The trauma of freezing is avoided and a three-dimensional impression of immuno-stained structures (e. g., nerves and their connections) is obtained. Areas suitable for electron microscopy can be selected from thick sections pre-stained by an immunoper-oxidase technique. The DAB reaction product can be osmicated to make it electron-dense; the area of interest can then be dehydrated and embedded in resin for ultrathin sectioning. However, caution in interpreting the fine structural localization of the Ag is necessary because the reaction product tends to move away from the original site [9] and the detergent treatment described below that is needed to make thick sections permeable to Abs is deleterious to ultrastructure.

Permeabilization procedure

1. Soak pre-fixed unmounted preparations in buffer containing detergent (e. g., 0.2% v/v Triton X-100) before immunostaining, and include detergent in the Ab diluent.
2. If solvents will not damage the Ag, dehydrate the preparations through graded alcohols to a solvent such as xylene and rehydrate again through the alcohols to buffer before immunostaining [10].
3. For these very thick preparations, long periods of washing and incubation with Ab are needed at all stages (cf. 5.5.2).

5.2.5   Unfixed Material

5.2.5.1   Fresh Frozen Tissue

Frozen sections are mainly used for immunostaining of epitopes that are destroyed by fixation, e. g. some lymphocyte surface markers, or the nuclear proliferation marker. Ki 67.

Rapid freezing preserves the architecture of a small block of tissue with its constituents in place. Thin sections (3–10 μm) can then be cut in a cryostat and picked up on slides. Immunostaining can be carried out after drying without further processing if the Ag is insoluble, but the structure will be better preserved if the sections are post-fixed (i. e., fixed after sectioning). Fresh frozen cryostat sections are not suitable for staining very soluble substances such as small peptides. A cryostat section thaws briefly with the heat of cutting, even if it freezes again immediately, and thaws again as it is picked up on a slide (which has to be warmer than the section to attract it). Very soluble substances dissolve and diffuse from their proper location during this process.

Freezing tissues

Freezing must be rapid to prevent formation of ice crystals which disrupt tissue structure. Use tissue blocks not thicker than 5 mm to ensure rapid freezing without cracking. A freezing medium with good conducting properties is essential. Liquid nitrogen, although very cold, is a poor conductor of heat but can be used if the mounted tissue block is held by the mount with forceps and moved around rapidly in the nitrogen during the freezing process to disperse the coat of warm nitrogen gas that forms around the immersed block. It is better to use *iso*pentane or the liquefied form of one of the inert gases such as Arcton, which can be solidified in a beaker suspended in liquid nitrogen, then allowed to warm up and used at its melting point. Prepare blocks from fresh tissue in the same way as for fixed tissue (cf. 5.2.3) but do not pre-soak in buffer or cryoprotectant.

Store frozen blocks in liquid nitrogen or a deep freeze below $-40\,°C$. Take care that they do not dry out in storage or they will be impossible to cut.

Sections

Cut 5 µm sections in a cryostat and pick them up from the surface of the knife on uncoated or *poly*-L-lysine-coated slides.

Dry them at room temperature for a period of 30 min to a day, or even longer if that is convenient, then fix and immunostain.

Drying denatures tissue proteins but is not deleterious to most Ags. However, the effect of long drying on the Ag of interest should be determined experimentally.

1. For long-term storage, wrap sections (unfixed or after brief fixation in acetone) back-to-back in foil or cling-film and seal them in a plastic bag containing silica gel or other dessicant.
2. Store the bag in a deep-freeze ($-20\,°C$ is adequate).
3. When the sections are to be immunostained allow the entire bag to reach room temperature before opening it.

The dessicant ensures that water of condensation does not come into contact with the sections. It is important that sections are not wet until they are to be immunostained and that thereafter they are not allowed to become dry throughout the procedure or drying artefacts will affect the structure. Some antigens become denatured in stored frozen sections; check this experimentally.

5.2.5.2   Fixatives for Frozen Sections

Choice depends on the Ag. Usually protein-precipitating fixatives such as acetone, alcohol or combinations of these with or without the addition of chloroform are used. Acetone and chloroform break down the lipids of cell membranes, increasing the permeability of the section. Cross-linking fixatives such as formalin may also be used. Protease digestion is never necessary for fresh-frozen sections.

1. Use short fixation times of 30 s to 15 min for these thin sections.
2. Fix in acetone or alcohol, allow the fixative to evaporate from the section or place the section directly in buffer.
3. After fixation in an aqueous solution such as formalin, rinse the section in buffer and keep it wet thereafter.

5.2.6   Freeze-dried Material

Rapid freezing, followed by dehydration of the tissue under vacuum while it is still frozen, then exposure of the dried tissue to vaporized fixatives preserves a labile Ag perfectly *in situ*. The dry, fixed block is impregnated with paraffin or resin under vacuum without being passed through solvents and is sectioned as usual.

5.2.6.1   Procedure

As for all procedures requiring tissue to be frozen, use small blocks and a good heat-conducting freezing medium. A tissue freeze-dryer is essential equipment.

1. Arrange the block of fresh tissue on a flat, friction-reduced surface such as the end of a metal spatula that has been sprayed with Teflon or a rigid piece of plastic.
This provides the tissue block with a flat surface to be placed in contact with the cold plate of the tissue dryer.
2. Plunge the tissue on its support into melting freezing medium (cf. 5.2.3). When frozen the tissue block will float off the support or can be dislodged from it easily.
3. Transfer it with pre-cooled forceps to the pre-cooled plate of the freeze dryer and evacuate the chamber.

The correct temperature for tissue freeze-drying is about $-40\,°C$. This is cold enough to prevent ice-crystal formation but still warm enough for water to sublime from the tissue and be removed by the vacuum pump of the dryer or trapped by the dessicant in the apparatus. Freeze-drying will be complete after about 16 h under these conditions.

4. Allow the apparatus to warm up to room temperature before releasing the vacuum to prevent condensation on the dry tissue.
5. For vapour fixation, transfer the tissue to a perforated basket or folded filter-paper in a pre-heated jar containing a dish of powdered *para*formaldehyde, crystalline *para*benzoquinone dissolved in toluene (about 0.07% w/v), or an alcoholic solution of diethylpyrocarbonate, as supplied commercially.
6. Seal the jar and place it in an oven at 60 °C for 1–3 h.
7. Remove the lid in a fume cupboard and transfer the tissue to melted paraffin in a vacuum oven.

Paraffin containing a plasticizer to improve penetration is recommended (e. g. RALwax I from *BDH*). Fatty tissue is not suitable for this method.

8. After 30 min to 1 h under vacuum, depending on the size of the block, embed the block in fresh paraffin of the same type and section as for conventional blocks.

5.2.6.2   Uses for Freeze-dried Vapour-fixed Sections

This method preserves substances that are particularly soluble, or diffuse easily, and prevents re-location of substances within cells by diffusion during fixation. Freeze-drying followed by formaldehyde fixation induces fluorescence in catecholamines. This property can be used to compare the localization of catecholamines with immuno-stained substances. However, separate, serial sections have to be used as the fluorescent catecholamines are likely to dissolve out of the de-waxed section when aqueous solutions are applied. The yellow/green fluorescence of residual fluorescent catecholamines might be confused with that of fluorescein: therefore, use a differently emmitting label if immunofluorescence methods are carried out on freeze-dried formaldehyde vapour-fixed material that contains catecholamines. Alternatively, fix in *para*benzoquinone or diethylpyrocarbonate instead of formaldehyde.

Fixation of freeze-dried tissue in acetone followed by paraffin embedding has been recommended for lymphocyte membrane Ags, providing better morphological preservation than frozen sections [11].

5.2.7   Live Cells

5.2.7.1   Use and Handling

The most frequent applications are in preparative and analytical flow cytometry and for counting populations of cells in a mixture in which some cells have surface Ags stained by immunofluorescence. In addition, surface Ags that are fixation-labile may be stained immunocytochemically before fixation. Cell surface receptors may be identified by immunostaining the receptor-bound ligand: preferably fix the cells after the ligand is bound. Internalization of receptor-bound ligand may be a subject for study. The identification of an Ag as on the outer surface (stained in living cells) or within the cytoplasm (only stained after permeabilization of the membrane) is another application. The secretion products of living cells deposited on a slide, gel or membrane may be immunostained, measured and identified with individual cells in the reverse haemolytic plaque, RELISPOT or cell blot assays (cf. 7.1 and 7.2).

Although the binding of Ab to a cell will not kill it, only cell surface Ags can be identified in this way, which limits the use of the technique. However, it ensures that the Ag is completely undamaged at the time of reaction. In any case, the cells will be killed by fixation and preparation for microscopy after immunostaining, unless the purpose of immunostaining is for separation of cell populations. For visualization of internal Ags, the cell membrane must be made permeable by drying, detergent, fixation or freezing and thawing, and these processes kill the cell.

Living cells can be immunostained attached to a slide or coverslip (adherent) or in suspension (non-adherent) and subsequently attached to a substrate for microscopy. Whether the firm substrate for adherent cells is glass or plastic will depend on the nature of the cells, but a glass slide or coverslip is preferable for light microscopical immunocytochemistry since plastics may be clouded by precipitant fixatives and solvents used in making permanent preparations, and are therefore not ideal for transmitted-light microscopy of subsequent immuno- or other stains. Some plastics are not inherently fluorescent and can be used for epi-illuminated fluorescence microscopy. Glass slides or coverslips may be coated with *poly*-L-lysine, which was originally used for cytological preparations and can be of a lower molecular weight than that used for sections [12]. Other coatings such as fibronectin may also be suitable. A plastic substrate is preferable if immunostained cells are subsequently to be examined by electron microscopy, provided that solvents of the plastic are avoided, as the plastic can be peeled away from the polymerized resin block leaving the cells ready for sectioning. Glass coverslips are snapped off after freezing in liquid nitrogen. Cell preparation methods have been described in the previous Sections of this Volume. General principles only are provided here because the individual requirements of different cell types are very varied.

5.2.7.2   Procedures

Adherent cells
Immunocytochemistry can be carried out on cultures of cells or organs grown on coverslips, or on deposits of dissociated cells on slides or attached to a membrane as in the cell blot assay [13].

Dispersed cell cultures

1. Use sterile conditions throughout.
2. Prepare cells by digestion of a tissue sample with trypsin or collagenase, and culture them appropriately to allow them to recover.
3. Re-trypsinize to detach and separate the cells, centrifuge and resuspend in culture medium. Count the cells in a haemocytometer, dilute appropriately in culture medium and dispense in drops on a suitably coated substrate.
4. Allow the cells to settle and attach to the substrate under the usual culture conditions.
5. Wash in protein-free medium.
6. Apply fluorescein-conjugated Ab in complement-free medium; carry out the reaction at 0 °C to avoid aggregation of surface Ags leading to "capping". If the Fab fraction of the Ab is used, the reaction can be caried out at room temperature and complement will not be activated. If an indirect method is used the second Ab must also be a Fab fraction.
7. Wash in protein-free medium, examine in UV microscope.
8. Continue culture as required.

Non-dispersed cell or organ cultures

Treat cell or explant cultures grown on coverslips in the same way as dispersed cells. Immunostaining is most effective when cells are not densely packed. Isolated cells in culture should not be allowed to grow to confluence and only the growing edges of organ explants should be considered.

Non-adherent Cells

Cells in a mixed population may be stained in suspension by immunofluorescence then separated from the rest by flow cytometry into a cell type-enriched population for further culture. Use immunostaining conditions the same as those for adherent live cells with the exception that the preparation must be centrifuged after each washing or incubation step and the cells resuspended in medium. Add Ab to the suspension to a predetermined optimal dilution.

If the purpose of staining live cells is not to keep them alive but merely to avoid fixation damage to the Ag, conditions need not be so rigorous. Azide may be included in the medium to prevent capping instead of carrying out the reactions at 0 °C. Cells may be fixed after application of the first Ab and deposited on a coated slide for the remaining steps of the method, or the immunocytochemical method may be finished with the cells in suspension before they are fixed and deposited on a slide or pelleted for processing and embedding, and sectioning for light- or electron microscopy.

5.2.7.3 Limitations

Some of these have already been mentioned. Cell surface Ags only can be labelled. Fc receptors on living cells may bind Ab nonspecifically. This can be avoided by using Fab fractions which are also required to avoid activation of the complement cascade if the medium contains complement. Use of complement-free medium and reaction at 0 °C avoids these problems. Fab (but not $F(ab)_2$) fractions also prevent the aggregation of Ab-bound cell surface Ags at one pole of the cell ("capping"). Some intractable problems are that Abs may sometimes be internalized by pinocytosis rather than being bound to their Ags, while dead cells with damaged membranes will absorb Abs nonspecifically, giving rise to nonspecific staining. However, the latter would not continue to be a problem if culture of the cells is continued.

5.2.8 Non-living Cells

5.2.8.1 Use and Handling

Diagnostic cytopathology relies on fixed cell preparations from suspensions, smears and imprints. In non-diagnostic studies, fixed preparations are less exacting to deal with than living cells, provided that no distinction need be made between antigens on the cell surface and within the cytoplasm.

This refers to cell preparations fixed before being immunostained. As for living cells, they may be in suspension, mechanically dissociated and dispersed on slides, or grown as organ or cell cultures. In addition, they may be made into cytospin preparations, smeared onto slides or attached to slides by imprinting from a cut surface of tissue. Immunostaining after fixation allows cytoplasmic as well as cell surface Ags to be identified. The fixative itself may provide adequate permeabilization or it may be necessary to follow it with a detergent rinse.

5.2.8.2   Preparing the Cells

Cells in suspension

1. For blood cells or cells aspirated through a fine needle from a tumour, wash in protein-free medium and purify or concentrate by density gradient sedimentation if necessary.
2. Centrifuge (500 ×g for 5 min), resuspend in an appropriate fixative, then repellet by centrifugation.
3. Either snap-freeze the pellet for cryostat sectioning (this is also a pre-fixation possibility), or treat as a tissue block for processing, embedding and sectioning. The pellet may be embedded in a small quantity of agar (1% w/v) and solidified before fixation so that the preparation does not need to be centrifuged after each step.
4. Treat sections subsequently in the same way as sections from blocks of tissue.

Cells on slides

Suspended cells from fine needle aspirates, mechanically dissociated, or from fluids such as cerebrospinal fluid, may be washed then driven onto coated slides (e. g. *poly*-L-lysine, cf. 5.2.10) by cytocentrifugation before or after fixation. This procedure deposits the cells evenly on a defined area of the slide which makes immunostaining easier than smearing the cells onto the slides. Another possibility is merely to place a drop of the cell suspension on a coated slide, allow the cells to settle for 30 sec then decant off the fluid. If the cells are suspended in a large volume they should be centrifuged and resuspended before being applied to slides by any of the above methods. Imprints from the freshly cut surface of a tissue block touched to a coated slide provide whole cell preparations that may give a rapid diagnostic answer while the remaining tissue is treated as a block.

5.2.8.3   Fixation and Storage

Unfixed cell preparations are usually allowed to dry thoroughly on the slide and, for some insoluble Ags, further fixation is unnecessary because the drying process denatures the cells enough to allow penetration of Abs.

Another "non-chemical" method of permeabilizing cells deposited or growing on a coverslip or slide is by freezing and thawing. The coverslip or slide is placed on a block of silid carbon dioxide to freeze, then withdrawn immediately to thaw. The process is repeated several times. If the Ag is soluble and fixation is unsuitable, the freezing and thawing can be carried out in a drop of primary Ab solution.

Depending on the Ag, and the preference of the investigator, dried cell preparations may be fixed briefly in acetone or alcohol or a combination of fixatives, e.g., methanol:acetone. 1:1, or 10% buffered formalin in acetone [14], before being immunostained. Some Ags are preserved better by fixation in alcohol or formalin before or immediately after deposition of the cells on slides without an intermediate drying step.

Preparations dried before or after fixation can be stored in the same way as fresh-frozen sections on slides (cf. 5.2.5).

5.2.8.4   Immunostaining

Cell preparations may be immunostained by any of several methods. Alkaline phosphatase (EC 3.1.3.1) is a particularly suitable marker for blood smears as the endogenous POD-like enzyme of erythrocytes and some leucocytes does not have to be taken into account. Immunogold methods, particularly with epipolarized illumination (cf. 5.3.4), are also useful as they can be combined easily with conventional stains.

If a POD-linked method is used, endogenous POD should be blocked by one of the milder methods (cf. p. 5.3.8.1).

The precautions against drying during the immunostaining procedure recommended for fresh frozen sections apply also to whole cell preparations.

5.2.9   Fixatives

The period of fixation depends partly on the size of the tissue block. Fresh cryostat sections or monolayers of cells will need only minutes of fixation while $5 \times 5 \times 3$ mm tissue blocks will need 6 to 24 h.

The cross-linking, antigen-blocking effects of formaldehyde-based fixatives may be partially reversed by rinsing the tissue for several hours in water or buffer after fixation. Protease treatment may be useful for paraffin sections (cf. 5.5.2).

Formol saline

Mix 10 ml concentrated commercial formalin (38% (w/v) aq. formaldehyde) and 90 ml sodium chloride, 0.15 mol/l.

Neutral buffered formalin

Mix 10 ml concentrated commercial formalin and 90 ml phosphate buffer, 0.1 mol/l, pH 7.0.

Buffered paraformaldehyde

Heat 8 g *para*formaldehyde in 90 ml water to 60 °C (in a fume cupboard). Clear by adding sodium hydroxide, 0.1 mol/l, dropwise with stirring and make up to 100 ml with distilled water. Add 100 ml phosphate buffer, 0.2 mol/l, pH 7.4.

Periodate lysine paraformaldehyde [2]

Solution A: L-lysine hydrochloride (0.1 mol/l, in phosphate buffer, pH 7.4, 50 mmol/l): Dissolve 1.827 g L-lysine hydrochloride in 50 ml water, adjust pH to 7.4 with disodium hydrogen phosphate, 0.1 mol/l, make up to 100 ml with phosphate buffer, 0.1 mol/l, pH 7.4. This solution may be stored at 4 °C for 10 days.

Solution B: Add 8 g *para*formaldehyde to 90 ml water, heat to 60 °C (in a fume cupboard). Clear by adding sodium hydroxide, 0.1 mol/l, dropwise and make up to 100 ml. Filter and store at 4 °C.

Just before use combine 3 parts of solution A with 2 parts of solution B; add sodium metaperiodate to 0.01 mol/l (0.0428 g in 20 ml). The final pH is about 6.2.

Periodate lysine paraformaldehyde dichromate [3]

Make as above using Tris, 0.2 mol/l, instead of phosphate buffer, and adjust pH to 7.5. Add an equal volume of 5% (w/v) potassium dichromate and polyethylene glycol $M_r =$ 400 to 10% (w/v). Adjust pH to 7.5.

1. Fix tissue blocks for 24–36 h in the dark (to retard reduction of dichromate).
2. After fixation, wash in running tap water for 6–18 h at room temperature, then process to paraffin.

Bouin's **fluid stock solution**

Stock solution
Mix 75 ml saturated aqueous, picric acid (filtered) and 25 ml commercial 38% (v/v) formalin.

Just before use add to 100 ml stock solution 5 ml glacial acetic acid.

A variant used in the author's laboratory contains a reduced quantity (1% v/v) of glacial acetic acid. This fixative retains well the antigenicity of (e. g.) the small regulatory peptides of the diffuse neuroendocrine system.

Zamboni's **(***Stefanini's***) fluid** [1]

Add 2 g *para*formaldehyde to 15 ml saturated aquous solution of picric acid, heat to 60 °C (in a fume cupboard), clear by adding sodium hydroxide, 0.5 mol/l, dropwise, filter and cool. Make up to 100 ml with phosphate buffer (0.331 g $NaH_2PO_4 \cdot 2\,H_2O$, 3.377 g $Na_2HPO_4 \cdot 7\,H_2O$ in 100 ml water, pH 7.3.

This solution may be stored at room temperature. After fixation for 6 h to overnight, rinse blocks (mammalian tissue) in PBS containing 15% (w/v) sucrose and 0.01% (w/v) sodium azide at 4 °C for several hours (cryoprotection) then freeze for cryostat sectioning as in 5.2.3.

Carnoy's fixative

Mix 60 ml ethanol, 30 ml chloroform and 10 ml glacial acetic acid.

1. Fix small tissue blocks for 1 h.
2. Dehydrate through 70%, 90% and 100% alcohol, then solvent.
3. Impregnate and embed in paraffin wax for sectioning.

Fix cryostat sections or whole cell preparations for 10 min.

5.2.10   Coating Slides with *Poly*-L-lysine

For whole cell preparations. Slides used for attachment of cells from suspension may be dipped in a solution of *poly*-L-lysine, $M_r = 30000$, and allowed to dry [12].

For attachment of fixed frozen sections or paraffin sections to be treated with a protease, a higher M_r (> 150,000) is advisable [5].

5.2.10.1 Procedure

1. Dissolve *poly*-L-lysine ($M_r = 150000$–300000) in water at 0.1% (w/v). Divide the solution into aliquots of about 1 ml and store frozen at −20 °C.
2. When required, thaw an aliquot completely and mix well. Unused solution may be re-frozen.
3. Place a drop of about 10 µl at one end of a clean slide.
4. Rock the edge of a second slide in the drop to spread the liquid along the edge of the slide. With the second slide at an angle of 25–40°, spread the *poly*-L-lysine solution over the first slide, using more pressure than for a blood smear, to give an even layer thin enough for interference colours to be seen as the liquid coats the surface. The coating dries rapidly and coated slides may be used immediately or stored at room temperature for several weeks.

5. Mark the coated side because the dried coating is not visible. The dipping method avoids this problem.

References

[1] *M. Stefanini, C. De Martino, L. Zamboni,* Fixation of Ejaculated Spermatozoa for Electron Microscopy, Nature London *216,* 173–174 (1967).

[2] *I. W. McLean, P. K. Nakane,* Periodate-Lysine-Paraformaldehyde Fixative. A New Fixative for Immunoelectron Microscopy, J. Histochem. Cytochem. *22,* 1077–1083 (1974).

[3] *K. Pollard, D. Lunny, C. S. Holgate, P. Jackson, C. C. Bird,* Fixation, Processing and Immunochemical Reagent Effects on Preservation of T-Lymphocyte Surface Membrane Antigens in Paraffin-Embedded Tissue, J. Histochem. Cytochem. 35, 1329–1338 (1987).

[4] *A. G. E. Pearse, J. M. Polak,* Bifunctional Reagents as Vapour and Liquid Phase Fixatives for Immunohistochemistry, Histochem. J. *7,* 179–186 (1975).

[5] *W. M. Huang, S. J. Gibson, P. Facer, J. Gu, J. M. Polak,* Improved Section Adhesion for Immunocytochemistry Using High Molecular Weight Polymers of L-Lysine. Histochemistry 77, 275–279 (1983).

[6] *G. I. Murray, S. W. B. Ewen,* Enzyme Histochemistry on Freeze-Substituted Glycol Methacrylate-Embedded Tissue, J. Histochem. Cytochem. 38, 95–101 (1990).

[7] *B. P. Lane, D. L. Europa,* Differential Staining of Ultrathin Sections of Epon-Embedded Tissue for Light Microscopy, J. Histochem. Cytochem. *13,* 579–582 (1965).

[8] *S. Semoff,* Light and Electron Microscopic Immunocytochemistry Combined through Cryomicrotomy, Opt. Electron Microscopy *10,* 4–7 (1984).

[9] *A. B. Novikoff, P. M. Novikoff, N. Quintana, C. Davis,* Diffusion Artifacts in 3,3′-Diaminobenzidine Cytochemistry, J. Histochem. Cytochem. *20,* 745–749 (1972).

[10] *M. Costa, R. Buffa, J. B. Furness, E. Solcia,* Immunohistochemical Localization of Polypeptide in Peripheral Autonomic Nerves Using Whole Mount Preparations, Histochemistry *6,* 157–165 (1980).

[11] *H. Stein, K. Gatter, H. Asbahr, D. Y. Mason,* Use of Freeze-Dried Paraffin-Embedded Sections for Immunohistologic Staining with Monoclonal Antibodies, Lab. Invest. 52, 676–683 (1985).

[12] *O. A. N. Husain, J. A. Millett, J. M. Granger,* Use of Polylysine-Coated Slides in the Preparation of Cell Samples for Diagnostic Cytology with Special Reference to Urine Samples, J. Clin. Pathol. *133,* 309–311 (1980).

[13] *M. E. Kendall, W. C. Hymer,* Measurement of Hormone Secretion from Individual Cells by Cell Blot Assay, Methods Enzymol. *168,* 327–338 (1989).

[14] *D. Y. Mason, C. Farrell, C. R. Taylor,* The Detection of Intracellular Antigens in Human Leucocytes by Immunoperoxidase Staining, Br. J. Haematol. *31,* 361–370 (1975).

5.3   Labels for Immunocytochemistry

Susan Van Noorden

A label, in the context of immunocytochemistry, is defined as a substance attached to an Ab or other reagent, by chemical, immune or other means, that is microscopically visible or can be made to produce microscopically visible evidence of its presence, in order to identify the Ab bound to the tissue Ag.

5.3.1   Fluorescent Labels

5.3.1.1   General

A good fluorescent label will absorb light efficiently and emit the resulting energy as visible light. It will not absorb light at the wavelength at which it emits, or no fluorescence would be seen, and it will give stable, non-fading fluorescence. The colour of the emitted light should be easily distinguishable from tissue autofluorescence. The relatively small molecular size of fluorescent labels means that a conjugated Ab retains much of its immunoreactivity, in contrast with an enzyme-conjugated Ab, provided that the immunoglobulin: fluorophore ratio is not much greater than 1:2. Fluorescent Abs can therefore achieve greater detectability than enzyme-labelled Abs in direct immunolabelling [1].

Immunofluorescence allows the site of a tissue Ag to be seen in sharp contrast against a dark background. The quality of the microscope and illumination are all-important, but can be discussed only briefly here. Fluorescence microscopy is reviewed in [2, 3]. A high-pressure mercury vapour lamp provides light from the shortest wavelengths in the ultraviolet, and appropriate filters ensure that the specimen is excited by the correct wavelength for maximum absorption by the fluorophore. Illumination of the specimen by incident light (epi-illumination) is more efficient than illumination from below (trans-illumination) because exciting light is not lost by passage through the microscope slide, and through the lower part of the preparation which may not have been exposed to immunoreagents. The objective lens also acts as a condenser. Background fluorescence, due to autofluorescence, fluorescence of tissue components due to nonspecific or unwanted immunoreactions and, in particular, fluorescence induced after formalin fixation, must be kept low. However, the filter bandpass must be wide enough to allow retention of enough background fluorescence for the immunofluorescent structures to be seen in context. A counterstain emitting fluorescence of a contrasting colour may be used to alter background fluorescence and thus enhance the visibility of the tissue structure (cf. 5.3.7).

All fluorescent labels tend to lose their fluorescence on dehydration through solvents: therefore, aqueous mountants are preferred, though these, unfortunately, are not entirely permanent. They also all fade to a variable extent under the exciting illumination, but the use of "non-fade" mountants is a help (cf. 5.3.7.2).

Fluorescent labels, which do not have to be treated further for identification, do not kill living cells and may therefore be used in fluorescent cell sorting.

5.3.1.2   Selected Labels

The following labels are the fluorochrome derivatives which are in most use today, having superseded earlier compounds.

Fluorescein isothiocyanate (FITC)

The maximum absorption occurs at an excitation wavelength of 495 nm, and emitted light is bright apple-green (520 nm). Contrast with background is reasonably good but red-fluorescing counterstains such as Pontamine Sky Blue [4] can be advantageous. The fluorescence of the label might be confused with the formaldehyde-induced green to yellow fluorescence of biogenic amines such as adrenaline, noradrenaline and serotonin. In some formaldehyde-fixed, amine-containing tissues, therefore, fluorescein may not be the label of choice, although much of the induced fluorescence will be removed by washing during the immunostaining procedure.

Tetrarhodamine isothiocyanate (TRITC)

This compound fluoresces red with an excitation maximum at 530 nm. A combination of fluorescein- and rhodamine-labelled Abs in double direct immunocytochemistry gives excellently contrasting fluorescence.

Texas Red [5]

This is another rhodamine derivative with similar fluorescence properties. It is superior to the isothiocyanate in that it fades less rapidly.

Lissamine rhodamine B [6]

This rhodamine derivative fluoresces orange-red, more weakly than TRITC but it is less visible through wide-band fluorescein emission filters (520–560 nm) and may therefore be more suitable than TRITC for some multiple labelling purposes [7].

Phycoerythrin [8]

Although the reddish orange fluorescence from this substance is less intense than that of the rhodamine fluorophores, phycoerythrin fluorescence is produced in the same excitation band as fluorescein and can be seen with the same filter combinations. Thus, it can be useful for double immunofluorescence, provided that the Ags to be located are in different tissue compartments.

DAMC (7-diethylamino-3-)4-isothiocyanotophenyl)-4-methylcoumarin) [9]

This compound fluoresces blue and has been used in double staining methods.

AMCA (7-amino-4-methylcoumarin-3 acetic acid) [10]

This is a similar label emitting blue fluorescence (448 nm) after maximal excitation at 349 nm. This label has been used in multiple immunofluorescence [7].

5.3.2   Enzyme Labels

5.3.2.1   Horseradish Peroxidase (POD)

This enzyme (EC 1.11.1.7) was the first to be used as a marker for Abs and fulfils the criteria outlined in 5.1.3 The soluble substrate provided is hydrogen peroxide, but a chromogen must also be present. One of the most frequently used chromogens is 3,3'-diaminobenzidine (DAB) (use as the tetrahydrochloride, since the free base is not soluble) which becomes oxidized to form a dark brown, insoluble polymer [11]. The enzyme is restored to its original state at the end of the reaction cycle and continues to act on the hydrogen peroxide substrate, bringing down more polymerized DAB until a point is reached at which the precipitate prevents the substrate from reaching the enzyme. Although the optimal pH for POD activity is about 5, the histochemical reaction is carried out at pH 7–7.6 to retard it and give more control (cf. 5.3.8.2).

The brown end-product can be converted to black by including salts of heavy metals such as nickel or cobalt in the reaction mixture [12, 13] (cf. 5.3.8.2) or by post-reaction deposition of metallic silver which gives an even greater intensification [14, 15]. Some of these silver intensification methods can produce blackening of argyrophilic components in the tissue such as reticulin fibres and enterochromaffin cells. This problem can be avoided by various pre-incubation treatments [16, 17] or by shortening the time in the silver solution. An extremely intense black stain can be achieved by developing the POD with nickel-enhanced DAB and post-silvering in a low pH solution [18].

The DAB reaction product may also be made electron-dense by osmication; this property is still occasionally used for electron microscopical immunocytochemical reactions, even since the introduction of colloidal gold as a more satisfactory marker.

Other chromogens often used in POD immunocytochemistry include 3-amino-9-ethyl carbazole, which gives a red reaction product, and 4-chloro-1-naphthol, which gives a dark grey-blue reaction product [19] (cf. 5.3.8.2). Both these products are soluble in alcohol and aqueous mountants are needed.

All the above POD development reagents might be carcinogenic and care should be taken when handling them. *Hanker* et al. [20] proposed a non-carcinogenic development reagent, a mixture of 1–4 benzendiamine hydrochloride and pyrocatechol, which produces a dark brown insoluble precipitate in the presence of hydrogen peroxide and POD. The reagent is said to be specific for plant peroxidase and thus blocking endogenous POD should be unnecessary. Despite these apparent advantages, the quality of available components has not been reliable and the method has not been widely used.

5.3.2.2   Alkaline Phosphatase (AP)

Routine use of AP (EC 3.1.3.1) as a label for Abs in immunocytochemistry was established in the late 1970s, although the enzyme had already been used in ELISA techniques with a soluble, coloured end-product for some years. The first immunocytochemical use was for double staining [21] (cf. 5.4.6), taking advantage of the different colours that could be achieved through different chromogens, and their contrast with the brown colour derived from an immunoperoxidase reaction on the same preparation.

AP is a readily available enzyme (from calf intestine) and provides stable Ab conjugates that give an intense bright red (or blue) immunostain. When the monoclonal AP anti-AP (APAAP) technique was developed [22], on principles similar to those of the PAP technique, AP became widely used for immunostaining, particularly in fresh tissues such as cryostat sections of lymphoid tumours and blood smears, where many monoclonal Abs were available to characterize the cells that did not react with paraffin-embedded tissues. The great advantge of AP as a marker, in addition to the brilliant colours of its reaction products, is that there is no need to block endogenous enzyme before carrying out the immunoreaction, and thus no danger of damaging susceptible Ags. Endogenous AP can present a problem, at least in fresh tissues (processing and embedding destroys the activity), but all isoenzymes of AP except the intestinal form can be inhibited by addition of levamisole to the developing medium after the immunoreaction has been completed [23]. Since the enzyme used to label the Abs is from the intestine, it is not affected by the inhibitor and allows the site of Ag-Ab reaction to be seen without confusion. This is not a suitable method for immunostaining fresh preparations of intestinal tissue.

The APAAP reagent is not cyclic, unlike PAP, and probably consists of two molecules of AP to one of Ab. Since the anti-AP is monoclonal, it does not have to be purified, and the APAAP reagent is made simply by adding about 10 mg of a crude preparation of AP to each ml of monoclonal antibody supernatant. This provides enough Ag to give an excess over the Ab and keep the complex in solution.

AP is usually developed by its action on one of the naphthyl phosphates at pH 8.0–9.0 in the presence of a diazonium salt: for example, naphthol AS-BI phosphate and Fast Red TR [24] (cf. 5.3.9.2). This yields a bright red precipitate. Fast Blue BB gives a bright blue colour. Both end-products are alcohol-soluble and aqueous mountants must be used. A less soluble end-product, also red, is given by hexazotised New Fuchsin [25]. A permanent blue-brown product results from a reaction based on a different principle, using 4-chloro-5-bromo-indolyl phosphate, which is a rather expensive substrate, and tetra nitro blue tetrazolium [26]. The intensity of the stain can be increased by repeating the second and third steps of the APAAP reaction, thus building up enzyme on the tissue site of Ag-Ab binding.

5.3.2.3   Glucose Oxidase (GOD)

This enzyme (EC 1.1.3.4) has two advantages as a label: it gives an intensely dark blue reaction product (formazan) which is insoluble [27] (cf. 5.3.10) and it is absent from animal tissue so that there is no need to block endogenous enzyme. It is not a suitable label for plant tissue. GOD-anti-GOD complexes are available, as are avidin-biotin complexes with GOD. However, labelling does not reach the same intensity as with peroxidase, even during a long incubation period, and the deposit tends to be crystalline in nature.

5.3.2.4   β-D-Galactosidase

The bacterial form of the enzyme (EC 3.2.1.23) is used for labelling Abs or immunoglobulin complexes. Its activity is optimal at a pH different from that of the mammalian enzyme: therefore, in mammalian tissue, no blocking is needed. The end-product of reaction in an indoxyl method (cf. 5.3.11) with β-D-galactoside is a bright turquoise blue and it is insoluble so it can be permanently mounted [28]. Unfortunately, the development period is long with this method.

5.3.3   Radioactive Labels

Radioisotopes have been used as labels for Ags as well as for Abs (cf. 5.4.5). The most usual label is ^{125}I, but ^{3}H has also been used. The Ab, or avidin or biotin for an ABC method, can be directly iodinated or tritiated [29], or, if the Ab is monoclonal, it can be produced *in vitro* in the presence of a radiolabelled amino acid, thus incorporating the radioactive element into the Ab [30]. This method of internally labelling Ab has the advantage of causing less damage to the activity of both reagents. The radioactivity of the immunocytochemical reaction is visualized by production of an autoradiograph, by dipping the preparation in radiation-sensitive emulsion or by exposing it to suitable film. The main advantages of these methods are that a) the density of the resulting autoradiograph is directly proportional to the amount of label bound to the preparation, and b) the label can be objectively quantified by grain-counting over individual cells at electron microscopical level or by densitometry at light microscopical level. The use of radiation-sensitive film makes it easy to measure a large area such as an entire transverse section through a spinal cord. Radioimmunocytochemistry can also be combined with immunoperoxidase methods to give double labelling.

The disadvantages include the intrinsic dangers of using radioactive substances, the short half-life of some isotopes (60 days for ^{125}I), the long exposure time needed to develop the autoradiographs, which could be several weeks, and the poor resolution at cellular level of the final result. Thus, these methods are recommended only when more convenient methods are unsuitable.

5.3.4   Colloidal Gold

5.3.4.1   Properties and Use

Abs labelled with colloidal gold were at first used only in electron microscopical immunocytochemistry [31]. In this application the extremely dense gold particles provided a much clearer immunolabel than the rather diffuse product, tending to obscure the underlying structure, that resulted from osmication of polymerized DAB after an immunoperoxidase reaction. An additional advantage for electron microscopical immunocytochemistry is that the gold particles can be made in several different sizes, with diameters ranging from 1 to 40 nm. Thus, different immune reagents can be labelled with gold of different sizes for multiple labelling methods. However, the intrinsic red colour of the gold allows it to be used in light microscopical immunocy-tochemistry also, the first application being to label B-lymphocytes in combination with development of endogenous POD to identify some of the non-lymphocytes [32].

Gold particles bind to proteins by non-covalent bonds at charged sites. Many protein molecules can be adsorbed to a single gold particle, but the proteins must be soluble in buffers of high ionic strength. Protein A, from *Staphylococcus aureus,* has the property of binding to the Fc portions of Abs. The protein is easily adsorbed to colloidal gold and is more soluble than IgG at its isoelectric point in buffers of low salt concentration. Protein A is thus often a better marker for a primary Ab than a gold-adsorbed second Ab, in that it is more stable and problems of species cross-reactivity do not apply. A similar molecule, Protein G, has greater affinity than Protein A for the immunoglo-bulins of some species. A combined "universal" Protein A/G has now been produced [33]. However, as proteins A and G bind to the Fc portion of Abs, it is important that background blocking, if any, is done with albumin only, and not with serum which contains immunoglobulins. Protein A-gold reagents have been used mainly for electron microscopical immunocytochemistry.

Gold-adsorbed Abs have to be used at relatively high concentrations or in multiple applications (see build-up methods, 5.4.4) in order to accumulate enough gold over the reaction site to be visible in a transmitted-light microscope. The efficiency of the reaction is increased if the preparation is viewed in dark field or with epi-polarization when the back-scattering of light makes the metallic particles shine brightly, but only very thin (1–2 µm) sections are suitable for this.

These problems were overcome when *Holgate* et al. [34] adapted a silver precipitation technique to amplify the immunogold reaction. The gold-labelled preparations were immersed in a silver lactate solution in the presence of a reducing agent (hydroquinone). Silver was precipitated from the solution onto the gold particles, which catalysed the reaction, building up a self-perpetuating and enlarging shell of metallic silver, and converting the barely visible red colour of the immunoreaction to an extremely dense black. This immunogold-silver staining increased the detectability of the immunogold reagents enormously, allowing the light chains of lymphocyte surface immunoglobulins to be identified in formalin-fixed paraffin sections for the first time [35]. The smallest size gold particles are most appropriate since they penetrate best and offer the largest surface area for silver deposition, and highly diluted primary Abs can be used. The method has since found many applications, particularly to amplify the reaction in cases where other techniques produce only a faint result. An improvement has been the substitution of light-insensitive silver acetate for silver lactate, allowing the final silver amplification to be monitored under the microscope [36] (cf. 5.3.8.2). Light-insensitive silver reagents are also available commercially. An aspect of the technique is the need for iodine treatment of formalin-fixed paraffin sections before application of the Ab sequence. This step, originally intended to remove pigment from sections after fixation in mercuric chloride, is not always necessary, but the rationale for its use has not yet been explained.

5.3.4.2   Advantages and Disadvantages

Among the advantages of the immunogold methods is their use of non-toxic reagents. In addition, the deposited black silver is very stable allowing the method to be combined with histological or histochemical stains. With epipolarized illumination combined with transmitted light, the silver deposit shines out white against the counterstained background, allowing easy identification of cell types, particularly in haematological or cytological preparations. The method also lends itself to some techniques of multiple immunostaining (cf. sequential staining without elution, 5.4.6).

There are also some disadvantages: it is hard to avoid background deposits of gold particles on tissue sections, perhaps because there is competition for the gold between charged sites on the Ab and in the tissue. The best way to avoid this is to wash the preparations rigorously with detergent, to include a high concentration of salt in the buffer, and to block with a concentrated serum. In electron microscopical immunocytochemistry, the large size of the gold particles means that immunoreactions, except for cell surface Ags, cannot be carried out prior to fixation and embedding because of the low penetrating ability of the gold-adsorbed Ab. However, the excellence of the marker in on-grid staining compensates for this limitation.

5.3.5   Bridging Labels

5.3.5.1   Haptens

Primary or secondary Abs can be labelled with small, antigenic molecules (haptens) that then act as Ags for bridging Abs to the haptens. Applied in excess, these permit the further attachment of a hapten-labelled Ab-enzyme complex or an anti-hapten Ab labelled with a marker that can be made visible [37, 38]. Nonspecific binding is blocked by non-immune serum from the species that provided the primary hapten-labelled Ab; thereafter, the identity of the species donating the Abs is unimportant since it is *via* the hapten that subsequent labelling takes place. By choosing a hapten that does not occur naturally, such as arsanilic acid or dinitrophenyl, only the specifically bound primary Ab can be detected. Primary Abs, even from the same species, labelled with different haptens, thus provide a useful method in double immunostaining. The price paid for a possible increase in specificity is that the primary Ab and the visible label-carrying reagent must both be labelled with the hapten and a bridging anti-hapten must be available.

5.3.5.2   Biotin

Biotin is a small water-soluble vitamin ($M_r = 44$) which has a high affinity for avidin [39–41] and can be attached to Abs in a high molecular ratio (cf. 5.4.3.2). Although biotin is not itself detectable, the combination of biotinylated Abs with avidin and a biotinylated label (eg. POD) provides an immunostain of high intensity and efficiency.

5.3.6   Methods of Labelling Antibodies

These have been described in Chapter 5 of Volume 2. This section therefore gives only a brief description of labelling procedures. Further information may also be found elsewhere [1, 2, 42, 43], and in references given below.

5.3.6.1   Fluorescent Labels

Fluorescein isothiocyanate

FITC is easily bound covalently to Ig molecules and provides a stable conjugate. The essentials of labelling are to incubate the FITC with a purified Ig in alkaline buffer, then to remove unreacted fluorescein on a Sephadex column and elute, dialyse and concentrate the conjugated Ig. Unreacted fluorescein must be removed and the fluorescein-protein ratio must be kept to a minimum because FITC is negatively charged and can itself bind to positively charged proteins in tissue, or increase the negative charge of the conjugate with the same effect. A globulin fraction is required because fluorescein would otherwise bind additionally to serum albumin and make it difficult to calculate the amount of FITC required.

Equipment needed

– 3 cm × 15 cm Sephadex G25 column, equilibrated with PBS;
– Similar column of DEAE cellulose;
– UV spectrometer.

Materials needed

1. Ig fraction of antiserum (e.g. ammonium sulphate-precipitated and (optional) affinity purified);
2. FITC (crystalline);
3. PBS;
4. sodium carbonate buffer 0.05 mol/l, pH 9.5, containing sodium chloride, 0.15 mol/l.

Method

1. Dissolve the Ig (1) in carbonate buffer (4) to give a concentration of 10–20 mg/ml. The final volume should be less than 8 ml for the column described.
2. Add 15–20 μg FITC (2) per mg protein and stir for 1 h at 4 °C.
3. Centrifuge 2000 × g for 10 min.
4. Place the supernatant on the Sephadex column and elute with PBS [3]. The first fraction is the fluorescein-protein conjugate. The second is the unreacted fluorescein which is discarded.
5. Concentrate the conjugated Ab by pressure dialysis.
6. Carry out further purification by gradient elution on a DEAE-cellulose column to rid the conjugate of unreacted Ig and conjugated molecules with too high a ratio of FITC to protein. The best proportion of FITC to protein is 1 or 2 FITC groups: 1 molecule of Ig.
7. Select the fraction by measuring the absorbance A of the conjugate at 280 nm (protein) and 495 nm (fluorescein) [1, 43].

   Molar ratio of fluorescein to protein is $\dfrac{2.87 \times A_{495}}{A_{280} - 0.35 \times A_{495}}$

Rhodamine (tetramethylrhodamine isothiocyanate)

TRITC is conjugated in a similar way but may need a higher label: protein ration (50 μg TRITC per mg protein) to take account of impurities in the fluorochrome [42]. Absorbance is measured at 280 and 550 nm.

AMCA, cf. [7]

5.3.6.2   Enzyme Labels

There are numerous methods for conjugating POD to Abs. Two methods using glutaraldehyde to cross-link the enzyme with the Ig in one [43] or two [1] stages are given here.

One-stage conjugation of POD

Equipment needed

- 1 cm × 30 cm Sephadex G 25 column equilibrated with PBS,
- spectrometer.

Materials needed

1. Ig fraction of antiserum (cf. fluorescent labelling, above);
2. sodium phosphate buffer, 0.1 mol/l, pH 7.0;
3. POD; Type XII, affinity purified, essentially salt-free 250–330 U/mg (using pyrogallol), RZ > 3.0 (*Sigma*)
4. glutaraldehyde, 0.02 % (w/v), freshly prepared in the phosphate buffer;
5. PBS.

Method

1. Dialyse or dissolve the Ig (1) in the phosphate buffer (2) to a final concentration of 2 mg/ml.
2. Dissolve 5 mg POD in 0.5 ml buffer (2) and add it to 0.5 ml Ig solution (1) and 1 ml glutaraldehyde solution (4). Mix at room temperature for 1 h.
3. Place the mixture on the Sephadex column and elute with PBS (5).
4. Monitor the absorbance of the eluant at 280 nm. The conjugate and any free protein are eluted together in the exclusion volume.

Two-stage conjugation of POD

This method provides excess peroxidase to ensure all Ab is labelled.

Equipment needed

- 0.7 cm × 12 cm Sephadex G 50 column equilibrated with sodium chloride, 0.15 mol/l.

Materials needed

1. POD, as above;
2. carbonate buffer, 0.05 mol/l, pH 9.5;
3. glutaraldehyde, 0.25 % (w/v), in carbonate buffer (2);
4. sodium chloride, 0.15 mol/l;
5. affinity-purified Ab;
6. lysine.

Method

1. Dissolve 80 mg POD (1) in 1 ml glutaraldehyde solution (3). Mix for 2 h at room temperature.
2. Separate excess glutaraldehyde from the glutaraldehyde-POD conjugate (void volume) on the Sephadex G50 column by eluting with sodium chloride (4).
3. Mix the glutaraldehyde-POD conjugate with 20 mg affinity-purified Ab, in a molar ratio of 1 Ab: 20 POD, for 23 h at room temperature.
4. Stop the reaction by adding lysine to 0.02 mol/l.
5. Use the fraction with the greatest absorbance at 280 nm.

Peroxidase anti-peroxidase

For preparation cf. [44].

AP and glucose oxidase

For conjugation cf. [45]

APAAP

For preparation cf. [22]

β-D-Galactosidase

For procedures cf. [46]

5.3.6.3   Adsorption of Protein to Colloidal Gold

Full details of the preparation of colloidal gold sols with particles of different sizes and determination of the minimal amount of protein to be added can be found in [47]. The amount of protein to be added, the centrifugation conditions and the final protein concentration vary with the size of the gold particles. The conditions set out here apply to particles of 5 nm diameter which is a suitable size for light-microscopical immunocytochemistry. Even smaller particles (1 nm diameter) are now available. The pH at which the reaction is carried out should be 0.5 pH units above the pI of the protein (e.g. pH 9.0 for purified Ig, pH 6.4–6.6 for streptavidin).

Adsorption to Ab

Materials needed

1. Bovine serum albumin (BSA) (globulin-free), 10 % (w/v) in doubly distilled water, pH adjusted to 9.0 with sodium hydroxide, 1 mol/l. Store frozen in suitable aliquots and microfilter (0.2 μm) just before use;
2. Tris buffer containing Tris 0.02 mol/l, sodium chloride 0.15 mol/l. Sodium azide 0.02 mol/l, 1 % BSA, pH 8.2;
3. colloidal gold sol of defined particle size (5 nm);
4. affinity-purified Ab;
5. 10–30 % (w/v) continuous sucrose or glycerol gradient (10.5 ml, 8 cm) in Tris buffer (2);
6. potassium carbonate, 0.1 mol/l.

Method

1. Adjust pH of the gold sol (3) to 9 with potassium carbonate (6).
2. Add slowly the minimal protecting amount of Ab (4) (pre-determined) with stirring.
3. After 2 min add the BSA solution (1) to a final concentration of 1 % (w/v).
4. Centrifuge at $60\,000 \times g$ for 1 h.
5. Aspirate and discard the supernatant leaving about 10 % of the initial volume.
6. Decant the loose part of the sediment and the remaining supernatant and layer it over the density gradient.
7. Centrifuge at $200\,000 \times g$ 45 min (for 5 nm gold).
8. Collect the upper half of the gradient in 1 ml fractions and examine them for particle size distribution and clusters by electron microscopy [48]. Pool the cluster-free fractions with uniform particle size.
9. Measure the absorbance at 520 nm (1 % (w/v) BSA-Tris (2) as blank) and dilute with 1 % BSA-Tris (2) to an A_{250} of 2.5 (for 5 nm gold).

5.3.6.4   **Biotinylation of Ab** [41, 49]

Materials needed

1. Affinity-purified Ab;
2. sodium hydrogen carbonate, 0.1 mol/l, pH 8.3 ± 0.2;
3. biotin-N-hydroxy succinimide ester;
4. dimethyl sulphoxide (DMSO);
5. PBS.

Method

1. Dialyse the Ab (1) against sodium hydrogen carbonate (2).
2. Adjust protein concentration to 1 mg/ml.
3. Dissolve biotin-*N*-hydroxy succinimide ester (3) in DMSO (4) to a final concentration of 1 mg/ml.
4. To each ml of Ab solution add immediately 150 μl biotin DMSO solution.
5. Mix for 4 h at room temperature in the dark.
6. Dialyse against PBS (5).
7. Concentrate by vacuum dialysis and add sodium azide to 0.02 % for storage.

5.3.6.5   Further Labelling Methods

Biotinylation of peroxidase or other label: cf. [50]
Labelling an Ab with a hapten: cf. [51]
Labelling an Ab with a radioisotope: cf. [52]
Labelling an Ag with a radioisotope: cf. [53]
Labelling an peptide Ag with colloidal gold: cf. [54]

5.3.7   Visualization of Fluorescent Labels

5.3.7.1   Microscope

This should be provided with a high pressure mercury vapour lamp and epi-illumination system. Appropriate filters ensure that light of the correct excitation wavelength for the fluorophore reaches the specimen. Secondary filters ensure that only the emitted light reaches the eye.

5.3.7.2   Mountants

1. Mount in buffered glycerine: glycerine: PBS, 9:1 (v:v). Fading is retarded by a) a high pH (8.6), and b) addition of 2.5 % (w/v) 1,4-diazobicyclo-(2,2,2)-octane (DABCO) [55].
2. Permafluor (*Lipshaw*) is a water-miscible mountant that sets hard and preserves fluorescence well. Seal the edges of the coverslip with nail varnish to prevent the mountant drying back.

3. Dry the preparations, dip briefly in xylene or other solvent (optional) and mount in a permanent non-fluorescent mountant. This procedure can produce a non-fading permanent preparation but results are not predictable.

5.3.7.3   Storage

Keep fluorescent preparations in the dark and (if in aqueous mountant) at 4 °C.

5.3.7.4   Restoration of Fluorescence

A preparation that has faded either through time or through exposure to light in the microscope may sometimes be restored by removal of the coverslip and re-application of the fluorescent Ab [56]. Presumably the second application replaces the original fluorescent Ab that has become detached and/or the first application failed to saturate the available binding sites.

5.3.7.5   Fluorescent Counterstains

These can be used to mask background staining or autofluorescence and enhance visibility of tissue in relation to immunofluorescence (of fluorescein).

Methyl Green

This gives a red nuclear fluorescence [57].

Materials needed

1. 0.1 % (w/v) methyl green (C. I. 42590) in distilled water;
2. PBS.

Method

1. Add 4 ml methyl green (1) to 36 ml PBS (2).
2. After completing the immunofluorescence staining procedure, immerse the preparations in the above solution for 5 min.
3. Wash in PBS (2) for 5 min with gentle agitation.
4. Mount as preferred.

Pontamine Sky Blue

This gives a red tissue fluorescence [4].

Materials needed

1. Pontamine Sky Blue (PSB);
2. dimethylsulphoxide (DMSO);
3. PBS.

Method

1. After completing the immunofluorescence stain, immerse the preparations in 0.05% PSB (1) in DMSO (2) for 30 min.
2. Wash in PBS (3).
3. Mount in aqueous mountant.
   The counterstain may be carried out before the primary Ab is applied, lessening the risk of obscuring specific immunofluorescence.

5.3.8   Visualization of Peroxidase

5.3.8.1   Blocking Endogenous POD Reactions

Blocking with excess substrate is usually carried out before the immunostaining method, but if the Ag sought is likely to be damaged by hydrogen peroxide the blocking step should be carried out after application of the primary Ab or at any stage before application of a POD linked reagent.

Paraffin sections and epoxy resin sections

Materials needed

1. Solvent for removing paraffin;
2. saturated solution of sodium hydroxide in alcohol for removing epoxy resin. Make the solution by adding solid sodium hydroxide pellets to absolute alcohol. Shake at intervals for a week. The solution is ready when it is pale yellow to dark brown and will remain effective for several months [58];
3. 100%, 90%, 70% (v/v) alcohol for hydrating sections;

4. 30 % (w/v) hydrogen peroxide stock solution. If higher dilutions only are available, adjust quantity accordingly;
5. 0.3 % (w/v) hydrogen peroxide: add 1 ml 30 % hydrogen peroxide (4) to 100 ml distilled water.

Method

1. Remove the wax from paraffin sections in solvent and bring them to water through graded alcohols. Remove the resin from epoxy resin sections by soaking in alcoholic sodium hydroxide (2) for 10–20 min, rinse in several changes of alcohol and bring to water [58].
2. Immerse for 30 min in 0.3 % hydrogen peroxide (5) in water or buffer (PBS or TBS). Rinse in buffer and proceed with the immunostaining method. Methanol (itself a partial inhibitor of POD) may be used instead of water or buffer; in this case, do not hydrate the sections but de-wax and take them to alcohol, then immerse in methanolic hydrogen peroxide. After 30 min, bring to water through graded alcohols.

Frozen sections, cell preparations

A less harsh method is required; two are given here.

Procedure A
Hydrogen peroxide in 70% (w/v) methanol in buffer

Materials needed

1. 30 % (w/v) H_2O_2;
2. methanol;
3. PBS (TBS);

Method

1. Mix 70 ml methanol and 30 ml PBS (TBS).
2. Add 1 ml H_2O_2 (1) (final concentration 0.3 %).
3. After fixation, immerse preparations in the above mixture for 30 min.
4. Rinse in PBS (TBS).

Procedure B
Nascent hydrogen peroxide from addition of glucose oxidase on glucose with sodium azide (another peroxidase inhibitor) [59].

Materials needed

1. PBS (pre-warmed to 37 °C);
2. 18 % (w/v) β-D-glucose;
3. 0.65 % (w/v) sodium azide;
4. glucose oxidase 1000 U/ml at 35 °C (*Sigma*, G 6891).

Method

1. Add 1 ml glucose (2) and 1 ml sodium azide (3) to 100 ml warm PBS.
2. Just before use add 100 U glucose oxidase (4).
3. Incubate preparations for 1 h at 37 °C.
4. Wash in PBS.

5.3.8.2   Development Methods

Note that many chromogens used are potentially carcinogenic. Wear gloves; make solutions and carry out reactions in a fume cupboard; dispose of solutions carefully (see below).

Storage of reagents

DAB in aqueous solution (e.g. 25–50 mg/ml) may be stored safely in frozen aliquots [60]. A 1 ml aliquot is sufficient for 100 ml of incubating medium. Thaw the aliquot completely before use (put container in hot water) as DAB particles may precipitate on storage.

Make enzyme development solutions just before use. H_2O_2 solutions keep well for several months at 4 °C but eventually deteriorate. Ensure supply is fresh enough. If stock solution is less than 30 % adjust volume added accordingly.

Procedure A: DAB/H_2O_2 [11]

Materials needed

1. PBS (pH 7.0–7.2) or TBS (pH 7.6);
2. DAB 25–50 mg/ml in 1 ml aliquots;
3. 30 % (w/v) H_2O_2.

Method

1. Add 25–50 mg DAB (2) to 100 ml PBS (TBS) (1). The solution should be clear or very light brown.

2. Just before use add 10–100 µl H_2O_2 (3) to the DAB solution (final concentration 0.01–0.03 %).
   (The quantities of DAB and H_2O_2 used vary among authors but are to be found within the range given. Decide on a standard for your own preparations).
3. Incubate preparations for 5–15 min (7–10 min is usually optimal) at room temperature.
4. Wash in buffer, examine microscopically.
   Reaction product is dark brown. If inadequate, preparations may be returned to the incubation medium but over-incubation may produce brownish background staining.
5. Wash in water, counterstain nuclei lightly in haematoxylin (blue) or methyl green (green) if required. The reaction product is insoluble, so the haematoxylin may be differentiated in acid alcohol if necessary and "blued" in alkaline solution.
6. Dehydrate through graded alcohols to solvent (e.g. xylene) and mount in permanent mountant.

Disposing of the DAB solution: add a few drops of household bleach (sodium hypochlorite). The solution will turn black (oxidized DAB) and may be flushed down the drain with water. Wash all glassware very throughly in water to remove all traces of bleach which would prevent future POD/DAB/H_2O_2 reactions.

Procedure B: 3-amino-9-ethylcarbazole/H_2O_2 [61]

Materials needed

1. Acetate buffer 0.05 mol/l, pH 5.0;
2. 4% (w/v) 3-amino-9-ethylcarbazole in dimethyl formamide (AEC stock solution);
3. 30 % (w/v) H_2O_2.

Method

1. Pre-incubate preparations in acetate buffer (1) for 5 min.
2. Mix incubation solution:
   0.5 ml AEC stock solution (2),
   9.5 ml acetate buffer (1),
   10 µl H_2O_2 (3).
3. Filter onto the preparations and incubate for 5–10 min at room temperature. The reaction product is red. It is alcohol-soluble; therefore, if haematoxylin is used to counterstain the nuclei blue, differentiation must be with aqueous 1 % HCl. Mount in a water-miscible mountant.

Procedure C: 4-chloro-1-naphthol/H$_2$O$_2$ (modified from [19])

Materials needed

1. 4-Chloro-1-naphthol;
2. alcohol;
3. PBS (TBS);
4. 30 % (w/v) H$_2$O$_2$.

Method

1. Dissolve 30–40 mg 4-chloro-1-naphthol (1) in 0.2–0.5 ml alcohol (2).
2. Add quickly with stirring 100 ml PBS (TBS).
3. Heat the mixture to 50 °C (not higher, to avoid inhibiting POD) to dissolve most of the white precipitate.
4. Filter rapidly through coarse filter-paper.
5. Add 50–100 µl H$_2$O$_2$ (4).
6. Incubate preparations in the warm filtrate for 5–15 min. The reaction product is blue-grey. It is alcohol-soluble.
   Methyl green would be a suitable nuclear counterstain. Use a water-miscible mountant.

Other Procedures

α-Naphthol/H$_2$O$_2$ and basic dye [62] (colour of end-product depends on the dye; products are variably alcohol-soluble).

Hanker's reagent/H$_2$O$_2$ [20]

Phenol-tetrazolium method [61] The end-product is an insoluble blue formazan. The pseudo POD of erythrocytes does not react with this substrate but endogenous POD and (in fresh preparations) NADH dehydrogenase must be inhibited.

Intensification of DAB/H$_2$O$_2$ reaction product

All methods described below result in a very dark reaction product. The post-DAB treatments can be used to "improve" a poor stain. If any background staining is present it, too, will be intensified.

Imidazole incorporated in the standard incubating medium [64]

This darkens the brown of the reaction product.

Materials needed

1. Imidazole;
2. PBS (TBS);
3. HCl, 1 mol/l;
4. DAB, 25–50 mg/ml in 1 ml aliquots;
5. 30 % (w/v) H_2O_2.

Method

1. Dissolve imidazole (1) in a small volume of PBS (2).
2. Adjust pH to 7.0 with HCl [3]
3. Add 25–50 mg DAB (4) to 100 ml PBS (TBS) (2).
4. Add imidazole solution to DAB solution to a final concentration of 0.01 mol/l.
5. Add 10–100 µl H_2O_2 (5).
6. Incubate preparations and finish as for procedure A.

Incorporation of heavy metal salt in incubation medium [64]

– Cobalt [12]

Materials needed

1. DAB, 50 mg aliquot;
2. PBS (TBS);
3. 0.5 % (w/v) cobalt chloride;
4. 30 % (w/v) H_2O_2.

Method

1. Dissolve 50 mg DAB (1) in 100 ml PBS (TBS) (2).
2. Add with stirring 1 ml $CoCl_2$ (3).
3. Incubate preparations in the above medium for 5 min.
4. Mix in 10 µl H_2O_2 (4).
5. Continue to incubate for a further 1–5 min, checking microscopically. The reaction product should be blue-black and the background clear.
6. Rinse in water, counterstain as required, dehydrate, clear and mount in permanent medium.

-Nickel [65]

Materials needed

1. Acetate buffer, 0.1 mol/l, pH 6.0;
2. nickel sulphate;
3. DAB 25 mg aliquot;
4. 30 % (w/v) H_2O_2.

Method

1. Pre-incubate preparations in acetate buffer (1).
2. Dissolve 1–2.5 g nickel sulphate (2) in 100 ml acetate buffer (1).
3. Add 25 mg DAB (3). Solution becomes cloudy but clears on stirring. Filter if necessary.
4. Add 23 µl H_2O_2 (4) (final conc. 0.007 %).
5. Incubate preparations for 5–15 min. Reaction product is dark blue-black.
6. Counterstain nuclei red in 1 % Neutral Red, or green in 2 % Methyl Green, 2 min. Wash briefly in water, blot dry with damp absorbent paper, dehydrate rapidly through two changes of absolute alcohol to solvent, mount in permanent mountant.

Note. Avoid haematoxylin, as blue nuclei detract from the contrast, and acid, which may remove the stain.

-Nickel with nascent H_2O_2 [13]

This method can provide a strong stain with a very low background, but the reaction starts slowly and increases in rate as the concentration of H_2O_2 increases. It requires careful microscopical monitoring to prevent over-reaction that results in background staining.

Materials needed

1. Acetate buffer, 0.1 mol/l, pH 6.0;
2. ammonium nickel sulphate;
3. DAB 30–50 mg/ml aliquot;
4. β-D-glucose;
5. ammonium chloride;
6. glucose oxidase, GOD (specifications cf. 5.3.8.1, procedure B).

Method

1. Pre-incubate preparations in acetate buffer (1).
2. Dissolve 2.5 g ammonium nickel sulphate (2) in 100 ml acetate buffer.
3. Add 50 mg pre-dissolved DAB (3). Solution becomes cloudy but clears on stirring.
4. Just before use add
   200 mg β-D-glucose (4),
   40 mg ammonium chloride (5),
   100 U GOD (6).
5. Incubate preparations for 5 to 20 min, checking microscopically.
   Reaction product is black and background should be clear.
6. Finish as in 5.3.8.1.

Intensification of DAB reaction product after standard development

Silver deposition on the reaction product provides a black stain and may be achieved in several ways. It may be necessary to prevent reaction of argyrophilic tissue elements (e.g. reticulin fibres) by pre-treatment [16, 17]. All glassware must be well washed in distilled water.

Silver-gold intensification [14]

The physical developer consists of two stock solutions which can be stored at room temperature away from light. All solutions are made in distilled water of high purity.

Materials needed

1. Solution A: 5 % (w/v) sodium carbonate;
2. Solution B: add to 1 l distilled water in the following order
   2 g ammonium nitrate, 2 g silver nitrate, 10 g tungstosilicic acid and 5 ml 37 % (w/v) formaldehyde;
3. 2% sodium acetate;
4. citric acid/ammonium acetate buffer, 0.1 mol/l, pH 5.5;
5. 1 % (v/v) acetic acid;
6. 0.05 % (w/v) gold chloride ($HAuCl_4$);
7. 3 % (w/v) sodium thiosulphate.

Method

1. Wash DAB-reacted preparations very well in distilled water.
2. Wash well in sodium acetate (3).
3. Transfer to citric acid/ammonium acetate buffer (4).
4. Just before use, add 20 ml solution B (2) to 20 ml solution A (1), dropwise with stirring.
5. Develop in the silver solution for 5–15 min, checking microscopically. Stop the reaction by immersion in 1 % acetic acid (5).
6. Wash in 3 changes of citric acid/ammonium acetate buffer (4), 5 min each.
7. Transfer to 0.05 % gold chloride (6) for 10 min.
8. Wash in citric acid/ammonium acetate buffer (4) for 5 min.
9. Treat with sodium thiosulphate (7) for 30 min.
10. Wash in water, counterstain as required, dehydrate, clear and mount in permanent medium

Silver methenamine intensification [15]

This is a simpler method than the preceding one but nevertheless effective [66]

Materials needed

1. Stock solution A: mix 100 ml 3% (w/v) hexamine and 5 ml 5% (w/v) silver nitrate;
2. 5% (w/v) sodium tetraborate;
3. silver development solution: mix 25 ml solution A with 25 ml distilled water and 2 ml sodium tetraborate, (2);
4. 0.2% (w/v) gold chloride;
5. 2.5% (w/v) sodium thiosulphate.

Method

1. Heat the development solution (3) to 60 °C protected from light.
2. Wash the DAB-reacted preparations very well in distilled water.
3. Immerse the preparations in the hot silver solution for 3–15 min, checking microscopically. The reaction is usually adequate after 5 min, converting a light DAB reaction product to dark brown to black. If a nickel-DAB reaction was used initially, silver intensification takes an even shorter time [42].
4. Wash in distilled water.
5. Tone in gold chloride (4) (to remove some background).
6. Wash in water.
7. Transfer to sodium thiosulphate (5) for 1 min.
8. Wash, counterstain as required, dehydrate, clear and mount in permanent medium.

Silver intensification after nickel/DAB development [18]

This method uses a low pH silver solution to prevent tissue argyrophilic reactions. It cannot be used on DAB alone: nickel enhancement is necessary. Coating slides with gelatin before silver development protects the preparations from nonspecific silver deposits which are washed away with the gelatin after the reaction [67].

Materials needed

1. Glycerinated gelatin: dissolve 15 g gelatin in 100 ml distilled water with heating. Add 100 ml glycerine and filter while hot through glass wool. Store at 4 °C. Melt for use. 0.5% (w/v) gelatin would be a suitable substitute;
2. sodium acetate, 3H$_2$O;
3. acetic acid glacial;
4. 1% (w/v) cetylpyridinium chloride;
5. 1% (v/v) Triton X-100;
6. silver nitrate;
7. 5% (w/v) sodium tungstate (can be kept at room temperature);
8. 0.2% (w/v) ascorbic acid (freshly prepared);
9. 1% (v/v) acetic acid;
10. photographic fixer (diluted 1:4), or 5% (w/v) sodium thiosulphate.

Method

1. Coat DAB/nickel-developed preparations with glycerinated gelatin (1) or 0.5 %
   gelatin and allow to dry at room temperature for at least 2 h.
2. Stock solution A: add 45 g sodium acetate (2) and 7.5 ml acetic acid (3) to 400 ml
   distilled water. Add 15 ml cetylpyridinium chloride (4), 5 ml Triton X-100 (5), 1.1 g
   silver nitrate (6) dissolved in a few ml distilled water.
   Make up to 800 ml with distilled water. Filter through Millipore filter (0.45 μm pore
   size). Store in dark bottles at room temperature (keeps for several weeks).
3. To 80 ml solution A add dropwise with vigorous stirring 10 ml sodium tungstate (7)
   and 10 ml ascorbic acid (8).
4. Immerse preparations in silver solution for 3–6 min, checking microscopically.
5. Stop the reaction by immersing slides in 1 % acetic acid (9).
6. Wash in gently running warm tap water for 45 min to remove the gelatin.
7. Fix in photographic fixer or sodium thiosulphate (10) for a few minutes.
8. Wash in running tap water 5 min.
9. Counterstain as required, dehydrate, clear and mount. Canada balsam has been
   recommended as a mountant that preserves silver stains well: others may also be
   suitable.

To remove excessive silver staining, *Farmer's* solution may be used. Silver is removed in
seconds, so use a cautious approach.

Farmer's solution:

Mix 90 ml 10 % (w/v) sodium thiosulphate and 10 ml 10 % (w/v) potassium ferricyanide.

Other methods

Intensification may be carried out with gold chloride alone, copper sulphate [68],
osmium tetroxide [11], ferric-ferricyanide [69].

5.3.9   Visualization of Alkaline Phosphatase

5.3.9.1   Blocking Endogenous Enzyme

This is necessary only in fresh or frozen preparations and is done by the addition of
levamisole to 1 mmol/l to the development medium [23].

5.3.9.2   Development Methods

Procedure A: Development to give a blue end-product; modified from [24]

Materials needed

1. Naphthol AS-MX phosphate;
2. dimethyl formamide;
3. Tris/HCl buffer, 0.1 mol/l, pH 8.2;
4. Fast Blue BB.

Method

1. Stock substrate solution (use a glass vessel – plastic may dissolve in dimethylfor-mamide): dissolve 2 mg naphthol AS-MX phosphate (1) in 0.2 ml dimethyl formamide (2); add quickly with stirring 10 ml Tris buffer (3).
   The stock substrate solution may be made in bulk and stored at 4 °C for several weeks or made more concentrated and stored in frozen aliquots of 1 mg naphthol phosphate per ml of buffer and diluted for use.
2. Just before use, add 1 mg Fast Blue BB (4) per ml stock substrate solution (1).
3. Filter and incubate preparations for 5–20 min. If reaction seems slow, place the preparations at 37 °C. The reaction product is bright blue. It is alcohol-soluble.
4. Wash the preparations well in water and mount them in a water-miscible mountant.

   For the development of a bright red end-product use Fast Red TR instead of Fast Blue BB.

Procedure B: Development for a red end-product less soluble in alcohol [25]

Materials needed

1. Naphthol AS-TR phosphate;
2. dimethyl formamide;
3. Tris/HCl buffer, 0.2 mol/l, pH 9.2;
4. stock substrate solution (glass vessel and storage as above): dissolve 2 mg naphthol AS-TR phosphate in 40 µl dimethyl formamide; add quickly with stirring 8 ml Tris buffer (3);
5. 4 % (w/v) New Fuchsin in HCl, 2 mol/l, (store indefinitely at 4 °C);
6. 4 % (w/v) sodium nitrite (keeps for 4 days at 4 °C);
7. hexazotized New Fuchsin (freshly made just before use): mix equal volumes of (5) and (6) and allow to react; the dark red solution will become yellowish brown and bubbles will form. After 1 min add the correct volume to the stock solution;
8. Levamisole (for fresh preparations).

Method

1. Just before use, add to 8 ml stock substrate solution, 100 µl freshly made hexazotized New Fuchsin (7).
3. Add levamisole (8) to 1 mmol/l if required to inhibit endogenous alkaline phosphatase.
4. Filter onto the preparations and incubate for 5–20 min at room temperature or 37 °C. Reaction product is red.
5. Wash in water, counterstain nuclei in haematoxylin (differentiating in aqueous 1 % HCl). Blot dry with damp absorbent paper, dehydrate rapidly and mount in permanent mountant.

Procedure C: Development for a permanent blue-brown end-product [26]

This is reported to be the most sensitive of the alkaline phosphatase development methods. It is also the most expensive.

Materials needed

1. 5-Bromo-4-chloro-3-indolyl phosphate (BCIP);
2. dimethyl formamide (DMF);
3. tetra nitro blue tetrazolium (TNBT);
4. Tris/HCl buffer, 0.2 mol/l, pH 9.5;
5. magnesium chloride · 10 H_2O;
6. solution A: dissolve 5 mg BCIP (1) in 100 µl DMF (2);
7. solution B: dissolve 10 mg TNBT (3) in 200 µl DMF (2), add 100 ml Tris buffer (4);
8. solution C: 30 ml Tris buffer (4) containing magnesium chloride (5), 10 mmol/l.

Method

1. Incubation solution: add solutions A (6) and B (7) to solution C (8).
2. Filter and incubate preparations for 15–30 min at room temperature or 37 °C.
3. Wash in water, counterstain nuclei with neutral red (1 % w/v) for 2 min. Wash in water, blot dry. Dehydrate rapidly in two changes of absolute alcohol, clear and mount in permanent medium.

5.3.10 Visualization of Glucose Oxidase [27]

Materials needed

1. β-D-Glucose;
2. Nitro Blue Tetrazolium (NBT);
3. phenazine methosulphate (PMS);
4. Tris HCl buffer, 0.05 mol/l, pH 8.3.

Method

1. Heat Tris buffer (4) containing glucose, 6.7 mg/ml (1) and NBT, 0.67 mg/ml, (2) to 37°C.
2. Add PMS (3) to 0.0617 mg/ml.
3. Incubate preparations for 1 h at 37 °C protected from light. The reaction product is dark blue.
4. Counterstain nuclei with neutral red (as previous method), dehydrate rapidly, clear and mount in permanent medium.

Suitable aliquots of NBT may be stored frozen in aqueous solution. PMS must be freshly added.

Glucose oxidase may be developed to give a permanent brown reaction product by substituting Tetra NBT for NBT [70].

5.3.11 Visualization of β-D-Galactosidase

Materials needed

1. 5-Bromo-4-chloro-indolyl-β-D-galactoside (BCIG);
2. dimethyl formamide (DMF);
3. PBS, pH 7.0–7.5 containing 1 mmol/l magnesium chloride;
4. potassium ferricyanide 50 mmol/l;
5. potassium ferrocyanide 50 mmol/l;
6. solution A: dissolve 50 mg BCIG (1) in 0.5 ml DMF (2);
7. solution B: add 0.5 ml potassium ferricyanide (4) and 0.5 ml potassium ferrocyanide (5) to 7 ml PBS (3).

Method

1. Add 0.05 ml solution A (6) to 2.276 ml solution B (7).
2. Incubate preparations for 1 h at 37 °C. Reaction product is turquoise blue.
3. Counterstain nuclei with neutral red (as previous methods), dehydrate, clear and mount in permanent medium.

Solutions A and B and the final incubation solution may be stored frozen.

5.3.12 Visualization of Colloidal Gold Labels

The deep magenta colour of colloidal gold is microscopically visible if present in high concentration, e.g., after a multi-layer immunoreaction. It may also be visualized in much lower amounts by the back scattering of yellow light when the preparation is viewed under dark field illumination or, better, by epi-polarized illumination which can be combined with transmitted light microscopy [71]. However, the great sensitivity of immunogold methods derives from the highly intensified black product of the deposition of metallic silver on the gold particles at the site of the immunoreaction; this, too, can be viewed with epi-polarized light, emitting brilliant white light. Apart from commercial silver intensification solutions, two methods are commonly used.

Procedure A: Intensification by silver lactate [34, 35]

The silver development solution is prepared just before use. Glassware must be thoroughly washed with distilled water, as must the immunogold-reacted preparations before incubation.

Materials needed

1. Solution A (citrate buffer, pH ca. 3.5): 2.35 g trisodium citrate dihydrate and 2.55 g citric acid in 85 ml distilled water;
2. solution B (hydroquinone): dissolve 0.85 g hydroquinone in 85 ml citrate buffer (solution A);
3. solution C: dissolve 0.11 g silver lactate in 15 ml distilled water; protect from light;
4. 5 % (w/v) sodium thiosulphate.

Method

1. Just before use add C (3) to B (2).
2. Incubate preparations in the dark for 4–8 min. Support the preparations vertically in the solution (e.g., in a *Coplin* jar) to prevent nonspecific deposits on the surface.
3. Check the reaction microscopically on well rinsed preparations. If it is weak, rinse the preparations well in distilled water and repeat the silver intensification with freshly made solution. The final result should be an intense, black silver deposit.
4. When the reaction is satisfactory, wash the preparations in distilled water.
5. Transfer to photographic fixer (diluted 1:4) or sodium thiosulphate (4) for 2 min.
6. Wash in running tap water for 10 min. Counterstain as required, dehydrate, clear and mount in permanent medium.

Some synthetic mountants may cause fading of the silver. If this is a problem, Canada balsam is recommended.

Control of non-specific deposition of silver grains on the sections.

Two methods are available.
1. Include gum arabic in the medium. For maximum effect (reaction will take up to 1 h, but is easier to control microscopically) replace 60 ml of citrate buffer with 60 ml of gum arabic (gum acacia), 500 g/l. A smaller proportion of gum arabic solution will retard the reaction less.

   Stock solution of gum arabic: dissolve 500 g gum arabic in 1 litre distilled water Stir for 4 h, then occasionally for 4 days at room temperature, filter through several layers of gauze and store frozen in aliquots.
2. Coat the preparations with 5 % (w/v) gelatin and allow them to dry before immersion in the silver solution. After the reaction the gelatin is removed in running warm tap water [36].

Procedure B: Intensification by silver acetate [36]

This development medium is not sensitive to light and is much less expensive than the silver lactate or commercial alternatives.

Materials needed

1. Silver acetate (should be finely crystalline – a suitable grade is supplied by *Fluka*);
2. hydroquinone;
3. citrate buffer (Solution A, previous method), pH 3.8 (approx);
4. solution A: 100 mg silver acetate (1) in 50 ml distilled water;
5. solution B: 250 mg hydroquinone (2) in 50 ml citrate buffer (3).

Method

1. Just before use mix solutions A and B (4 and 5).
2. Incubate as above.

Preparations may be checked microscopically while in the medium at a low level of illumination.

5.3.13 Autoradiographic Development

The procedure for developing autoradiographs will depend on the isotope and the amount of radioactivity incorporated in the labelled reagent. ^{3}H or ^{125}I are the most commonly used isotopes (note: the half-life of ^{125}I is only 60 days). It may be necessary to try a variety of exposure times to attain the optimum. Choice of the dipping/stripping film technique or exposure to an apposed radiation-sensitive film depends on whether a preparation is to be viewed in the microscope or whether a measure is required of the gross amount of radiation (equivalent to amount of antigen) in one area compared with another. Two methods are quoted as examples, but see [72] for details of autoradiographic technique. On sectioned material, the thinner the section, the better the microscopical resolution.

^{125}I antigen in the RICH technique – dipping or stripping film [53]

After carrying out the immunoreaction:
1. Fix preparation in 2.5 % (w/v) glutaraldehyde in cacodylate buffer, 0.2 mol/l, pH 7.2, for 5–15 min (optional).
2. Wash in distilled water, for 5–15 min.
3. Dip in emulsion (e.g. *Kodak* NTB-2), or coat slides with stripping film under safelight. Allow to dry and pack in a light-tight box.
4. Leave at 4 °C.
5. Develop samples after 2 days, 1 week, 3 weeks respectively using *Kodak* D19 developer. Fix in sodium thiosulphate.
6. Counterstain with haematoxylin and eosin.

Avidin-[^{3}H]Biotin Complex – film technique [71]

As an example, large sections of rat mid-brain treated with anti-substance P, biotinylated second Ab and [^{3}H] ABC.

1. Appose sections to *LKB* tritium-sensitive Ultrofilm in a light-tight casette.
2. Expose for up to 8 weeks at $-20\,°C$ and develop in Kodafix (*Kodak*).

Contact prints or image analysis from the developed film allow semi-quantitative analysis of the relative amounts of radiation from different areas.

References

[1] *L.A. Sternberger*, Immunocytochemistry, 3rd Ed. John Wiley and Sons, New York (1986)

[2] *R.C. Nairn*, Fluorescence Microscopy and Photomicrography, in: *R.C. Nairn* (ed.), Fluorescent Protein Tracing, 4th Ed., Churchill Livingstone, Edinburgh (1976) pp. 68–108.

[3] *F.W.D. Rost*, Fluorescence Microscopy, in: *A.G.E. Pearse* (ed.), Histochemistry, Theoretical and Applied, Volume 1, 4th Edn., Churchill Livingstone, Edinburgh (1980) pp. 346–378.

[4] *T. Cowen, A.J. Haven, G. Burnstock*, Pontamine Sky Blue: A Counterstain for Background Autofluorescence in Fluorescence and Immunofluorescence Histochemistry, Histochemistry *82*, 205–208 (1985).

[5] *J.A. Titus, R. Haugland, S.O. Sharrow, D.M. Segal*, Texas Red, A Hydrophilic Red-Emitting Fluorophore for Use with Fluorescein in Dual Parameter Flow Microfluorometric and Fluorescence Microscopic Studies, J. Immunol. Methods *50*, 193–204 (1982).

[6] *C.S. Chadwick, M.G. McEntegart, R.C. Nairn*, Fluorescent Protein Tracers: A Trial of New Fluorochromes and the Development of an Alternative to Fluorescein, Immunology *1*, 315–327 (1958).

[7] *M.W. Wessendorf, N.M. Appel, T.W. Molitor, R.P. Elde*, A Method for Immunofluorescence Demonstration of Three Coexisting Neurotransmitters in Rat Brain and Spinal Cord, Using the Fluorophores Fluorescein, Lissamine Rhodamine and 7-Amino-4-Methylcoumarin-3-Acetic Acid, J. Histochem. Cytochem. *38*, 1859–1877 (1990).

[8] *V.T. Oi, A.N. Glazer, L. Stryer*, Fluorescent Phycobiliprotein Conjugates for Analyses of Cells and Molecules, J. Cell Biol. *93*, 981–986 (1982).

[9] *W.A. Staines, T. Yamamoto, P.E. Daddona, J.I. Nagy*, Adenosine Deaminase-Containing Hypothalamic Neurons Accumulate 5-Hydroxytryptophan: A Dual Color Immunofluorescence Procedure Using a New Fluorescence Marker, Neurosci. Lett. *70*, 1–5 (1986).

[10] *H. Khalfan, R. Abuknesha, M. Rand-Weaver, R.G. Price, D. Robinson*, Aminomethyl Coumarin Acetic Acid: A New Fluorescent Labelling Agent for Proteins, Histochem. J. *18*, 497–499 (1986).

[11] *R.C. Graham, M.J. Karnovsky*, The Early Stages of Absorption of Injected Horseradish Peroxidase in the Proximal Tubules of Mouse Kidney. Ultrastructural Cytochemistry by a New Technique, J. Histochem. Cytochem. *14*, 291–302 (1966).

[12] *S.M. Hsu, E. Soban*, Color Modification of Diaminobenzidine (DAB) Precipitation by Metallic Ions and Its Application to Double Immunohistochemistry, J. Histochem. Cytochem. *30*, 1079–1082 (1982).

[13] *S. Shu, G. Ju, L. Fan*, The Glucose Oxidase – DAB – Nickel Method in Peroxidase Histochemistry of the Nervous System, Neurosci. Lett. *85*, 169–171 (1988).

[14] *F. Gallyas, T. Görcs, I. Merchenthaler*, High Grade Intensification of the End-Product of the Diaminobenzidine Reaction for Peroxidase Histochemistry, J. Histochem. Cytochem. *30*, 183–184 (1982).

[15] *C.S. Peacock, I.W. Thompson, S. Van Noorden*, Silver Enhancement of Polymerised Diaminobenzidine. Increased Sensitivity for Immunoperoxidase Staining, J. Clin. Pathol. *44*, 756–758 (1991).

[16] *F. Gallyas*, Suppression of the Argyrophil III Reaction by Mercapto Compounds. (A Prerequisite for the Intensification of Certain Histochemical Reactions by Physical Developers.), Acta Histochem. *70*, 99–105 (1982).

[17] *F. Gallyas, J.R. Wolff,* Metal-Catalyzed Oxidation Renders Silver Intensification Selective. Applications for the Histochemistry of Diaminobenzidine and Neurofibrillary Changes, J. Histochem. Cytochem. *34,* 1667–1672 (1986).

[18] *B. Frigo, L. Scopsi, C. Patriarca, F. Rilke,* Silver Enhancement of Nickel-Diaminobenzidine as Applied to Single and Double Immunoperoxidase Staining, Biotechnic and Histochemistry *66,* 159–166 (1991).

[19] *P.K. Nakane,* Simultaneous Localization of Multiple Tissue Antigens Using the Peroxidase-Labeled Antibody Method: a Study in Pituitary Glands of the Rat, J. Histochem. Cytochem. *16,* 557–560 (1968).

[20] *J.S. Hanker, P.E. Yates, C.B. Metz, A. Rustioni,* A New Specific, Sensitive and Non-Carcinogenic Reagent for the Demonstration of Horseradish Peroxidase, Histochem J. *9,* 789–792 (1977).

[21] *D.Y. Mason, R.E. Sammons,* Alkaline Phosphatase and Peroxidase for Double Immunoenzymatic Labelling of Cellular Constituents, J. Clin. Pathol. *31,* 454–462 (1978).

[22] *J.L. Cordell, B. Falini, W.N. Erber, A.K. Ghosh, Z. Abdulaziz, S. MacDonald, K.A.F. Pulford, H. Stein, D.Y. Mason,* Immunoenzymatic Labeling of Monoclonal Antibodies Using Immune Complexes of Alkaline Phosphatase and Monoclonal Anti-Alkaline Phosphatase (APAAP) Complexes, J. Histochem. Cytochem. *32,* 219–222 (1984) .

[23] *B.A. Ponder, M.W. Wilkinson,* Inhibition of Endogenous Tissue Alkaline Phosphatase with the Use of Alkaline Phosphatase Conjugates in Immunohistochemistry, J. Histochem. Cytochem. *29,* 981–984 (1981).

[24] *M.S. Burstone,* Histochemical Demonstration of Phosphatases in Frozen Sections with Naphthol AS-Phosphates, J. Histochem. Cytochem. *9,* 146–153 (1961).

[25] *N.J. Malik, M.E. Damon,* Improved Double Immunoenzymatic Labelling Using Alkaline Phosphatase and Horseradish Peroxidase, J. Clin. Pathol. *35,* 1092–1094 (1978).

[26] *A.S.H. De Jong, M. Van Kessel-Van Vark, A.K. Raap,* Sensitivity of Various Visualisation Methods for Peroxidase and Alkaline Phosphatase Activity in Immunoenzyme Histochemistry, Histochem. J. *17,* 1119–1130 (1985).

[27] *S.C. Suffin, K.B. Muck, J.C. Young, K. Lewin, D.D. Porter,* Improvement of the Glucose Oxidase Immunoenzyme Technique, Am. J. Clin. Pathol. *71,* 492–496 (1979).

[28] *A. Bondi, G. Chieregatti, V. Eusebi, E. Fulcheri, G. Bussolati,* The Use of β-Galactosidase as a Tracer in Immunohistochemistry, Histochemistry *76,* 153–158 (1982).

[29] *S.P. Hunt, J. Allanson, P.W. Mantyh,* Radioimmunocytochemistry, in: *J.M. Polak, S. Van Noorden* (eds.), Immunocytochemistry, Modern Methods and Applications, 2nd Ed., John Wright and Sons, Bristol 1986, pp. 99–114.

[30] *A.C. Cuello, J.V. Priestley, C. Milstein,* Immunocytochemistry with Internally Labeled Monoclonal Antibodies, Proc. Natl. Acad. Sci. U.S.A. *79,* 665–669 (1982).

[31] *W. Faulk, G. Taylor,* An Immunocolloid Method for the Electron Microscope, Immunochemistry *8,* 1081–1083 (1971).

[32] *W.D. Geoghegan, J.J. Scillian, G.A. Ackerman,* The Detection of Human B-Lymphocytes by both Light and Electron Microscopy Utilizing Colloidal Gold-labeled Anti-Immunoglobulin, Immunol. Commun. 7, 1–12 (1978).

[33] *L. Ghitescu, Z. Galis, M. Bendayan,* Protein AG – Gold Complex: An Alternative Probe in Immunocytochemistry, J. Histochem. Cytochem. *39,* 1057–1065 (1991).

[34] *C.S. Holgate, P. Jackson, P.N. Cowen, C.C. Bird,* Immunogold-Silver Staining: New Method of Immunostaining with Enhanced Sensitivity, J. Histochem. Cytochem. *31,* 938–944 (1983).

[35] *C.S. Holgate, P. Jackson, I. Lauder, P.N. Cowen, C.C. Bird,* Surface Membrane Staining of Immunoglobulins in Paraffin Sections of *Non-Hodgkin's* Lymphomas Using Immunogold-Silver Staining Technique, J. Clin. Pathol. *36,* 742–746 (1983).

[36] *G.W. Hacker, L. Grimelius, G. Danscher, G. Bernatzky, W. Muss, H. Adam, J. Thurner,* Silver Acetate Autometallography: An Alternative Enhancement Technique for Immunogold-Silver Staining (IGSS) and Silver Amplification of Gold, Silver, Mercury and Zinc in Tissue, J. Histotechnol. *11,* 213–221 (1988).

[37] *S. Cammisuli, L. Wofsy,* Hapten-Sandwich Labelling. III. Bifunctional Reagents for Immunospecific Labelling of Cell Surface Antigens, J. Immunol. *117,* 1695–1704 (1976) .

[38] *B. Jasani, D. Wynford Thomas, E.D. Williams,* Use of Monoclonal Anti-Hapten Antibodies for Immunolocalisation of Tissue Antigens, J. Clin. Pathol. *34,* 1000–1002 (1981).

[39] *M.H. Heggenes, J.F. Ash,* Use of the Avidin-Biotin Complex for the Localization of Actin and Myosin with Fluorescence Microscopy, J. Cell Biol. *73,* 783–788 (1977).

[40] *J.L. Guesdon, T. Ternynck, S. Avrameas,* The Use of Avidin-Biotin Interaction in Immunoenzymatic Techniques, J. Histochem. Cytochem. *27,*(1979) 1131–1139.

[41] *S.M. Hsu, L. Raine, H. Fanger,* Use of Avidin-Biotin-Peroxidase Complex (ABC) in Immunoperoxidase Techniques: A Comparison between ABC and Unlabeled Antibody (PAP) Procedures, J. Histochem. Cytochem. *29,* 577–580 (1981).

[42] *L.-J. Larsson,* Immunocytochemistry: Theory and Practice, C.R.C. Press, Boca Raton 1988.

[43] *A. Johnstone, R. Thorpe,* Immunochemistry in Practice, 2nd edn., Blackwell Scientific Publications, Oxford 1982.

[44] *L.A. Sternberger, P.H. Hardy, Jr., J.J. Cuculis, H.G. Meyer,* The Unlabeled Antibody-Enzyme method of Immunohistochemistry. Preparation and Properties of Soluble Antigen-Antibody Complex (Horseradish Peroxidase – Antihorseradish Peroxidase) and Its Use in Identification of Spirochetes, J. Histochem. Cytochem. *18,* 315–333 (1970).

[45] *S. Avrameas,* Coupling of Enzymes to Proteins with Glutaraldehyde. Use of the Conjugates for the Detection of Antigens and Antibodies, Immunochemistry *6,* 43–52 (1969).

[46] *M.T. O'Sullivan, E. Gnemmi, D. Morris, G. Chieregatti, M. Simmons, A.D. Simmonds, J.W. Bridges, V. Marks,* A Simple Method for the Preparation of Enzyme-Antibody Conjugates, FEBS Lett. *95,* 311–313 (1978).

[47] *J. De Mey,* The Preparation and Use of Gold Probes, in: *J.M. Polak, S. Van Noorden* (eds.), Immunocytochemistry, Modern Methods and Applications, 2nd Ed., John Wright and Sons, Bristol 1986, pp. 115–145.

[48] *J.W. Slot, H.J. Geuze,* Gold Markers for Single and Double Immunolabelling of Ultrathin Cryosections, in: *J.M. Polak, I.M. Varndell* (eds.), Immunolabelling for Electron Microscopy, Elsevier Science Publishers, Amsterdam 1984, pp. 129–142.

[49] *C.C. Czerkinsky,* Antibody-Secreting Cells, in: *H.U. Bergmeyer, J. Bergmeyer, M. Grassl* (eds.), Methods of Enzymatic Analysis, 3rd Ed., Volume X, Antigens and Antibodies, 1, VCH, Weinheim 1986, pp. 23–34.

[50] *E.A. Bayer, A. Wilchek,* The Use of the Avidin-Biotin Complex as a Tool in Molecular Biology, in: *D. Glick,* (ed.), Methods of Biochemical Analysis, Vol. 26, John Wiley and Sons, New York 1980, pp. 1–45.

[51] *E.F. Wallace, L. Wofsy,* Hapten-Sandwich Labelling IV. Improved Procedures and Non-Cross-Reacting Hapten Reagents for Double-Labelling Cell Surface Antigens, J. Immunol. Methods *25,* 283–289 (1975).

[52] *E.J. Glazer, J. Ramachandran, A. Basbaum,* Radioimmunocytochemistry Using a Tritiated Goat Anti-Rabbit Second Antibody, J. Histochem. Cytochem. *32,* 778–782 (1984).

[53] *L.-I. Larsson, T.W. Schwartz,* Radioimmunocytochemistry – A Novel Immunochemical Principle, J. Histochem. Cytochem. *25,* 1140–1146 (1977).

[54] *L.-I. Larsson,* Simultaneous Ultrastructural Demonstration of Multiple Peptides in Endocrine Cells by a Novel Immunocytochemical Technique, Nature (London) *282,* 743–746 (1979).

[55] *G.D. Johnson, R.S. Davidson, K.C. McNamee, G. Russell, D. Goodwin, E.J. Holborow,* Fading of Immunofluorescence. During Microscopy: A Study of the Phenomenon and Its Remedy, J. Immunol. Methods *55,* 231–242 (1982).

[56] *W.M. Weinstein, J. Lechago,* A Restaining Method to Restore Fluorescence in Faded Preparations of Tissues Treated with the Indirect Immunofluorescence Technique, J. Immunol. Methods *17,* 375–378 (1977).

[57] *E.A. Schenk, C.J. Churukian,* Immunofluorescence Counterstains, J. Histochem. Cytochem. *22,,* 962–966 (1974).

[58] *B.P. Lane, D.L. Europa*, Differential Staining of Ultrathin Sections of Epon-Embedded Tissue for Light Microscopy, J. Histochem.Cytochem. *13*, 579–582 (1965).

[59] *S. Andrew, B. Jasani*, An Improved Method for the Inhibition of Endogenous Peroxidase Non-Deleterious to Lymphocyte Surface Markers. Application to Immunoperoxidase Studies on Eosinophil-Rich Tissue Preparations, Histochem. J. *19*, 426–430 (1987).

[60] *L.J. Pelliniemi, M. Dym, M.J. Karnovsky*, Peroxidase Histochemistry Using Diaminobenzidine Tetrahydrochloride Stored as a Frozen Solution, J. Histochem. Cyotchem. *28*, 191–192 (1980).

[61] *R.C. Graham, U. Ludholm, M.J. Karnovsky*, Cytochemical Demonstration of Peroxidase Activity with 3-Amino-9-Ethylcarbazole, J. Histochem. Cytochem. *13*, 150–152 (1965).

[62] *A. Mauro, I. Germano, G. Giaccone, M.T. Giordano, D. Schiffer*, 1-Naphthol Basic Dye (1-NBD). An Alternative to Diaminobenzidine in Immunoperoxidase Techniques, Histochemistry *83*, 97–102 (1985).

[63] *G.I. Murray, C.O. Foster, S.W.B. Ewen*, A Novel Tetrazolium Method for Peroxidase Histochemistry and Immunohistochemistry, J. Histochem. Cytochem. *39*, 541–544 (1991).

[64] *W. Straus*, Imidazole Increases the Sensitivity of the Immunocytochemical Reaction for Peroxidase with Diaminobenzidine at a Neutral pH, J. Histochem. Cytochem. *30*, 491–493 (1982).

[65] *M.B. Hancock*, A Serotonin-Immunoreactive Fiber System in the Dorsal Columns of the Spinal Cord, Neurosci. Lett. *31*, 247–252 (1982).

[66] *L. Scopsi, L.-I. Larsson*, Increased Sensitivity in Peroxidase Immunocytochemistry. A Comparative Study of a Number of Peroxidase Visualization Methods Employing a Model System, Histochemistry *84*, 221–230 (1986).

[67] *G. Danscher, J.O.R. Nørgaard*, Ultrastructural Autometallography: A Method for Silver Amplification of Catalytic Metals, J. Histochem. Cytochem. *33*, 706–710 (1985).

[68] *J.S. Hanker, W.W. Ambrose, C.J. James, J. Mandelkorn, P.E. Yates, S.A. Gall, E.H. Bossen, J.W. Fay, J. Laszlo, J.O. Moore*, Facilitated Light Microscopic Cytochemical Diagnosis of Acute Myelogenous Leukaemia, Cancer Res. *39*, 1635–1639 (1979).

[69] *Z. Nemes*, Intensification of 3,3'-Diaminobenzidine Precipitation Using the Ferric Ferricyanide Reaction and Its Application in the Double Immunoperoxidase Technique, Histochemistry *86*, 415–419 (1987).

[70] *H. Gay, W.R. Clark, J.J. Docherty*, Detection of Herpes Simplex Virus Infection Using Glucose Oxidase-Antiglucose Oxidase Immunoenzymatic Stain, J. Histochem. Cytochem. *32*, 447–451 (1984).

[71] *J. De Mey, G.W. Hacker, M. De Waele, D.R. Springall*, Gold Probes in Light Microscopy, in: *J.M. Polak, S. Van Noorden* (eds.), Immunocytochemistry, Modern Methods and Applications, 2nd ed., John Wright and Sons, Bristol 1986, pp. 71–88.

[72] *A.W. Rogers*, Techniques in Autoradiography, 3rd Ed Elsevier, Amsterdam 1979.

[73] *S.P. Hunt, P.W. Mantyh*, Radioimmunocytochemistry with [^{3}H]Biotin, Brain Res *291*, 203–217 (1984).

5.4   Range and Scope of Immunocytochemical Methods

Susan Van Noorden

In this section the principles of the various methods will be described and their applications, advantages and disadvantages discussed. Protocols are given in 5.5.

Any of the methods can be adapted for the localization of any Ag. The ultimate aim is to achieve intense labelling of the Ag with negligible background staining and well preserved tissue structure. The method of choice will depend on the nature and quantity of the Ag, which will also determine the way in which the tissue is prepared, and on the quality of the Ab.

In describing these methods, all Abs are assumed to be at suitable predetermined dilutions in buffer, such as phosphate-buffered saline (PBS) or Tris-buffered saline (TBS), which is also used for washing the preparations. Details of buffers and Ab dilution and testing are given in 5.5. The control of background staining is discussed in 5.6.

5.4.1   Direct Method

This is a one-step method in which the primary Ab bears the label, whether fluorescent, enzyme or other. After preliminary steps (e. g., blocking of endogenous peroxidase if necessary, blocking of nonspecific binding by application of normal serum from the same species as that used to raise the Ab) the primary Ab at a suitable dilution is applied to the preparation and allowed to react. Excess Ab is thoroughly washed off, the label is developed if appropriate, and the preparation is mounted for microscopy, after counterstaining if required (Figure 1).

Advantages

The method is rapid, since only one Ab is employed, and is particularly suitable for immunostaining fragile tissue such as frozen sections which may not withstand multiple washes and Ab applications. However, the quantity of available Ag must be great enough to compensate for the relatively low sensitivity of the method. It is a highly specific method, since only one Ab is involved, and there is no possibility of unwanted binding of conjugated components of a second-layer anti-Ig. It is also useful for double staining in which two differently labelled primary Abs raised against separate tissue Ags are applied simultaneously to stain two Ags in a single preparation. For the double direct method, it does not matter if the two Abs are raised in the same species as there can be no danger of cross-species immunoreactivity which is a potential hazard of double indirect staining.

Disadvantages

Each Ab that is used must be individually labelled, probably by the investigator since commercial preparations may not be available. The method cannot produce more than a

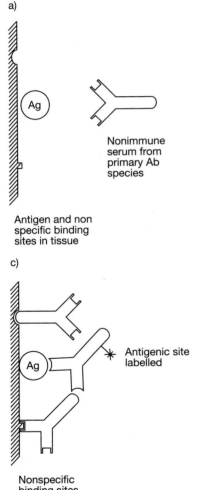

a)

Nonimmune
serum from
primary Ab
species

Antigen and non
specific binding
sites in tissue

c)

Antigenic site
labelled

Nonspecific
binding sites
blocked

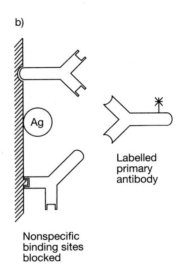

b)

Labelled
primary
antibody

Nonspecific
binding sites
blocked

Fig. 1. Direct immunocytochemical method with labelled primary antibody.
a) In the first stage, nonspecific sites in the tissue section are blocked by Ig in normal serum from the same species that will next provide the primary antibody.
b) The labelled primary antibody is added, preferably at a saturating concentration. The label can be an enzyme, a fluorochrome, an isotope or biotin; the principle of the assay is the same.
c) The specific antibody binds to the antigen. Binding is detected by a method appropriate to the label used.

1:1 ratio of labelled Ab molecules to Ag molecules, and primary pAbs to diverse Ags may not be of particularly high titre; thus its detectability is limited and a relatively high concentration of Ab will be needed. This disadvantage may be overcome by use of mAbs that can be produced in quantity.

5.4.2   Indirect Method

This two-step method consists of application of an unlabelled primary Ab which is detected by a secondary, labelled Ab, raised against the Ig of the species providing the primary Ab. Nonspecific binding of Abs to tissue is prevented by preincubation with nonimmune serum from the species providing the second Ab (Figure 2).

Advantages

There is usually greater efficiency with this method than with the direct method, perhaps due to amplification of the signal. Because there are at least two Ab binding sites on the Fc portion of the primary Ab, two molecules, or more, of the second Ab can bind to each molecule of primary Ab, thus doubling the potential maximum quantity of label. However, *Sternberger* [1] sugests that the increased signal is due to the high titre of the anti-Igs that arise from hyperimmunisation of the host species with such readily available Ag. Whatever the reason, the primary Ab can usually be used at a dilution at least ten times greater than for the direct method, which conserves precious Ab and ensures that any unwanted reactants in the primary Ab serum are diluted out giving a cleaner result.

Only the second Ab, the anti-species Ig, is labelled, and will serve to detect a primary unlabelled Ab of that species raised against any Ag. A laboratory keeping a stock of labelled Abs against-human, rabbit, mouse, rat, goat or sheep Igs should be well equipped to detect most primary Abs.

Fig. 2. Indirect immunocytochemical method with unlabelled primary antibody and labelled ▶ second antibody.
a) Nonspecific binding sites in the tissue are first blocked by normal serum from the same species that later provides the second antibody.
b) Unlabelled specific primary antibody added in saturating concentration.
c) After this has bound to the antigen in the section, excess antibody is washed away and the labelled second anti-species Ig antibody reagent is added.
d) The binding of the second antibody is detected by a method appropriate to the label (cf. Fig. 1).

a)

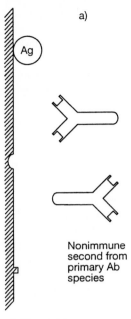

Nonimmune
second from
primary Ab
species

Antigen and
nonspecific
binding sites
in tissue

b)

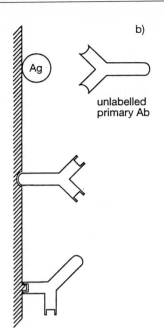

unlabelled
primary Ab

Nonspecific
binding sites
blocked

c)

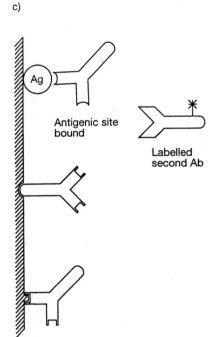

Antigenic site
bound

Labelled
second Ab

d)

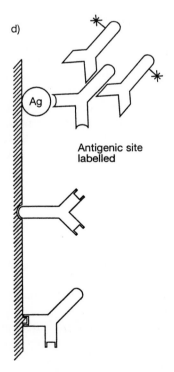

Antigenic site
labelled

Disadvantages

The greater effort and longer time required to carry out the two-step procedure may be disadvantageous, but this is outweighed by the benefits.

The use of two Abs in place of one doubles the chance of nonspecific or unwanted reactions with tissue components, but these reactions can normally be blocked by an application of nonimmune serum (cf. 5.5).

Second Abs are usually polyclonal and care must be taken that they are species-specific, so that they react only with Ig from the species providing the first Ab without any cross-reaction with Ig from the species in which the Ag is being localized. Igs from related species are inherently cross-reactive. For example, Abs raised in rabbit to rat Igs will also bind to mouse Igs. If a primary rat monoclonal Ab is being used to label an Ag in mouse tissue, the detecting rabbit anti-rat Ig must be preabsorbed with mouse Igs to prevent binding and labelling of Igs in the mouse tissue substrate in addition to the specific primary rat Ab. If unabsorbed antisera are to be used the problem can usually be overcome by adding to the diluted detecting antiserum 1% of normal serum from the species of origin of the tissue.

5.4.3   Three-layer Techniques

5.4.3.1   Unlabelled Enzyme Anti-enzyme Method

This method [2] provides a cleaner and more intense immunocytochemical reaction of greater detectability than an indirect method. The primary Ab (e. g., rabbit anti-Ag) is unlabelled, as is the second, anti-Ig (e. g., goat anti-rabbit Ig). The third layer is a soluble, stable, cyclic peroxidase anti-peroxidase (PAP) complex consisting of three molecules of POD immunologically complexed to two molecules of an Ab against POD raised in the same species as the primary Ab (rabbit, in this example). Provided that the second, linking, Ab is in excess so that only one of its Ag-binding sites is occupied by the primary Ab and the other is available for the PAP, a large amount of POD is built up over the Ag in the tissue (Figure 3).

Advantages

The signal-to-noise ratio of this method is greater than that of an indirect immunope-roxidase method for several reasons:
1. None of the reagents is chemically conjugated. Thus the Abs and enzyme all retain their full activity.
2. Contaminating Abs in the unconjugated (goat) antiserum to (rabbit) Ig in the second layer cannot cause unwanted staining of the tissue because any molecules that do

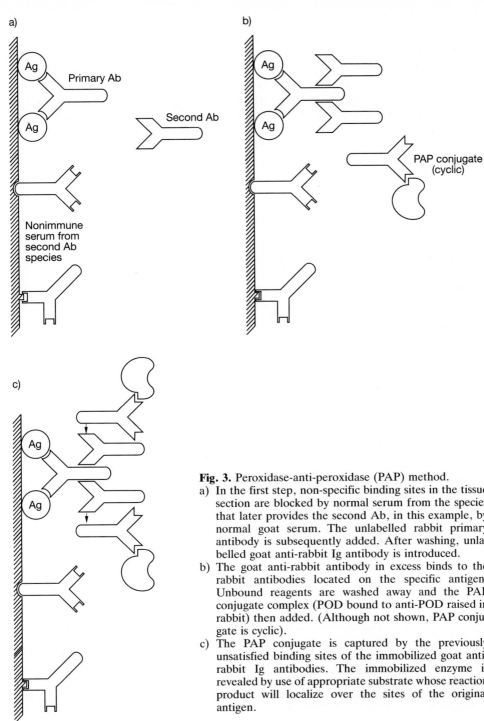

Fig. 3. Peroxidase-anti-peroxidase (PAP) method.

a) In the first step, non-specific binding sites in the tissue section are blocked by normal serum from the species that later provides the second Ab, in this example, by normal goat serum. The unlabelled rabbit primary antibody is subsequently added. After washing, unlabelled goat anti-rabbit Ig antibody is introduced.

b) The goat anti-rabbit antibody in excess binds to the rabbit antibodies located on the specific antigen. Unbound reagents are washed away and the PAP conjugate complex (POD bound to anti-POD raised in rabbit) then added. (Although not shown, PAP conjugate is cyclic).

c) The PAP conjugate is captured by the previously unsatisfied binding sites of the immobilized goat anti-rabbit Ig antibodies. The immobilized enzyme is revealed by use of appropriate substrate whose reaction product will localize over the sites of the original antigen.

bind are not labelled. Nonspecific binding of first and second layers is prevented by prior incubation of the tissue with normal serum from the species providing the second Ab.

3. The (rabbit) PAP complex is affinity purified during production by virtue of precipitation of the anti-peroxidase with peroxidase added in the correct proportion. Contaminating Abs and unreacted POD do not precipitate and are discarded. The precipitate is resuspended with excess POD which at pH 2.3 combines with it to form the soluble PAP complex. After neutralization the Ig complex is reprecipitated with ammonium sulphate, then redissolved in water and dialysed. The complex will act as an Ag only to the specifically reacted anti-(rabbit) Ig of the second layer, and will not detect any unwanted contaminating Abs that may have bound to the tissue, since these will not be anti-(rabbit) Ig.

4. The cyclic form of the PAP complex gives it stability and prevents detachment of the POD during the washing stages.

5. Partly because of the increased amount of available label and partly because of the necessity for the linking Ab to be in excess so as to retain a free binding site for the PAP, the primary Ab can and must be very highly diluted, usually at least ten times more diluted than for the two-layer method. This means that any contaminating Abs in the primary antiserum are diluted out to a negligible level. Even if the primary Ab is a mAb (the PAP complex then being made with mouse or rat anti-peroxidase, as appropriate), a high dilution must be used. The use of a too-concentrated primary Ab results in the prozone effect [3]; all Ag binding sites on the linking anti-Ig are occupied by the primary Ab and the PAP complex cannot attach (Figure 4).

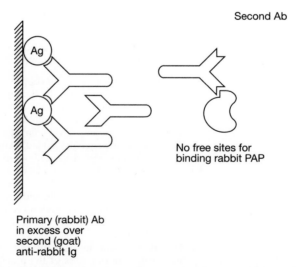

Fig. 4. Prozone effect. Typically as seen in the PAP method illustrated in Fig. 3. In this case if the primary (rabbit) antibody is in excess with respect to the second goat anti-rabbit Ig reagent, then the latter will be bound without leaving unsatisfied binding sites needed to capture the subsequent PAP reagent.

6. A further consequence of the high dilution of the primary Ab is that both Ag-binding sites are likely to be occupied by Ag, and dissociation from the Ag during the procedure due to the reversibility of the Ag-Ab reaction is unlikely to occur for both sites at once, decreasing potential loss of the first Ab, despite the fact that some high affinity Abs may have been diluted out of the antiserum.

Disadvantages

The third step increases the time taken to complete the reaction. The PAP complex must be from the same species as the primary Ab, (or a cross-reacting one) so PAPs from several species may have to be obtained to allow for primary Abs raised in different species. PAP complexes tend to be expensive.

5.4.3.2 Avidin-Biotin Methods

Avidin is a large glycoprotein ($M_r = 67000$) extracted from chicken egg white, whereas biotin is present in large quantity in egg yolk, as well as in several tissues such as liver and kidney. Avidin has four binding sites for biotin and can also be directly conjugated to all types of label in the same way as Igs. The biotin molecule, while not itself a label in that it cannot be visualized directly, has one binding site for avidin and one carboxyl group which, after activation, allows it to react with other proteins (e. g., enzymes) *via* their NH_2 groups [4]. The reaction between avidin and biotin is of extremely high affinity (K_a 10^{-15} l/mol). Several molecules of biotin can be conjugated to one Ab molecule, or to immunocytochemical labels such as enzymes (but not fluorochromes or colloidal gold): the small size of the biotion molecule allows retention of the full bioactivity of the Ab or enzyme. If a multi-biotinylated Ab is used in the second layer of the reaction, a large number of directly labelled avidin molecules can bind to the biotin, building up a very high level of label at the site of the primary Ab-Ag reaction (Figure 5).

In an alternative method [5] an avidin-biotinylated label complex (ABC) is made in advance, using excess avidin so that some biotin-binding sites are left free to accomodate the biotin molecules on the biotinylated second Ab (Figure 6). An even higher ratio of label to Ag is achieved by this method.

Because of the large size of the avidin molecule and the even larger ABC, steric hindrance can prevent attachment of the maximun number of labelled third reagents. To overcome this, at least in part, biotin molecules are often not attached to the second Ab directly but somewhat distanced from it by a spacer molecule [6].

The immunostaining procedure with avidin-biotin reagents is carried out in the same way as with enzyme-anti-enzyme complexes. A primary Ab is followed by a biotinylated second Ab to the species in which the first Ab was raised, and the third layer is labelled avidin or an ABC. Nonspecific staining is blocked in advance by nonimmune serum from the species providing the second Ab. However, there is no need for the second

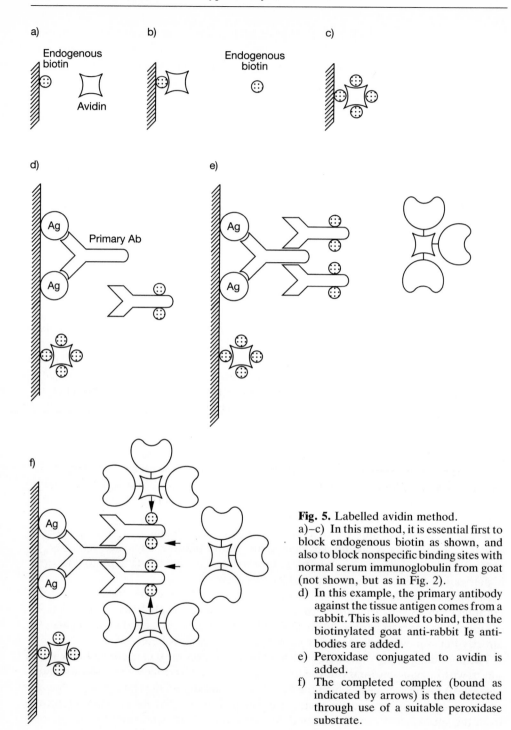

Fig. 5. Labelled avidin method.

a)–c) In this method, it is essential first to block endogenous biotin as shown, and also to block nonspecific binding sites with normal serum immunoglobulin from goat (not shown, but as in Fig. 2).

d) In this example, the primary antibody against the tissue antigen comes from a rabbit. This is allowed to bind, then the biotinylated goat anti-rabbit Ig antibodies are added.

e) Peroxidase conjugated to avidin is added.

f) The completed complex (bound as indicated by arrows) is then detected through use of a suitable peroxidase substrate.

a)

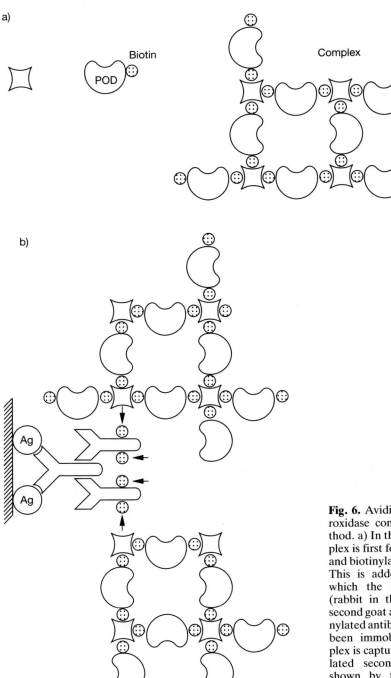

Fig. 6. Avidin-biotinylated peroxidase complex (ABC) method. a) In this method, a complex is first formed from avidin
and biotinylated peroxidase. b)
This is added to sections in
which the primary antibody
(rabbit in this case) and the
second goat anti-rabbit Ig biotinylated antibodies have already
been immobilized. The complex is captured by the biotinylated second antibodies (as
shown by the arrows), and
detected with an appropriate
substrate.

(biotinylated) Ab to be in great excess over the primary Ab as the binding of the labelled avidin or ABC to the biotin does not depend on an immunological reaction.

Advantages

These methods result in an even higher ratio of visible label to Ag than the enzyme-anti-enzyme methods and can often be used with even greater dilutions of the primary Ab. They also have greater versatility since there is no need to consider the species of the primary Ab except for the biotinylated anti-Ig. One type of ABC can identify any type of biotinylated Ab, including a directly biotinylated primary Ab. This can be an advantage when an Ab is used against an Ag in the species in which it was raised. If a second, anti-species, Ig has to be used, much unwanted staining can result from reactions with Igs but if the first Ab is biotinylated, labelled avidin or ABC can be used as the second layer (cf. 5.4.6.3).

Disadvantages

Avidin is a glycoprotein and may bind to lectin-like molecules in the tissue through its oligosaccharide groups, giving unwanted staining. These carbohydrate groups may also give rise to nonspecific adherence to the tissue substrate. In addition, avidin has an isoelectric point of 10.5 which favours binding to negatively charged sites in the tissue, including mast cells. Sometimes this can be prevented by adjusting the buffer used to dilute the avidin to pH 9.0 [7], but all these problems can be avoided by the use of streptavidin in place of avidin. Streptavidin, produced by the bacterium *Streptomyces avidinii*, is a protein ($M_r = 60000$), not a glycoprotein, with a neutral isoelectric point, but in its capacity to bind biotin or carry labels it is identical to avidin [8]. It thus has the advantages of avidin without the problems of unwanted binding to tissue and is widely used in consequence. It must be said, however, that many manufacturers successfully modify avidin to prevent these problems.

A further problem concerns endogenous biotin, particularly in tissues such as liver. Binding of labelled avidin or ABC can be prevented by preincubation with unlabelled avidin, followed by unlabelled biotin which blocks any remaining biotin-binding sites on the applied avidin. Since biotin molecules have only one binding site for avidin, there will be no further danger of attachment of applied avidin [9]. If biotin-rich tissues are to be stained, the enzyme-anti-enzyme technique may be more suitable.

Because of their high detectability, avidin-biotin methods may be less suitable than enzyme-anti-enzyme methods for distinguishing between large and small amounts of Ag and thus, paradoxically, less sensitive. This is discussed further in 5.4.7.

5.4.4   Build-up Methods

Any of the methods discussed can be amplified by insertion of extra layers.

A direct method may be converted to an indirect method by a labelled second Ab, and further to a three-layer method. This, of course, requires additional Abs. After the second Ab (e.g., POD-labelled goat anti-rabbit Ig) of the indirect method, another application of the first rabbit Ab could be used (Figure 7). This would bind to any unoccupied antigenic sites in the tissue, from which low-affinity Abs might have been washed off during the staining procedure. It would also bind to any free rabbit Ig-binding sites on the second Ab, if the optimal amount had been used originally so that one arm of each anti-Ig molecule would not be attached to the primary Ab. Any rabbit Ig could be used, but it would be safer to re-use the original Ab to avoid identifying unwanted tissue Ags. A fourth layer would be a repeat of the second, labelled anti-rabbit Ig. Thus, extra label would be built up over the site of reaction. In the absence of suitable third layer complexes, this is a useful alternative.

An enzyme-anti-enzyme method can similarly be amplified. After the third layer, the linking anti-Ig and the enzyme-anti-enzyme complex are re-applied [10, 11]. This is a standard method of increasing the signal in the alkaline phosphatase-anti-alkaline phosphatase method [12] (Figure 8).

Even ABC methods can be amplified, provided that the original combination of avidin and biotinylated label is adjusted to leave some spare biotin-binding sites on the avidin. A second application of biotinylated anti-Ig and ABC can then be used [13]. A simpler method involves combining a PAP method with an ABC method [14]. A biotinylated anti-Ig is used (in excess) as the second Ab, reacted with PAP in the third layer, re-applied, reacted again with PAP, and finally with POD ABC. A lower level of amplification could be achieved by mixing PAP and ABC in the third layer and omitting the re-application. These methods are recommended only if the level of Ag to be detected is low; otherwise, steric hindrance might become a problem.

5.4.5   Labelled Antigen

This is another method that increases the specificity of immunolabelling. Certain of its variations are abbreviated to RICH (radioimmunocytochemical) [15] or GLAD (gold-labelled Ag detection) [16]. In both methods, nonspecific binding sites are first blocked by normal serum or inappropriate Ig from the same species supplying the Ab (Figure 10). In the RICH method a radioiodinated antigen is mixed with antibody in such proportion that one of the two agbinding sites of each antibody molecule is'occupied by labelled Ag. When applied to the tissue, the specifically labelled Ab will

a)

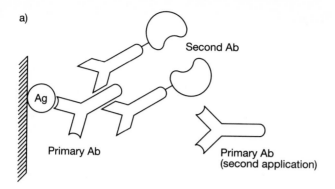

Second Ab

Ag

Primary Ab

Primary Ab
(second application)

b)

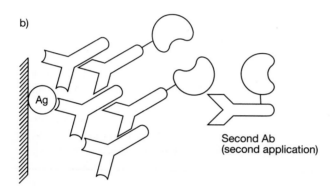

Ag

Second Ab
(second application)

c)

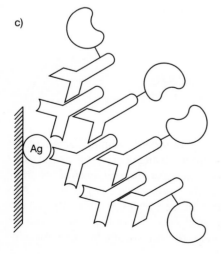

Ag

Fig. 7. Build-up of label by repeated application
of reagent layers.
a) In the first place, after blocking of nonspecific
   binding sites (as Fig. 2), the unlabelled primary antibody and the enzyme-labelled second
   antibody are added as in the conventional
   indirect method (Fig. 2). Another application
   of primary antibody is then made.
b) A second application of the labelled second
   antibody follows.
c) The resulting many-layered complex is
   detected in the usual manner with an appropriate substrate.

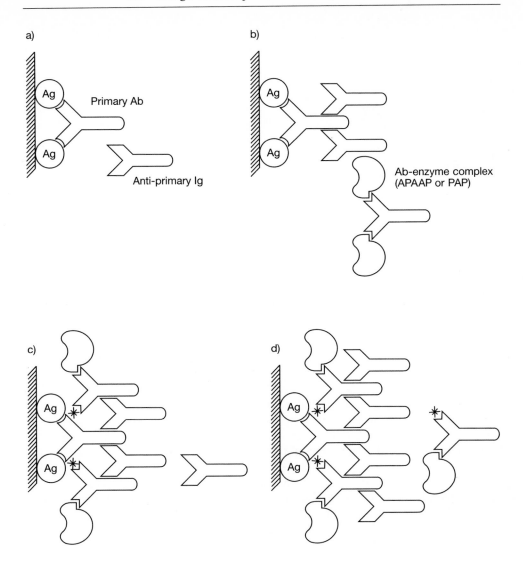

Fig. 8. Alkaline phosphatase anti-alkaline phosphatase (APAAP) method with repetition of the second and third layers. This greatly amplifies the amount of enzyme immobilized over the sites of antigen localization. Initially, nonspecific binding sites are blocked by normal goat serum (cf. Fig. 2).

a) In this example, a mouse mAb against the tissue antigen is bound and then an excess of an unlabelled goat anti-mouse Ig reagent added.

b) Mouse APAAP complex is added and is captured by the immobilized goat anti-mouse Ig antibodies.

c) A second application of unlabelled goat anti-mouse Ig antibodies is then made.

d) Further mouse APAAP complex is added.

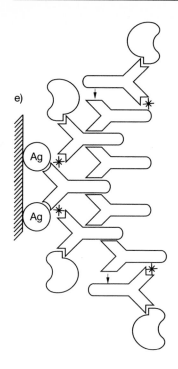

Fig. 8 (continued)
e) The amplified binding of enzyme is detected by use of an
    appropriate substrate.
In this example, no difference is shown between use of POD
or AP. The former, however, forms a cyclic PAP complex,
the latter a non-cyclic complex (APAAP) with maximal Ab
bound. Sites available for enzyme binding are indicated
(*).

bind to the tissue Ag. The radiolabel is developed by autoradiography. In the GLAD
method an unlabelled primary Ab is applied in excess to react with the tissue Ag. A
colloidal gold-adsorbed Ag is then added, and binds to the free arm of the primary Ab.
Provided that the Ab of interest does not find unoccupied nonspecific binding sites, only
specifically bound primary Ab is detected. The gold-labelled Ag was designed for
electron microscopical immunocytochemistry, but might be made visible at light
microscopical level with silver enhancement (cf. 5.3.8.2). POD-labelled Ags have also
been used and the enzyme is identified in any conventional way [17]. Despite the fact
that the primary Ab must have free binding sites available, its dilution is about the same
as used for a PAP method.

Fig. 9. Combined PAP and ABC method. This is a combination of methods illustrated in Figs. 3 and ▶
6. Initial stages of blocking nonspecific sites as in Fig. 2 and endogenous biotin as in Fig. 5 are
necessary but are not illustrated here.
a) The PAP reaction with immobilized biotinylated second antibody is followed by application of
    more biotinylated antibody.
b) Further enzyme is introduced to the immobilized complex in the form of peroxidase-labelled
    avidin.
c) The peroxidase-avidin complex binds to the biotinylated second antibody at all the biotin sites
    indicated by arrows to amplify amount of bound label. The enzyme is detected in the usual
    manner.

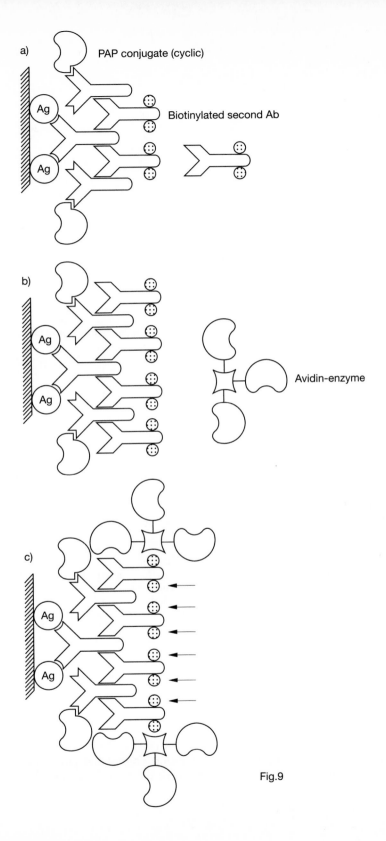

a) PAP conjugate (cyclic)

Biotinylated second Ab

b)

Avidin-enzyme

c)

Fig.9

a)

b)

c)

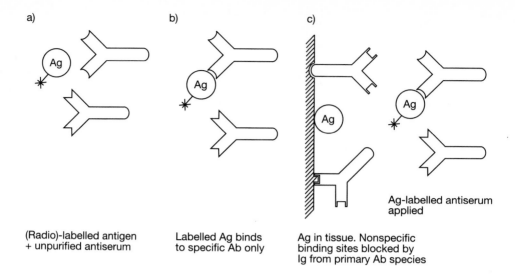

(Radio)-labelled antigen
+ unpurified antiserum

Labelled Ag binds
to specific Ab only

Ag-labelled antiserum
applied

Ag in tissue. Nonspecific
binding sites blocked by
Ig from primary Ab species

d)

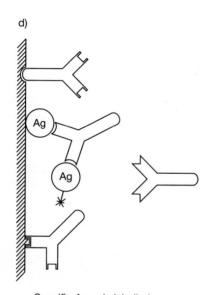

Specific Ag only labelled

Fig. 10. Labelled antigen (RICH) method.
a) This uses a soluble preparation of tissue antigen that can be labelled, e.g. isotopically. This is allowed to react with antiserum against the antigen in question.
b) Complexes are formed, but only with specific antibody in the serum.
c) The complex is applied to a section in which nonspecific binding sites have already been blocked with appropriate normal serum.
d) Provided the complexes of antigen-antibody were made in antibody excess, they will bind to the antigen in the tissues. In this example, binding would be detected autoradiographically.

The advantage of this method is its high specificity. The disadvantages are the need to label each Ag separately, the time taken to develop a radiolabel and, in the case of the GLAD method, the need to amplify with silver for light microscopy.

5.4.6   Multiple Immunostaining

The identification of two or more Ags in a single preparation is of obvious importance in analysing the spatial and quantitative relationships between Ags present in different structures and in showing co-localization of Ags in the same structure. Several methods are able to show multiple Ags unequivocally and simultaneously. They depend on specific and non-cross-reacting Abs, both primary and secondary, and on clearly differentiated end-products of reaction.

5.4.6.1   Serial Sections

Immunostaining of adjacent sections with Abs to different Ags avoids problems of crossover reactions and comparison of the results will show whether the same structure contains more than one Ag. The sections must be less than 2 μm thick to ensure that adjacent sections pass through the same structures. Paraffin sections of small blocks and semithin resin sections are ideal. The tissue must contain recognisable "landmarks" such as vessels, cysts or connective tissue strands to aid identification of individual cells. A homogeneous tumour mass, for example, is not suitable for study by this method.

5.4.6.2   Mirror-Image Sections

When thicker sections are necessary (e.g., prefixed frozen sections), reverse-face sections should be used. When cutting pairs of cryostat sections, the second section of the pair is turned over on the cryostat knife blade after cutting, so that when it is picked up on a slide the common cut surfaces of both sections are uppermost, the structures on one section being mirror images of those on the other. Thus, even in 20 μm sections, the same immunoreactive nerve could be identified with two different Abs. Photomicrographs of one of the pair may be printed laterally transposed so that the sections appear as conventional serial sections for easier identification of the same structure.

5.4.6.3   Single Preparations

Neither of the above methods is suitable for nonsectioned material such as cell preparations, and comparison of adjacent sections is a tedious process. Methods for multiple staining on the same preparation require non-cross-reacting detection systems or, if the Ags are known to be in different structures, very intense development of the first immunoreaction product to mask any crossover and also different or differently developed labels.

5.4.6.4   Double Direct Immunostaining

Two (or more) differently labelled primary Abs, raised in the same or different species, are applied to the same preparation, sequentially or simultaneously, at their predetermined optimal dilutions. This method avoids crossover reactions since primary Abs only are involved, but has the disadvantages that each Ab must be separately labelled and that the method is relatively insensitive.

Double direct immunofluorescence staining

Two primary Abs are labelled with different fluorochromes such as TRITC, seen as red fluorescence with a green filter and FITC, seen as green fluorescence with a blue filter. Switching filters shows whether the same or different structures are fluorescent with the different Abs. Double exposure photography can be used to show red and green fluorescence in the same field. If the two Ags are present in the same structure the combination of red and green fluorescence will appear orange. Phycoerythrin could be seen as orange fluorescence with the filter used for fluorescein but the distinction is not as clear as with the red of rhodamine. A third Ag could be localized using the blue fluorescence of AMCA, for example (cf. 5.3.1.2).

Double direct immunoenzyme staining

Two enzymes may be used as labels, e. g. POD and AP. The development colours are chosen so that, if two Ags are present in the same structure, a mixed colour is obtained. Thus POD might be developed in brown or red and AP in blue (cf. 5.3.8 and 5.3.9) to give a purple mixed colour.

If the Ags are known to be in separate structures it is possible for both Abs to be labelled with POD, and the reactions carried out and developed sequentially. The first reaction product is developed black with an intensified DAB reaction (e. g. DAB-nickel) and the second, brown or red (cf. 5.3.8.2). This method would be unsuitable for colocalized Ags as the second, lighter reaction product would not show up on the same structure as the first, black reaction product. The first reaction, when highly developed, might in any case mask the second tissue Ag and prevent its reaction with the Ab.

Other labels

Other suitable label combinations include colloidal gold with silver intensification (cf. 5.3.12): (a) in combination with a fluorescent label, viewed either with transmitted light (for the black silver/gold) combined with epi-illuminated fluorescence, or with epipolarized light (white back-scatter from the silver) combined with fluorescence; or (b) in combination with an enzyme label. A biotinylated primary Ab could be localized by a second layer of avidin labelled in any suitable way, combined with another, differently labelled primary.

5.4.6.5   Double Indirect (2-Step) Immunostaining

When sensitivity is increased by an amplified immunoreaction, and two primary Abs raised in the same species are used, problems of crossover reactions occur. Even when the reactions are carried out sequentially, the second primary Ab (e. g. rabbit anti-Ag 2) could bind to unoccupied anti-rabbit Ig sites on the second Ab of the first reaction. The second anti-rabbit Ig could then bind not only to the rabbit anti-Ag 2 on the tissue substrate, but also to that on the second Ab of the first reaction. Thus a mixed reaction would be seen on the first Ag site and a single reaction on the second Ag site. This would be acceptable (though not aesthetic) if the two Ags were known to be present in different structures but would not be helpful in determining their presence in the same structure. Various methods have been devised for overcoming this problem.

Sequential staining without elution

Provided the two Ags are known to be in different structures, the label of the first immunoreaction is developed in a very dark colour so that any build-up of the second reaction on top of the first is not noticeable. Heavy metal-intensified DAB-POD or silver-intensified colloidal gold would be suitable labels for the first reaction, with any label for the second reaction.

It has been suggested [18] that reactive sites on the first set of Abs are physically masked by intense development of the (POD) label.

Sequential staining with elution [19]

If two Ags are suspected of being present in the same structure and the only available primary Abs are both raised in the same species, the problem of potential crossover may be overcome by a sequential immunoenzyme method, eluting the first set of Abs (after develping the enzyme reaction) so that the reaction product remains on the preparation. The second immunoreaction is then carried out and the second enzyme label developed in a contrasting colour. Mixed colours will show colocalization of the two Ags.

Method

Elution is performed by soaking the preparation in a low pH buffer, e. g. glycine/HCl buffer, 0.1 mol/l, pH 2.2. Before the second set of Abs can be applied, control staining must be done to find the length of time needed to detach the entire first set of Abs from the preparation, as outlined below.

1. Immunostain up to 10 preparations but develop the label on one only to check that the reaction is satisfactory.
2. Treat the remaining preparations with several changes of glycine/HCl, 0.1 mol/l, buffer, pH 2.2, removing preparations at intervals of 1, 2, 4, 8, 16 and 24 h.
3. Wash the acid-treated preparations well in PBS.

4. Repeat the immunostaining procedure from the second Ab stage and develop the POD reaction.

If staining occurs, the acid treatment has not been long enough. If the primary Ab has been removed (with its bound second- (and third-) layer reagents, no staining will occur.

Optimal elution times should be established for each primary Ab as avidities differ, and it is easiest to use the Ab with the shortest elution time as first Ab in the double stain. High avidity Abs may be eluted more efficiently by electrophoresis [20] or by acidified potassium permanganate [21] (although this treatment might damage some Ags). DAB and 4-chloro-1-naphthol are suitable chromogens for a double immunoperoxidase stain by these methods. A third Ag may be localized on the same preparation after a second elution step. A soluble reaction product (e. g. from 4-chloro-1-naphthol) may be photographed then dissolved before the second immunoreaction is carried out (provided that all Abs are also removed) to ensure that a colocalized second Ag is not masked by the first reaction product. Photographs of the first and second reactions may then be compared.

Sequential staining with blocking of spare antibody binding sites [22]

After the first (rhodamine immunofluorescence) reaction, preparations are dried (by dehydration through alcohols to xylene) and exposed to formaldehyde vapour from paraformaldehyde powder at 80°C for 3–4 h. This effectively blocks any unused Ig-binding sites on the first set of reactions and prevents crossover of the second set of Abs, localized by fluorescein immunofluorescence. There are two essential controls: the first is to ensure that the second Ag is not damaged by treatment with the formaldehyde vapour (single-immunostain a treated positive control preparation) and the second, to check that all potential binding sites on the first reaction have been blocked by staining with an irrelevant second primary Ab raised in the same species as the test Abs. If free sites are available, a second immunofluorescence reaction will occur, otherwise no staining will be detected. This reaction is suitable for multiple immunogold labelling at electron-microscopical level.

Simultaneous double 2-step immunostaining

This method, pioneered by several groups [23, 24], relies on simultaneous application at their predetermined optimal dilutions of two primary Abs to different Ags, raised in different species, e. g., rabbit and mouse, and revealed with simultaneously applied, differently labelled, non-crossreacting, anti-species Igs (e. g., goat anti-rabbit Ig and goat anti-mouse Ig, but not goat anti-rabbit Ig and rabbit anti-mouse Ig which would react with each other). Where POD and AP are the labels, POD developed in brown and AP in blue will show separate (blue and brown) or colocalized (purple) Ags.

Simultaneous double 3-step immunostaining

The method may be used with 3-layer techniques such as rabbit PAP and mouse APAAP or rabbit PAP and mouse ABC, etc. With the increasing range of mAbs available it is now easy to find suitable pairs of Abs and detecting reagents. With mAbs, it is also possible to use primary Abs of different Ig subclass, revealed with subclass-specific second-layer anti-Igs.

5.4.6.6   Triple Immunostaining

Provided that at least one of the Ags to be localized is in a separate structure from the other two, triple immunostaining [25] can be carried out by immunostaining the first Ag by any method that can be developed in an intensely black colour, then a simultaneous double immunoenzyme stain by one of the methods outlined above. Provided that the first reaction colour is strong enough, any crossover from the other reactions will not be noticed. Other methods of triple and even quadruple staining have been devised with many different colour combinations [25]. Triple immunofluorescence was achieved with three non-cross-reacting systems [26].

5.4.7   Quantification

5.4.7.1   Limits to Quantification

Immunocytochemistry is not an exact technique. It is currently impossible to determine the amount of Ag present in a preparation using immunocytochemical procedures (cf. 5.8). The reasons for this are manifold:

1. The relation between the amount of Ag in a preparation and the amount of Ab that binds to it is dependent on the preparation procedure (fixation, embedding, thickness of section) which determines how much Ag is available.
2. The ability of the Ab to penetrate the preparation is another variable, dependent on the preparative technique and on the size of the label molecule.
3. The concentration of Ag may vary across a preparation and at sites of particularly high concentration it could prevent the theoretical maximum binding of Ab by steric hindrance.
4. A pAb may contain Abs to several different epitopes on the Ag molecule.
5. The amount of label incorporated in an Ab is not easily standardized.
6. The end-points of enzyme development are not standardized and small variations in technique could lead to large variations in amount of product.

For absolute quantification to be a possibility Ags should be unfixed and unaltered by any processing; a one-layer direct method would be required, with mAbs carrying a fixed amount of label in a known molecular relationship to the antibody, able to penetrate the preparation and react fully with the Ag in a 1:1 ratio. The optical density of the reaction product should be measurable and bear a direct relationship to its concentration. Alternatively, the amount of (soluble) reaction product extracted from the preparation could be measured. Although this would move an essentially morphological discipline into the realms of biochemistry, the advantage over measuring the amount of antigen by radioimmunoassay (e.g.) in the first place would be that the cellular localization of the antigen would be known.

5.4.7.2   Image Analysis

Computerized image analysis has revolutionized morphometry, making the process of measurement more accessible. Under carefully controlled conditions it is possible to count the number of immunostained structures in a preparation or to measure the area occupied by immunostained structures in test and control specimens and to measure the integrated density of an immunostained area, subtracting the density of the "background". Using these methods it is certainly possible to determine whether one preparation has "more" or "much more" Ag than another and to give a numerical level to the results. The principles of image analysis are covered in 5.9.

Attempts have been made to assess the amount of Ag in a tissue structure by comparing the density of the DAB reaction product of an immunoperoxidase stain with standard concentrations of antigen dotted onto nitrocellulose paper treated similarly [27]. Provided that all stages of the procedure are controlled carefully, this method allows a range of antigen levels in the tissue to be calibrated against the standards, and can be used to compare one tissue with another. Nevertheless, the difference in thickness between the nitrocellulose paper and the tissue sections, among other inevitable variables, precludes absolute quantification. It is accepted that quantification in immunocytochemistry can, at present, be comparative only.

5.4.7.3   Antigen Concentration and Antibody Dilution

Even without the use of image analysis, much can be learnt about the levels of Ag within a preparation by judicious choice of the immunocytochemical detection method. *Sternberger* [1] has pointed out that, of the most sensitive three-layer techniques, PAP but not ABC can be used to differentiate between high and low concentrations of Ag. This is because, even at high concentrations of Ag, the PAP system has access to the primary Ab while with the ABC system, because of the large size of the complex, steric hindrance prevents binding of the maximum possible quantities of ABC, even when much primary Ab is available to react. Thus an ABC method would give a stronger reaction than a PAP method when localizing very small quantities of Ag but would be less effective in a comparing Ag concentrations.

The difference between low and high concentrations of Ag can also be shown (with a PAP technique) by using higher than usual dilutions of Ab – the supraoptimal dilution technique [28]. A high concentration of Ag will be revealed easily by both optimal and supraoptimal dilutions, but a low concentration will be much less detectable by the supraoptimal dilution because of the lower Ab:Ag ratio.

References

[1] *L. A. Sternberger*, Immunocytochemistry, 3rd Edn. John Wiley and Sons, New York 1986.
[2] *L. A. Sternberger, P. H. Hardy, Jr., J. J. Cuculis, H. G. Meyer*, The Unlabeled Antibody-Enzyme Method of Immunohistochemistry. Preparation and Properties of Soluble Antigen-Antibody Complex (Horseradish Peroxidase – Antihorseradish Peroxidase) and Its Use in Identification of Spirochetes, J. Histochem. Cytochem. *18*, 315–333 (1970).
[3] *J. W. Bigbee, J. C. Kosek, L. E. Eng*, The Effects of Primary Antisera Dilution on Staining of "Antigen"-Rich Tissue with the Peroxidase Antiperoxidase Technique, J. Histochem. Cytochem. *25*, 443–447 (1977).
[4] *E. A. Bayer, A. Wilchek*, "The Use of the Avidin-Biotin Complex as a Tool in Molecular Biology", in: *D. Glick* (ed.), Methods of Biochemical Analysis, Vol. 26, John Wiley and Sons, New York 1980, pp. 1–45
[5] *S. M. Hsu, L. Raine, H. Fanger*, Use of Avidin-Biotin-Peroxidase Complex (ABC) in Immunoperoxidase Techniques: a Comparison between ABC and Unlabeled Antibody (PAP) Procedures, J. Histochem. Cytochem. *29*, 577–580 (1981).
[6] *S. M. Costello, R. T. Felix, R. W. Giese*, Enhancement of Immune Cellular Agglutination by Use of an Avidin-Biotin System, Clin. Chem. *25*, 1572–1580 (1979).
[7] *G. Bussolati, P. Giugliotta*, Non-Specific Staining of Mast Cells by Avidin-Biotin-Peroxidase Complexes (ABC), J. Histochem. Cytochem. *31*, 1419–1421 (1983).
[8] *L. Chaiet, F. J. Wolf*, The Properties of Streptavidin, a Biotin-Binding Protein Produced by Streptomycetes, Arch. Biochem. Biophys. *106*, 1–5 (1964).
[9] *G. S. Wood, R. Warnke*, Suppression of Endogenous Avidin-Binding Activity in Tissues and Its Relevance to Biotin-Avidin Detection Systems, J. Histochem. Cytochem. *29*, 1196–1204 (1981).
[10] *P. Ordronneau, P. Petrusz*, Immunocytochemical Demonstration of Anterior Pituitary Hormones in the Pars Tuberalis of Long-Term Hypophysectomized Rats, Am. J. Anat. *158*, 491–506 (1980).
[11] *L. L. Vacca, S. J. Abrahams, N. E. Naftchi*, A Modified Peroxidase-Antiperoxidase Procedure for Improved Localization of Tissue Antigens: Localization of Substance P in Rat Spinal Cord, J. Histochem. Cytochem. *28*, 297–307 (1980).
[12] *D. Y. Mason*, Immunocytochemical Labeling of Monoclonal Antibodies by the APAAP Immunoalkaline Phosphatase Technique, in: *G. R. Bullock, P. Petrusz* (eds.), Techniques in Immunocytochemistry, Vol. 3, Acad. Press, New York 1985, pp. 25–42.
[13] *G. Cattoretti, E. Berti, R. Schiro, L. D'Amato, C. Valeggio, F. Rilke*, Improved Avidin-Biotin-Peroxidase Complex (ABC) Staining, Histochem. J. *20*, 75–80 (1988).
[14] *M. Davidoff, W. Schultze*, Combination of the Peroxidase Anti-Peroxidase (PAP)- and Avidin-Biotin-Peroxidase Complex (ABC)-Techniques: an Amplification Alternative in Immunocytochemical Staining, Histochemistry *93*, 531–536 (1990).
[15] *L.-I. Larsson, T. W. Schwartz*, Radioimmunocytochemistry – a Novel Immunocytochemical Principle, J. Histochem. Cytochem. *25*, 1140–1146 (1977).

[16] *L.-I. Larsson*, Simultaneous Ultrastructural Demonstration of Multiple Peptides in Endocrine Cells by a Novel Immunocytochemical Method. Nature, London, *282*, 743–746 (1979).

[17] *D. Y. Mason, R. Sammons*, The Labeled Antigen Method of Immunoenzymatic Staining, J. Histochem. Cytochem. *27*, 823–840 (1979).

[18] *L. A. Sternberger, F. A. Joseph*, The Unlabeled Antibody Method. Contrasting Color Staining of Paired Pituitary Hormones Without Antibody Removal, J. Histochem. Cytochem. *29*, 1424–1429 (1979).

[19] *P. K. Nakane*, Simultaneous Localization of Multiple Tissue Antigens Using the Peroxidase-Labeled Antibody Method: a Study in Pituitary Glands of the Rat, J. Histochem. Cytochem. *16*, 557–560 (1968).

[20] *F. Vandesande, K. Dierickx*, Identification of the Vasopressin Producing and Oxytocin Producing Neurons in the Hypothalamic Magnocellular Neurosecretory System of the Rat, Cell Tissue Res. *164*, 153–162 (1975).

[21] *G. Tramu, A. Pillez, J. Leonardelli*, An Efficient Method of Antibody Elution for the Successive or Simultaneous Localization of Two Antigens by Immunocytochemistry, J. Histochem. Cytochem. *26*, 322–324 (1978).

[22] *B. L. Wang, L.-I. Larsson*, Simultaneous Demonstration of Multiple Antigens by Indirect Immunofluorescence or Immunogold Staining. Novel Light and Electron Microscopical Double and Triple Staining Method Employing Primary Antibodies from the Same Species, Histochemistry *83*, 47–56 (1985).

[23] *D. Y. Mason, R. E. Sammons*, Alkaline Phosphatase and Peroxidase for Double Immunoenzymatic Labelling of Cellular Constituents, J. Clin. Pathol. *31*, 454–462 (1978).

[24] *G. T. Campbell, A. S. Bhatnagar*, Simultaneous Visualization by Light Microscopy of Two Pituitary Hormones in a Single Tissue Section Using a Combination of Indirect Immunohistochemical Methods, J. Histochem. Cytochem. *24*, 448–452 (1976).

[25] *S. Van Noorden, M. C. Stuart, A. Cheung, E. F. Adams, J. M. Polak*, Localization of Pituitary Hormones by Multiple Immunoenzyme Staining Procedures Using Monoclonal and Polyclonal Antibodies, J. Histochem. Cytochem. *34*, 287–292 (1986).

[26] *M. W. Wessendorf, N. M. Appel, T. W. Molitor, R. P. Elde*, A Method for Immunofluorescence Demonstration of Three Coexisting Neurotransmitters in Rat Brain and Spinal Cord, Using the Fluorophores Fluorescein, Lissamine Rhodamine and 7-Amino-4-Methylcoumarin-3-Acetic Acid, J. Histochem. Cytochem. *38*, 1859–1877 (1990).

[27] *R. Peretti-Renucci, C. Feuerstein, M. Manier, P. Lorimier, M. Savasta, J. Thibault, N. Mons, M. Geffard*, Quantitative Image Analysis with Densitometry for Immunohistochemistry and Autoradiography of Receptor Binding Sites – Methodological Considerations, J. Neurosci. Res. *28*, 563–600 (1991).

[28] *L. L. Vacca Galloway*, Differential Immunostaining for Substance P in Huntington's Diseased and Normal Spinal Cord: Significance of Serial (Optimal, Supra-Optimal and End-Point) Dilutions of Primary Antiserum in Comparing Biological Specimens, Histochemistry *83*, 561–569 (1985).

5.5   Immunostaining Procedures

Susan Van Noorden

5.5.1   General Aspects

The protocols given here are examples in common use. Most may be used on any type of tissue preparation. Some selected applications are described. Timing of the various steps depends on the preparation, on the quality and dilution of the reagents and on the temperature of reaction. It is for the user to decide on PBS or TBS as buffer medium, blocking reagents, timing, etc., so it is important to establish standard methods for each laboratory.

The materials and apparatus listed below are needed for all methods.

5.5.1.1   Materials Needed

1. Phosphate-buffered saline, PBS (phosphate, 10 mmol/l; NaCl 0.15 mol/l; pH 7.0–7.2):
   dissolve 14.1 g Na_2HPO_4, $2H_2O$, 2.72 g KH_2PO_4 and 87 g NaCl in 10 l distilled water.
2. Tris-buffered saline (TBS) (50 mmol/l Tris, 10 mmol/l NaCl; pH 7.6):
   may be used instead of PBS and is preferred for AP-linked reagents.
3. Ab diluent (PBS/TBS containing 0.1 % w/v BSA and, for dilution and storage of Abs but NOT for POD-linked reagents, 0.1 % (w/v) NaN_3).
4. Hydrogen peroxide (30 % w/v):
   keeps for several months at 4 °C but may deteriorate; ensure fresh supply. If a solution of lower concentration is used, adjust volume to be added accordingly.
5. Endogenous POD blocking solution (0.3 % (w/v) H_2O_2):
   dilute 1 ml 30 % hydrogen peroxide (4) with 100 ml water, PBS (1), TBS (2), methanol, or 70 % methanol in PBS/TBS.
6. Protease solutions as required (cf. Enzyme digestion, 5.3).
7. Background blocking protein, e.g., serum from species providing primary Ab (in direct method) or second Ab (in two- or three-layer method), diluted 1/20 in (3).
8. Primary Ab, second Ab and third reagents diluted at predetermined optimal dilutions in (3), without sodium azide if POD-linked.
9. Substrates, chromogens, intensification media, mountants according to the label to be revealed (cf. 5.3).

10. Humid chamber for incubating preparations (e.g., 22 cm diameter *Petri* dish containing rack made from wooden orange sticks or glass rods cut to fit the dish and wads of tissue moistened with distilled water – takes four slides).
11. *Pasteur* pipettes and rubber teats.
12. Vials for diluting Abs.
13. Fibre-free paper tissues for wiping slides.
14. Hydrophobic isolating pen (optional).
15. *Coplin* jars or slide carriers in suitable dishes for rinsing preparations.

In the following protocols it is assumed that the preparations have been mounted on poly-L-lysine-coated slides (except for pre-fixed, free-floating preparations), that fresh or frozen preparations have been suitably fixed and placed in buffer, and that embedding medium has been removed from wax or resin sections and that they have been hydrated.

PBS is quoted as the buffer throughout, except where TBS is specified, but TBS could be be used in its place.

5.5.1.2   Application of Reagents

Reagents are applied to the preparations with a *Pasteur* pipette. The absolute quantity applied is not important but the preparation must be completely covered, with the drop of reagent extending beyond its edges to avoid artefacts from drying of the reagent. In general, 50–100 µl is adequate to cover an average section but smaller amounts may suffice. Since reagents are expensive, economy is important.

5.5.1.3   Hydrophobic Pen

Encircling the preparation with a hydrophobic pen helps to contain the reagent over the preparation and facilitates the slide-wiping procedure. The pen should be used on the dry slide before fixation for cell preparations and frozen sections, or after removal of embedding medium but before hydration for paraffin or resin sections. However, if a hydrophobic pen is not available, wiping carefully round the area is usually sufficient to create a surface-tension barrier between the dry slide and the wet area of the preparation, allowing a drop of reagent to spread evenly over the preparation but no further.

5.5.1.4   Establishing Antibody Standard Working Dilutions

Each newly acquired Ab must be tested in a series of dilutions on a positive control preparation under the conditions of its intended use, in order to find a standard dilution.

A primary Ab is most easily tested with known second/third reagents at their standard dilutions. Second/third reagents should be tested with a standard dilution of primary Ab. The dilution range depends on the immunostaining method: for two-layer methods the dilution of a primary Ab is usually about ten times higher than for a one-layer method, and increases again for a three-layer technique. The incubation period also influences the degree of dilution. As a rough guide, test primary mAbs, supplied in culture medium, in doubling dilutions from neat to 1/256. Monoclonal Abs supplied in ascites fluid will usually dilute in the range of 1/1 000 to 1/10 000. Polyclonal Abs supplied as antisera should be tried from 1/50 to 1/6 400. The preferred dilution is that which gives a strong immunoreaction and low background. A standard dilution for (commercial) labelled second Abs (anti-Igs) is usually within the range of 1/10 to 1/500.

5.5.2   Cell Preparations and Frozen Sections

It is helpful to scratch a line with a diamond pen on the UNDERSIDE of the slide around the area occupied by the cells or sections, preferably while the preparations are dry, before fixation. When the back of a wet slide is wiped dry the engraved line shows where the preparations are: they are difficult to see when the slide is wet.

It is particularly important that fresh cells or frozen sections are not allowed to become dry at any stage of the procedure after they have been wetted with the first aqueous solution. Drying results in damaged tissue structure and immunostaining that cannot be interpreted. Leave preparations in buffer until the next reagent is ready to apply. Treat preparations singly.

Incubation periods are best kept short when fresh preparations are used, as long periods in aqueous solutions may damage tissue structure, but may be extended to overnight for pAbs requiring high dilutions: mAbs are preferred because long incubation times and high dilutions are not necessary.

5.5.2.1   Direct Immunofluorescence

1. Wipe slide dry except for the area of the preparation and place it on a rack in a damp chamber.
2. Apply normal serum from the species providing the primary Ab diluted 1/20 in PBS/BSA (3). Cover and leave for at least 10 min at room temperature.
3. Drain off the serum or soak it up with a tissue (taking care not to touch the preparation) but do not rinse (low affinity binding to non-specific sites may be reversed by rinsing). Wipe the slide dry around the preparation.
4. Apply primary fluorescent label-conjugated Ab at predetermined dilution in PBS/BSA (3) to cover the preparation. The drop should spread easily over the area left wet by the blocking serum. Cover and leave for 1 h at room temperature.

5. Drain off the Ab and wash in three changes of PBS, 5 min each.
6. Dry around the preparation and mount in a water-miscible mountant (PBS/glycerine or Permafluor, cf. 5.3.7.2).
7. Examine in fluorescence microscope.

Controls: A negative control preparation in which an irrelevant fluorescent Ab is substituted in step 4 (to confirm specificity of binding), a preparation not treated with Ab (to show autofluorescence) and a positive control preparation (to show that the Ab is effective) should be carried through at the same time as the specifically labelled preparation.

5.5.2.2   Indirect (2-Layer) Immunoperoxidase Staining

1. Block endogenous POD reactions, if necessary, using a method suitable for fresh preparations. (cf. blocking methods, 5.3.8.1) If blocking damages the Ag, it may be carried out after reaction with the primary Ab.
2. Wash briefly in PBS.
3. Wipe the slide dry except for area of the preparation and apply normal serum from the species supplying the second-layer Ab, diluted 1/20 in diluent (3). Cover and leave for at least 10 min.
4. Drain off or soak up the serum, but do not rinse. Wipe slide dry around the preparation and apply unlabelled primary Ab at pre-determined optimal dilution in PBS/BSA (3). Cover and leave for 1 h at room temperature.
5. Wash in 3 changes of PBS, 5 min each.
6. Wipe the slide dry except for the area of the preparation and apply the second, POD conjugated Ab at pre-determined optimal dilution in diluent (3) without azide. Cover and leave for 1 h at room temperature.
7. Wash in 3 changes of PBS, 5 min each.
8. Develop POD in DAB/H_2O_2 or other medium (cf. development methods, 5.3.8.2) Counterstain as appropriate, dehydrate, clear and mount in permanent medium.

Controls: suitable negative controls include omission of the primary Ab or its substitution by an irrelevant Ab.

5.5.2.3   Alkaline Phosphatase Anti-Alkaline Phosphatase (APAAP) Staining

1. Wipe slide dry except for area of preparation and apply normal serum from the species supplying the second-layer Ab, diluted 1/20 in diluent (3). Cover and leave for at least 10 min at room temperature.

2. Drain off or soak up serum but do not wash. Apply primary mouse mAb at pre-determined dilution in diluent (3). Cover and leave for 1 h at room temperature.
3. Wash in 3 changes of PBS, 5 min each.
4. Wipe slide dry except for area of preparation and apply unlabelled second Ab (to Ig of species (mouse) providing the primary Ab) at pre-determined dilution in diluent (3). Cover and leave for 30 min–1 h at room temperature.
5. Wash in 2 changes of PBS and 1 of TBS, 5 min each.
6. Wipe slide dry except for area of preparation and apply (mouse) APAAP at pre-determined dilution in TBS. Cover and leave for 30 min–1 h at room temperature.
7. Wash in 3 changes of TBS, 5 min each.
8. (Optional – to increase the intensity of the reaction). Repeat application of 2nd Ab and APAAP, 10 min each, washing in TBS between the layers and after the APAAP.
9. Develop AP by chosen method, adding levamisole 1 mmol/l to the incubating medium to inhibit endogenous AP (cf. enzyme methods, 5.3.9).
10. Counterstain and mount as appropriate.

Controls: as for indirect immunoperoxidase staining.

5.5.3   Paraffin Sections

Paraffin-embedded tissue has already been dehydrated and taken through solvents; drying affects sections less drastically than fresh material but should, nevertheless, be avoided. Some Ags in formalin-fixed preparations require protease treatment to reveal antigenic sites (cf. enzyme digestion, below).

Remove wax from paraffin sections by soaking them in two changes of a solvent (e.g. xylene). Hydrate through alcohol (two changes of 100 %, one of 70 %) and rinse in water.

5.5.3.1   Peroxidase Anti-Peroxidase (PAP) Staining

1. Block endogenous POD in 0.3 % (w/v) H_2O_2 in water for 30 min at room temperature.
2. Wash in water.
3. Treat with protease if necessary (cf. 5.5.3.3).
4. Wash in water then PBS.
5. Wipe slide dry except for the area of the section and apply normal serum from the species providing the second Ab, diluted 1/20 in diluent (3) (an alternative blocking

agent such as 1 % (w/v) BSA or chicken egg albumin may be used). Cover and leave for at least 10 min at room temperature.

6. Drain off or soak up the serum but do not rinse. Wipe the slide dry round the section and apply unlabelled primary (polyclonal, rabbit) Ab at pre-determined high dilution in diluent (3). Cover and leave overnight at 4 °C.
7. Bring to room temperature and wash in three changes of PBS, 5 min each.
8. Wipe slide dry except for area of the section and apply unlabelled second Ab (against Ig of species (rabbit) providing primary Ab) at pre-determined optimal dilution in diluent (3). Cover and leave for 30 min–1 h at room temperature.
9. Wash in three changes of PBS, 5 min each.
10. Wipe slide dry except for area of the section and apply (rabbit) PAP at pre-determined optimal dilution in diluent (3) without azide. Cover and leave for 30 min–1 h at room temperature.
11. Wash in 3 changes of PBS, 5 min each.
12. Develop POD by chosen method. Counterstain and mount as appropriate (cf. 5.3.8.2).

Controls: as for indirect immunoperoxidase staining.

5.5.3.2   Avidin-Biotinylated POD Complex (ABC) Staining

1.–4. As PAP method (above).
5.   Block with normal serum, NOT chicken egg albumin because it contains avidin.
6.–7. As PAP method (above).
8.   As PAP method, except that second Ab is biotinylated.
9.   Prepare ABC reagent by mixing avidin and biotinylated POD with PBS (no azide) in the proportions recommended by the manufacturer. The components of the complex must be allowed to react together for at least 30 min before being applied to the preparation. Once made, the reagent may survive storage for a few days, but if the complex becomes too large, steric hindrance will prevent it from binding effectively. Therefore, it is best to make only the amount that is needed for one day.
10.   Wash in 3 changes of PBS, 5 min each.
11.   Wipe slide dry except for area of section. Apply preformed ABC-POD. Cover and leave for 30 min–1 h.
12.   Wash in 3 changes of PBS, 5 min each.
13.   Develop POD by chosen method. Counterstain and mount as described in Section 5.3.8.2.

Controls: as for indirect staining method.

5.5.3.3   Enzyme Digestion

Aldehyde fixation can "over-fix" some proteins and block their antigenic groups. Protease treatment of sections is said to reverse the cross-linking and reveal the antigenic groups [1, 2]. That this is really the mechanism has not yet been established but, in practice, protease digestion can certainly help to make some tissue Ags more available to Ab. Experience dictates which Ags require such treatment, but the protease only exceptionally affects adversely the reactivity of Ags (eg. leucocyte common Ag) in the tissue preparation. Igs are among the molecules "over-fixed" by formalin that can be made more immunoreactive by proteases. If precipitant fixatives are used alone (e.g. *Carnoy's* fixative, which consists of ethanol, chloroform and acetic acid) or in combination with formaldehyde (e.g. *Bouin's* fluid, which contains picric acid and formalin), protease digestion is not usually necessary or effective.

Each new batch of protease must be tested to determine the appropriate time for digestion. Incubate preparations with the protease solution at 20–37 °C at the enzyme's optimal pH, for a time ranging from 1 to 75 minutes depending on the Ag and the length of fixation time. Over-digestion, leading to disintegration of the tissue, must be avoided. A "standard" procedure can be arrived at for each type of Ag but if variable fixation times are encountered the incubation time may have to be altered accordingly. A range of proteases should also be tried if a "new" Ag is to be studied.

Trypsin, in crude from containing some chymotrypsin, is cheap and is usually effective, but some Ags may give better results with other enzymes. Only trial can decide this. The incubation time must be established for each batch of enzyme and for each Ag. It is usually (for trypsin) within the range of 10–20 min but some Ags may require longer.

Trypsin (EC 3.4.21.4)

Materials needed

1. Trypsin (crude, porcine) 1000–5000 BAEE U/mg; contains chymotrypsin (*EC* 3.4.21.1) 500–1000 ATEE U/mg (*ICN* cat. no 150213).
2. Calcium chloride 0.1 % (w/v), kept at 37 °C.
3. Sodium hydroxide 0.1 mol/l.

Method

1. Mix 0.1 g trypsin (1) into 100 ml warm calcium chloride solution (2). The solution will be cloudy, and the pH about 5.5.
2. Working quickly (to avoid cooling the solution), bring to pH 7.8 with NaOH (3). Most of the trypsin will dissolve.
3. Incubate sections for a standard time at 37 °C.
4. Wash well in cold running water then in distilled water.

Protease

Materials needed

1. Protease Bacterial type XXIV 7–14 U/mg (*Sigma*, cat. no. P 8038)
2. PBS pre-warmed to 37 °C

Method

1. Make an 0.05 % (w/v) solution of protease (1) in warm PBS (2).
2. Incubate preparations for 5 to 20 min at 37 °C.
    The optimal incubation times must be pre-determined as for trypsin.
    As this enzyme is considerably more expensive than trypsin, use it as drops on the
    preparation, rather than by immersing the preparations in a large volume.

Pepsin (EC 3.4.23.1)

Materials needed

1. Pepsin from porcine stomach mucosa, 600–1 000 U/mg (*Sigma*, ca. no. P 7129)
2. HCl, 0.01 mol/l, at 37 °C.

Method
1. Dissolve 4 mg pepsin (1) in 1 ml HCl (2).
2. Place drops on sections and incubate at 37 °C for 20–30 min.

Pronase E

Materials needed

1. Pronase from *Streptomyces griseus* 4 U/mg (*Sigma,* cat. no. P 6911)
2. Tris/HCl buffer, pH 7.5 at 37 °C.

Method

1. Make a 0.1 % solution of pronase (1) in Tris buffer (2).
2. Incubate preparations at 37 °C for 15–30 min.

Neuraminidase (EC 3.2.1.18)

Materials needed

1. Neuraminidase (Type V) from *Clostridium perfringens* 0.5–2 U/mg (*Sigma*, cat. no.
    N 2876)

2. Sodium acetate buffer, 0.1 mol/l, pH 5.5, at 37 °C.
3. Calcium chloride 0.1 % (w/v).

Method

1. Dissolve 0.1 U neuraminidase in 1 ml acetate buffer (2).
2. Add 100 µl calcium chloride solution (2).
3. Incubate in drops on preparations at 37 °C for 5–20 min.

Neuraminidase may be dissolved in buffer or water and stored frozen in 0.1 U aliquots.

5.5.3.4   Antigen Retrieval by Microwave Treatment

Several antigens previously immunoreactive only in fresh-frozen tissue have been demonstrated in formalin-fixed paraffin sections after microwave treatment. The timing, power and number of applications of the microwaves must be assessed for individual antigens and methods.

The method given below was used to reveal the Ki 67 antigen in the nuclei of proliferating cells for detection by mAbs MIB 1 and 3 [3].

Materials needed

1. Microwave oven.
2. Plastic *Coplin* jars.
3. Citrate buffer. (Dissolve 2.1 g citric acid monohydrate in 1 l water. Adjust pH to 6.0 with NaOH.)

Method

1. Remove wax from paraffin sections and rehydrate.
2. Place in plastic *Coplin* jar (2) and cover with citrate buffer (3).
3. Microwave for 2 × 5 min at maximum power (700 W) in a domestic microwave oven (or 450 W in a laboratory microwave processor (eg. *Bio Rad* H2500). The sections must remain immersed in the buffer throughout.
4. Cool to room temperature in the buffer, wash with PBS and continue with the chosen immunostaining method.

5.5.4   Pre-fixed Frozen Sections, Vibratome Sections, Whole-Mount Preparations

Sections or other preparations that are more than 10–15 μm thick and have not been processed through lipid solvents may need to be made permeable to Abs. The use of detergents and dehydration-rehydration procedures has been discussed in 5.2.4.

Long incubation periods in Ab solutions and washing buffers are advised for free-floating thick Vibratome sections and whole-mount material (e.g., iris membrane, stripped muscle layers of gut wall). The Abs are placed in wells of culture plates or small beakers or dishes that can accommodate the preparations, and are removed and replaced by pipetting with a *Pasteur* pipette. Reagents may thus penetrate the specimen from all surfaces. Higher concentrations of Ab are required than for thin sections because of the larger amount of available Ag. Sample schedules for PAP and fluorescence methods are given below.

5.5.4.1   Pre-fixed Thick Preparations, PAP Method

1. Dehydrate the sample through graded alcohols, 30 min in each, to xylene (1 h) then rehydrate through the same series, or treat the sample with detergent, e.g. 0.2–0.5 % (v/v) Triton X-100 in PBS for 1 h. Detergent may be included in the subsequent washing steps and in the Ab solutions.
2. Block endogenous POD activity with 0.3 % H_2O_2 for 30 min.
3. Wash in 2 changes of PBS, 30 min each.
4. Incubate overnight in normal serum from the species providing the second Ab, diluted 1/10 in PBS with 0.2 % (v/v) Triton X-100.
5. Incubate in primary Ab at a suitable dilution in PBS diluent (3) for 72 h at 4 °C.
6. Wash in several changes of PBS over 10–12 h.
7. Incubate 6–8 h in suitably diluted second Ab.
8. Wash in several changes of PBS over 10–12 h.
9. Incubate in PAP complex, suitably diluted (no azide) for 6–8 h.
10. Wash in several changes of PBS over 10–12 h.
11. POD development: Immerse the preparations in 0.05 % (w/v) DAB in PBS for 10 min, then transfer to 0.05 % DAB containing 0.015 % (w/v) H_2O_2 for a further 10 min. This ensures even development of the enzyme through the thickness of the specimen.
12. Wash several times in PBS, then flatten and stretch the preparation onto a poly-L-lysine-coated slide, or pick it up unstretched if a frozen section, and allow to dry.
13. Rinse in distilled water, dehydrate through graded alcohols, clear and mount in permanent medium.

5.5.4.2 Pre-fixed Thick Preparations, Immunofluorescence

1.–7. as 1–8 above, omitting step 2, blocking of endogenous POD, and using a fluorescein-conjugated second Ab.
8. Pick up or flatten and stretch the preparation on a poly-L-lysine-coated slide.
9. Mount in PBS-glycerine or Permafluor.

5.5.5 Immunogold Staining with Silver Intensification (IGSS) (Paraffin Sections)

Note. Best results are obtained if the colloidal gold particles adsorbed to the second Ab are of small diameter, 5 nm or less.

Solutions needed

1. *Lugol's* iodine: 1 % (w/v) iodine in 2 % (w/v) potassium iodide.
2. 2.5 % (w/v) sodium thiosulphate.
3. IGSS buffer I. Tris/HCl buffer 0.05 mol/l, pH 7.4, containing 2.5 % (w/v) sodium chloride and 0.2 % (v/v) Triton X-100.
4. IGSS buffer II. Tris HCl buffer, 0.05 mol/l, pH 8.2, containing 0.87 % (w/v) sodium chloride.
5. Ab diluent for primary Ab: TBS containing 0.1 % (w/v) BSA and 0.1 % (w/v) sodium azide.
6. Ab diluent for gold-adsorbed second Ab: IGSS buffer II (4) containing 0.8 % (w/v) BSA.
7. Reagents for silver intensification (cf. 5.3.8.2).

Method

1. Bring paraffin sections to water, encircling sections with hydrophobic pen after removing the wax and rinsing in alcohol. Since there is detergent in the buffer this helps to prevent the Ab solution from spreading over the slide. Alternatively, take particular care to wipe the slide dry around the section, or paint a ring of mountant around the section.
2. Immerse in *Lugol's* iodine (1) for 5 min (may not be necessary for all preparations) then wash in water.
3. Bleach in sodium thiosulphate (2).
4. Wash well in tap water, then in 2 changes of IGSS buffer I (3), 5 min each.
5. Wipe slides dry around the section and apply undiluted normal serum from the species supplying the second (gold-adsorbed) Ab. Cover and leave for 15 min.

6. Drain off or soak up serum but do not wash.
7. Apply primary Ab diluted in TBS/BSA (5). The dilution is usually in the range of that used for a PAP method with overnight incubation. Cover and leave for 90 min.
8. Wash in 2 changes of IGSS buffer I (3), 10 min each.
9. Wash once in IGSS buffer II (4) for 10 min.
10. Wipe slide dry around the section and apply normal serum as in 5. Cover and leave for 10 min.
11. Drain off or soak up serum but do not wash.
12. Apply gold-adsorbed second Ab (to Ig of species providing the primary Ab) at pre-determined optimal dilution in IGSS diluent (6). Cover and leave for 1 h.
13. Wash in 3 changes of IGSS buffer II, 5 min each.
14. Wash briefly in several changes of distilled water, then in 4 changes of distilled water of 5 min each.
15. Intensify with silver by one of the methods outlined in 5.3.8.2.

References

[1] *S. Huang, H. Minassian, J.D. More,* Application of Immunofluorescent Staining in Paraffin Sections Improved by Trypsin Digestion, Lab. Invest. *35,* 383–391 (1976).
[2] *J.C.W. Finley, P. Petrusz,* The Use of Proteolytic Enzymes for Improved Localization of Tissue Antigens with Immunocytochemistry, in: *G.R. Bullock, P. Petrusz* (eds.), Techniques in Immunocytochemistry, Vol. 1., Academic Press, London, (1982) pp. 239–249.
[3] *G. Cattoretti, M.H.G. Becker, G. Key, M. Duchrow, C. Schlüter, J. Galle, J. Gerdes,* Monoclonal Antibodies Against Recombinant Parts of the Ki 67 Antigen (MIB 1 and MIB 3) Detect Proliferating Cells in Microwave-Processed Formalin-Fixed Paraffin Sections, J. Pathol. *168,* 357–363 (1992).

5.6   Problem Solving and Practical Aspects

Susan Van Noorden

5.6.1   Unwanted Staining

This may be due to nonspecific binding of antibodies to various components of tissues or to the activity of endogenous enzymes, as well as to properties of the reagents or even to errors in technique.

5.6.1.1   Fc Receptors

Problem

Certain cells (macrophages, granulocytes) carry on their plasma membranes receptors for the Fc portion of Abs. These receptors are destroyed by formalin fixation and embedding but in fresh tissue preparations, such as frozen sections or blood smears, they may be an important cause of Ag-independent binding to the tissue of Igs from the applied Ab.

Solutions

a) Preincubation of the preparation with non-immune serum (5–20 % (v/v) solution), containing Igs, from the species providing the second Ab in an indirect method, or the same species as the labelled Ab in a direct method, will occupy the Fc receptors and prevent the applied Ab from reacting.
b) Reagent Abs may be used as Fab or F(ab)$_2$ fractions, with the Fc portion removed by papain or pepsin digestion. It may be necessary to use an anti-Fab reagent as second Ab and the second and third reagents should themselves also be Fab fractions.

5.6.1.2   Complement Binding

Problem

Complement factors (C1q) in the antiserum may become bound to the tissue and provoke deposition of Ig which will subsequently be identified by a labelled Ab [1].

Solution

C1q is not inactivated by heating sera to 56 °C but could be removed from serum by adding an irrelevant Ag-Ab complex. However, the problem applies only to concentrated antisera. Use of highly dilute sera should solve it.

5.6.1.3   Hydrophobic or Charged Tissue Sites

Problem

In fixed tissues, negatively charged Abs may be bound to positively charged sites.

Solutions

a) Blocking with normal serum, as for Fc receptors, solution (a). *Note.* Serum should not be used for blocking when protein A reactions are involved since binding of this protein to the extra Fc portions of serum Igs will produce extra unwanted staining. Other proteins such as BSA (1 % w/v), egg white or oralbumin (not in ABC methods as it contains avidin) or non-fat dried milk may also be used to block nonspecific tissue sites, and are usually cheaper than serum.

b) Use buffers with a high salt content (NaCl, 0.5 mol/l) or high pH (8–9) [2] or containing detergent such as 0.2 % (w/v) Triton X-100 or 0.1 % (w/v) saponin, which is less likely to extract membrane proteins [3].

5.6.1.4   Aldehyde Groups in Tissue

Problem

Formaldehyde or glutaraldehyde fixation may leave residual aldehyde in the tissue which interacts with Igs *via* amino groups.

Solution

Reduce the aldehyde groups to alcohol by pre-treatment with freshly prepared 0.02 % (w/v) sodium borohydride for 2 minutes [4] or add to the blocking protein substances containing non-interfering amino groups such as ammonium chloride (50–100 mmol/l) [5] or ethanolamine (100 mmol/l) [6].

5.6.1.5   Endogenous Enzyme

Problem

POD in macrophages and catalase in red blood cells or AP, particularly in unfixed preparations, may be confused with applied enzyme-linked immune reagents (cf. 5.3.8.1 and 5.3.9.1).

Solutions

a) Block POD with hydrogen peroxide 0.3 % (w/v) in methanol or buffer or water for 30 min or with phenylhydrazine [7] or, for delicate Ags in fresh material, with nascent hydrogen peroxide and sodium azide [8] before beginning the immunostain or at any stage before application of the enzyme-linked reagent. Block non-intestinal AP by including levamisole (1 mmol/l) in the enzyme development medium [9].

b) Use an alternative enzyme as label.

5.6.1.6   Endogenous Biotin

Problem

Some tissues, e.g., liver and kidney, contain biotin which can bind labelled avidin or ABC.

Solution

Pre-incubate the preparation with unlabelled avidin (1 g/l for 20 min) to occupy the biotin, then, after washing in buffer, with unlabelled biotin (0.1 g/l for 20 min) to block remaining biotin-binding sites on the avidin [10].

5.6.1.7   Avidin Binding

Problem

Avidin may bind to lectin-like molecules in the tissue through its carbohydrate groups, or to charged sites because of its high isoelectric point. It also binds to mast cells.

Solutions

a) Use a high pH buffer (pH 9.0) [11].
b) Use modified avidin (commercially available) that avoids these problems
c) Use streptavidin instead of avidin.

5.6.1.8   Binding of Aggregated Igs to Basic Peptide Sequences

Problem

Certain basic amino acid sequences often found in peptides (e.g. lysine) attract Igs (and other proteins) that may have become aggregated in a stored Ab solution. Aggregates in any layer of an immunocytochemical reaction could thus bind and produce nonspecific staining [12].

Solution

Pre-absorb antisera with a basic amino acid, e.g., low molecular weight poly-L-lysine ($M_r = 3\,000–6\,000$) 1–2 mg per ml of diluted antiserum, at 4 °C for 24 h. This blocks the binding capacity of the aggregates and does not affect specific immunoreactions [12].

5.6.1.9   Free Label

Problem

Unreacted label present in the labelled Ab solution may bind to the tissue. This may also be a problem if the label becomes detached from the Ab during storage.

Solution

a) Remove free label from the Ab solution by column chromatography.
b) Do not store labelled Ab in highly diluted solutions.

5.6.1.10 Poorly Preserved Tissue

Problem

Poorly fixed or necrotic tissue will result in leakage of proteins from the cells and a high level of non-specific and diffuse specific binding of Abs.

Solution

Ensure that tissue is fixed or otherwise preserved promptly.

5.6.1.11 Contaminating Antibodies

Problem

The primary Ab (polyclonal) may contain Abs, in addition to the specific Ab, that can react specifically or nonspecifically with the tissue.

Solutions

a) Dilute the Ab as far as possible to remove the contaminating Ab population.
b) Affinity-purify the primary Ab.
c) Use a monoclonal primary Ab.

5.6.1.12 Cross-reactions of Immunoglobulins

Problem

The detecting anti-Ig may cross-react with Igs in the tissue of the species to be stained as well as identifying those of the species providing the primary Ab.

Solution

Add to the second Ab, serum or Igs from the species in which the Ag is to be stained. Usually 1 % (v/v) is adequate to absorb out the cross-reacting Abs. Test by using the anti-Ig as primary Ab to identify Igs in peripheral blood or spleen cells (of the host species) prepared in the same way as the tissue to be immunostained.

5.6.1.13 Cross-reactions of Primary Antibody

Problem

The primary Ab may cross-react with molecules that share antigenic groups with the Ag under investigation. If substances structurally related to the Ag are present in the tissue they too will be immunostained by the "specific" Ab.

Solution

Use an Ab specific to an unshared region of the molecule under investigation. With pAbs it may be possible to absorb out the cross-reacting population using the shared fragment of the molecule. Genuine cross-reactivity is otherwise impossible to avoid and great care must be taken to establish specificity when the Ag is one of a family of related substances.

5.6.1.14 Method Factors

All aspects of the chosen method must be carefully controlled. Using the wrong pH, temperature, time of incubation, constitution of enzyme development medium, Ab dilution, excessive or incomplete washing as well as human error at any stage can adversely affect the achievement of a good immunocytochemical reaction.

5.6.2   Lack of Staining

5.6.2.1   Unavailable Antigen

Problem

Cross-linking fixation with aldehydes may block antigenic groups on some proteins. This applies in particular to the sections from formalin-fixed paraffin-embedded tissues that are routinely used in histopathological diagnosis.

Solutions

a) Treatment with a protease such as trypsin before applying the Ab may reverse the cross-linking and reveal antigenic groups (cf. enzyme digestion, section 5.5.3.3).
b) Shortening the fixation time, using non-cross-linking fixatives or adding precipitants to aldehyde fixatives may be tried.

5.6.2.2   Incorrect Tissue Treatment

Problem

Incorrect treatment of tissue, such as over-fixation, over-heating or harsh methods of blocking endogenous enzymes, can damage some Ags. Over-stringent washing or the use of very low pH buffers can remove bound Abs from their sites of reaction.

Solution

No universal solution applies. Attention to detail is recommended.

5.6.2.3   Prozone Effect

Problem

In a technique using an enzyme-anti-enzyme complex as the third layer, the relative concentrations of the primary and secondary Abs must be such that the second Ab is in excess, leaving one anti-Ig binding site free for reaction with the third-layer complex. If the primary Ab is too concentrated with respect to the second Ab, no free sites will be available and no identification of the reaction can take place (see unlabelled enzyme anti-enzyme method section 5.4.3).

Solutions

a) Dilute the primary Ab further.
b) Increase the concentration of the second Ab.
c) Use a two-step or ABC method.

5.6.3   Controls

In immunocytochemistry, as in any experimental procedure, controls are obligatory for correct interpretation of the results. They are of three kinds: control of specificity of the primary (and other) Abs (specificity controls); controls to show that the method is working (positive/method controls), and controls to show that the reaction is due to the applied Ab (negative controls).

5.6.3.1 Specificity Controls

In the first instance, the primary Ab must be shown to react only with the Ag under investigation. Known positive tissue is used to assess the specificity of the Ab, and as a control when unknown tissue is being tested for the presence of an Ag. The simplest test is to add excess pure, preferably synthetic, Ag to the Ab in solution so that all the Ag-binding sites on the Ab are occupied. When the absorbed Ab is applied to the tissue no reaction should take place. A similar absorption with a related or unrelated molecule should have no effect. Graded reduction of the quantity of Ag added should show a gradual return of immunocytochemical staining. It is convenient to use nanomolar quantities of Ags so that absorption data from different Ags can be compared.

Test the Ab at the maximum dilution that gives consistent immunostaining in order to economize on the amount of Ag needed. Incubate pure, preferably synthetic, Ag with aliquots of the diluted Ab in graded amounts from 10 to 0.01 nmol per ml of the diluted Ab.

The time required for pre-incubation of Ag with Ab may be quite short (e.g. 30 min at 37 °C) but overnight incubation at 4 °C and storage of absorbed Abs is acceptable.

This approach is usually successful but a number of cautions apply.

5.6.3.2 Importance of Antigen Purity

Problem

If an extracted Ag was used for the initial immunization and contained some contaminants, there is a possibility that the Ab under test is in fact reacting with a contaminant and not with the desired Ag. If the tissue contains the contaminant an immunocytochemical reaction will be obtained. If the absorption test is then done with the immunogen, containing the same contaminant, no staining will occur and "specific absorption" will have been shown.

Solution

If pure or synthetic Ag is used no absorption would occur, showing the reaction to be not specific for the Ag under investigation

5.6.3.3 Receptor Sites for the Antigen May Be Present in the Same Tissue as the Stored Antigen

Problem

The soluble Ab-bound Ag used as an absorption test may bind to the receptor sites, resulting in the detection of the "absorbed" Ab in the subsequent immunocytochemical staining steps.

Solution

If this is an expected problem, occupation of the receptor sites before applying the absorbed Ab should avoid it.

5.6.3.4   Destruction of the Antigen

Problem

Enzymes in an antiserum may digest the Ag being used for absorption, resulting in no absorption.

Solution

Add a protease inhibitor to the antiserum, eg. Trasylol 4000 KIU/ml (*Bayer*).

5.6.3.5   Nonspecific Binding of Ig-or Ag-Ab Complexes

Problem

Ag-Ab complexes formed in solution when an antigen is added for an absorption test may find tissue binding sites that did not attract the smaller Igs in the original antiserum.

Solution

Use solid-phase absorption. In this approach pure Ag is adsorbed to a solid matrix such as cyanogen bromide-activated Sepharose^R beads. Diluted Ab is mixed with the beads for 24 h. Specific Ab remains bound to them while the rest of the solution is collected by centrifugation and, Ab-free, is used to immunostain the tissue. If the original staining was specific to the Ag under investigation, no staining will occur.

Solid-phase absorption avoids many of the problems outlined above, but is more complicated to carry out. Much more Ag is required than for liquid-phase absorption and it is also very difficult to assess the quantity of Ag required and to compare different amounts.

5.6.3.6   Cross-reacting Antibodies

Problem

Absorption tests can only identify Abs that react with shared structures of related molecules if repeated absorptions are carried out with the different related Ags. This may well have to be done, but although it will identify the problem it cannot identify the Ag in the tissue which may be one or more of several capable of reacting with the Ab.

Solution

The only remedy is to use region-specific, non-cross-reacting Abs and use the relevant fragments of the molecule for the absorption test. In cases where the related Ag is unsuspected or undiscovered there is no solution. Cross-reacting Abs may be more easily characterized by *in vitro* tests on blots of different Ags or by ELISA.

Absorption tests are less necessary for monoclonal Abs than for polyclonal antisera, since the unique specificity of a mAb can be tested *in vitro* by ELISA, Ag blots or RIA. However, such tests will not assess how well the Ab will bind to the Ag in tissue, nor necessarily its cross-reactivity which may present worse problems than pAbs. With pAbs there is hope that, even if the greater population of Abs in the serum is cross-reactive, there may be a residual population to an unshared region of the molecule that could be retrieved by region-specific absorption or affinity purification and used as a specific Ab. If a mAb cross-reacts, nothing can be done.

Specificity problems are discussed in greater detail in [12].

Once an Ab has been proved to be specific (by immunocytochemistry) there is no further need to carry out absorption controls, although they are advisable when a new type of location or preparation is being investigated.

5.6.3.7 Positive/Method Controls

A positive control preparation for each primary Ab must be taken through each staining run to ensure that all steps have been carried out correctly. Many errors can be made, but is is reasonable to assume that if the result on the control positive preparation is as normally found, the results on the test material can be trusted.

5.6.3.8 Negative Controls

It is also essential to carry through a negative control for each type of preparation being used in each staining run. The control consists of substituting for the primary Ab an irrelevant Ab, or a non-immune serum (at the same concentration as the primary Ab), or an irrelevant anti-Ig, or buffer alone for one of the other reagents, or of omitting one or more of the steps of the method. Any of these substitutions should give no immunostaining, any "positive" result being nonspecific, or due to cross-reaction of Igs with those of the host species, or to endogenous enzyme. Careful investigation will show which factors are responsible for any such staining.

5.6.4   Other Important Factors

5.6.4.1   Concentration/Dilution of Antibodies

In order to achieve the highest possible signal, the applied Ab should always be in excess of the Ag to be localized. However, when polyclonal antisera are being used they should be diluted as far as possible in order to limit effects of unwanted components. Adequate incubation time must be allowed so that the most avid Abs in the polyclonal mixture can compete successfully for the antigenic sites. Even highly diluted Abs achieve maximal binding within four to eight hours of incubation with a tissue section. A primary antiserum at low dilution (e.g. 1/20) may react adequately within 30 min but there is a danger of nonspecific attachment.

Overnight incubation may not increase the binding but will not decrease it and is more convenient in daily practice. The dilution of the primary Ab is also dependent on the method used and the amount of amplification. For example, a direct, one-step method with a labelled primary Ab diluted 1/10 might be complete in 30 min. The same Ab might be used at 1/100 if the incubation was for 4 h or longer, at 1/1 000 if used unlabelled for an indirect, two-step method and 1/3 000–1/5 000 for a three-step PAP or ABC method. If speed is important, e.g., for rapid diagnosis, short incubation times with concentrated Abs may have to be used.

One way of increasing the chances for avid Abs in a polyclonal antiserum to compete successfully for the tissue Ag is to rinse the preparations half-way through the incubation period and re-apply the primary Ab. Low-affinity Abs will be washed off, making their Ag again available for binding by the avid population in the second application of antiserum [13].

Monoclonal Abs are not subject to the above strictures since only one Ab and no contaminants are present. However, mAbs may be diluted for economy. A concentration of about 10 µg/ml is usually satisfactory, even for a short incubation period, as only clones yielding high-avidity Abs will be selected for immunocytochemistry. In practice, this amounts to a 1/10 to 1/100 dilution of the original culture medium, but may be nearer 1/1 000–1/10 000 if the Ab is in the form of concentrated Ig or ascites fluid.

The second Ab in a two- or three-step method is usually a hyperimmune antiserum, prepared and purified commercially. Dilution is not required to remove contaminants as tissue nonspecific binding sites will have been blocked. The Ab is therefore usually applied in low dilution (1/20–1/500) for 30 min to 1 h which is adequate to provide an excess of anti-Ig to bind to the first Ab. Increasing the incubation time will often allow further dilution, but care must be taken that an excess is present for an enzyme-anti-enzyme reaction (cf. section 5.4.3).

Optimal dilutions of all Abs must be pre-determined by titration in a known Ag-containing preparation of the type to be used in the experiment. The reaction must be immunocytochemical, not another system such as RIA or ELISA, in order to take account of nonspecific, cross-reacting or unwanted binding which would not otherwise be recognized.

5.6.4.2   Temperature

The reaction rate of Ag-Ab binding may be increased by incubating at 37 °C, but nonspecific binding will also be increased. Unless a result is required urgently, immunocytochemical staining is best carried out at room temperature (20 °C) or, if overnight incubation is being used, at 4 °C to avoid the drying hazard. A humid chamber should always be used.

5.6.4.3   Diluent for Antibodies

Abs are usually diluted in phosphate or Tris buffers varying in molarity from 0.01 to 0.1 mol/l, and in pH from 7.0 to 7.6, containing the physiological concentration (0.85 % w/v) of sodium chloride. To prevent attachment of weakly binding contaminants or low-affinity Abs a higher concentration of sodium chloride (up to 0.5 mol/l) or a higher pH (8.0–9.0) may be used [2], but a higher concentration of Ab may be needed in this case to increase the proportion of avid Abs that can take advantage of the increased number of available binding sites.

5.6.4.4   Storage of Antibodies

Abs in high dilution can bind to the glass or plastic walls of the storage vessel, considerably reducing the real concentration of the solution. To prevent this, irrelevant protein such as BSA or normal serum (from the species providing the second Ab) is added to the buffer to compete with the Ab for the nonspecific binding sites. For long-term storage of diluted antisera or monoclonal Abs in their original culture medium, a preservative such as sodium azide (0.01–1.0 % w/v) is added. Some Abs can be kept in this way for several years at 4 °C. Solutions containing azide must not be used to dilute peroxide-associated reagents as sodium azide is an inhibitor of peroxidase.

An alternative method of long-term storage of Abs is to snap-freeze (in liquid nitrogen) small aliquots at low dilution (up to 1/100) or undiluted, depending on what is a convenient amount to provide the working dilution for short-term storage, and keep them at or below −20 °C. A fairly high concentration of (serum) protein is needed to protect the Ab so high dilutions should not be frozen. The original volume in the vial should be noted so that, even if some drying out occurs, the correct final dilution can still be made. Slow freezing of large volumes is not recommended, and Abs should not be repeatedly thawed and frozen.

Occasionally, freezing destroys the reactivity of an Ab and, although a polyclonal antiserum will probably contain enough surviving Ab populations, a mAb of this kind will, of course, be rendered useless. It is therefore advisable to test a sample of Ab after freezing and thawing before committing the entire stock to the freezer. Abs can be stored at $-20\,°C$ without freezing by diluting them $1:1$ (v/v) with glycerol. The glycerol will not affect the immunoreaction, but the doubled volume must be allowed for when the working dilution is made.

Lyophilization (freeze-drying) is a good way of preserving Abs. The original volume and dilution of the antiserum or mAb should be recorded.

5.6.5   Apparatus

5.6.5.1   General

Very little apparatus is required for conventional immunostaining techniques. The essentials are a humid chamber in which the preparations, mounted on slides or coverslips, can be laid flat. Large, covered *Petri* dishes are suitable, although more complicated Perspex dishes with inbuilt racks are available commercially. *Pasteur* pipettes are used for applying drops of Ab solutions and adjustable-volume micropipettes are used to make dilutions of reagents. Preparations on slides can be placed in a slide carrier for rinsing in a large volume of buffer, or buffer can be squirted onto them from a wash-bottle (this is less satisfactory, because more handling of the slides is involved and preparations may be washed off). Non-fluff paper tissue is used to wipe the slides dry (except for the area of the preparation) after washes. Peroxidase blocking and development and silver enhancement methods are conveniently and safely carried out in bulk with the slides in a slide carrier, but for small numbers of preparations and other enzymes, drops of solution on the preparations can be used as for the immune reagents.

5.6.5.2   Automation

Several companies produce equipment for automated or semi-automated immunostaining. The principles of design vary, but in all cases the slide carrying the preparation is supported in a chamber, and measured amounts of reagents are supplied in sequence from pre-charged reservoirs and washed out with buffer. Fully automated apparatus uses electronically controlled delivery while the much less expensive semi-automated variety requires the operator to apply the solutions, but avoids the need for handling the preparations and drying the slides between steps. These devices are certainly labour-saving but the question of cost-effectiveness must be considered.

5.6.6 Photomicrography

As for any morphological method, results must be recorded as photomicrographs. Many laboratories possess a photomicroscope with an automatic exposure meter, requiring the operator only to set up the microscope and focus the specimen correctly, set the film speed and press a button.

Fluorescence photomicrography requires very sensitive, fast films, since long exposure of fluorescent preparations to UV light results in fading. "Daylight" films are used for colour recording.

For preparations that can be viewed in a standard light microscope, photomicrography of immunostained preparations does not differ from that for conventional histological staining. "Tungsten" films are suitable. In black-and-white photography, appropriately coloured filters might be necessary to emphasize the immunostained area.

For discussion of the theoretical and practical aspects of photomicrography see [14, 15].

References

[1] R. Buffa, E. Solcia, R. Fiocca, O. Crivelli, A. Pera, Complement-Mediated Binding of Immunoglobulins to Some Endocrine Cells of the Pancreas and Gut, J. Histochem. Cytochem. 27, 1279–1280 (1979).

[2] D. Grube, Immunoreactivities of Gastrin (G) Cells. II. Nonspecific Binding of Immunoglobulins to G-Cells by Ionic Interactions, Histochemistry 66, 149–167 (1980).

[3] K.I. Goldenthal, K. Hedman, J.W. Chen, J.T. August, M.W. Willingham, Postfixation Detergent Treatment for Immunofluorescence Suppresses Localization of Some Integral Membrane Proteins, J. Histochem. Cytochem. 33, 813–820 (1985).

[4] A.S. Craig, Sodium Borohydride as an Aldehyde Blocking Reagent for Electron Microscope Histochemistry, Histochemistry 42, 141–144 (1974).

[5] C. Tougard, R. Picart, Use of Pre-Embedding Ultrastructural Immunocytochemistry in the Localization of a Secretory Product and Membrane Proteins in Cultured Prolactin Cells, Am. J. Anat. 175, 161–177 (1986).

[6] L.-I. Larsson, Immunocytochemistry: Theory and Practice, C.R.C. Press, Boca Raton 1988, pp. 51.

[7] W. Straus, Phenylhydrazine as Inhibitor of Horseradish Peroxidase for Use in Immunoperoxidase Procedures, J. Histochem. Cytochem. 20, 949–951 (1972).

[8] S. Andrew, B. Jasani, An Improved Method for the Inhibition of Endogenous Peroxidase Non-Deleterious to Lymphocyte Surface Markers. Application to Immunoperoxidase Studies on Eosinophil-Rich Tissue Preparations, Histochem. J. 19, 426–430 (1987).

[9] B.A. Ponder, M.W. Wilkinson, Inhibition of Endogenous Tissue Alkaline Phosphatase with the Use of Alkaline Phosphatase Conjugates in Immunohistochemistry, J. Histochem. Cytochem. 29, 981–984 (1981).

[10] G.S. Wood, R. Warnke, Suppression of Endogenous Avidin-Binding Activity in Tissues and Its Relevance to Biotin-Avidin Detection Systems, J. Histochem. Cytochem. 29, 1196–1204 (1981).

[11] *G. Bussolati, P. Giugliotta,* Non-Specific Staining of Mast Cells by Avidin-Biotin-Peroxidase Complexes (ABC), J. Histochem. Cytochem. *31*, 1419–1421 (1983).

[12] *L. Scopsi, B.-L. Wang, L.-I. Larsson,* Unspecific Immunocytochemical Reactions with Certain Neurohormonal Peptides and Basic Peptide Sequences, J. Histochem. Cytochem. *34*, 1469–1475 (1986).

[13] *J. Gu, K. Islam, J.M. Polak,* Repeated Application of Primary Antibody Improves Immunofluorescence Staining, Histochem. J. *15*, 475–482 (1983).

[14] *S. Bradbury,* Photomicrography, in: *J.M. Polak, S. Van Noorden* (eds.), Immunocytochemistry, Modern Methods and Applications, 2nd Edn., John Wright and Sons, Bristol pp. 225–242 (1986).

[15] *D. J. Thomson, S. Bradbury,* Introduction to Photomicrography. Royal Microscopical Society Handbook, Oxford University Press, Oxford 1987, pp. 1–74.

5.7　Immunogold Methods for Electron Microscopy

F. B. Peter Wooding and Marion D. Kendall

5.7.1　Special Considerations and Choice of Method

In common with all other immunocytochemical methods, the accurate localization of an antigen by electron microscopy (EM) depends critically upon its accessibility to specific antibody. In EM sections, only epitopes on molecules at the cut surface are available for reaction with the identifying antibody, so that the thickness of the section is not as critical as the ability to recognize subcellular compartments over which the label is localized. Several good general reviews are available [1–6].

The labelling protocols have many steps, each with alternatives, so that ideally quantitative comparisons are necessary to choose between the alternatives but unfortunately these are rarely available [cf. 2, 7, 8]. All known published studies are cited here, but many of the opinions that follow are based only on the experience of the authors in a specific area and must be treated with suitable caution.

All treatment processes, freezing, fixation and embedding, potentially can modify molecular structure. Antibodies normally recognize native (unaltered) epitopes: therefore, it is crucial to minimize such changes, but this requirement is in direct conflict with the need to preserve and visualize the fine structure. This is the main reason for the variety of detail in the various published methods. The aim here is to present a simple procedure which is capable of modification to suit specific needs.

In brief, the requirement for post-embedding localization is to fix the relevant tissue, which is subsequently frozen or embedded in resin. Sections are then cut, an antibody labelling regime is chosen, controls are run and the gold particle label localized and quantitated (Fig. 1).

It is the general experience that pAbs are more successful for EM studies than mAbs, but there is no way of predicting this except to compare the relevant antibodies in an immunocytochemical context. Light microscope immunocytochemistry with the use of silver-enhanced gold label (cf. section 5.3) is usually the best indicator of possible EM success, but results from RIA and Western blots can also be used as partial indicators. Initially, it is best to use the antibody giving the highest titre but other available antibodies should not be ignored.

Since a 3mm EM grid with cryo or resin sections sits comfortably on 5 µl drop of liquid on Parafilm or Nescofilm, high concentrations of scarce antibody can be used initially, e.g. 1/10 and 1/100. The first requirement is to establish conditions for a reproducible label. For screening use light microscopy with gold to purple sections from the same block that will be used for the EM localization. Such sections can be picked up on pieces of cover slip (5–10 mm^2) and handled exactly as EM grids are, using similarly small quantities of equivalent reagents but finishing with silver enhancement of the primary gold label [9].

If the 1/10 or 1/100 dilution produces an apparently nonspecific deposit of label over the entire section, the dilution should be increased until an acceptable background level is achieved. The high concentration of primary (or secondary) antibody can mask a specific localization so it should be diluted until only a background level of label is seen before assuming a negative result.

A positive methodological control is always advisable as described for light microscopic methods (cf. 5.4 and 5.5). The several steps, transfers between drops and washing variability make reproducibility difficult to achieve. To counter this always include one section of material for which the optimal labelling protocol has been established previously. The expected result from the control section validates the run. Inexperienced workers are advised to obtain a block and some antibody from an established practitioner, or to prepare their own; rodent pituitary tissue and commercial anti-growth hormone or prolactin antibodies make a reliable system.

Once a reproducible localization has been established, absorption controls using purified antigen are the best test of specificity. If the antigen is not available, the use of an unrelated antibody, preferably of the same isotype, and omission of each of the reagents in turn provides the necessary checks.

5.7.2   Antibody Labelling Regimes

To reduce nonspecific, i.e. background, deposition, all antibodies should be as pure as possible. However, relatively impure reagents may be effective because the system can act as its own affinity matrix (Fig. 1).

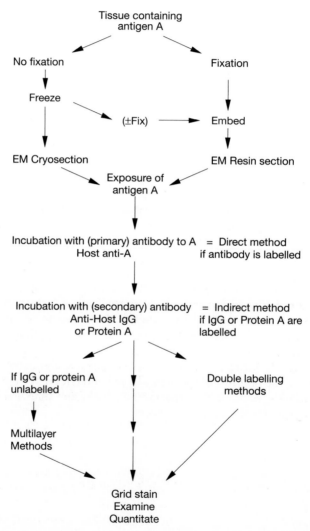

Fig. 1. Approaches to postembedding tissue labelling with antibodies for EM immunocyto-chemistry.

5.7.2.1   Direct Labelling of the Primary Antibody with Colloidal Gold

The main drawback is loss of reactivity of the antibody because of absorption onto the gold colloid of the relevant epitope, also each antibody must be labelled separately which is expensive and the absorption efficiency differs with each protein.

5.7.2.2   Indirect Labelling

The primary antibody is detected with a secondary antibody or protein A molecule, both of which react with the Fc portion of the primary antibody.

Antibodies (IgG and IgM)

The second antibody preparation is raised by injecting purified IgG from the species in which the primary antibody was raised (e.g. mouse) into a second species (e.g. rabbit) and purifying and labelling the resultant anti-mouse IgG antibodies. Then the mouse mAb is localized with the labelled rabbit anti-mouse IgG. This can be prepared by the individual researcher or is commercially available in various gold colloid sizes. Broad spectrum commercial anti-mouse IgG + IgM reagents are recommended but preparations specific for the various immunoglobulin isotypes are available.

Proteins A and G

Proteins A and G bind avidly and specifically to the Fc portion of vertebrate IgG molecules [10]. They can be absorbed to gold colloid and retain their reactivity with Fc [11]. Again, several sizes are commercially available. Although they do react with IgGs from all species, the avidity of the reaction varies considerably: for example, polyclonal rabbit IgG is several times as reactive as polyclonal mouse IgG with protein A. Reactivity with mAbs is usually very poor [3].

The advantages of the indirect method are the possibility of tailoring the secondary antibody to suit the primary antibody; use of the secondary antibody to detect several different antibodies from the same species, and most important, the potential increase in sensitivity, since more than one labelled secondary antibody molecule can react with the primary antibody so that higher dilutions are possible. This indirect method is the one that is generally found to be most useful. In some cases labelled IgG gives on average twice as much label as protein A or G but in others [6] the labels from the two indirect systems are equivalent and IgG produces small clusters, rather than the individual gold particles resulting with the use of protein A. In one study, protein G has been shown to be quantitatively better than protein A with cryosections [10] but the species of origin of the antibody is equally important [3].

5.7.2.3   Multilayer Techniques

As noted above, the indirect method (two layers) is potentially more sensitive than one layer and this applies to the use of even more layers. The problems are that background labelling and nonspecific deposits from each layer also increase and the reproducibility is low [12]. Both antibody and protein A [13] multilayers can be used. It is recommended to use a multiple layer for mouse mAbs (mAb – rabbit anti-mouse IgG – goat-anti-rabbit gold colloid) since the commercial goat anti-rabbit gold produces a significantly higher label than a monoclonal-goat anti-mouse gold sequence. However, unless the labelling with the indirect method is very weak, the drawbacks of background dirt and non-reproducibility may not justify the use of multilayer methods.

5.7.2.4   Co-Localization of Antigens on the Same Section

Using different sized gold colloid probes it is possible to localize two antigens on the same section. This can be very useful for checking granule contents, for example, or the relationship between the enzymes in a biochemical synthetic sequence. The major problem is to devise a labelling programme which avoids cross-reactions and interference during application of the second label. See [14] for references and a useful comparison of methods.

Simultaneous labelling

If the antibodies are sufficiently different, e.g., a mouse mAb and rabbit pAb, the primary antibodies can be mixed, as can the different secondary detectors, each with a different size of gold colloid. The level of labelling is never as high as can be attained with either antibody alone but good results can obtained. If the antibodies do cross-react or are too similar, e.g., two rabbit pAbs or two mouse mAbs, the following strategies are available.

Sequential label on opposite sides of sections mounted on marked grids

The same labelling regime is used on each side in turn. Care must be taken not to sink the grids into the drops of the reagents during either sequence. The sections need to be without any holes or tears to avoid seepage of reagents and spurious cross-reactions when the second side is labelled. Labelling at the edges of each section is usually unreliable because of seepage. There is a complex method for covering the first side with a Formvar film after the first run to eliminate this problem [15]; carbon coating of the side labelled initially has also been recommended [16].

Sequential label on the same side of a section

This necessitates masking the first label so that it cannot subsequently react with any of the second-run reagents.

1. Formaldehyde vapour masking. After the first labelling run, expose the section to formaldehyde vapour at 60 °C for 2 h [14]. This blocks potential sites of cross-reaction between the secondary antibodies.

2. Use unlabelled secondary antibody or protein A at high concentration to react with those Fc portions of the primary antibody which failed to attract a labelled IgG or protein A in the initial labelling step. The second labelling run then follows.

The second of these methods is probably the least effective. In all methods a high percentage of grids with nonspecific dirt and cross-reactions are usually produced and reproducibility is low. Good, clear results are possible, as shown in Fig. 2a, b, c demonstrating localization of growth hormone and prolactin in separate sectors of the same anterior pituitary cell granule [17]. However, these processes are time-consuming and often very similar information can be achieved by means of serial or adjacent sections stained with different antibodies.

5.7.3   Fixation

Fixation stabilizes tissue components with minimal cyto-architectural disruption and prevents diffusion and loss of peptides, lipids, nucleic acids and carbohydrates by cross-linking these macromolecules in a three dimensional network (cf. 5.2.1) [18, 19]. A good fixative for immunocytochemistry provides adequate tissue fixation without undue loss of antigenicity, diffuses rapidly into the tissue and causes little shrinkage. Cross-linking of macromolecules may potentially alter or mask the target epitopes so that optimal preservation of ultrastructure, i.e., maximal cross-linking, is usually inimical to retention of adequate antigenicity. All these modifiers indicate that nothing in this area is universally applicable and optimal fixation conditions for each antigen should be considered theoretically and separately, but there are some guide lines which may be applied generally.

Experiments involving the treatment of pure antigens with various fixatives and estimation of the residual antigenicity [20] seldom predict the behaviour of the antigens *in vivo* where the fixation conditions are so much more complex. It would be useful to have more quantitative studies comparing the effect of different fixation regimes in the same tissue with the same antigen. Most published comparative studies agree in outline but the detail is usually contradictory.

Fixation of tissue for EM is better with aldehydes which are cross-linking fixatives, rather than with precipitating fixatives such as alcohol, acetone or picric acid [3]. The latter group produce too coarse a fine-structure for unequivocal identification of subcellular organelles and can cause unacceptable distortion, notably shrinkage, of the tissue, but for another opinion cf. [21].

Mixtures of fixatives can combine the benefits of both; formaldehyde with glutaraldehyde is commonly used, and mixing a cross-linker with a precipitant produces a wide range of fixatives based on formaldehyde and picric acid in various concentrations [4, 26, 29] (cf. Table 1). Uranyl acetate after aldehyde fixation is generally considered to improve the retention of antigenicity and membrane preservation [22] and periodate with lysine [23], sodium borohydride after glutaraldehyde [24] or microwave treatment [25] have all been suggested to be useful additions to aldehyde processing but with no quantitation of the improvement claimed.

Formaldehyde is the most widely used but, having only one reactive group, its cross-linking action is said to be reversible: storage in dilute (0.01 %) formaldehyde is recommended [26] to preserve structure and antigenicity but there is no published quantitated justification for this. Storage of samples in cacodylate buffer for up to one month may preserve antigens effectively. It may be advisable to embed, which stabilizes the antigen permanently, within two or three days of fixation with formaldehyde if the antigen is initially soluble or sensitive.

For any tissue, perfusion fixation is better than immersion of fragments. This is because of the homogeneity produced by rapid delivery of fixative to each cell virtually simultaneously, and the firmness attained before the tissue is cut into the small pieces essential for further processing.

There are no comparative studies on the optimal temperature for fixation for immunocytochemistry; cold fixative would favour retention of antigenicity but 37 °C would be better theoretically for fine-structure preservation. Room temperature may provide a convenient compromise. If perfusion is not possible it is essential to divide the tissue into slices less than 0.5 mm thick with a sharp razor blade and transfer material to the fixative as quickly as possible. Once the blood supply is interrupted, redistribution of soluble and other antigens as a result of division of the tissue and hypoxic change is extremely rapid. Choice of fixative for immunocytochemistry thus depends on a variety of considerations. Table 1 is a summary of published [1, 2, 4, 7, 17, 18, 21, 26] and unpublished approaches to fixation.

Times given for fixation vary widely: use a basic 30 min (perfusion) or 60 min (immersion), with 10 min as a minimum to produce coherence for subsequent processing. Choice of buffer does not seem critical: use cacodylate to allow subsequent histochemical processing (with phosphate trapping) but phosphate, Tris, PIPES, and barbiturate-acetate buffers, all at around pH 7.2, can be used.

Use hypertonic fixatives [27]: 3 % (w/v) formaldehyde in cacodylate buffer 0.1 mol/l plus 5 % (w/v) sucrose (with 1 % (v/v) glutaraldehyde if the antigen is more resistant). Many workers use iso-osmotic fixatives successfully.

If formaldehyde is used, this must be freshly de-polymerized from paraformaldehyde. To start an investigation, use 3 % formaldehyde in phosphate buffer for 30 min and modify the regime from the results: addition of glutaraldehyde will improve membrane-preservation and visualization; osmium post-fixation is even better for this but both usually reduce antigenicity, osmium drastically. After aldehyde fixation it is usual to rinse in ammonium chloride or glycine. This is said to block free carbohydrate groups

Table 1. Comparative features of fixation procedures for EM immunocytochemistry

Fixative	%	Immerse fix speed of penetration	Speed of cross-linking	Dis-tortion/ shrinkage	Preserva-tion of antigenicity	Visualization of ultrastruc-tural detail	Storage after fix
Single							
Formaldehyde freshly made from paraformaldehyde	1–4	++	+	–	++++	+	+
Glutaraldehyde	1–2	+	++++	–	+	+++	+++
	0.2	+	+++	–	++	++	+
Acetone	100	+++	–	++	++	++coarse	
Osmium Tetroxide	1	+	–	++	+	++++	
Mixtures							
Formaldehyde+ Glutaraldehyde	1–3 0.1–1	+	++	–	++	+++	+++
Formaldehyde+ Picric Acid	2–3 0.1–0.2	++	+	–	+	+	
Freeze substitution							
Osmium tetroxide	0.4–4	++	–	–	+	++	
Glutaraldehyde	0.3–1	++	++	–	++	+	

remaining in the tissue from the fixative and thereby to reduce background [1]. There are no quantitative studies to substantiate this claim.

5.7.4 Processing of Tissues

Thin sectioning is essential for EM. The tissue has to be either frozen or embedded in resin before thin sections can be cut. The various procedures are outlined in Fig. 1. Theoretically, maximum antigenicity is retained by ultra-rapid cooling of untreated tissue so that the tissue water is replaced by vitrified, crystal-free ice.

Vitrification preserves intact the three-dimensional matrix that water provides for the cell and, in particular, the shell of water molecules around surface epitopes on molecules. The disruption normally produced by crystal formation on freezing is eliminated. Vitrification is technically very difficult to achieve and sections of such material are usually impractically fragile. However, the vitrified water can be replaced while frozen by organic solvents (freeze substitution) and the material then embedded in resin. Routine cryosectioning uses 'gentle' fixatives and anti-freezes to prepare the tissue, losing some antigenicity but achieving notable sections, and completely avoids the use of the harsh organic solvents necessary for conventional resin embedding.

5.7.4.1   Freezing

The most rapid method of freezing is achieved by slamming the tissue against a polished copper block cooled in liquid helium in a special apparatus. Fresh tissue can be vitrified by this method but the expense is only justified if the events under investigation occur very rapidly or the antibody is exceptionally sensitive. Normally fixed and cryopro-tected (usually with sucrose) tissue can be frozen by immersion in liquid nitrogen, propane or Freon. Ice-crystal damage is always present but areas relatively free from it can normally be found.

Freeze Substitution

Even with slam freezing, vitrification is restricted to a depth of about 15–20 mm from the copper surface. The vitrified water layer can then be replaced at low temperature (usually about −80 °C) by an organic solvent (usually acetone) over 1 to 2 days and this 'freeze substitution' is said to preserve antigenicity and ultrastructure better than other fixation methods [7, 28, 29]. The tissue is then gradually warmed either to −35 °C to −45 °C for low temperature acrylic resin embedding, or to room temperature for conventional embedding.

Tissue can be processed in this way with no chemical fixative [30]; the final image on an acrylic resin section lacks contrast but is essentially similar to material treated conventionally. Most workers use a chemical fixative, e.g., 1–4 % osmium or 0.3 % glutaraldehyde in the substituting acetone to increase membrane contrast. In an excellent comparative quantitative study of various freeze substitution regimes, conventional chemical fixation and both acrylic and epoxy embedding were compared [7]. Glutaraldehyde in acetone freeze substitution followed by Araldite embedding gave the highest label, but the antigen was unusually resistant to epoxy embedding. It is a general experience, however, that conventional glutaraldehyde and K4M acrylic resin processing gives 2–4 times more label than glutaraldehyde-osmium-Araldite.

5.7.4.2   Cryosectioning

Some fixation and use of sucrose as anti-freeze is necessary prior to freezing, otherwise the sections are too fragile to survive the labelling manipulations. Frozen sections are picked up on a drop of sucrose, allowed to thaw and are then transferred to filmed grids [26]. Subsequent labelling procedures are common to all sections on grids, whether in resin or 'frozen'. After labelling, the 'frozen' sections have to be stabilized before they can be examined by EM. A combination stain and embedding medium, uranyl acetate and methyl cellulose, is normally used [26], but dilute acrylic or expoxy resins [31] or polyvinylalcohol have also been employed [32]. Osmium tetroxide is often used to improve membrane definition prior to the uranyl acetate embedding step. It must be remembered that the evidence for any significant penetration into the cryosection by gold label (however small) is very limited [cf. 5.33].

5.7.4.3   Resin Embedding

Both acrylic and epoxy resins can be used.

Acrylic resins

Acrylics preserve antigenicity better because they can be processed and cured at $-20\,°C$ and below and, probably more important, most are hydrophilic. Thus the environment on the section surface is more suited to epitope display than on the hydrophobic epoxy resins. It must be remembered that antibodies and gold labelled reagents are always on the surface of the section, only penetrating down holes or splits, even on frozen sections. The major drawback of tissue in acrylics is the difficulty of visualizing the fine structure, particularly membranes, and this is also true of frozen sections. However, use of aqueous or alcoholic uranyl acetate and dilute lead for general stains, with aqueous phosphotungstic acid for glycoproteins and possibly osmium [34], singly or in combination, can normally produce a satisfactory result. The acrylics are mixtures of methyl, butyl and glycol methacrylates with small percentages of special additives, normally cross-linkers such as DMP or benzoyl peroxide. They can be tailored to cure with ultraviolet light (K4M, K11M, LR White or Gold) or spontaneously (GMA). The Lowicryl range can be cured at $-20\,°C$ (K4M) or $-70\,°C$ (K11M) as long as careful precautions are taken [35] and this supposedly preserves even more antigenicity than curing at room temperature [36], although there are few quantitative studies clearly demonstrating this [cf. 37, 38]. LR White or LR Gold resins can be cured at room temperature or LR Gold at $-20\,°C$ and have been shown to be as good as K4M where direct quantitative comparisons have been made [39–41]. Processing or curing at low temperature may only be advantageous with some antigens, so it is recommended to experiment at room temperature first. The strength and/or duration of the fixation process may be more important.

Epoxy resins

Epoxy resins potentially provide consistently better ultrastructural preservation and visualization, but this can only be fully exploited after fixation in glutaraldehyde followed by osmium which unfortunately destroys many antigens. If the antigen does survive, the label can be localized very precisely. This is usually limited to antigens in high concentration, e.g., in pituitary granules or crystalline arrays. Antigen availability on osmicated epoxy sections can be improved by chemical treatment of the section surface, often called etching, although there is little evidence for any significant loss of epoxy resin [cf. 42]. The oxidizing agents sodium metaperiodate or hydrogen peroxide are most widely used and are believed to act by removing osmium from the surface of the section [43]. This pre-treatment undoubtedly can increase the label two or three fold but the improvement varies with antigen and the individual block. Periodate and peroxide can be used successfully but have no effect on non-osmicated sections of either epoxy or acrylic resin, supporting their direct effect on osmium. Alcoholic sodium ethoxide (NaOH pellets in absolute ethanol) is a much stronger oxidizing agent than periodate or peroxide and can completely dissolve the resin from 1–5 μm epoxy sections. Dilute solutions have been used to treat EM sections before labelling and are said to increase it significantly [44–46]; it is very difficult to prevent sodium ethoxide damaging sections extensively.

There are many commercial epoxy resins available. Most of the quantitative evidence [39] indicates that all provide a similar retention of antigenicity [47] so that ease and familiarity of use are probably more important than considerations of low viscosity, or unquantitated claims of better preservation of antigens. In general, frozen sections preserve antigens best giving, for comparison, 20 gold particles per square micron; followed by acrylics 10; non-osmicated epoxies 4; and osmicated epoxies 1 or 0 [4, 8, 37, 48, 49].

5.7.5   Colloidal Gold

Comprehensive ranges of secondary antibodies and proteins A or G absorbed to gold colloids are available commercially. Preparation of a gold colloid and absorption of a protein are simple chemical procedures but purification and exact size selection are more complex. There are several good reviews giving full details of preparation methods if an unusual colloid is required [10, 50–52]; cf. [53] for 0.8 nm gold. Commercial products have sizes from 1 to 40 nm diameter; for scale drawings of the complexes, see Figs. 2d–g.

5.7.5.1   Size Considerations

Assuming a uniform antigen distribution on a section, the number of gold particles that can be localized per unit area is related to their size [54–57] as shown in Figs. 2 and 3. The smallest particles give the highest number, but considerations of ease of visualization and photography after section staining are also important and 10 nm gold particles (subsequently refered to as G10) are a good general compromise [54–56].

For co-localisation, G5 and G15 give an unequivocal result, G5 and G10, or G10 and G15, can look very similar on a photomicrograph.

Gold colloids are remarkably stable and long-lived. However, there is recent evidence that antibody may not be irreversibly adsorbed to the gold colloid but is in equilibrium with free antibody [56]. It is therefore advisable to keep a standard tissue block which has been shown to produce a good level of label on sections. Dubious old or new colloid can then be checked against this known standard. Acrylic or epoxy blocks show no diminution in section label after up to 7 years storage.

Another way of balancing the sensitivity, i.e., size of the colloid, against visibility is to use the smallest (1 nm) gold colloid. Each particle is then used as a focus for deposition of silver ions in a cascade process. This is the method used very successfully for light

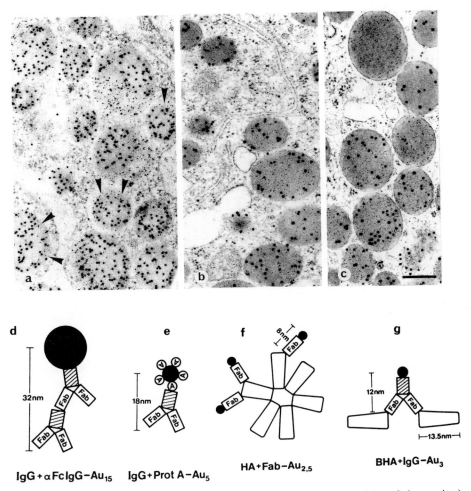

Fig. 2. a–c) Post-embedding immunogold co-localization (on opposites sides of the section) of prolactin (17 nm gold particles) and growth hormone (5 nm gold particles) on glutaraldehyde/osmium/epoxy sections of cow anterior pituitary. Individual granules may contain a uniform distribution of one (c) or both (b) hormones. Growth hormone is frequently restricted to a rim (arrowheads in a) or to one sector of a granule. From [16] with permission. Bar = 0.3 μm.
d–g) Scale drawings showing the relative sizes of gold colloid and adsorbed proteins. IgG: immunoglobulin, Fab: fragment of immunoglobulin, protein A, and HA bovine haemagglutinin or BHA; subunit. From [90] with permission.

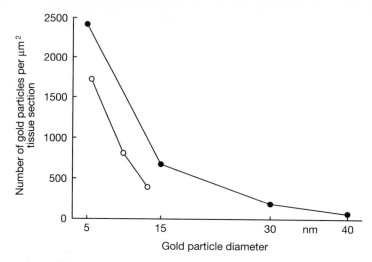

Fig. 3. Comparison of the antigen detecting sensitivities of different sizes of labelled gold particle. The data are from different papers [50, 51 with permission] so no direct numerical comparisons between protein A (○) and IgG (●) are valid. The common feature is the very similar rapid decrease in sensitivity with increasing size of particle.

microscope sections. Good EM labelling in this manner may be very sporadic because of the rapid nonspecific deposition of silver, but the technique has been used successfully [30, 59].

5.7.5.2   Variants of Gold Colloid Labels

Other gold labelled reagents available include cationic gold colloid, which can be used to assess the negative charge density on unfixed or fixed surfaces [60], and gold colloids coated with lectins [61] which will localize specific carbohydrates or carbohydrate sequences, just as directly labelled antibodies localize their epitopes. Another ingenious use of gold colloid is to coat it with a pure enzyme; the marker can then potentially recognise the substrate of the enzyme on a section provided that the active site is not masked by absorption to the colloid. For example, phospholipase from cobra venom has been used to localize phospholipids on osmicated epon sections [62, 63], hyaluronidase (EC 3.2.1.35) to localize hyaluronic acid [64], and DNAase (EC 3.1.21.1) and RNAse (EC 3.1.27.5) to localize nucleic acids [65].

Gold colloid has also been used successfully to localize intra-membrane antigens (in either intracellular or surface membranes) exposed by freeze-fracture methods [66, 67] a variation on the pre-embedding label-epoxy sectioning procedure. A further method allows localization of antigen on the cytoplasmic surface of the plasmalemma by peeling this membrane from a living cell [68].

In addition, gold colloids can mark sites of nucleic acid hybridization after a biotin-labelled nucleic acid probe has been used on sections. The probe can then be localized using a gold-labelled molecule binding specifically to biotin, either an antibody or streptavidin [69]. The smallest gold colloid particles (0.8–1.2 nm) have been used to localize active sites or receptors directly on individual large enzymes or other proteins visualized by negative staining [70].

5.7.6   Quantitation

Several studies have demonstrated in model systems that the number of gold particles per square micron of section is directly proportional to the concentration of a soluble antigen as demonstrated, for example, when an antigen is mixed with gelatin to provide a tissue equivalent which is fixed and processed in the normal way [5, 20, 71].

Membrane antigens can be quantitated on tissue sections but the calculations and controls are more complex [72]. The technique of post-embedding gold labelling is therefore suitable for quantitative comparative studies of antigen distribution over organelles on a frozen [49] or resin-embedded section. However, this is a lengthy process and variability is unavoidable. For determination of absolute concentrations, include a standard slice of a known concentration of antigen in gelatin alongside the specimen. The label on the test tissue can then be directly related to the label over the standard processed on the same section [73].

Fixation and embedding for subsequent quantitation need to be kept as uniform as possible; the particle distribution can then be counted per square micron of the relevant organelle or area and these numbers used for statistical evaluation.

There are two main approaches to quantitation: strict stereological methods or counting over standard areas in the electron microscope. The former involves precise rules for taking micrographs in random array and analysing these with superimposed grids by counting intercepts over the chosen organelles [49, 72]. This produces both relative percentage areas of all the organelles included and also the number of superimposed gold particles. It is comprehensive, but expensive in cost of micrographs and very time-consuming. For most labelling studies this is unnecessarily detailed, if there is a need only to establish that the particular area or organelle of interest has a significantly higher label than another structure or background. For this purpose a system of rapid but accurate counting on the EM, without taking micrographs can be used. The system can be validated by two independent observers counting the same area of a grid. A circle of wire attached to a pointer (which is present within many EM columns) can be swung over the image screen when required. This circle defines a small area of the screen at a magnification selected to allow easy counting of the gold particles within the circle. It is positioned over a relevant area, e.g. a granule, at a magnification at which the label cannot be seen. This is to eliminate unconscious selection of well-labelled areas. The magnification is then increased to the level selected for counting. The area of the circle and magnification give the absolute area counted for subsequent conversion to uniform square microns and statistical manipulation. For linear measurement, the diameter of the circle can be used as a standard length to estimate the number of particles per micron, e.g., along a plasmalemma. The system also allows for a rapid check over say ten 'relevant' and ten 'background' areas to obtain an estimate of the density of label.

5.7.7   Alternatives to Post-embedding Labelling

5.7.7.1   Pre-embedding Labelling

Intracellular and tissue antigens

The main problem is to allow penetration of the primary antibody and labelled secondary antibody or protein A to the site of the antigen while retaining sufficient recognizable fine structure.

Freezing and/or detergents are used to permeabilize the cells, either added to the fixative or employed after the fixative step. If the detergent and primary antibody incubation are carried out before fixation, there is usually too much damage to the fine structure. The initial fixation can be gentle (1–2 % formaldehyde) and short with a stronger fixation (3 % glutaraldehyde) after the incubation with the primary antibody since this antibody is resistant to glutaraldehyde modification. The method can be used with isolated cells, monolayers (usually to localize microfilaments or microtubules) [74, 75] and thin (5–10 μm sections, usually frozen) slices of tissue [76]. These preparations are taken through the usual indirect labelling sequence after fixation and permeabilization. Some authors add detergent to all the solutions of the labelling sequence. Rather than the whole IgG molecule, the secondary labelled antibody can be a labelled Fab fragment of IgG which, being smaller, should penetrate better [73, 74].

Surface labelling

There is no problem with penetration here since the target antigen is on the surface of the membrane or particle. The technique is suitable for isolated cells, monolayers and isolated subcellular membrane fractions or particles. No initial fixation is usually necessary because the primary antibody can be added to the solution in which the cells or fractions are suspended without deleterious effect, but mild pre-fixation may be required to prevent 'capping' and internalization of label in some cells. After the antigen has reacted with the primary antibody, strong (3 % glutaraldehyde) fixation is possible, especially as the primary antibody IgG is resistant to glutaraldehyde whereas the target antigen may not have been. The labelling sequence and reagents are the same as for sections but the reactions are carried out in cell or organelle suspensions. Thorough washing between steps is necessary and the usual controls should be included. Post-fixation in osmium tetroxide and epoxy embedding is best for good ultrastructural preservation. This technique is very useful since it allows investigation of very sensitive antigens, but only those at membrane surfaces exposed to the suspending solution.

5.7.7.2 Scanning EM Labelling

Colloidal gold can be used as a surface marker for Scanning EM (SEM), usually on isolated cells or surface epithelia labelled before processing. The problem is that, for the gold marker particle to be large enough to be unequivocally recognizable against background irregularity and cell surface projections, it needs to be at least 30 nm in diameter. The drawback of this considerable decrease in sensitivity of detection can be circumvented if a small (1–5 nm) gold marker is subsequently enlarged chemically by silver intensification Fig. 4 [77]. However, the gold particles, after the essential carbon coating, look just the same as any other surface irregularity and the unique shape and electron density which makes the gold so uniquely recognizable on transmission EM (TEM) is lost. The problem can be overcome for particles of 15 nm and over by using a back-scattered electron image (BEI) [77–79]. This visualizes only the gold particles as it gives atomic number contrast and the image can be superimposed on the conventional SEM image (Fig. 4). However, not all scanning microscopes are suitably equipped, and BEI cannot be used with osmicated tissue. SEM processing is the same as that described under pre-embedding-surface labelling but, after fixation, the tissue is critical-point dried and carbon-coated before SEM examination. TEM after pre-embedding-surface labelling is more sensitive and can provide similar and more conclusive evidence of surface distribution of label by careful, though time-consuming, use of serial or adjacent sections. Full details of SEM preparation can be found in references [50, 78, 79].

5.7.8 Basic Indirect Method for K4M Acrylic Resin

Method

1. Fix in 3 % paraformaldehyde in cacodylate buffer (0.1 mol/l, pH 7.2) with 5 % sucrose (w/v) for 30 min.
2. Rinse in buffer and leave in 10 % (w/v) ammonium chloride in cacodylate buffer for 30 min.
3. Store in cacodylate buffer at 4 °C.
4. Transfer to 50 % ethyl alcohol at room temperature.

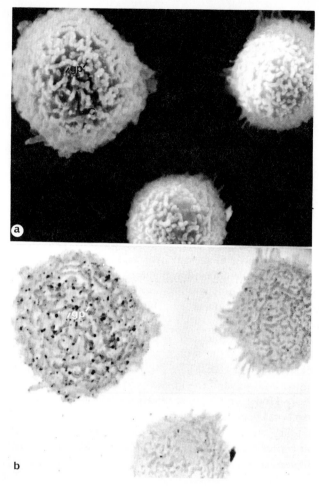

Fig. 4. Scanning electron micrographs of 3 murine leucocytes, only one of which is labelled. a) Using conventional secondary emission imaging considerable surface detail is apparent but the label is not visible, whereas the back-scattered electron image (in reverse polarity) of the same field in b) clearly demonstrates the label (gp) but the structural detail is lacking. The primary antibody was donkey anti-rabbit IgG on 10 nm gold colloid, subsequently enhanced for 3 min with silver (a and b × 45 000).

5. Dehydrate in an alcohol series to 100 % including 75 % alcohol with 1 % (w/v) Eosin to make specimen easy to see during subsequent processing.
6. Infiltrate with 50 % alcohol: 50 % K4M acrylic resin at room temperature for 30 min.
7. Infiltrate with 33 % alcohol: 66 % K4M acrylic resin at room temperature for 30 min.
8. Infiltrate with 100 % K4M overnight.

9. Transfer to *Beem* capsule filled with K4M. Orient the tissue suitably; use a flat-bottomed *Beem* capsule if necessary.
10. Cure for 8 h with a UV light placed under, and 10 cm from, a transparent plastic rack holding the *Beem* capsules with the tissue at the end pointing towards the UV light. Cover this with a box lined with aluminium foil to reflect maximum UV light onto the samples for optimum curing.
11. Cut sections 80–150 nm thick, pick up on naked 300 mesh nickel grids (copper reacts with the reagents).
12. Float the grid, section side down, for 10 min on drops of 1 % (w/v) bovine serum albumin (BSA) in phosphate buffer, 0.1 mol/l, pH 7.2 with 0.05 % (w/v) of bacteriostatic Thimerosal (DBSBT). Dispense DBSBT in 10–20 µl drops onto a piece of Nescofilm (Parafilm) in the bottom of a glass *Petri* dish. The BSA blocks all sites on the section which might react nonspecifically with the primary antibody. The antibody will displace any BSA molecule over its target epitope.
13. Remove excess DBSBT by touching edge of grid to filter-paper, do not wash. Dry back of grid if necessary.
14. Float on drops of primary antibody diluted in DBSBT. The *Petri* dish is placed in a plastic box with a tightly fitting lid with wet filter-paper in the bottom. Leave for 120 min at room temp (20 °C) or overnight at 4 °C.
15. Wash grid in jet of PBS from a plastic wash-bottle. Direct the jet across, not through, the grid.
16. Blot off excess PBS at edge of grid, dry back of grid.
17. Float on drops of secondary gold-labelled antibody diluted in DBSBT for 30 min.
18. Wash as 15.
19. Wash with jet of glass-distilled water (GDW) for 10 s.
20. Float on GDW drop for 10 min.
21. Dry, check labelling on two grid squares on the EM before staining grid.
22. Stain with saturated uranyl acetate in 50 % ethylalcohol for 4–15 min depending on level of label seen in 21.
23. Wash with jet of 50 % ethylalcohol for 5 s.
24. Wash with jet of GDW for 5 s.
25. Dry and examine in EM. If ultrastructure is still not adequately visualized, try 1/10 diluted lead citrate for 5–30 s. This should stain nuclei and mitochondria but it coarsens the image and it may be difficult to get the optimal level of lead staining. However it is possible to remove most of a lead over-stain with a second uranyl acetate incubation for 10 min without affecting the gold labelling which is comparatively tenacious. There is a problem here with the increase in staining 'dirt' (even more tenacious) with every round of staining. Proper visualization of both label and ultrastructure is vital and it is worth spending some time optimizing this. Aqueous uranyl acetate (2 %, w/v) can be used if the alcoholic uranyl solution gives too uniform a stain, and 1 % (w/v) phosphotungstic acid in 3 % HCl (PTA) gives a good stain for nuclei, collagen fibres, glycoprotein granules and lysosomes in a very different pattern to uranyl acetate, again without affecting the gold label.

5.7.9   Variations of Basic K4M Method

5.7.9.1   K4M Embedding at −20 °C

1. Steps 1–3 of basic protocol.
2. Step 4 of basic protocol but at 4 °C.
3. Steps 5–10 of basic protocol but at −20 °C.
4. Steps 11–25 of basic protocol as above.

5.7.9.2   Cryoprocessing

1. Steps 1–3 of basic protocol.
2. Infiltrate with Sucrose, 2.3 mol/l, in PBS overnight.
3. Freeze tissue on tip of cryo-ultratome holder in Freon 22 cooled in liquid nitrogen and store in liquid nitrogen as long as necessary.
4. Cut cryosections, remove them from the cryochamber on the bottom of a drop of sucrose, 2.3 mol/l, held in a wire loop. Sections thaw out at this stage.
5. Touch sections in loop onto filmed grid on bench. Invert loop, with sections now adherent to the grid, onto a large DBSBT drop on Nescofilm, withdraw loop.
6. Transfer sections on the grids to two more drops of DBSBT to dilute out the sucrose. Sections can then be left at this stage for 2–3 days at 4 °C in a wet-box without deleterious effect if initially fixed with glutaraldehyde. Formaldehyde-fixed sections are more fragile and it is advisable to process those on the day of cutting. Sections must not be allowed to dry before being processed for labelling.
7. Steps 12–19 from basic protocol. If the sections are particularly fragile, jet washing may be too vigorous. The gentler alternative is to transfer the grid onto three successive drops of PBS leaving it for 5 min on each drop.
8. Float grid on 1 % aqueous osmium tetroxide for 15 mins.
9. Wash with GDW.
10. Float grid on 4 % aqueous uranyl acetate for 20 min.
11. Do not blot, carry over small amount of uranyl acetate on grid.
12. Float grid on 0.3 % (w/v) methyl cellulose (viscosity 400 cps) for 15 min. Blot off excess and allow to dry. This step is critical since too much uranyl acetate will obscure detail on the section, too little will produce too fragile a specimen to survive the EM beam. An alternative is to use uncured dilute acrylic or epoxy mixtures instead of methyl cellulose to provide coherence for the section, cf. [31].

5.7.9.3   Osmium-Fixed Epoxy Embedded Material

EM Protocol

1. Conventional glutaraldehyde and osmium fixation and epoxy embedding.
2. Float sections on nickel grids on a drop of saturated sodium metaperiodate (~5 % w/v) or 10 % (v/v) hydrogen peroxide for 30 min.
3. Jet wash grids with GDW, place on drops of GDW for 10 min.
4. Steps 12–21 from basic protocol.
5. Steps 22–25 from basic protocol but grid staining will need to be longer for osmicated Epon material, e.g., 20 min in alcoholic uranyl acetate and 1–5 min in full strength lead citrate.

5.7.9.4   Light Microscopy Protocol

1. Steps 1–10 from basic protocol.
2. Cut 1–2 µm thick sections from an acrylic or epoxy block and pick up at least two on a small (3–6 mm^2) square of coverslip produced by chequer board scoring of glass coverslip with a diamond pen. Dry the pieces of glass with sections uppermost at room temperature for 10 min then in a 60 °C oven for at least 30 min. This ensures that the sections remain on the glass during processing.
3. Steps 12–16 from basic protocol.
   When washing, avoid contact between filter-paper and the section side of the glass. Blot with filter-paper at the edge of glass and only dry *non*-section side.
4. In step 17 from basic protocol use 1/40 diluted commercial 1 nm gold-labelled IgG.
5. Steps 18–20 from basic protocol.
6. Float glass pieces on drops of freshly mixed A and B solutions of silver intensification reagents (*Amersham Plc*) on multi-well slides, *not* parafilm.
7. Monitor development of silver deposition on the sections using the light microscope. Stop the reaction by washing with GDW, float glass on water drop for 10 min. Dry.
8. Sections can be stained lightly (try 20 °C or 60 °C) with 1 % (w/v) aqueous fast green or 0.1 % (w/v) toluidine blue in 10 % borate or haematoxylin in acid alcohol without effect on the silver label. Choice of stain depends on the tissue, the first two are general stains, haematoxylin can give excellent nuclear definition.

5.7.9.5   Absorption Control Protocols

Establish the optimal dilution (say 1:100) of primary antibody for reproducible labelling. Take two 50 µl aliquots of a 1:50 dilution of antibody, add 50 µl of DBSBT to one and 50 µl containing five times excess of the primary antigen required to neutralize the antibody to the other. Incubate for two hours at 37 °C, centrifuge at > 10 000 × g for 5 min and use supernatants for coincident comparable labelling runs, preferably on adjacent or serial sections. Label should be reduced by at least 75 % on the section treated with absorbed antibody. If the decrease is less than this, increase the amount of antigen used. If the concentration of antigen required to neutralize the antibody is unknown, gradually increase the amount of antigen added until the desired inhibition of labelling is achieved. Failure significantly to inhibit labelling indicates that the labelling is nonspecific.

References

[1] *J. Roth*, Postembedding Cytochemistry with Gold Labelled Reagents: A review, J. Micros. Lond. *143*, 125–137 (1986).

[2] *M. Bendayan, A. Nanci, F.W.K. Kan*, Effect of Tissue Processing on Colloidal Gold Cytochemistry, J. Histochem. Cytochem. *35*, 983–996 (1987).

[3] *M. Bendayan, S. Garzon*, Protein G-gold Complex: Comparative Evaluation with Protein A-Gold for High Resolution Immunocytochemistry, J. Histochem. Cytochem. *36*, 597–607 (1988).

[4] *M.L. Kann, J.P. Fouquet*, Comparison of LR White Resin, Lowicryl K4M and Epon Postembedding Procedures for Immunogold Staining of Actin in the Testis, Histochemistry *91*, 220–226 (1989).

[5] *J.W. Slot, G. Posthuma, L.Y. Chang, J.D. Crapo, H.J. Geuze*, Quantitative Aspects of Immunogold Labeling in Embedded and Nonembedded Sections, Am. J. Anat. *185*, 271–281 (1989).

[6] *J.W. Stirling*, Immuno and Affinity Probes for Electron Microscopy: A Review of Labeling and Preparation Technique, J. Histochem. Cytochem. *38*, 145–157 (1990).

[7] *M. Ichikawa, K. Sasaki, A. Ichikawa*, Optimal Preparative Procedures of Cryofixation for Immunocytochemistry, J. Electron Micros. Techn. *12*, 88–94 (1989).

[8] *S.R. Walker, M.C. Williams, B. Benson*, Immunocytochemical Localisation of the Major Surfactant Apoproteins in Type II Cells, Clara Cells and Alveolar Macrophages of Rat Lung, J. Histochem. Cytochem. *34*, 1137–1148 (1986).

[9] *G. Danscher, J.O.R. Norgaard*, LM Visualisation of Colloidal Gold on Resin Embedded tissue, J. Histochem. Cytochem. *31*, 1394–1398 (1983).

[10] *Y. Balslev, G.H. Hansen*, Preparation and Use of Recombinant Protein G-gold Complexes as Markers in Double Labelling Immunocytochemistry, Histochem. J. *21*, 449–454 (1989).

[11] *M. Bendayan*, Protein A-Gold Electron Microscope Immunocytochemistry: Methods, Applications and Limitations, J.Electron. Micros. Techn. *1*, 243–270 (1984).

[12] *E.J. Gosselin, G.D. Sorenson, J.C. Dennelt, C.C. Care*, Unlabeled Antibody Methods in Electronmicroscopy: A Comparison of Simple and Multi-step Procedures Using Colloidal Gold, J. Histochem. Cytochem. *32*, 799–804 (1984).

[13] *M. Bendayan, M.A. Duhr*, Modification of the Protein A-Gold Immunocytochemistry Technique for the Enhancement of its Efficiency, J. Histochem. Cytochem. *34*, 569–575 (1986).

[14] *R. Holm, J.M. Nesland, M. Altramand, A.Vincents Johanessen*, Double Staining Methods at the Ultrastructural Level Applying Colloidal Gold Conjugates, Ultrastruc. Pathol. *12*, 279–290 (1988).

[15] *I. Shore, J. Moss*, The Use of Formvar Films on Both Sides of a Section to Facilitate the Selected Surface Technique for Double Immunostaining at the EM level, Histochem. J. *20*, 183–184 (1988).

[16] *J.N. Skepper, J.M. Woodward, V. Navaratnam*, Immunocytochemical Localisation of Natriuretic Peptide Sequences in the Human Right Auricle, J. Mol. Cell. Cardiol *20*, 343–351 (1988).

[17] *G. Fumagalli, A. Zanini*, In Cow Anterior Pituitary Growth Hormone and Prolactin Can be Packed in Separate Granules of the Same Cell, J. Cell Biol. *100*, 2019–2024 (1985).

[18] *C.H. Fox, F.B. Johnson, J. Whiting, P.P. Roller*, Formaldehyde Fixation, J. Histochem. Cytochem. *33*, 845–853 (1985).

[19] *D. Hopwood*, Cell and Tissue Fixation 1972–1982, Histochem. J. *17*, 389–442 (1985).

[20] *G.D. Gagne, M.F. Miller*, An Artificial Test Substrate for Evaluating Electron Microscopic Immunocytochemical Labeling Reactions, J. Histochem. Cytochem. *35*, 909–916 (1987).

[21] *V. Glezerov, B. Dorsett*, Lymphocytic Membrane Antigens in GMA Embedded Tissues, Stain Technol. *64*, 105–112 (1989).

[22] *P.A. Erickson, D.H. Anderson, S.K. Fisher*, Use of Uranyl Acetate en Bloc to Improve Tissue Preservation and Labelling for Post Embedding Immuno-Electronmicroscopy, J. Electron Micros. Techn. *5*, 303–314 (1987).

[23] *I.W. McLean, P.K. Nakane*, Periodate-lysine-paraformaldehyde Fixation. A New Fixative for Immuno-Electronmicroscopy, J. Histochem. Cytochem. *22*, 1072–1083 (1974).

[24] *T. Kosaka, I. Nagatsu, J.Y. Wu, K. Hama*, Use of High Concentrations of Glutaraldehyde for Immunocytochemistry of Transmitter Synthesizing Enzymes in the CNS, Neuroscience Oxford *18*, 975–990 (1986).

[25] *S.R. Shi, M.E. Key, K.L. Kalra*, Antigen Retrieval in Formalin Fixed Paraffin Embedded Tissues: An Enhancement Method for Immunohistochemical Staining Based on Microwave Oven Heating of Tissue Sections, J. Histochem. Cytochem. *39*, 741–748 (1991).

[26] *K.T. Tokuyasu*, Application of Cryoultramicrotomy to Immunocytochemistry, J. Micros. London *143*, 139–149 (1986).

[27] *B. Arborgh, P. Bell, K.U. Brun, V.P. Collins*, The Osmotic Effect of Glutaraldehyde During Fixation. A Transmission Electronmicroscopy and Cytochemical Study, J. Ultrastruct. Res. *56*, 339–350 (1976).

[28] *P.W. Dudek, A.F. Boyne*, An Excursion Through the Ultrastructural World of Quick Frozen Pancreatic Islets, Am. J. Anat. *175*, 217–243 (1986).

[29] *M.T. Nicolas, G. Nicolas, C.H. Johnson, J.M. Bassot, J.W. Hastings*, Characterisation of the Bioluminescent Organelles in Gonyaulax Polyedra (Dinoflagellates) after Fast Freeze Fixation and Antiluciferase Immuno-gold Stain, J. Cell Biol. *105*, 723–735 (1987).

[30] *P. Monaghan, D. Rovertson*, Freeze Substitution without Aldehyde or Osmium Fixatives: Ultrastructure and Implications for Immunocytochemistry. J. Micros. Oxford *158*, 355–363 (1990).

[31] *G.A. Keller, K.T. Tokuyasu, A.H. Dutton, S.J. Singer*, An Improved Procedure for Immunoelectronmicroscopy Ultrathin Plastic Embedding of Immunolabeled Ultrathin Frozen Sections, Proc. Nat. Acad. Sci. U.S.A. *81*, 5744–5747 (1984).

[32] *K.T. Tokuyasu*, Use of PVP and PVA for Cryoultramicrotomy, Histochem. J. *21*, 163–171 (1989).

[33] *Y.D. Stierhof, H. Schwarz, H. Frank*, Transverse Sectioning of Plastic Embedded Immuno-labeled Cryosections: Morphology and Permeability to Protein A-Colloidal Gold Complexes, J. Ultrastruct. Res. *97*, 187–196 (1986).

[34] *M.A. Berryman, R.D. Rodewald*, An Enhanced Method for Post Embedding Immunocytochemical Staining which Preserves Cell Membranes, J. Histochem. Cytochem. *38*, 159–170 (1990).

[35] *A.M. Glauert, R.D. Young*, The Control of Temperature during Polymerisation of Lowicryl K4M: There is a Low Temperature Embedding Method, J. Micros. London *154*, 101–113 (1989).

[36] *J.D. Acetarin, E. Carlemalm, W. Villiger*, Development of New Lowicryl Resins for Embedding Biological Specimens at even Lower Temperature, J. Micros. London *143*, 81–88 (1986).

[37] *G. Mahrle, H.J. Schulze, A. Kuhn, A. Wevers*, Immunostaining of Keratin and Vimentin in Epidermis. Comparison of Different Post-embedding Immunogold Techniques for Electronmicroscopy, J. Histochem. Cytochem. *37*, 863–868 (1989).

[38] *B.L. Armbruster, R.M. Garavito, E. Kellenberger,* Dehydration and Embedding Temperatures Affect the Antigenic Specificity of Tubulin and Immunolabeling by the Protein
A-Colloidal Gold Technique, J. Histochem. Cytochem. *31,* 1380–1384 (1983).

[39] *H. Shida, R. Oliga,* Effect of Resin use in the Post Embedding Procedure on Immunoelectronmicroscopy of Membrane Antigens with Special Reference to Sensitivity, J. Histochem.
Cytochem. *38,* 1687–1691 (1990).

[40] *H.C.F. Mutasa,* Applicability of Using Acrylic Resins in Post Embedding Ultrastructural
Immunolabeling of Human Neutrophil Granule Proteins, Histochem. J. *21,* 249–258
(1989).

[41] *G.R. Newman, J. Hobot,* Modern Acrylics for Post Embedding Immunostaining Techniques,
J. Histochem. Cytochem. *35,* 971–981 (1987).

[42] *S. Enestrom, B. Kniola,* Quantitative Visual Comment Using a Computerised Image Analysis
System, Stain Technol *65,* 263–278 (1990).

[43] *M. Bendayan, M. Zollinger,* Ultrastructural Localisation of Antigenic Sites on Osmium Fixed
Tissues Applying the Protein A-Gold Technique, J. Histochem. Cytochem. *31,* 101–109
(1983).

[44] *A.B. Johnson, A. Bettica,* On Grid Immunogold Labeling of Glial Intermediate Filaments in
Epoxy Embedded Tissue, Am. J. Anat. *185,* 335–341 (1989).

[45] *C.E. Somers, D.E. Battaglia, B.M. Shapiro,* Localisation and Developmental Fate of
Ovoperoxidase and Proteoliasin, Two Proteins Involved in Fertilisation Envelope Assembly,
Dev. Biol. *131,* 226–235 (1989).

[46] *J.A. Litwin, K. Beier,* Immunogold Localisation of Peroxisomal Enzymes in Epon Embedded
Liver Tissue. Enhancement of Sensitivity by Etching with Ethanolic Sodium Hydroxide,
Histochemistry *88,* 193–196 (1988).

[47] *C.B. Rodning, S.L. Evlandsen, H.D. Coulter, I.D. Wilson,* Immunohistochemical Localisation
of IgA Antigens in Sections Embedded in Epoxy Resin, J. Histochem. Cytochem. *28,*
199–205 (1980).

[48] *M.P. Wenderoth, B.R. Eisenberg,* Ultrastructural Distribution of Myosin Heavy Chain mRNA
in Cardiac Tissue: A Comparison of Frozen and LR White Embedding, J. Histochem.
Cytochem. *39,* 1025–1033 (1991).

[49] *G. Griffiths, H. Hoppeler,* Quantitation in Immunocytochemistry: Correlation of Immunogold Labeling to Absolute Numbers of Membrane Antigens, J. Histochem. Cytochem. *34,*
1389–1398 (1986).

[50] *M. Horisberger,* Evaluation of Colloidal Gold as a Cytochemical Marker for Transmission and
Scanning Electronmicroscopy, Biochem. Cell *36,* 253–258 (1979).

[51] *J.W. Slot, H.J. Geuze,* A New Method of Preparing Gold Probes for Multiple Labeling
Cytochemistry, Eur. J. Cell. Biol *38,* 87–93 (1985).

[52] *C. Deroe, P.J. Courtoy, P. Baudhuin,* A Model of Protein-Colloidal Gold Interactions, J.
Histochem. Cytochem. *35,* 1191–1198 (1987).

[53] *J.F. Hainfeld,* A Small Gold Conjugated Antibody Label: Improved Resolution for
Electronmicroscopy, Science *236,* 450–454 (1987).

[54] *L. Ghitescu, M. Bendayan,* Immunolabelling Efficiency of Protein A-Gold Complexes, J.
Histochem. Cytochem. *38,* 1525–1530 (1990).

[55] *J. Gu, M. Dandrea,* Comparison of Detecting Sensitivities of Different Sizes of Gold Particles
with EM Immunogold Staining Using Atrial Natriuretic Peptide in Rat Atria as a Model, Am.
J. Anat. *185,* 264–270 (1989).

[56] *S. Yokota,* Effect of Particle Size on Labelling Density for Catalase in Protein A Gold
Immunocytochemistry, J. Histochem. Cytochem. *36,* 107–109 (1988).

[57] *P.M.P. Vanbergenenhenegouwen, J.L.M. Emmissen,* Controlled Growth of Colloidal Gold
Particles and Implications for Labeling Efficiency, Histochemistry *85,* 81–87 (1986).

[58] *N.R. Kramarcy, R. Sealock,* Commercial Preparations of Colloidal Gold Antibody Complexes Frequently Contain Free Active Antibody, J. Histochem. Cytochem. *39,* 37–39
(1991).

[59] *P.M. Lackie, R.J. Hennessy, G.W. Hacker, J.M. Polak,* Investigation of Immunogold-Silver
Staining by Electron Microscopy, Histochemistry *83,* 545–550 (1985).

[60] *E. Skutelsky, J. Roth,* Cationic Colloidal Gold, A New Probe of Anionic Cell Surfaces by Electron Microscopy, J. Histochem. Cytochem. *34,* 693–696 (1986).

[61] *J. Roth,* Application of Lectin-Gold Complexes for Electron Microscope Localisation of Glycoconjugates on Thin Sections, J. Histochem. Cytochem. *31,* 987–999 (1983).

[62] *S. Girod, C. Fuchey, C. Galabert, S. Lebouvallet, N. Bonnet, D. Ploton, E. Puchelle,* Identification of Phospholipids in Secretory Granules of Human Submucosal Respiratory Cells, J. Histochem. Cytochem. *39,* 193–198 (1991).

[63] *P.A. Coulombe, F.W.K. Kan, M. Bendayan,* Introduction of a High Resolution Cytochemical Method for Studying the Distribution of Phospholipids in Biological Tissues, Eur. J. Cell. Biol. *46,* 569–576 (1988).

[64] *I. Londono, M. Bendayan,* High Resolution Cytochemistry of Neuraminic and Hexuronic Acid Containing Macromolecules Applying the Enzyme-Gold Approach, J. Histochem. Cytochem. *36,* 1005–1014 (1988).

[65] *S. Berger, H.G. Schweiger,* Perinuclear Dense Bodies: Characterisation as DNA containing Structures Using Enzyme Linked Gold Granules, J. Cell Sci. *80,* 1–11 (1986).

[66] *M.R. Torrisi, P. Pinto da Silva,* Compartmentalisation of Intracellular Membrane Glycocomponents is Revealed by Fracture Label, J. Cell. Biol. *98,* 29–34 (1984).

[67] *P. Pinto da Silva, F.W.K. Kan,* Label Fracture: A Method for High Resolution Labelling of Cell Surfaces, J. Cell. Biol. *99,* 1156–1161 (1984).

[68] *D.A. Susan, R.G.W. Anderson,* Simultaneous Visualisation of LDL Receptor Distribution and Clathrin Lattices on Membranes Torn from the Upper Surface of Cultured Cells, J. Histochem. Cytochem. *39,* 1017–1024 (1991).

[69] *E.R. Unger, M.L. Hammer, M.L. Chenggis,* Comparison of ^{35}S and Biotin as Labels for in situ Hybridisation: Use of an HPV Model System, J. Histochem. Cytochem. *39,* 145–150 (1991).

[70] *W. Baschong, N.G. Wrigley,* Small Colloidal Gold Conjugated to Fab Fragments or to IgG as High Resolution Labels for Electron Microscopy, J. Electron Micros. Techn. *90,* 313–323 (1990).

[71] *G. Posthuma, J.W. Slot, H.J. Geuze,* Usefulness of Immunogold Techniques in Quantitation of a Soluble Protein in Ultrathin Sections, J. Histochem. Cytochem. *35,* 405–410 (1987).

[72] *K.E. Howell, U. Reuter-Carlson, E. Devancy, J.P. Luzio, S.D. Fuller,* One Antigen, One Gold? A Quantitative Analysis of Immunogold Labeling of Plasma Membrane 5'-Nucleotidase in Frozen Thin Sections, Eur. J. Cell. Biol. *44,* 318–327 (1987).

[73] *G. Posthuma, J.W. Slot, T. Veenendaal, H.J. Geuze,* Immunogold Determination of Amylase Concentration in Subcellular Compartments, Eur. J. Cell. Biol *46,* 327–335 (1988).

[74] *Y. Shiomura, N. Hirokawa,* The Molecular Structure of Microtubule Associated Protein 1A (MAP1A) in vivo and in vitro. An Immuno-EM and Quick Freeze Deep Etch Study, J. Neuro. Sci. *7,* 1461–1469 (1987).

[75] *J.C.R. Jones, A.E. Goldman, H. Yang, R.D. Goldman,* The Organisation and Fate of the Intermediate Filament Network in Two Epithelial Cell Types During Mitosis, J. Cell. Biol *100,* 93–102 (1985).

[76] *N. Rooney, C. Day, T. Gray, J.C.E. Underwood,* Electronmicroscopic Localisation of Cell Surface Markers in Tissue Sections Using Monoclonal and Gold Conjugated Antibodies, J. Pathol *148,* 29–34 (1986).

[77] *R.F. Stump, J.R. Pfeiffer, M.C. Schnecbeck, J.C. Seagrave, J.M. Oliver,* Mapping Gold Labeled Receptors on Cell Surfaces by Backscattered Electron Imaging and Digital Image Analysis: Studies of the IgE Receptor on Mast Cells, Am. J. Anat. *185,* 128–141 (1989).

[78] *E. de Harven, R. Lecung, H. Christensen,* A Novel Approach for Scanning Electronmicroscopy of Colloidal Gold Labeled Cell Surfaces, J. Cell. Biol. *99,* 53–57 (1984).

[79] *E. de Harven, D. Soligo, H. Christensen,* Should We Be Counting Immunogold Marker Particles on Cell Surfaces with the SEM? J. Micros. London *146,* 183–189 (1987).

5.8   Quantitative Histochemistry

Joseph Chayen and Lucille Bitensky

Initially, histochemistry was considered to be merely another way of staining cells or sections. This was made explicit by *Barka* and *Anderson* [1] who stated that histochemistry is "a system of chemical morphology that adds another dimension to histology. ... Its contribution cannot be assessed in the dynamic, physiological terms of biochemistry ... finite measurement is not the immediate goal of microscopic histochemistry. Deriving its theoretical foundations from chemistry, histochemistry remains essentially a morphological tool". However, it has developed into a quantitative form of cellular biochemistry involving localization of activity as well as its quantification [2]. It is this form of quantitative histochemistry that will now be considered.

The special features of quantitative histochemistry are as follows:

Sensitivity: treatment might affect only a small proportion of the cells of a given population. Conventional biochemical methods generally require up to 10^6 cells [3]. In contrast, histochemical procedures can be applied to individual cells. Consequently, if a response doubles a particular activity in 10% of the cells, biochemical procedures might not be able to detect this change whereas quantitative histochemistry, measuring the activity in individual cells, would easily distinguish a 100% change in each of the affected cells.

Localization within individual cells: if an activity was quantitatively unchanged but altered its location inside the affected cells (which comprised 10% of the whole population), for example, from the cell membrane to the cytosol, this altered location would be very obvious measured histochemically or by immunocytochemical staining.

Latent activity: there are many examples of active moieties, or enzymes, which occur in a latent form. In well preserved cells, their presence cannot be detected by an activity but may be detectable by the binding of a labelled antibody. Such binding may occur irrespective of whether the moiety is in a biologically active or inactive form. Latency may be due to the fact that the active moiety is sequestered behind a membrane. Typical examples of this are the lysosomal enzymes which are not available to react with exogenously added substrates until the lysosomal membrane is disrupted, as it may be by fixation. Other examples, such as ornithine decarboxylase, can be detected immunologically [e.g. 4] but there is no evidence that what is so detected has any biological activity; the half-life of the biologically active form is only 8–30 min [5].

5.8.1 Basic Procedures

5.8.1.1 Problems in Preparing the Specimen

In considering such problems, it is assumed that the specimen has to be sectioned; however similar considerations will apply, where pertinent, to suspensions of cells.

Chemical fixation [6] or freeze-substitution procedures [7, 8] may result in loss of material, even from solid pieces of tissue. Treatment with alcohol or with acetone, whether for fixation or for embedding in wax, may also cause denaturation and so reveal previously cryptic antigenic sites. The use of solvents will not only remove fatty material but will also influence lipid-protein bonds, which stabilize membranes [as discussed in 9, 10], and so disclose otherwise protected antigens. Conventional biochemical extraction procedures, by their very nature, will uncover otherwise unreactive sites.

To avoid the deleterious effect of fixation, many workers use frozen tissue, but freezing may also damage tissue and cells as has been well illustrated by *Passay* and *Dmochowski* [11] and *Luyet* [12]. The structure of the tissue may become reconstituted, to some extent, on thawing in a suitable medium, so obscuring the damage that had been done.

5.8.1.2 Effect of Other Histochemical Procedures

Immersion of unfixed sections in an aqueous medium, for disclosing antigenic sites, can cause up to 50% of the dry mass of unfixed sections to be lost into the reaction medium. The operator may therefore be faced with losing material either by fixation or from unfixed sections into the reaction medium. The procedures of chilling, sectioning and flash-drying described below have overcome these difficulties [13, 14]. Examples of the value of such methods are that they can be used in sensitive cytochemical bioassays of polypeptide hormones in which the sections respond with the same sensitivity as the intact tissue, and also in electron microscopical analyses of such sections [15].

5.8.1.3 Preparation of Sections

Chill small pieces of the tissue (up to 5 mm^3) by precipitate immersion in n-hexane at $-70\,°C$. Thermocouple traces [16] should show no formation of ice, thus implying that the tissue is supercooled. Section the tissue in a refrigerated cryostat with the cabinet temperature not higher than $-25\,°C$ (i. e., below the lowest ice-water transition point) and with the knife cooled with solid carbon dioxide to about $-70\,°C$. Flash-dry the section by bringing a glass slide, at room temperature, up to it. There is then a gap of about 2 mm between the warm slide and the cold knife and the section should jump off the knife onto the slide, leaving a imprint of water on the knife. This flash-drying is essential to avoid the formation of ice.

5.8.1.4   Reactions

The medium used for the reactions, or the immunological staining, must contain a suitable concentration of a colloid stabilizer that will prevent loss of material into the aqueous medium. It has been shown [17] that a suitable concentration of a form of polyvinyl alcohol (e.g. 30% (w/v) of GO4/140: *Wacker Chemical Co.*) or of a commercial polypeptide derived from collagen (Polypep 5115, *Sigma* [18]) will retain all the measurable content of sections immersed in an aqueous medium.

Although the use of these tissue stabilizers was developed for sections, Polypep 5115 has also been found to be of use with isolated cells. The concentration required may depend on the type of cell to be investigated.

5.8.1.5   Measurement

Coloured reaction-products, as with peroxidase or alkaline phosphatase methods, are measured in individual cells by microdensitometry. Simple photometry is suitable only where the coloured reaction-product is distributed homogeneously throughout the cell [19, 20]. Otherwise, and therefore in almost all cases, the measurement must be done with a microdensitometer such as the *Vickers* M85A. In this, the cell is first selected by normal microscopy. Then a scanning spot, which can be as small as $0.25\ \mu m$ (the limit of resolution of the light microscope and therefore optically homogeneous), is sent across the cell and the absorption of light at each point is transmitted to the detecting system. The absorption of all these points of light is integrated to give a value for the cell. By suitable calibration against filters of known extinction, this value of *relative absorption* can be converted into an absolute absorbance value.

Measurement of the value obtained by fluorescence microscopy is more difficult. The amount of fluorescence in a cell can be measured if a suitable photomultiplier is mounted above the microscope. However, a single reading is meaningless. It is first necessary to determine that the amount of fluorescence measured falls within the linear, or relatively linear, response of the photomultiplier. Often this can be arranged by altering the voltage applied to the photomultiplier. Some estimate of the real intensity of the fluorescence can be obtained if a range of samples of the pure reaction-product can be used to generate a calibration graph: x units of fluorescence in the specimen corresponds to y units of the pure product. However, even this is only an approximation because conditions in the cell may modify the precise nature of the fluorescence.

5.8.2 Procedures for Localizing the Antibody-Antigen Reaction

5.8.2.1 Immunological Methodology

Basically two types of methods have been described for the cytological demonstration and localization of antigens [e. g. 21, 22] (cf. 5.4). The first involves the direct interaction between a labelled antibody and the tissue antigen. For the second type, which includes the indirect, three-layer and build-up methods, the primary antibody is not labelled but its localization is demonstrated by the application of a labelled secondary antibody, or other reagent, which detects the presence of the primary antibody. What follows concerns solely the demonstration of the enzymatic label, irrespective of which immunological method is used.

Two enzymatic labels in the commonest current use are peroxidase and alkaline phosphatase and the object of their use is to demonstrate the localization of antigen.

Peroxidase activity

Method of *Van Norden,* [22]. The activity is demonstrated by a solution of DAB (up to 0.5 g/l in PBS). Just before it is to be used, hydrogen peroxide is added to give a final concentration of between 0.015 and 0.03% (w/v). The sections are immersed in this solution. The colour developed is measured after an incubation period that is less than 5 min in some cases.

Consideration of the method

The DAB reaction product is not totally insoluble in water (cf. alkaline phosphatase method following). Consequently, its location may reflect the general region rather than the exact site of the antigen-antibody reaction. The precise site at which the reaction product becomes insoluble may depend on the rate at which it is generated: the slower its production, the further it is likely to move before becoming absorbed. This question of diffusion of reaction product has been discussed in detail [9, 23–25], and should be considered in the interpretation of experiments on the quantitative measurement of antigen expression by the peroxidase-DAB method.

Alkaline phosphatase activity

In the normal method of *Van Noorden* [22], 1 mg of a naphthol phosphate, such as naphthol AS-MX phosphate or naphthol AS-TR phosphate, is dissolved in a small volume of dimethyl formamide which, just before use, is dispersed into 4 or 5 ml (according to the substrate) of a Tris-HCl buffer at pH 8.2 or 9.0. Free naphthol, liberated by the enzymatic reaction, is visualized by its becoming coupled simultaneously by a dye, such as Fast Blue BB or hexazotized New Fuchsin.

Consideration of the method

Many critical cytochemical studies have been made on the demonstration of this enzyme: it was almost a "test case" for the validity of cytochemistry (e.g *Danielli* [23, 24]). Most were done on the method in which calcium ions are used to trap the liberated phosphate; calcium phosphate is virtually insoluble. However, the insolubility of the product of the above method, which produces naphthol-Fast Blue BB or similar conjugate, is not known. As *Burstone* [26] wrote: "... although there is no actual knowledge about the submicroscopic nature of a 'capture reaction' involving a stain precursor (e. g. liberated naphthol), we can *assume* that the reaction should take place as rapidly as possible. A rapid capture reaction, however, does not necessarily preclude poor localizations. For example, β-naphthol may couple very rapidly with a suitable diazo reagent but may produce diffusion artefacts because the dyes are known in many instances to remain in a colloidal state following coupling". Studies on the diffusion (in sections) of the naphthylamine-Fast Blue B reaction product showed that this reatction-products could diffuse as far as 160 μm from the cell of its origin; other coupling reagents allowed the reaction product to diffuse up to 1000 μm [27].

Even with the phosphate-precipitation method, considerable diffusion-error can occur. It had been thought that, since calcium phosphate is very insoluble, localization of the enzyme should be very precise. However, it has been shown that the proposed nuclear localization of alkaline phosphatase [28] was artefactual due to insufficient calcium ions to insolubilize both the phosphate and the enzyme itself [29].

5.8.2.2   Possible Pitfalls

1. Chemical fixation and treatment can cause erroneous localization of the antigen in tissue sections.
2. The product of the DAB reaction is likely to be imprecisely localized. However, the fuzzy appearance of the DAB reaction product seen with cell membrane antigens in sections of frozen tissue is not seen with all antigens, suggesting that diffusion of unfixed antigen may also contribute to the imprecision of the system.
3. The naphthol method for localizing alkaline phosphatase activity is unlikely to demonstrate the precise location of this activity. However, if the localization is not critical, it yields a measurable product.
4. Alkaline phosphatase activity can be localized provided that the tissue is freeze-sectioned and the reaction is performed with a sufficiently high concentration of calcium ions [29].

5. The reaction product of the recommended alkaline phosphatase method is cobalt sulphide, which normally yields a product that is too intense for precise microdensitometric measurement. Very short reaction times may overcome this problem [20].
6. Immunocytochemical quantification is currently, at best, only comparative for the reasons outlined above.
7. Many histochemical studies deal with the effects, or lack of observed effects, on the metabolism or structure of cells consequent to an immunological reaction. It should be remembered that they are based on methods that may cause more damage than any immunological reaction is likely to induce. However, provided that the methods of preparing the tissue sections, or isolated cells, are those outlined here, then valuable quantifiable information on the response of cells to immunological events can be obtained. For example, this approach was used to investigate the intracellular response to an allo-immune reaction at the surface of ascites tumour cells [30–32] and the mechanism of T-cell cytolysis [33]. Some of the metabolic systems amenable to quantitative histochemical analysis are outlined in Table 1.

Table 1. Marker-enzyme activity

Marker	Relevance	Method	Target-site
DNA & RNA	Synthesis; freeing from binding	Methyl green pyronin [9, 25]	Nucleus and cytoplasm
Phospholipids	Dysjunction of lipid-protein complexes	Acid heamatein [34, 35]	Membranes
5′-Nucleotidase (EC 3.1.3.5)	Activation of membranes; purine synthesis	[36]	Membranes
Succinate dehydrogenase (EC 1.3.99.1)	Mitochondrial activity	[9, 25]	Mitochondria; no co-enzyme required
Glucose-6-phosphate dehydrogenase (EC 1.1.1.49)	Growth; synthesis of many constituents; NADP-dependent	[37]	Cytosol: pentose-phosphate pathway
Lactate dehydrogenase (EC 1.1.1.27)	Glycolytic activity; NAD-dependent	[38]	Cytosol
Hydroxyacyl dehydrogenase (EC 1.1.1.35)	Oxidation of fatty acids; particulate; NAD-dependent	[39]	Mitochondria or peroxisomes

References

[1] *T. Barka, P. J. Anderson,* Histochemistry, Harper and Row, New York 1963, pp. 341–343.
[2] *J. Chayen,* Quantitative Cytochemistry: a Precise Form of Cellular Biochemistry, Biochem. Soc. Trans. *12,* 887–898 (1984).

[3] *J. T. Dingle, A. J. Barrett*, Some Special Methods for the Investigation of the Lysosomal System, in: *J. T. Dingle, H. B. Fell* (eds.), Lysosomes in Biology and Pathology, Elsevier, Amsterdam 1969, Vol. 2, pp. 555–566.

[4] *L. Persson, E. Rosengren, F. Sundler*, Localization of Ornithine Decarboxylase by Immuno-cytochemistry, Biochem. Biophys. Res. Commun. *104*, 1196–1201 (1982).

[5] *A. M. Kaye*, Purification and Properties of Ornithine Decarboxylase, Cell Biochem. Funct. *2*, 2–6 (1984).

[6] *B. Sylvén*, Effects of Freezing and Drying Compared with Common Fixation Procedures, in: *R. J. C. Harris* (ed.), Freezing and Thawing, Institute of Biology, London 1951, pp. 168–176.

[7] *K. Ostrowski, J. Komender, H. Koscianek, K. Kwarecki*, Quantitative Investigation of the P and N Loss in the Rat Liver when Using Various Media in the "Freeze-substitution" Technique, Experientia *18*, 142–146, (1962).

[8] *K. Ostrowski, J. Komender, H. Koscianek, K. Kwarecki*, Quantitative Studies on the Influence of the Temperature Applied in Freeze-substitution on P, N, and Dry Mass Losses in Fixed Tissue, Experimentia *18*, 227–230 (1962).

[9] *J. Chayen, L. Bitensky, R. Butcher*, Practical Histochemistry, Wiley, London, New York 1973, 1st edn. pp. 80–87.

[10] *J. E. Lovelock*, The Denaturation of Lipid-protein Complexes as a Cause of Damage by Freezing, Proc. R. Soc. London B. *147*, 427–433 (1957).

[11] *R. D. Passey, L. Dmochowski*, Freeze-drying of Tumour Tissues, in: *R. J. C. Harris* (ed.), Freezing and Thawing, Institute of Biology, London 1951, pp. 63–75.

[12] *B. J. Luyet*, Survival of Cells, Tissues and Organisms After Ultra-rapid Freezing, in: *R. J. C. Harris* (ed.), Freezing and Thawing, Institute of Biology, London 1951, pp. 77–98.

[13] *J. Chayen*, The Cytochemical Approach to Hormone Assay, Int. Rev. Cytol. *53*, 333–396 (1978).

[14] *J. Chayen*, The Cytochemical Bioassay of Polypeptide Hormones, Springer, Berlin, Heidelberg, New York 1980, pp. 52–60.

[15] *F. P. Altman, R. J. Barrnett*, The Ultra-structural Localisation of Enzyme Activity in Unfixed Tissue Sections, Histochemistry *41*, 179–183 (1975).

[16] *R. Lynch, L. Bitensky, J. Chayen*, On the Possibility of Super-cooling in Tissues, J. R. Microsc. Soc. *85*, 213–222 (1966).

[17] *F. P. Altman, J. Chayen*, Retention of Nitrogenous Material in Unfixed Sections During Incubation for Histochemical Demonstration of Enzymes, Nature *207*, 1205–1206 (1965).

[18] *R. G. Butcher*, Tissue Stabilization During Histochemical Reactions: the Use of Collagen Polypeptides, Histochemie *28*, 231–235 (1971).

[19] *J. Chayen*, Microdensitometry, in: *T. F. Slater* (ed.), Biochemical Mechanisms of Liver Injury, Academic Press, London, New York 1978, pp. 257–291.

[20] *L. Bitensky*, Microdensitometry, in: *D. Evered, M. O'Connor* (eds.), Trends in Enzyme Histochemistry and Cytochemistry, Ciba Foundation Symposium, Excerpta Medica, Amsterdam 1980, pp. 181–202.

[21] *Ch. W. Pool, R. M. Buijs, D. F. Swaab, G. J. Boer, F. W. van Leeuwen*, On the Way to a Specific Immunocytochemical Localization, in: *A. C. Cuello* (ed.), Immunohistochemistry, Wiley, Chichester, New York 1983, pp. 2–46

[22] *S. Van Noorden*, Tissue Preparation and Immunostaining Techniques for Light Microscopy, in: *J. M. Pollak, S. Van Noorden* (eds.), Wright, Bristol 1986, 2nd edn., pp. 26–53.

[23] *J. F. Danielli*, Cytochemistry: A Critical Approach, Wiley, New York 1953, pp. 28–77.

[24] *J. F. Danielli*, The Calcium Phosphate Precipitation Method for Alkaline Phosphatase, in: *J. R. Danielli* (ed.), General Cytochemical Methods, Academic Press, New York 1958, pp. 423–443.

[25] *J. Chayen, L. Bitensky*, Practical Histochemistry, Wiley, London, New York, 1991, 2nd end., pp. 145–150.

[26] *M. S. Burstone*, Enzyme Histochemistry and its Application in the Study of Neoplasms, Academic Press, New York 1962.

[27] *M. McCabe, J. Chayen*, The Demonstration of Latent Particulate Amino-peptidase Activity, J. R. Microsc. Soc. *84*, 361–371 (1965).

[28] *M. Chèvremont, H. Firket*, Alkaline Phosphatase of the Nucleus, Int. Rev. Cytol. *2*, 261–288 (1953).

[29] *R. G. Butcher, J. Chayen*, Quantitative Studies on the Alkaline Phosphatase Reaction, J. R. Microsc. Soc. *85*, 111–117 (1966).

[30] *D. C. Dumonde, C. M. Walter, L. Bitensky, G. J. Cunningham, J. Chayen*, Intracellular Response to an Iso-immune Reaction at the Surface of Ascites Tumour Cells, Nature *192*, 1302 (1961).

[31] *D. C. Dumonde, L. Bitensky, G. J. Cunningham, J. Chayen*, The Effects of Antibodies on Cells, I. Biochemical and Histochemical Effects of Antibodies and Complement on Ascites Tumour Cells, Immunology *8*, 25–36 (1965).

[32] *L. Bitensky*, Cytotoxic Action of Antibodies, Br. Med. Bull. *19*, 241–244 (1963).

[33] *J. Chayen, A. A. Pitsillides, L. Bitensky, I. H. Muir, P. M. Taylor, B. A. Askonas*, T-cell Mediated Cytolysis: Evidence for Target-cell Suicide, J. Exp. Pathol. *71*, 197–209 (1990).

[34] *J. Chayen*, The Histochemistry of Phospholipids and its Significance in the Interpretation of the Structure of Cells, in: *S. M. McGee-Russell, K. F. A. Ross* (eds.), Cell Structure and Its Interpretation, Edward Arnold, London 1968, pp. 149–156.

[35] *B. Henderson, L. Bitensky, J. Chayen*, Altered Phospholipids in Human Rheumatoid Synoviocytes, Ann. Rheum. Dis. *37*, 24–29 (1978).

[36] *B. Henderson, J. J. Johnstone, J. Chayen*, 5'-Nucleotidase Activity in the Human Synovial Lining in Rheumatoid Arthritis, Ann. Rheum. Dis. *39*, 248–252 (1980).

[37] *J. Chayen, D. W. Howat, L. Bitensky*, Cellular Biochemistry of Glucose 6-phosphate and 6-phosphogluconate Dehydrogenase Activities, Cell Biochem. Funct. *4*, 249–253 (1986).

[38] *B. Henderson*, Quantitative Cytochemistry of Lactate Dehydrogenase Activity, Cell Biochem. Funct. *2*, 149–152 (1984).

[39] *D. J. Chambers, M. V. Braimbridge, G. T. B. Frost, A. M. Nahir, J. Chayen*, A Quantitative Cytochemical Method for the Measurement of β-Hydroxyacyl CoA Dehydrogenase Activity in the Rat Heart Muscle, Histochemistry *75*, 67–76 (1982).

5.9   Image Analysis

Don-Carlos Abrams and David R. Springall

5.9.1   General Considerations

A major problem that faces microscopists in the detailed examination of tissues, cells and organelles is visualizing and quantifying the spatial arrangement of cells in a tissue, of intracellular cellular constituents in the cytoplasm or of constituents of organelles. Many techniques have been developed to assist the investigator in observing these microscopic details: image processing is one of these techniques. The purpose of this section is to introduce the concept of image processing to those unfamiliar with this technique and to discuss its application to quantitative immunological methods.

Immunocytochemical techniques were initially used to identify microscopic structures by virtue of their immunoreactivity. In the past, many scientists have been content with the localization of antigens and have not been particularly interested in the quantification of immunoreactivity or cellular dimensions. Such localization is normally observed using some form of microscopy. By adding a video camera or some other photosensitive device, the microscope can be used to obtain images suitable for analysis by computers. The plethora of image analysis and image processing techniques, which originated in the 1960s as part of the space programme, can now be applied to images of biological material, allowing enhanced visualization, multidimensional quantification and multidimensional visualization. These methods have enabled scientists to measure rapid biological activity both spatially and temporally, to measure (in real units) the dimensions of cells and organelles and to identify changes in local concentrations of a variety of ligands and tissue markers.

However, the advances have brought problems that researchers are only now beginning to address, particularly standardization of sample preparation, software and hardware.

5.9.1.1   What is an Image?

A digital image is a two-dimensional graphical representation of an array of values. In a monochrome image (black and white), which is usually referred to as a grey scale image,

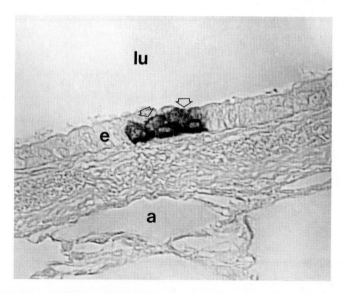

Fig. 1. An 8-bit 512 × 512 grey scale image of a section of rat lung showing alveoli (a) and a bronchiole with immunoreactivity for the vasoactive regulatory peptide CGRP in a group of endocrine cells (arrows) in the epithelium (e) of a bronchiole (lu = lumen).

each value codes for a single picture element, known as a pixel, that represents the brightness of the image at some predefined position within the picture. The digital image is comprised of rows and columns of pixels. The number of pixels that constitute an image row is known as the image width. Similarly, the number of pixels in an image column is termed the image height. Figure 1 shows a grey scale image of endocrine cells in bronchiolar epithelium of a rat. The image width consists of 512 columns of pixels, the height of 512 rows.

The quality of a digital image may be defined by the spatial resolution (i. e. the more pixels, the better) and the quantization of the image. Quantization is governed by the digitizing system and is related to the number of computer binary digits (bits) that are used to represent a pixel. An image that consists of single bit data is known as a binary image. Such an image contains only black and white information and is of limited use. In biology, most images are 8-bit and therefore consist of pixels whose values are integers in the range from 0 (pure black) to 255 (pure white). Intermediate values are shades of grey (Fig. 2).

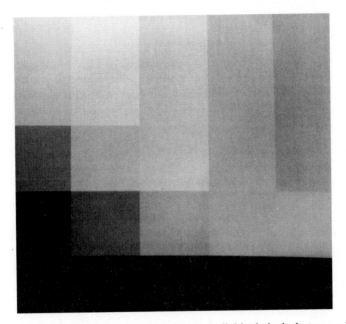

Fig. 2. A greatly enlarged part of figure 1 illustrating the individual pixels that comprise the image. The pixel values, representing shades of grey, are:

159	169	145	129	110
135	147	135	109	90
51	121	138	110	97
2	44	110	115	117
7	4	2	3	1

Conventionally, the coordinates of a pixel are specified relative to the top left hand corner of the image. Pixels are always stored sequentially in the image file and it is the position of the pixels within the stream of data that determines the position of the pixel in the final image. A square image consisting of 512 rows and 512 columns, would have 262 144 pixels. If each pixel was represented by 8 bits of data, then the size of the image file would be 256 kilobytes.

5.9.1.2   What is Image Analysis?

Having defined a digital image, it is now appropriate to describe the purpose of image analysis and image processing. Although these terms have different meanings they are often used interchangeably. Image analysis is concerned with the detailed examination of digital images to extract quantitative or qualitative information without having to modify the image. Typical examples include computerized quantitative histology [1] and pictorial information retrieval. Image processing is the technique of transforming one image into another, usually by mathematical manipulation of the pixel position or magnitude or both.

In biology, image analysis is extensively used to obtain quantitative information on structures or objects within images. To understand the limitations and capabilities of biological image analysis, the investigator must have a fundamental understanding of the stages involved in the processing of images. The remainder of this section describes basic image processing operations together with software and hardware requirements, and discusses a number of biological applications. Only grey scale image analysis will be described although colour image analysis is becoming established.

5.9.1.3   Hardware Requirements

Image processing systems are based on digital computers. They are commercially available as specialized or nonspecialized machines. For example, the ContextVision™ GOP 302 system is a multiprocessor computer system designed specifically for image processing. A fundamental component of this machine is the array processor. This device allows computer-intensive image operations to be performed extremely quickly. As well as these specialized image processing systems, it is also possible to base an image processing system around an industry-standard personal computer (PC). There are many commercially available packages that have been specifically designed to be used with PCs. The three principle hardware elements necessary for an image processing system are concerned with image capture, image display and image storage (Fig. 3).

5.9.1.4   Image Capture

Image capture, or "digitization", involves converting the image into a numerical representation suitable for interpretation by the computer. For conventional microscopy, image capture is usually performed with a television camera. Other devices may be used; for example, photosensitive devices such as the photomultiplier tubes in the confocal scanning laser microscope (cf. 5.10), or digital scanners.

The television signal is digitized by a "frame grabber". Most frame grabbers are equipped with on-board memory that is capable of holding several images simultaneously. Image processing systems are capable of digitizing images at TV rates; i.e., approximately 30 images per second. The spatial resolution of the digitized image is usually expressed as a matrix: the image width by the image height. The quantization is determined by the resolution of the analogue-to-digital (AD) converters that capture the image. Colour frame grabbers have three 8-bit AD converters; one for the red component, one for the green component and one for the blue component.

5.9.1.5 Display

The output device converts the digital image into an analogue signal and displays the image at a video device. Television and computer monitors (Fig. 3) are the most common devices used to display images. The typical monitor which is supplied with the personal computer is a high resolution device. The resolution of these displays is

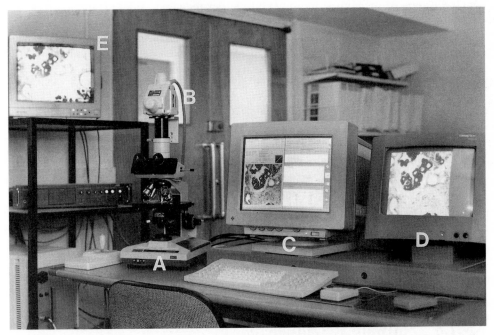

Fig. 3. A typical system suitable for biological image processing. The microscope (A) and the camera (B) are attached to the *Sun* computer (not shown) via a frame grabber. The two monitors (C and D) are used for computer control and image display respectively. A further monitor (E) displays a live image directly from the camera.

user-configurable with a maximum resolution of 1024×768 pixels. For displaying larger images, Unix workstations are often employed. The monitors attached to these computers tend to be 19-inch display units with a typical resolution of 1200×800 pixels or higher (Fig. 3).

5.9.1.6   Storage

Digital images occupy large amounts of space. It is not uncommon for a set of confocal images to require 30 or 40 megabytes of disk storage space. Consequently, mass storage is one of the most important prerequisites for any image processing system. The main storage media for images are magnetic disks, magnetic tapes, optical disks and WORM (Write Once Read Many) disks.

The choice of storage device is primarily dictated by the total storage space required although access speeds are often taken into consideration. Magnetic tapes, which are the cheapest storage media, are ideal for archival purposes. However, accessing information from magnetic tape can be time-consuming and impractical. The computer disks (magnetic, optical and WORM) are more practical as information may be written and read from them at reasonable speeds. Although recent advances in disk technology have led to substantial reductions in the cost of these devices, magnetic disks remain about 3 orders of magnitude more expensive per megabyte than magnetic tapes. At present we are witnessing the introduction of large magnetic *Winchester* disks which are capable of storing in excess of 2 gigabytes of computerized data. These devices are ideal for image storage and allow vast amounts of data to be accessible immediately.

5.9.1.7   Networks

Computer networks provide investigators with the ability to transfer data between computers efficiently. The advantages of these systems are too numerous to mention in detail, but they are primarily concerned with the sharing of resources. In particular, different stages of the image processing procedure may be performed by different machines. For example, image capture may be performed by a standard desktop computer. The images may then be transferred to more powerful and specialized machines for processing. At the *Royal Postgraduate Medical School,* London, images are captured using one of many data acquisition stations. All images are stored centrally on a large fileserver and are accessible by local and remote computers *via* an efficient computer network. These images are continuously available to scientists and clinicians for research, diagnostic and development purposes.

5.9.1.8   Software Requirements

Following the image capture stage, the images are usually processed using computer software. It is the software that dictates whether a particular analysis can be performed automatically, semiautomatically or not at all. To date, very few of the problems that we wish to address, using image processing, have not required manual intervention. This is primarily due to difficulties in programming the computer to interpret the images satisfactorily.

Image processing may be divided into two categories depending on the complexity of the analysis that is required. First, low-level image processing which is concerned with the processing of individual pixels and is the type of processing that most life scientists adopt. Examples of low-level image processing include thresholding and edge detection, which will be discussed later. The second image processing category is high-level image processing, also termed machine vision. Machine vision is concerned with the manipulation and description of other structures in the image rather than individual pixels. These structures are usually whole entities, for example cells or nuclei. High-level knowledge is required to interpret images in this manner.

Image processing and image analysis software may be classified into four partially overlapping categories. First, there are specific image analysers which are usually supplied with their own hardware and perform a limited number of specific tasks efficiently and well. Such machines include the Seescan™, Cires™ and the Ivos™. Although these systems are usually very robust and require little or no computer knowledge to operate, they lack flexibility.

The second category of image processing software includes packages such as Optimas™, MicroGOP™ and Vidas™. These systems are general purpose image processing packages. They have their own command language which allows the user to record image processing sequences and to execute these sequences whenever necessary. They are not usually tied to one application and therefore may be used to address a number of image processing problems for developmental and routine work. The manufacturers of these systems usually supply programs tailored to the user's requirements. However, the user requires a basic understanding of computer technology in order to operate these packages.

The third category of programs were designed for computer literate users with an understanding of image processing and image analysis techniques. These systems are similar to the second category of software, but include a library of image processing programs that may be incorporated, by the users, into their own programs. The user requires a thorough understanding of computer programming, image processing and image analysis. Semper™, X-IMAGE and the Context Vision GOP 302 Image Processing System fall into this category. The advantage of these systems is flexibility, in that the user can create programs to address in-house problems and exchange data with other similar systems to solve specific tasks.

Finally, the fourth category comprises those systems that are designed totally in-house. These set-ups can be designed to do precisely what is required and can also be developed to process the results using specified techniques. This system can be very labour-intensive to produce, requiring close collaboration of programmers and users, but may be the only solution to a particular problem.

5.9.2   Stages in Image Analysis

This section is not a complete overview of the image processing stages that must be performed on digital images. Instead, it is a brief insight into some of the stages that can be considered. The interested reader requiring additional information on image processing should consult one of the standard texts [2–4] or a general survey [5].

Prior to image processing there are a number of stages that must be considered. These include sample preparation, image capture, noise removal, image segmentation, geometric correction, feature detection and mensuration.

5.9.2.1   Sample Preparation

Sample preparation is often the most important stage in a biological experiment involving digital image processing. This step often dictates how successful image analysis will be at extracting the required information from images of tissues and cells. The reproducibility of such information is critical if this technology is to succeed. Sample preparation techniques must be standardized and optimized for image analysis. The importance of standardization has been extensively reviewed by *Wittekind* [6]. The whole sample preparation regime should be examined. Fixation, staining and mounting techniques [7] that yield images suitable for human observation may be inappropriate for image analysis.

Whereas human vision can easily contend with low-contrast structures, especially when these elements appear as different colours, a camera cannot, and low contrast structures may be lost during the digitization procedure or in the following image processing stages. The digital image is always degraded when compared with the image seen with the microscope and therefore it is important that the structures of interest are clearly visible in the image. Finally, reproducibility of the adapted sample preparation techniques is also important particularly if samples are to be compared over long time periods.

5.9.2.2   Image Quality

In biology, we are fortunate to be able to optimize our image capture to obtain good quality images. This usually involves altering the light intensity on the microscope and the black level on the camera control unit to obtain images that utilize the full dynamic range of the grey scale. Random noise may be suppressed by capturing many frames of the same image. These frames are then averaged to produce the final image which is stored to disk. This process is known as frame averaging. To remove background shading, background subtraction is often performed on the captured images [3, page 62]. Good quality images can improve the efficiency of subsequent image processing stages.

5.9.2.3   Segmentation

Segmentation is a critical step that determines which objects are extracted from the image for the next stage of the image processing procedure. It is the process of subdividing an image into objects of interest and background. For example, if we are interested in the volume relationship between the nucleus and cytoplasm of a particular cell type, it would be necessary to segment the image twice. The first segmentation procedure would extract information relating to the nuclei and the second segmentation would extract cytoplasmic information.

Segmentation is a very difficult aspect of image processing. There are many specific and general purpose computer algorithms that perform segmentation. They differ according to the methods they employ and the results they produce. The common approaches to segmentation include thresholding [8], edge detection [9], line detection [10] and relaxation [11] although segmentation has also been performed using texture [12] and region-growing algorithms [13].

Thresholding

If the objects in an image appear darker than the background, it is feasible to attempt to segment the image by identifying the grey level values which compose the object. The upper and lower thresholds of this grey level range are then used to construct a binary image. This is known as thresholding and is the simplest method of segmentation. The thresholds are usually obtained manually, although automatic and semiautomatic methods are available [14]. Figure 4 shows the result of thresholding applied to Figure 1. In general, variable thresholds, which depend upon the position of objects within the image and based on the local pixel values, or multiple thresholds are used, because individual thresholds will rarely include all the objects without any background.

Although manual thresholding is a simple and common method of segmentation, intra- and inter-operator variations are very high and thus the procedure should be repeated several times on the same image. It has been suggested that many observers should be used to threshold images of immunochemically stained tissues [15].

Line detection

In segmentation, it is often important to determine the characteristics of boundaries. For example, is a boundary a straight line or is it curved? Often such features would be concealed behind other objects, distorted due to the digitization process or otherwise

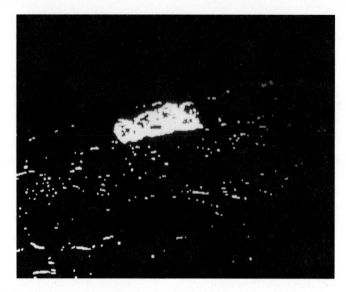

Fig. 4. A single threshold has been applied to Figure 1. Although the cells have been selected at this threshold level, some of the background has also been detected.

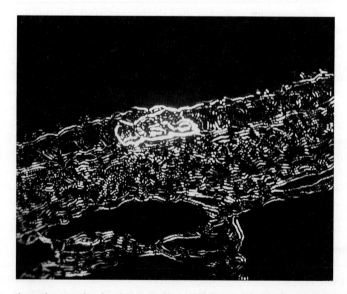

Fig. 5. An edge detection routine has been applied to Figure 1. The cells, airway wall and the walls of the alveoli have been detected.

incomplete. Under these conditions it is essential that image processing algorithms are capable of detecting such objects. Straight lines in images may be detected using the *Hough* transform [10]. This method is based on extracting information from parameterized features such as lines and circles.

Edge detection

Edge detection algorithms attempt to identify components of a boundary. This may be achieved by examining the rate of change of pixel intensities (gradient) near a given pixel. If the gradient is high, then the pixel could be interpreted as belonging to an edge. Similarly, if the gradient is low, then the converse is true. This approach is a common method for detecting meaningful interruptions in the grey level pattern (Fig. 5).

Region growing techniques

Both edge detection and line detection algorithms segment images by attempting to localize the boundaries of structures. Region growing techniques attempt to localize objects by identification of their interiors. The concept behind these algorithms is to identify features that separate one region from another. These features are grey level-related and allow pixels to be grouped into regions with distinct boundaries. The simplest method of region growing is pixel aggregation where points within the image are selected as seed points; neighbouring pixels are added to the seed only if they have similar characteristics (i.e., grey level value, colour or texture).

There are many more algorithms available for image segmentation, some of which are very simple while others make assumptions; interested readers are referred to *Haralick* [16].

5.9.2.4   Mensuration

The final stage in image analysis is usually concerned with mensuration. The aim of this stage is to extract meaningful quantitative information from the digital images. There are two main problems associated with mensuration. Firstly, tissues, cells and organelles occupy 3-dimensional space. Therefore, the investigator should consider thoroughly which measurement parameters would provide useful information and, in particular, what aspect of the tissues or cells are being measured. The common profile area measurement is a simple method for obtaining volumetric data from histological sections. However, if this technique is to provide meaningful data from 2-dimensional images, certain prerequisites must be met. These prerequisites include appropriate collection of raw data and the correct sectioning of tissues, and have been described in detail elsewhere [17]. The second problem, which has also been addressed by *Weibel*, is that of sampling. The overall aim of a quantification experiment is to extract representative data: that is, data that represent the entire structure that is being investigated. It is impractical to observe a whole organ or to analyse every cell within a smear. Therefore, the material must be sampled in such a way that the resulting sample is representative of the whole population. This may be achieved by selecting random histological sections or randomly selecting cells from a smear. Histological samples are usually larger than the field of view observable with a microscope. Further sub-sampling is often required to prevent bias entering the sampling strategy.

Having obtained representative samples, it is then possible to estimate lengths, areas and volumes using the correct stereological techniques [18]. The area of a structure may be obtained by counting the number of pixels that represent that structure. The result is usually converted to real units or expressed as a percentage of the total area as in the case of immunoreactivity quantification described below.

5.9.3   General Applications of Image Analysis

Image analysis and image processing have been employed in many areas of cell and tissue biology. The purpose of this section is not to cite every image processing application that as been published, but to mention the types of analysis that can and can not be performed. In the 1960s, automated systems were developed for human white blood cell recognition [19], automatic chromosome analysis [20] and for the estimation of the number of neurones in brain tissue [21]. The major research programmes in image analysis throughout the 1950s, 1960s and 1970s were mainly concerned with the analysis of blood smears, cervical smears, chromosome analysis and the flow systems [22]. Image analysis is now used routinely in a wide range of specialities including DNA ploidy analysis [23] and sperm assessment [24].

5.9.4   Quantification of Immunostaining

Image analysis has been used to quantify immunocytochemical reactions in two principal ways: by measuring the area or number of stained structures, or measuring the intensity of staining. The former is usually performed to give an estimate of changes in the tissue density of the stained structure or, if that density does not change, as a measure of the amount of antigen present. The latter is used to estimate antigen concentration, although it should be emphasized that only comparative and not absolute values are obtained (cf. 5.8). Both methods have their relative merits for antigen quantification. Area estimation or counting is relatively simple but does not measure the magnitude of differences. This can be achieved by staining intensity measurement, but it is time-consuming and exacting in technical requirements for producing immunostained preparations.

5.9.4.1   Area Measurement

This requires that the stained structures are present at a moderate density, i. e. within every microscope field. Data are obtained by interactively thresholding random images of the immunostained tissue section such that all pixels with an intensity greater than the threshold represent the specific staining. The number of these pixels thus represents the area of stained structures; it may be expressed in absolute units (e. g. mm^2), or as a ratio to a base such as field area or area of tissue. It has been used for neural quantification [25–27], either to show changes in nerve density, when staining for an anatomical marker of nerves, or to determine the release of neurotransmitters or modulators by the resultant decrease in the number of nerves that remain immunoreactive for those antigens. A corollary of this method is the so-called "supraoptimal dilution" technique [28]. It relies on the reduction in antigen detectability when the primary antiserum is diluted beyond its normal range. This causes a decrease in staining intensity overall that puts low levels of antigen below the limit of detection, so that structures containing them do not stain, and it increases the discriminating capability of the method. Thus, a qualitative measure of quantitative differences in antigen concentrations can be obtained, allowing the comparison of test and control groups of tissues. The method has been used to show differences in neurotransmitter levels [28] and in concentrations of a bioactive peptide, calcitonin gene-related peptide (CGRP), in pulmonary endocrine cells (Fig. 1) following exposure *in vivo* to hypoxia [29].

5.9.4.2   Intensity of Staining

However, the most informative measurement for antigen quantification is intensity of immunostaining. In image analysis this is conventionally expressed as an optical density, rather than as an absorbance value used elsewhere in this volume. Quantification may be achieved by use of either fluorescence or enzyme labels, but the latter are probably easier. The general assumption is that the amount of a specific antibody that binds to a tissue section is proportional to the amount of antigen present. Within the limits of steric hindrance this is almost certainly true [30, 31]. Thus, provided that the effects of tissue fixation and processing on antigenicity are minimal, or at least equal between specimens being compared, the method can be reliable. Great care is necessary in standardizing

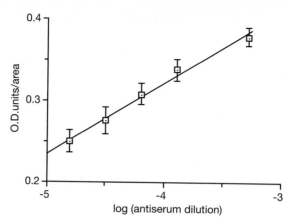

Fig. 6. Average optical density (integrated optical density per unit area of stain) of CGRP immunostaining in endocrine cells of rat lung at different dilutions of antiserum showing that there is a log-linear relationship.

the staining procedure, and it is necessary to validate the linearity of the relationship between antigen concentration and staining intensity, preferably using artificial standards such as antigen bound to agarose beads. Care is needed to select the appropriate dilution of primary and secondary antibodies and to ensure that the histochemical development of enzyme activity does not saturate for the highest antigen concentration in the tissues studied.

The method has been used to quantify the hypoxia-induced changes in pulmonary endocrine levels of CGRP mentioned above [32]. Initially, the effects of varying the conditions for the different steps in the staining procedure were tested using tissues from Wistar rats subjected to hypoxia for seven days. Sections were stained with doubling dilutions of anti-CGRP serum (1:2,000 to 1:64,000) using the peroxidase-antiperoxi-dase method. Further sections were stained with the 1:16,000 dilution and the peroxidase reaction was developed for various lengths of time (2.5 to 10 min). All incubation times and temperatures were rigidly standardized and sufficient quantities of all reagent solutions to complete the study were prepared in advance and stored appropriately. The optical density of the staining was measured using an IBAS 2000™ computerized image analysis system (*Zeiss Kontron,* UK). The stained area to be measured was outlined interactively and the optical density determined. A background value was obtained after moving the outline to an equivalent but unstained tissue area. The specific average optical density (total minus background) and area of staining were obtained and the integrated optical density calculated by multiplying them.

The immunostaining intensity was linearly related to the log of antiserum dilution (Fig. 6) and to times of development up to 6–8 min (Fig. 7). An antiserum dilution of 1:16,000, and a development time of 4.5 min was chosen. When used to stain a series of standards prepared from CGRP-coupled agarose beads, a linear relationship between CGRP concentration and optical density was obtained (Fig. 8).

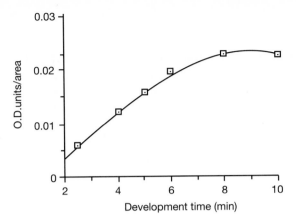

Fig. 7. Average optical density of staining as in Figure 6 after different times of development showing the increase in staining is linear up to 6 minutes under the conditions used.

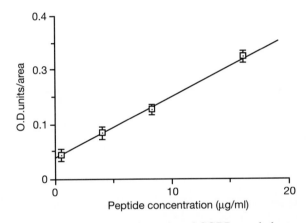

Fig. 8. Average optical density of staining of a series of CGRP-coupled agarose beads using an anti-CGRP serum diluted 1:16,000, showing a linear relationship with CGRP concentration in the solutions used to label the beads.

Using these conditions to measure a total of 556 cell groups, representing 2500 cells in 15 hypoxic and 15 control animals, CGRP staining intensity was shown to be increased ($p < 0.04$) by an average of 12%, corresponding on the standard curve to an increase of 15–20% in CGRP concentration in the endocrine cells of hypoxic animals [32].

Conclusions

The impact that computers have made in the quantitative and qualitative assessment of cells and tissues is irrefutable, despite their limited use in clinical practice. However, the success of computers in these areas of science depends not only on technical advancements in image processing but also on improvements in software engineering and preparative techniques. Quantitative study of cells and tissues can be very tedious and time-consuming but is becoming increasingly necessary because semi-quantitative visual estimation, with its associated subjective bias, becomes less acceptable to the scientific community. Image processing and image analysis have reduced the manual input required to perform such studies. As digital image processing and computer technology develop, the role of computers in research and diagnosis will expand.

References

[1] *R. P. Bolender*, Quantitative Morphology for Biologists and Computer Scientists, Microsc. Res. Tech. *21*, 338–346 (1992).

[2] *R. C. Gonzalez, P. Wintz*, Digital Image Processing, 2nd ed., Addison-Wesley, Publishing Company, Reading MA 1987.

[3] *A. Low*, Introductory Computer Vision and Image Processing, McGraw-Hill, London 1991.

[4] *W. Niblack*, An Introduction to Digital Image Processing, Prentice-Hall, London 1986.

[5] *A. Rosenfeld*, Survey – Image Analysis and Computer Vision: CVGIP, Image Understanding *55*, 349–380 (1992).

[6] *D. Wittekind*, Standardization of Dyes and Stains for Automated Cell Pattern Recognition, Anal. Quant. Cytol. Histol. *7*, 6–30 (1985).

[7] *T. D. Visser, J. L. Oud, G. J. Brakenhoff*, Refractive Index and Axial Distance Measurements in 3-D Microscopy, Optik *90*, 17–19 (1992).

[8] *P. C. Chen, T. Pavlidas*, Segmentation by Texture Using a Co-occurrence Matrix and a Split-and-Merge Algorithm, Comput. Graphics Image Proc. *10*, 172–182 (1979).

[9] *R. A. Kirsch*, Computer Determination of the Constituent Structure of Biological Images, Comput. Biomed. Res. *3*, 315–328 (1971).

[10] *P. V. C. Hough*, Method and Means for Recognizing Complex Patterns, U.S. Patent 3,069,654, 1962.

[11] *B. J. Schafter, A. Lev, S. W. Zucker, A. Rosenfeld*, Application of Relaxation Methods to Edge Reinforcement, IEEE Trans. Syst. Man Cybernet., SMC-7, 813–816 (1977).

[13] *S. W. Zucker*, Region Growing: Childhood and Adolescence, Comput. Graphics Image Proc. *5*, 382–399 (1976).

[14] *R. Kohler*, A Segmentation System Based on Thresholding, Comput. Graphics Image Proc. *15*, 319–338 (1981).

[15] *R. Jagoe, J. Steel, V. Vucicevic, N. Alexander, S. Van Noorden, R. Wootton, J. M. Polak*, Observer Variation in Quantification of Immunocytochemistry by Image Analysis, Histochem. J. *23*, 541–547 (1991).

[16] *R. M. Haralick, L. G. Shapiro*, Image Segmentation Techniques, Computer Vision, Graphics and Image Processing *29*, 100–132 (1985).

[17] *E. R. Weibel*, Stereological Methods, Vol. 1, Academic Press, London 1979.

[18] *L. M. Cruz-Orive, E. R. Weibel*, Recent Stereological Methods for Cell Biology: A Brief Survey, Am. J. Physiol. *258*, L148–L156 (1990).

[19] *M. Ingram, P. E. Norgren, K. Preston Jr.*, Image Processing in Biological Science, in: *D. M. Ramsey* (ed.), Image Processing in Biological Science: proceedings of a conference held November 1966 [Los Angeles], University of California Press, California 1968, pp. 97–117.

[20] *E. M. Nadel*, Computer Analysis of Cytophotometric Fields by CYDAC and Its Historical Evolution from the Cytoanalyzer, Acta Cytol. *9*, 203–207 (1965).

[21] *H. P. Mansberg, J. M. Segarra*, Counting of Neurons by Flying Spot Microscope, Ann. New York Acad. Sci. *99*, 309–322 (1962).

[22] *W. Coulter*, High-Speed Automatic Blood Cell Counter and Cell Size Analyzer, Proc. Natl. Electron. Conf., *12*, 1034–1042 (1956).

[23] *F. Giroud, M. P. Montmasson*, Re-Evaluation of Optimal *Feulgen* Reaction for Automated Cytology, Anal. Quant. Cytol. Histol. *11*, 87–95 (1989).

[24] *R. O. Davis, P. W. Niswander, D. F. Katz*, New Measures of Sperm Motion. I. Adaptive Smoothing and Harmonic Analysis, J. Androl. *13*, 139–152 (1992).

[25] *T. Cowen, G. Burnstock*, Image Analysis of Catecholamine Fluorescence, Brain Res. Bull. *9*, 81–86 (1982).

[26] *T. Cowen*, Image Analysis of FITC-Immunofluorescence Histochemistry in Perivascular Substance P-Positive Nerves, Histochemistry *81*, 609–610 (1984).

[27] *G. Terenghi, C. B. Bunker, Y. F. Liu, D. R. Springall, T. Cowen, P. M. Dowd, J. M. Polak*, Image Analysis Quantification of Peptide-Immunoreactive Nerves in Skin of Patients with *Raynaud's* Phenomenon and Systemic Sclerosis, J. Pathol. *164*, 245–252 (1991).

[28] *L. L. Vacca-Galloway*, Differential Immunostaining for Substance P in *Huntington's* Diseased and Normal Spinal Cord: Significance of Serial (Optimal, Supra-Optimal and End-Point) Dilutions of Primary Anti-Serum in Comparing Biological Specimens, Histochemistry *83*, 561–569 (1985).

[29] *D. R. Springall, G. Collina, G. Barer, A. J. Suggett, D. Bee, J. M. Polak*, Increased Intracellular Levels of Calcitonin Gene-Related Peptide-Like Immunoreactivity in Pulmonary Endocrine Cells of Hypoxic Rats, J. Pathol. *155*, 259–267 (1988).

[30] *R. H. Benno, L. W. Tucker, T. H. Joh, D. J. Reis DJ*, Quantitative Immunocytochemistry of Tyrosine Hydroxylase in Rat Brain. I. Development of a Computer Assisted Method Using the Peroxidase-Antiperoxidase Technique, Brain Res. *246*, a225–236 (1982).

[31] *R. R. Mize, R. N. Holdefer, L. B. Nabors*, Quantitative Immunocytochemistry Using an Image Analyzer. I. Hardware Evaluation, Image Processing, and Data Analysis, J. Neurosci. Methods *26*, 1–24 (1988).

[32] *J. T. McBride, D. R. Springall, R. J. D. Winter, J. M. Polak*, Quantitative Immunocytochemistry Shows Calcitonin Gene-Related Peptide-Like Immunoreactivity in Lung Neuroendocrine Cells is Increased by Chronic Hypoxia in the Rat, Am. J. Respir. Cell Mol. Biol. *3*, 587–593 (1990).

5.10   Confocal Microscopy

Vyvyan Howard, Arlene Hall and Mark Browne

5.10.1 General Considerations

A large volume of work has been written recently about confocal microscopy. Textbooks on the topic now exist [1, 2]. However, there still appears to be a large proportion of the microscope-using scientific community that remains uninformed about the considerable interest that the technology holds for biologists and material scientists. There have been some excellent review articles [3]. However, the objective of this account is to give an empirical description of the basic concepts behind the confocal microscope and to cite some key references for those who wish to read further [4–8].

The confocal microscope was first conceived over three decades ago. The earliest published account was a patent publication by *Marvin Minsky* [9]. Independently of *Minsky, Petran* and *Hadravsky* [10] were working on a different realization of the microscope. If you had asked any biologist at that time what he would ask of a microscope, he would probably have requested to be able to see living processes and, moreover, in three dimensions. As the confocal microscope can be rather good at both these activities, under the right circumstances, it is a question of some interest to the scientific community as to why it took so long for the technology to develop. It seems that there were three major factors:

1. At the time that *Minsky's* and *Petran's* work was beginning to appear, the electron microscope was emerging as an everyday, commercially available tool. This generated a massive wave of activity which had the effect of eclipsing developments in light microscopy.
2. Light sources of sufficient intensity to drive confocal microscopes were not readily available and were costly. The subsequent appearance of the laser, with virtually unlimited power, greatly accelerated the development of certain forms of confocal microscope.
3. Three-dimensional microscope images produce vast amounts of data. In many configurations the image signal from a detector such as a photomultiplier tube or similar device must be digitized at high speed. Computer technology thirty years ago simply could not cope. The advent of powerful microcomputers, with plentiful, low-cost memory and mass storage devices has been the major breakthrough which has facilitated 3-D image data handling and the explosion of research and development in confocal microscopy since 1984.

5.10.1.1 Conventional Light Microscopy

In the conventional light microscope, the condenser lens gives (with more or less success) a uniform flux of light energy through the specimen. If the specimen is of appreciable thickness the image will be blurred. This is because, in transmission, there will be multiple refractions above and below the plane of focus of the objective lens. The "in focus" information at the focal plane is present but the contrast is low because of the additional information from above and below (cf. Fig. 1). This is why thin sections are in general prepared for conventional light microscopy.

The objective lens, commonly the most expensive element, is frequently highly corrected for chromatic and spherical aberrations and may be specifically designed for use in one of the contrast techniques. A highly corrected imaging system can be said to be diffraction-limited and, as such, its resolving power is constrained by the following relationship [from 11, 12]:

$$d = 1.22\ \lambda/(NA_{obj.} + NA_{cond.}) \tag{a}$$

where d is the minimum distance to which the diffraction images of two points in the specimen can approach one another laterally before they merge and can no longer be separately resolved; λ is the wavelength *in vacuo* of the light used for observation; and $NA_{obj.}$ and $NA_{cond.}$ the numerical apertures (NA) of the objective and condenser lenses, respectively. The NA is the product of the refractive index of the medium between lens and specimen and the sine of the half angle of the cone of light either acceptable by the objective or emitted from the condenser. This relationship can be equally provided with reference to the *Rayleigh* criterion for resolution when the value for d is equal to the radius of the *Airy* disk, which is the first minimum of a unit diffraction pattern. The diffraction pattern can be thought of as a point spread function (PSF), which is ultimately convolved with all image features, and therefore constitutes a fundamental property of a given imaging system. The PSF is the image produced of an infinitely small point in the specimen space. In some forms of microscopy, such as dark field or differential interference contrast, features below the resolution limit can be visualized, but are presented as features described by the unit diffraction pattern.

The axial resolution of a microscope can be related to the "axial setting accuracy" ζ, which is defined as the distance one has to move the fine focus before the image of an infinitely thin object changes perceptibly.

Françon [13] gave the following relation:

$$2\ \zeta = \lambda/(4n \times \sin^2(u/2)) \tag{b}$$

where u is the angle of the half cone of light that is captured by the objective lens. The important thing to note from eqns. (a) and (b) is that axial resolution improves with the square of NA while lateral resolution is related only to the first power of NA.

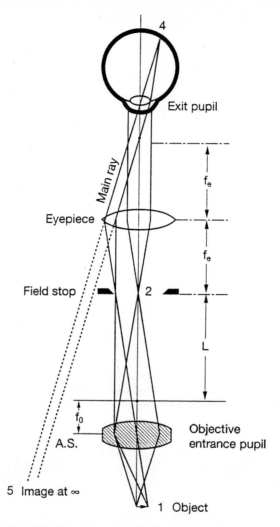

Fig. 1. A schematic representation of the compound light microscope. *fe* is the focal length of the eyepiece, *fo* the focal length of the objective and L the length of the tube.

Object (*1*) is located just outside the focal plane of the objective, *fo*, so a real magnified image is formed at (*2*) and this image becomes the object for the eyepiece. Acting as a magnifier, the eyepiece forms a large virtual image at (*3*). This image then becomes the object for the eye which forms the final real image on the retina (*4*).

a)

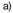
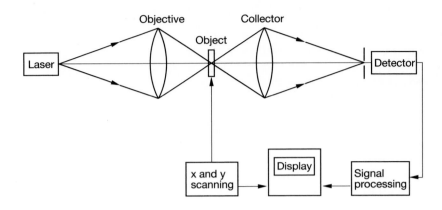

b)

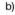
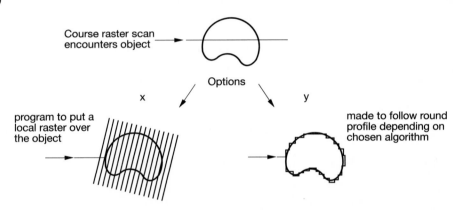

Fig. 2. a) A schematic diagram of the scanning optical microscope. A point source of light is focused by the objective to a spot within the object. b) In this configuration, the object is scanned in x and y as shown in Figure 2b. The detector sends its output to a signal processor which is displayed on a CRT, the position of the display on the CRT is dictated by the position of the xy scan. In this way, a 2-D image is built up as indicated in figure 2b.

5.10.1.2 Scanning Optical Microscopy

Scanning optical microscopes (SOM) exhibit a number of advantages over convention-ally illuminated forms, many of which are shared by video microscopy. However, some features are unique to the techniques in which the specimen is imaged by point-wise illumination in a raster scanning action (Fig. 2).

These include:
- reduction in scatter by virtue of localized illumination;
- variation in magnification can be achieved by control of the scanning raster;
- high sensitivity point detectors, such as photomultiplier tubes, can be used and hence the input energy to the specimen can be minimized;
- complex contrast effects can be achieved with simple equipment.

The first such microscope was developed in 1951 by *Young* and *Roberts*[14] [cf. 13], and used a scanned UV cathode ray tube (CRT) and focusing optics to provide illumination. The brightness of the scanned spot of light was modulated by the specimen and the transmitted beam was detected by a photomultiplier tube and amplified, prior to display, on another CRT scanned synchronously with the source. The inventors were aware of all the potential advantages of the technique, but it took significant technological developments before real exploitation could be achieved, and techniques such as flow cytometry became more important for rapid cell sorting and diagnosis.

5.10.2 Features of Confocal Microscopy

The confocal scanning light microscope (CSLM) can be seen as an extension of the SOM, but one important addition is made with respect to the detector scheme. In a CSLM, the source and detector apertures (the latter of those is known as the "confocal pinhole") are located in conjugate focal planes. By this construction, the detector is preferentially exposed to light emanating from the focal region in the specimen (Fig. 3). It is therefore something of a paradox that the confocal microscope, which is heralded as a 3-D microscope, in fact collects data as a series of thin 2-D "optical sections".

Contrast can be improved by rejection of light from out-of-focus planes, and, by reducing the field of view by scanning, the lateral resolution of the microscope can be improved by a factor of up to 2 [15, 16].

The light is emitted from a high intensity point source. This is often, but by no means always, from a laser. In transmission, the configuration can be likened to two microscopes with a common optical axis, both focused onto a common focal plane.

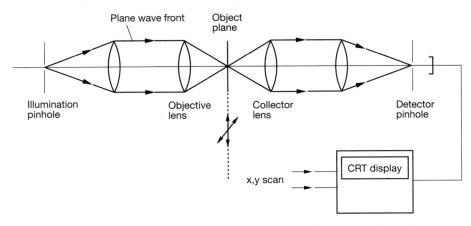

Fig. 3. A plane light wave is brought to a focal point by the objective lens. The collector lens is positioned so that the back-projected image of the detector pinhole exactly coincides with this focal point. The object is scanned mechanically through the common focal point, modulating the light intensity on the detector. The detector signal is amplified and used to produce an image, either by modulating the intensity of a CRT running in synchrony with the object scan or by acting as the input to produce a digital image. Both these techniques have been used and allow some signal processing to be performed on the image. The latter is preferred currently, due to the great propensity of powerful digital computers.

The light spot is imaged by the second microscope at the second pinhole situated at the back focal plane. This acts as a spatial filter, which means that the information above and below the focal plane does not get through the pinhole to any appreciable extent and therefore does not reach the detector, as shown in Figs. 4 and 5. At this stage, therefore, two cones of light are illuminated within the specimen which concentrate at a point at the shared focal plane. To build up a conventional 2-D image, this spot of light has to be scanned in some way. There are at least four ways of achieving this.

a) The specimen can be scanned past the spot on a stage that moves in x and y dimensions.
b) The optical system can be scanned so that the light spot is moved in x and y over the stationary specimen.
c) The focused light beam is scanned through the specimen using galvanic mirrors or similar devices.
d) Many spots of light can be simultaneously scanned across specimen with the use of a *Nipkow* type disc.

Techniques a) and b) are said to be "on axis" configurations, using only the central part of the objective lens. In c) and d) the configuration is "off axis" and here the design of the objective lens is much more critical [17].

It is therefore possible to build up an image point by point which is in effect an "optical section". This is achieved non-invasively. The lateral resolution and the thickness of the optical section (axial resolution) are dictated by the properties of the spot of light that is imaged at the detector. There are three basic factors controlling this, two affecting the actual physical size of the spot within the specimen and the third controlling how much of the spot is imaged at the detector. They are as follows.

a) The wavelength of the light: the shorter this is, the smaller the spot.
b) The NA of the objective lens: the higher this is, the smaller the point.
c) The size of the "confocal" pinhole: the smaller this is, the more restricted the information reaching the detector, particularly in the z axis (cf. Fig. 4).

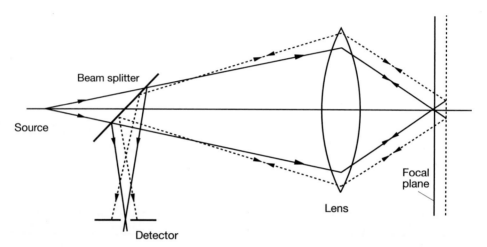

Fig. 4. The confocal microscope in epi-configuration with ray paths showing how light from the focal plane is imaged at the confocal pinhole in front of the detector while light from outside the focal plane is imaged in front (or indeed behind) the confocal pinhole, thus restricting the information appearing in the final image to a narrow focal plane.

To create a 3-D image, multiple optical sections are collected in a perfectly registered stack. Although each individual section is "thin", a projection through the stack leads to an image of a volume whose whole depth is in focus. If the stack is tilted, stereo pairs can be produced. The stack can be tilted physically [18], to produce the best stereo, or sections can be translated before projection to produce a synthetic stereo image.

In addition to conventional x–y scans, x–z or y–z visualization is possible. The arrangement is especially well suited to quantitative studies of the optical properties of the specimen but, to date, it has been primarily the imaging advantages which have been exploited. The price to be paid for confocal detection is a significant reduction in image brightness.

There are three basic forms of CSLM, characterized by the scanning mechanism employed; all offer the potential for various modes of contrast, including reflectance, phase, DIC, polarization and fluorescence. For example, by using split detectors and subtracting the signals electronically, a differential phase contrast image can be produced, which shows significant promise for imaging of birefringent specimens. Simultaneous multimode, epi-fluorescence confocal and conventional transmission imaging have been performed on specimens and the resultant images overlaid from computer stored data showing exact registration and localization of labelled species.

Most microscopes act in a reflective- or epi-mode, since this enables the detected light to traverse the same optical path as the transmitted beam, thereby simplifying de-scanning where necessary, and conjugate focal plane location of the detector. The first type of CSLM is the original form described by *Minsky*. In this instrument, the optical system remains on axis and fixed while the specimen is scanned on some form of mechanical stage. This construction achieves spatially invariant imaging performance and can therefore minimize optical aberrations. However, mechanical scanning may be disadvantageous to biomedical specimens and image formation is relatively slow. The technique has been developed and studied in great detail by *Sheppard* and *Wilson* in Oxford, though for biomedical applications it has been superseded by the beam scanned instruments.

Petran & Hadravsky conceived the second form of confocal microscope without knowledge of *Minsky's* device. The motivation was the study of living, unstained, nervous tissue, in which scatter and glare prevented adequate contrast for visualization in conventional modes. The tandem scanning microscope was thus conceived (cf. Figs. 5 and 6), and represents a direct viewing confocal microscope in which a rapidly spinning

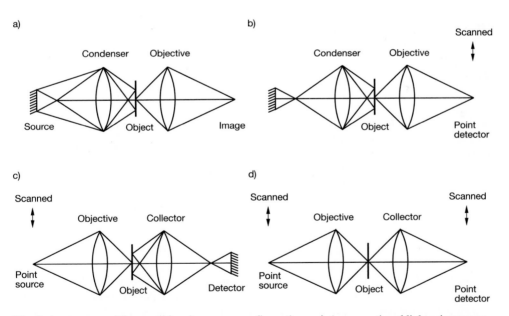

Fig. 5. A summary of the possible microscope configurations. a) A conventional light microscope. b) A conventional condenser illumination with a scanned objective with a point detector. c) The reverse of b) with a scanned point source. d) Confocal scanning configuration where the point source and point detector have to be scanned synchronously.

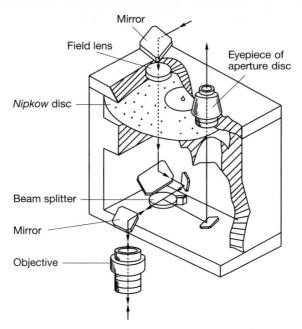

Fig. 6. The Tandem Scanning Reflected Light Microscope. The light beam enters the head *via* a field lens and then traverses one side of the *Nipkow* disc, which is rotating. After two reflections the light passes through a thin beam splitter and is reflected downwards through the objective and into the specimen, the focal plane being illuminated with a pattern of light spots that are moving to give a parallel scan. Reflected or fluorescent light is collected by the objective, reflected by the mirror above the objective, the beam splitter and a final inverting mirror so that the apertures on the input side of the disc are mapped perfectly onto the apertures on the output side. The final image is viewed through a *Ramsden*-type eyepiece which is focused onto the *Nipkow* disc.

Nipkow disk, with holes arranged in *Archimedean* spirals emanating towards its circumference, is broadly illuminated, and scans many spots of light simultaneously through the specimen space, thereby building many images per second (Fig. 7). In this arrangement, the reflected light is optically folded to return through conjugate holes placed symmetrically on the opposite radius of the disk for confocal detection. This image can be directly visualized by the eye, or video detection can be used. Using this microscope, living nervous tissue, hard tissues such as bone and dental enamel, and fluorescently labelled neurones have been observed, quantified and studied in 3-D. The microscope has been extensively exploited by *Boyde* [18] for these and other purposes, and is commercially available.

In the final form of the CSLM the light beam is tightly constrained and scanned or steered, by mirrors or electro-optic beam deflectors, e.g. acousto-optic deflectors (AOD). This form is now preferred by most commercial manufacturers, enabling easy use of laser illumination, fairly rapid image formation, flexibility of scanning, and combination with conventional transmission imaging. Objective performance becomes critical here in the determination of imaging plane characteristics, depth of field and

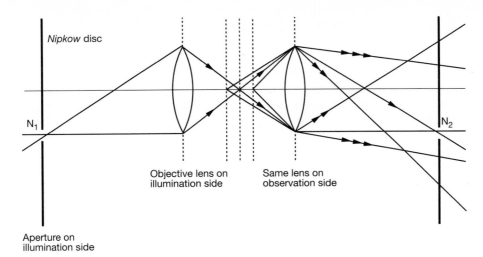

Fig. 7. The *Nipkow* disc arrangement and depth discrimination. Scanning is achieved based on the *Nipkow* disc, the holes in the disc are arranged in several *Archimedian* spirals. The configuration of the microscope is such that the almost hexagonal pattern of holes on the input side of the microscope are mapped onto the conjugate holes of the output side of the of the disc. This is shown in transmission in this figure. Light emanating from aperture N1 will only be imaged at the aperture N2 if the information comes from the focal plane. In fact, in reflectance, the two lenses in the diagram become the same lens and N1 and N2 are congruent holes on opposite sides of the same disc, the right hand side of the diagram representing the reflectance pathway.

chromatic effects. Even though laser illumination is used, when fluorescence imaging is employed, the image is detected at a different wavelength, and any chromatic aberration in the objective can lead to a focal plane mismatch and consequent loss of signal, though this latter point is relevant to all confocal microscopes.

Mirror scanned systems offer image acquisition at one to ten images per second while AODs can at least scan images at up to one hundred per second. Image formation, quality, resolution and contrast are all dependent on the photon fluxes available and each case is considered on its merits. In the case of fluorescence imaging, excessive illumination ($>$ a few mW) can result in photobleaching and, from the point of view of achieving high quality images, it is meaningful only to enhance collection efficiency and fluorophore delivery to target molecules.

5.10.3   Applications of Confocal Microscopy

The primary applications of confocal microscopy to biomedical research are currently in the elucidation of 3-D microstructure and in fluorescence imaging to study cell dynamics and biochemical processes. With regard to the exploitation of confocal microscopy, fluorochromated antibodies provide specific probes for cellular structures. The preparation of such probes and reagents is described elsewhere (cf. 5.3 and Volume 2, 5. See also Vol. 1, 3.4.3). Microstructure is considered both in the sense of morphology of isolated objects, e. g. cells, and in terms of connectivity and relational characteristics of structures such as dendritic processes in neurones and simple networks.

Fluorescent intensity and distribution can be used to quantify and localize the presence of selective, bright markers which can be attached by monoclonal antibodies, specific affinity ligand or covalent bonding to receptors with high specificity even in living cells. Fluorescent chemical indicators now provide measures of the chemical activity of Ca^{2+}, H^+ and Na^+ cations, membrane potential and enzyme activity.

New fluorophores are under development continuously but this is a slow, painstaking process. Two micrographs are shown to illustrate the major advantages of confocal microscopy in immunofluorescence imaging. In Fig. 8 a high power view of dual-

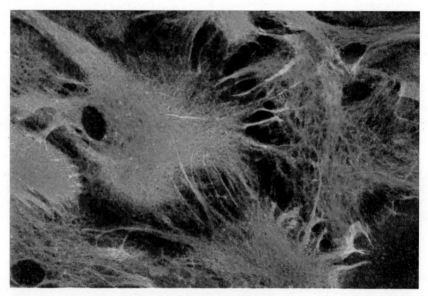

Fig. 8. This shows rat type 1 astrocytes stained with an FITC-conjugated antibody to a surface marker and TRITC antibody biotin-streptavidin to intermediate filaments. Superposition of two single images taken with different dichroic filters. x63 1.4 NA oil immersion lens. Field width 183 μm. (This image was kindly provided by *A Entwistle and P Noble,* Ludwig Institute for Cancer Research, University College, London, UK)

labelled astrocytes shows the increased resolving power of the confocal microscope, many very fine microfilaments being visible. The other noteworthy feature is the lack of "flare" and "image spread" which is inevitable with conventional light microscopy of specimens of any appreciable thickness. Therefore, although these cells are quite deep with respect to the optical section thickness (approx 0.5 µm) it is possible to obtain a clear image.

Fig. 9 illustrates the ability of the confocal microscope to produce 3-D images from intact, though admittedly small, animals. The non invasive nature of optical sectioning means that living specimens can be viewed, provided that non-toxic stains are used. Zero dimensional features such as particle number, spatial distribution and connectivity only make sense in three dimensions. The possibility of monitoring growth of a network in the same developing animal by sequential confocal microscopy should be feasible.

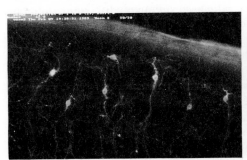 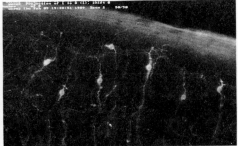

Fig. 9. Stereopair image of serotonergic neurons stained with a standard anti 5-HT streptavidin/biotin/FITC regime in an intact specimen of *Grillotia erinacaceus,* a shark parasite. Imaging was performed with a x20/0.75 NA dry objective. 8 optical sections, separated from one another by 10 µm, were each frame averaged with a *Kalman* filter 50 times before projection through the stack. Field width 300 µm. Field depth 80 µm. (This work was performed in collaboration with *Dr. George McKerr,* Biomedical Science Research Group, University of Ulster at Coleraine, Northern Ireland)

5.10.4 Measurement

There are two main approaches to unbiased 3-D measurement of geometrical features in microscopy:

Firstly, measurements can be made on suitably sampled 2-D images with random geometrical probes. This is the stereological approach [19, 20]. By employing sampling techniques such as these, efficient 3-D measurements of first order statistical properties can be made in conventional as well as confocal microscopy. The techniques can be applied in confocal microscopy either manually [21, 22], semi automatically [23] or, on suitably digitized 2-D images, fully automatically by "digital stereology" [24].

Secondly, confocal microscopy offers an additional possibility of being able to collect and measure a complete 3-D digitized image and analyse it automatically. Some form of objective measurement is necessary in 3-D microscopy. There are considerable problems associated with simply displaying 3-D images [25]. About 10% of the population cannot, for example, appreciate stereo vision from stereo-pair micrographs. Measurement of stereo-pairs is possible by stereophotogrammetry but this is tedious and some measures (typically surface and length) are not available without bias.

Automatic measurement of 3-D images carries with it all the problems associated with 2-D images. The criteria for segmentation are critical and can have a big effect on the result. By examining a small volume in great detail there are the usual problems of ensuring that the sample is representative. However, that is not an argument for not developing automatic 3-D image analysis; rather an argument for good sampling regimes. Efforts have now been made to produce software that will analyse 3-D binary images automatically [26]. Programs have also been produced that will analyse grey level 3-D images [27] and, although the latter study was made on images that were not obtained from a confocal microscope, the approach is directly applicable.

The development of microscopic imaging techniques has been a contributory factor to our understanding of the microstructure and function of most biomedical systems. Video and computer technology, laser scanning and the development of new specific chemical labels are ensuring that the multidisciplinary topic of microscopy will continue to be an important tool for biomedical science. The development of 4-D (x, y, z, time), chemically-sensitive microscopy promises new insights for the coming decades.

References

[1] *T. Wilson* (ed.), Confocal Microscopy, Academic Press, London 1990.
[2] *J. Pawley* (ed.), Handbook of Biological Confocal Microscopy, Plenum, London 1990.
[3] *M. Petran, M. Hadravsky, J. Benes, R. Kucera, A. Boyde*, The Tandem Scanning Reflected Light Microscope, Proc. Roy. Mic. Soc. 20, 125–139 (1985).
[4] *H. C. Claussen*, Mikroskope, in: *S. Fluegge* (ed.), Encyclopedia of Physics, Vol. 29, Springer-Verlag, Heidelberg 1967, pp. 343–425.
[5] *S. Inoue*, Video Microscopy, Plenum, New York 1986.
[6] *R. Mc. Jones*, Basic Microscopic Technics, University of Chicago Press, Chicago 1966.
[7] *M. Pluta*, Advanced Light Microscopy: Specialised Methods, Vol. 2, Elsevier, Warszawa 1989.
[8] *K. F. A. Ross*, Phase Contrast and Interference Microscopy for Cell Biologists, Arnold, London 1967.
[9] *M. Minsky*, Microscopy Apparatus, US Patent No. 3,013,467. Filed 7 November 1957.
[10] *M. Petran, M. Hadravsky, D. Egger, R. Galambos*, Tandem Scanning Reflected Light Microscope, J. Opt. Soc. Am. 58, 661–664 (1968).
[11] *E. Abbe*, Beiträge zur Theorie des Mikroskops und der mikroskopischen Wahrnehmung, Schultzes Archiv f. mikr. Anat. 9, 413–451 (1873).

[12] *E. Abbe*, Note on the Proper Definition of the Amplifying Power of a Lens or Lens-system, J. Roy. Microsc. Soc. *4*, 348–351 (1884).

[13] *M. Francon*, Progress in Microscopy, Row, Peterson, Evanson, Illinois 1961.

[14] *J. Z. Young, F. Roberts*, A Flying-spot Microscope, Nature *167*, 231 (1951).

[15] *G. Tolardo di Francia*, Resolving Power and Information, J. Opt. Soc. Am. *45*, 497–501 (1955).

[16] *E. Ingelstam*, Different Forms of Optical Information and Some Interrelations Between Them, Istituto Nazionale di Ottica, Arecetri-Firenze 1956, pp. 128–143.

[17] *C. J. Cogswell, C. J. R. Sheppard, M. C. Moss, C. V. Howard*, A Method for Evaluating Microscope Objectives to Optimize Performance of Confocal Systems, J. Microsc. *158*, 177–185 (1990).

[18] *A. Boyde*, Stereoscopic Images in Confocal (Tandem Scanning) Microscopy, Science *230*, 1270–1272 (1985).

[19] *H. J. G. Gundersen*, Stereology of Arbitrary Particles, J. Microsc. *143*, 3–45 (1986).

[20] *C. V. Howard*, The Confocal Microscope as an Instrument for Measuring Microstructural Geometry, in: *T. Wilson* (ed.), Confocal Microscopy, Academic Press, London 1990, pp. 285–303.

[21] *C. V. Howard, S. Reid, A. Baddeley, A. Boyde*, Unbiased Estimation of Particle Density in the Tandem-scanning Reflected Light Microscope, J. Microsc. *138*, 203–212 (1985).

[22] *A. Baddeley, C. V. Howard, A. Boyde, S. Reid*, Three-dimensional Analysis of the Spatial Distribution of Particles Using the Tandem-scanning Reflected Light Microscope, Acta Stereol. *6*, Suppl. II, 87–100 (1987).

[23] *M. C. Moss, M. A. Browne, C. V. Howard, D. Joyner*, An Interactive Image Analysis System for Mean Particle Volume Estimation Using Stereological Principles, J. Microsc. *156*, 79–90 (1989).

[24] *H. Q. Zhao et al.*, Digital Stereo – A Comparative Study of Digital Stereological Surface Density Estimators, Trans. RMS – Micro *90*, 315–318 (1990).

[25] *M. A. Browne, G. D. Jolleys and D. J. Joyner*, Comparison of surface and volume-based rendering of multislice biomedical images, Proc. Biomedical Processing of S.P.I.E. (1991), p. 1450.

[26] *V. Conan, S. Gesbert, C. V. Howard, D. Jeulin, F. Meyer, D. Renard*, Geostatistical and Morphological Methods Applied to Three-dimensional Microscopy, J. Microsc. *166*, 169–184 (1992).

[27] *P. Bhanu Prasad*, Use of the Shell Correction Method for Quantification of Three-dimensional Digitized Images, Trans RMS – Micro *90*, 297–300 (1990).

5.11   Flow Cytometry

Manfred Kubbies

5.11.1   Principles

Flow cytometry is a rapid, single cell analytical and preparative technique [1, 2]. Cells are hydrodynamically focused in a fluid stream to pass one after another through a laser beam (or through the focus of an arc or xenon lamp). Light scattered from cells or fluorescence emitted by cell-bound fluorochromes is registered by opto-electronic components such as photodiodes and/or photomultipliers. The electronic signals are processed and digitized in analogue/digital converters and transferred to a computer for data recording and analysis.

In principle, flow cytometers consist of: a *fluid system* (cells in suspension, sheath fluid; directs single cells through a laser beam or focus), a *light source* (laser, arc or xenon lamp; fluorochrome excitation and light scattering), *optics* (optical filters; separation of excitation light from emitted fluororescence or scattered light), *electronics* (photomultiplier, photodiodes, electronic amplifier; generation of electronic signal correlated with light intensity), *data acquisition/analysis* (analogue/digital converters, computer hard- or *software; data recording/storage/analysis)* [3].

Because of the rapid signal generation and data recording, up to several thousand cells and from one to six cellular parameters per single cell can be analysed within one second. Parameter acquisition and recording can be logically correlated *via* gating procedures (e. g. if cells show higher forward scatter but lower side scatter then acquire green fluorescence). The data can be stored either in histogram (1D) or cytogram (2D) mode, or list mode format (for subsequent re-analysis). Different phylo- and ontogenetic cellular pro- and eukaryotic cell systems can be analysed; however, the material must always consist of a single cell suspension. Numerous fluorochromes for labelling of various cellular and biochemical components or cell physiological parameters are available [4]. These include: for DNA, bisbenzimide (AT), chromomycin (GC) and propidium iodide; for RNA, acridine orange and pyronin Y; for membrane potential, rhodamine 123 and carbocyanine dyes; for proteins fluorescein, phycoerythrin and Texas red; as calcium probes, Indo-1 and Fluo-3; for pH ADB, BCECF and Snarf-1; for oxidative burst, dichlorofluorescein and dihydrorhodamine; for lipids, labelled lipids and nile red; for viability, propidium iodide and fluorescein diacetate.

In summary, flow cytometry offers several unique advantages: high speed analysis of single cells, multiparameter analysis of single cells, excellent statistics of heterogenous cell systems, objective data evaluation and recording, single or mass cell sorting capabilities.

In the following only analytical methods are described. For preparative applications of flow cytometry see section 4.2.2.5.

5.11.2 Analytical Applications

Flow cytometric analysis can be performed on viable, fixed or detergent treated cells. Depending on the nature of the cells under investigation the following parameters are amenable to analysis: *morphology* (e.g., size, granularity), *nucleic acids* (e.g., DNA-/RNA content, AT/GC ratio, chromatin structure), *proteins* (e.g., total protein content, specific proteins *via* intra-/extracellular Ab labelling), *glycosides* (e.g., lectin binding), *lipids* (e.g., membrane turnover, cell tracking), *functional parameters* (e.g., viability, glutathione, enzymes, drug uptake, cell proliferation/kinetics), *cell activation* (e.g., membrane potential, pH, ion flux, oxidative burst) [1, 2].

Alterations of cellular parameters may indicate pathological processes. Flow cytometric single cell analysis gives valuable diagnostic and/or prognostic factors for various clinical investigations: tumour diagnosis and prognosis (solid tumours and leukaemia: DNA content and cell proliferation), haematological disorders (phenotype analysis in immunodeficiency syndromes, anaemia diagnosis, various haematological diseases), infectious diseases (septic shock, bacteriuria), amongst others.

Phenotype analysis of leucocyte populations is described, although the cytochemical procedures are also applicable to other cell systems. Phenotype analysis is restricted to the use of labelled monoclonal or polyclonal antibodies specific for surface receptors or intracellular epitopes. It should be mentioned, however, that some cellular phenotypes can be evaluated by a number of non-Ab immunofluorescence-based procedures: e.g., different uptake rates of fluorochromes depend on cellular membrane potential (T-cells *vs* B-cells), RNA-content (thrombocytes *vs* reticulocytes), and scatter characteristics (lymphocytes, monocytes, granulocytes).

5.11.2.1 General Aspects

Phenotypes of leucocytes are characterized by lineage-specific receptors (e.g. T-cell, B-cell, monocyte) or activation markers (e.g. IL-2 or transferrin receptor) which are classified *via* the CD-nomenclature (cluster of differentiation or designation) [5]. However, the differentiation of non-leucocyte cells can also be examined (e.g., mesenchymal or epithelial cells: intermediate filaments, vimentin or cytokeratin) [6]. Proliferative activity, assessed by detection of intracellular proliferation markers or oncogene products, is often related to distinct cellular phenotypes (e.g., Ki67, PCNA or c-myc protein in cycling bone-marrow cells or tumour cells) [6–11]. To achieve a more elaborate phenotype analysis, various extra- and/or intracellular markers can be analysed in a multiparametric fashion.

Application of direct fluorochrome-labelled, antigen-specific monoclonal or polyclonal antibodies is called the direct immunofluorescence technique. For multiparametric analysis, each specific antibody must be labelled with a fluorochrome exhibiting a different emission wavelength [12]. In indirect immunofluorescence, the unlabelled, specific first-step antibodies are detected by fluorochrome-labelled second-step reporter molecules: first, mouse-Ab unlabelled, second, anti-mouse Ab-fluorochrome; first, mouse-Ab-biotin, second, streptavidin-fluorochrome; first, mouse-Ab-digoxygenin, second, anti-digoxygenin Ab-fluorochrome. Multiparametric analysis using indirect immunofluorescence is possible by applying either differently labelled first-step antibodies (unlabelled *vs* biotinylated *vs* digoxygeninated) and/or first-step antibodies generated in different species (e. g., mouse, rat, goat, rabbit). The second step reporter molecules must be labelled with different fluorochromes. The most common fluorochromes used in flow cytometry are: FITC (excitation max.: 488 nm, emission max.: 520 nm) and R-phycoerythrin (excitation max.: 495/564 nm, emission max.: 576 nm). Both fluorochromes are routinely excited by the 488 nm line of an argon laser. A full description of fluorescence antibody methods is given in 5.2, 5.3 and 5.4.

For identification of fluorescent labelled haematopoetic cell subpopulations, cell fractions of interest are distinguished by their forward *vs* right angle scatter characteristics (e. g., lymphocytes, monocytes, granulocytes) [13]. In cell lines, intact cells can be differentiated from dead cells by their scatter parameters [14]. Haematopoietic subpopulations are analysed by gating on the scatter cluster of cells and recording of the corresponding cellular immunofluorescence.

Various factors affect phenotype analysis by flow cytometry: technique (alignment of the instrument, instrument stability, etc.), cytochemistry (optimal staining and/or fixation procedure, antibody affinity, specificity and cross-reaction, specimen handling, etc.), and biological and environmental factors. The last comprise factors such as donor age, donor sex, stress, smoking, medication, disease state, time of day, exercise, etc. All factors must be considered carefully in interpreting phenotype analysis and in comparison to established normal control values [15–17]. Guidelines have been published for quality assurance and immunophenotyping of peripheral blood lymphocytes using flow cytometry [18].

5.11.2.2   Analysis of Surface Antigens

Direct immunofluorescence labelling of cells is simple and rapid. However, sensitivity of detection of low numbers of surface markers is lower in comparison to indirect labelling procedures. In addition, indirect immunofluorescence staining provides the opportunity of using a variety of second-step reporter molecules conjugated with different fluorochromes (e. g., testing new or commercially unavailable, unlabelled specific antibodies).

Isolation of lymphocytes by centrifugation on a Ficoll gradient results in loss of most of mono- and granulocytes (cf. section 2.2.2). On the contrary, erythrocyte lysis by an ammonium chloride procedure (see below) avoids loss of these cells which are then accessible for further analysis [19, 20]. Keep media and reagents cold, and perform cell labelling on ice; protect fluorochrome-labelled cells from intense light.

Direct immunofluorescence labelling

1. Use Ficoll-isolated PBL's or cell line cells.
2. Resuspend 1×10^6 cells in 2 ml RPMI1640/10% (v/v) FCS/0.1% (w/v) Na azide.
3. Centrifuge cells at $150 \times g$ for 5 min at 4 °C.
4. Resuspend pellet in 100 µl RPMI1640/10% FCS/0.1% Na azide.
5. Add fluorochrome-conjugated antibody/antibodies according to supplier's recommendation; mix and incubate for 30 min on ice.
6. Repeat steps 2 and 3.
7. Resuspend cell pellet in 1 ml RPMI1640/10% FCS/0.1% Na azide.
8. Analyse cells within 2 hours.

Notes: Instead of RPMI other basic media, PBS or HBSS, can be used. FCS concentration can be decreased to 2% or replaced by 0.1 to 1.0% (w/v) BSA. Incubation time in step 5 may be decreased to 15 min.

Indirect immunofluorescence labelling

1. Perform steps 1–4 of the direct immunofluorescence labelling method.
2. Add unlabelled first antibody according to supplier's recommendation or titrate for optimal antibody concentration; mix and incubate for 30 min on ice.
3. Repeat steps 2, 3 and 4 of the direct method.
4. Add fluorochrome-labelled second antibody (anti-first antibody/ or other reporter molecule (e.g., fluorochrome-labelled streptavidin) according to supplier's information; mix and incubate for 30 min on ice.
5. Repeat steps 2, 3 and 7 of the direct method.
6. Analyse cells within 2 hours.

Notes: See notes for direct method. Perform labelling procedure in PBS/0.1% Na azide in case of biotinylated antibodies (if necessary add 0.1 to 1.0% (w/v) biotin-free BSA to prevent non-specific staining).

Immunofluorescence labelling of PBL before erythrocyte lysis

1. Place 100 µl whole blood in test tube.
2. Add fluorochrome-labelled or unlabelled antibody/antibodies according to supplier's information; mix and incubate for 30 min on ice.
3. Add 3 ml PBS/0.1% Na azide, mix.
4. Centrifuge cells at $150 \times g$ for 5 min at 4 °C.
5. For direct immunofluorescence labelling proceed to step 8. For indirect labelling procedure, resuspend cells in 100 µl PBS/0.1% Na azide.
6. Add second-step antibody or reporter molecule according to supplier's information; mix and incubate for 30 min on ice.

7. Repeat steps 3 and 4.
8. Add 5–10 ml 1 × ammonium chloride lysis solution (20 °C; see below); mix and incubate for 3–5 min at room temperature.
9. Centrifuge cells at 150 × g for 5–10 min at 4 °C.
10. Repeat steps 3 and 4.
11. Resuspend cells in 1 ml RPMI1640/10% FCS/0.1% Na azide.
12. Analyse cells within 2 hours.

Notes: See indirect immunofluorescence labelling procedure. 10 × ammonium chloride lysis solution: dissolve 8.29 g. NH_4Cl, 1.09 g $KHCO_3$ and 37.0 mg Na_2 EDTA in 100 ml distilled water. Prepare 1 × solution by dilution in distilled water (check pH 7.2–7.4; filter solution; use within one week; keep solution at room temperature). Increasing time of exposure to ammonium chloride before centrifugation may alter subpopulation distribution due to cell death and differential loss.

Immunofluorescence labelling of PBL after erythrocyte lysis

1. Add 10 ml 1 × ammonium chloride lysis solution at room temperature to test tube.
2. Add 0.2–0.5 ml whole blood; mix and incubate for 3–5 min at room temperature.
3. Perform steps 9, 3 and 4 of the method for labelling before lysis (above).
4. Resuspend pellet in 100 µl ice-cold RPMI1640/10% FCS/0.1% Na azide.
5. For direct immunofluorescence labelling repeat steps 5–7 of the direct immunofluorescence protocol. For indirect immunofluorescence labelling repeat steps 2–5 of the indirect immunofluorescence protocol.
6. Analyse cells within 2 hours.

Notes: See notes of other labelling procedures.

Controls

In addition to daily instrument control and alignment, antibody controls must be chosen carefully to allow interpretation of results [21]. Minimum controls required are: 1. unstained, autofluorescent cells; 2. cells labelled with second-step reporter molecule; 3. labelling of cells with an irrelevant isotype-matched antibody (fluorochrome-labelled or unlabelled). Fluorescence gates for discriminating negative from positive cells should be adjusted according the control tests allowing for 0.1 to 1.0% unspecific positive cells.

Multi-colour immunofluorescence: spectral overlap and compensation

Different fluorochromes show distinct excitation maxima but most emission spectra overlap. Although narrow bandpass filters decrease recording of spectral overlap, there is inevitable fluorescence cross-talk. Electronic compensation is required according to the quantitative contribution of the unwanted cross-talk signals in photomultipliers. For example, more cross-talk signal is typically present in the PE-channel from emitted FITC fluorescence in comparison to the PE-fluorescence cross-talk into the FITC-channel. Electronic compensation between one or two pairs of photomultipliers might be required in cases of two- or three-colour analysis [22].

For minimum fluorescence cross-talk, antibody fluorochrome labels should be chosen carefully. Abundant receptors should be labelled with fluorochromes (e. g. PE) showing less spectral overlap into other fluorescence channels. Conversely, use FITC for lower receptor numbers. Dual colour labelled samples may be compensated directly. However, two single-colour labelled control samples should be used for adjustment of electronic compensation: the negative and positive populations should be aligned parallel to the X-axis and Y-axis of the cytogram, respectively. Electronic compensation needs re-adjustment if samples show significantly different fluorescence intensities. Software programs provided by manufacturers of flow cytometers handle these problems automatically.

Viability staining of antibody-labelled cells

After labelling, the viability of cells should be confirmed. A viability greater than 90% is desirable. This may be done: a) microscopically by trypan blue staining (cf. section 2.1), b) flow-cytometrically (1 µg propidium iodide per ml for 1 min; dead cells fluoresce red at 488 nm excitation; viable cells show autofluorescence only).

To improve analysis add 1 µg propidium iodide per ml to the stained sample. Gate on cells of interest, and on propidium iodide-negative (viable) cells, and record immuno-fluorescence from cells within both gates [23].

Paraformaldehyde fixation of labelled cells

If fixed, cells can be kept for several days before analysis. The most common procedure is paraformaldehyde fixation which preserves cell morphology satisfactorily [19].
1. Centrifuge labelled cells at $150 \times g$ for 5 min at 4 °C.
2. Resuspend $1-3 \times 10^6$ cells in 100 µl ice-cold PBS.
3. Vortex cells and add dropwise 1 ml of 0.5% paraformaldehyde solution (see below).
4. Fix cells for 1–4 h at 4 °C.
5. Repeat step 1.
6. Resuspend cells in 1 ml ice-cold PBS.
7. Analyse cells; alternatively cells may be analysed after step 4.

Notes: Paraformaldehyde fixed cells may be stored for up to 4 weeks without significant loss of fluorescence and alteration of cell morphology. Prepare 10% (w/v) paraformaldehyde stock solution (20 ×): disolve 10 g paraformaldehyde in 100 ml PBS, adjust to pH 7.4, and filter through 0.45 µm filter. Keep solution in the refrigerator in the dark. For use, dilute paraformaldehyde stock in PBS, and filter again through 0.45 µm filter to avoid contamination by paraformaldehyde crystals. Always use fresh 0.5% paraformaldehyde fixative. Determine the stability of different cell preparations to prolonged storage by experiment.

Blocking nonspecific Ig-binding

Nonspecific binding of antibodies to lymphocytes or other cells by Fc-receptors results in false positive staining of cells. The procedure described below minimizes this nonspecific binding effect.
1. Wash 1×10^6 cells (isolated PBLs or cell line cells) in 1 ml PBS/0.1% Na azide at room temperature.
2. Resuspend pellet in 100 µl PBS/0.1% Na azide supplemented with 5–20% normal rabbit, human or goat serum.
3. Incubate for 30 min at room temperature.
4. Cool cells on ice and add specific antibody(ies) according to direct or indirect immunofluorescence labelling procedure. Proceed as indicated in protocols.

Some pitfalls in immunofluorescence labelling

1. Preferably use fluorochrome-labelled F(ab) or F(ab)₂ antibody fragments for immunostaining to avoid nonspecific Fc-receptor binding (or block nonspecific Ig-binding sites, cf. above).
2. Antibodies conjugated with phycoerythrin may need longer incubation times for maximum binding.
3. In the case of different, unlabelled, antigen-specific antibodies from different animals, check cross-reactivity of anti-species specific, fluorochrome-labelled second antibody.
4. Staining of cells might alter their scatter characteristics; therefore check whether cells are still located in scatter gate.
5. Activation of cells might alter surface receptor density.

5.11.2.3 Analysis of Intracellular Antigens

Fixation procedures

Detection of intracellular antigens requires fixation of cells before their exposure to antibody. Two principal fixation protocols exist: a) fixation using denaturing alcohols, b) fixation using cross-linking fixatives (e. g., paraformaldehyde) with subsequent detergent treatment [9–11].

Alcohol fixation
1. Wash 1×10^6 cells once in 2 ml cold PBS.
2. Resuspend pellet in 300 µl cold PBS, vortex-mix cells and add dropwise 700 µl absolute ethanol or methanol.
3. Incubate for at least 1 h at -20 °C.
4. Centrifuge cells at $150 \times g$ for 5 min at 4 °C.
5. Resuspend cells in 100 µl PBS/10% FCS (4 °C).

Paraformaldehyde fixation
1. Wash 1×10^6 cells once in 2 ml cold PBS.
2. Resuspend pellet in 50–100 µl PBS, vortex-mix cells and add 1 ml 1% paraformaldehyde (4 °C).
3. Incubate for at least 1 h at 4 °C.
4. Centrifuge cells at $150 \times g$ for 5 min at 4 °C.
5. Resuspend pellet in 1 ml PBS/0.1% Triton X100 (or 0.1% NP40 or 0.5% Saponin) on ice for 15 min (mix two or three times).
6. Repeat step 4.
7. Resuspend pellet in 100 µl PBS/10% FCS (4 °C).

Notes: Vortex cells during addition of fixative to avoid cell clumping. Optimal fixative and non-ionic detergent concentrations and treatment duration might vary slightly for different cell types and should be established empirically [9–11].

Direct immunofluorescence

1. Add direct labelled antibody to fixed cell suspension (cf. above).
2. Incubate for 1 h on ice; keep cells in the dark.
3. Add 2 ml PBS/10% FCS, mix and centrifuge at $150 \times g$ for 5 min at 4 °C.
4. Repeat step 3.
5. Resuspend cells in 1 ml PBS/10% FCS.
6. Analyse cells.

Note: Refer to direct immunofluorescence surface staining method.

Indirect immunofluorescence

1. Add unlabelled antibody to fixed cell suspension (see above).
2. Incubate for 1 h on ice, keep cells in the dark.
3. Add 2 ml PBS/10% FCS, mix and centrifuge cells at 150 $\times$ g for 5 min at 4 °C.
4. Resuspend cell pellet in 100 µl PBS/10% FCS, and add fluorochrome-labelled second antibody.
5. Incubate for 30 to 60 min (FITC-F(ab)$_2$ or PE-F(ab)$_2$) on ice; keep cells in the dark.
6. Repeat step 3.
7. Resuspend pellet in 1 ml PBS/10% FCS.
8. Analyse cells.

Note: Refer to indirect immunofluorescence surface staining, and direct immunofluorescence labelling intracellular antigens.

5.11.2.4   Cell Proliferation and Cell Activation

Subpopulation-specific cell cycle analysis

1. Use 1×10^6 intracellular antigen labelled or surface-marker labelled, paraformaldehyde-fixed cells. Resuspend cells in cold PBS, add Tween 20 to a final concentration of 0.01% (v/v), and mix.
2. In the case of FITC-labelled cells add per ml 10–20 µg propidium iodide and 10 *Kunitz* units* RNase A, and incubate for at least 2 h at 4 °C in the dark. Analyse cells (488 nm excitation: propidium iodide (DNA cell cycle) and FITC (immunofluorescence)) [10].
3. In the case of FITC/phycoerythrin labelled cells, add per ml 10 µg 7-aminoactinomycin D (7-AAD) [24, 25] and 10 *Kunitz* units RNaseA, and incubate for at least 2 h at 4 °C in the dark. Analyse cells (488 nm excitation: 7-AAD (DNA cell cycle) and FITC/PE (immunofluorescence)).

Note: Check through a control assay (antibody staining only) that the mild detergent treatment has not removed antibody. Increased incubation time for DNA staining is required in fixed cells (possibly overnight incubation in paraformaldehyde-fixed populations).

---

* *Kunitz* unit is that amount of enzyme, which at 25 °C produces an increase in the absorbance of 0.001 per min with DNA as the substrate.

Subpopulation specific Ca^{2+} flux analysis

1. Use isolated leucocytes (whole blood erythrocyte lysis), Ficoll-isolated PBLs or permanent cell line cells. Resuspend cells in RPMI1640/10% FCS.
2. Load 5×10^6 cells/ml with indo-1 AM, 3 µmol/l, (Ca^{2+}-sensitive fluorochrome) for 45 min at 37 °C.
3. Centrifuge cells at $150 \times g$ for 5 min at room temperature.
4. Perform cell surface immunofluorescence staining as described above. Attention: perform staining without Na azide at room temperature.
5. Resuspend cells at 1×10^6 cells/ml in RPMI1640/10% FCS; keep cells at 20 °C and raise temperature to 37 °C before Ca^{2+} flux analysis.
6. Analyse cells within 2–3 hours.

Note: Do not use Na azide (cell membrane leaks Ca^{2+} ions; if necessary, dialyse antibodies). Do not resuspend cells in Ca^{2+}/Mg^{2+}-free PBS if extracellular Ca^{2+}-flux is to be studied. Because labelling might alter activation response [26, 27] use negative gating procedure: label all cells, except the population of interest, with antibodies, and gate for indo-1 fluorescence on unlabelled population.

References

[1] *M. R. Melamed, T. Lindmo, M. L. Mendelsohn*, Flow Cytometry and Sorting, 2nd. Ed., Wiley-Liss, New York 1990.
[2] *H. M. Shapiro*, Practical Flow Cytometry, 2nd Ed., Alan R. Liss, New York 1988.
[3] *M. A. Van Dilla, P. N. Dean, O. D. Laerum, M. R. Melamed*, Flow Cytometry: Instrumentation and Data Analysis, Academic Press, London 1985.
[4] *A. S. Waggoner*, Fluorescent Probes for Cytometry, in: *M. R. Melamed, T. Lindmo, M. L. Mendelsohn* (eds.), Flow Cytometry and Sorting, Wiley-Liss, New York 1990, pp. 209–226.
[5] *W. Knapp, B. Dörken, P. Rieber, R. E. Schmidt, H. Stein, A. E. G. Kr. von dem Borne*, CD Antigens 1989, Blood *74*, 1448–1450 (1989).
[6] *J. T. Bijman, D. J. T. Wagener, J. M. C. Wessels, P. van den Broek, F. C. S. Ramaekers*, Cell Size, DNA, and Cytokeratin Analysis of Human Head and Neck Tumors by Flow Cytometry, Cytometry *7*, 76–81 (1986).
[7] *D. R. Van Boeckstaele, J. Lan, H. W. Snoeck, M. L. Korthout, R. F. De Bock, M. E. Peetermans*, Abberant Ki-67 Expression in Normal Bone Marrow Revealed by Multiparameter Flow Cytometric Analysis, Cytometry *12*, 50–63 (1991)
[8] *G. Landberg, E. M. Tan, G. Roos*, Flow Cytometric Multiparameter Analysis of Proliferating Cell Nuclear Antigen/Cyclin and Ki-67 Antigen: A New View of the Cell Cycle, Exp. Cell Res. *187*, 111–118 (1990).
[9] *C. V. Clevenger, K. D. Bauer, A. L. Epstein*, A Method for Simultaneous Nuclear Immunofluorescence and DNA Content Quantitation Using Monoclonal Antibodies and Flow Cytometry, Cytometry *6*, 208–214 (1985).
[10] *H. Holte, T. Stokke, E. Smeland, R. Watt, H. K. Blomhoff, O. Kallhus, R. Ohlsson*, Levels of myc Protein as Analyzed by Flow Cytometry Correlate with Cell Growth Potential in Malignant B-cell Lymphomas, Int. J. Cancer *43*, 164–170 (1989).
[11] *C. C. Stewart*, Flow Cytometric Analysis of Oncogene Expression in Human Neoplasias, Arch. Pathol. Lab. Med. *113*, 634–640 (1989).

[12] R. Festin, A. Björkland, T. H. Tötterman, Single Laser Flow Cytometric Detection of
      Lymphocyte Binding Three Antibodies Labelled with Fluorescein, Phycoerythrin and a
      Novel Tandem Fluorochrome Conjugate, J. Immunol. Methods 126, 69–78 (1990).
[13] L. W. M. M. Terstappen, R. A. Mickaels, R. Dost, M. L. Loken, Increased Light Scattering
      Resolution Facilitates Multidimensional Flow Cytometric Analysis, Cytometry 11, 506–512
      (1990).
[14] B. Goller, Cloning Cells with a Cell Sorter, in: J. H. Peters, H. Baumgarten (eds.), Monoclonal
      Antibodies, Springer Verlag, Heidelberg – New York 1992, pp. 206–210.
[15] C. W. Caldwell, J. Maggi, L. B. Henry, H. M. Taylor, Fluorescence Intensity as a Quality
      Control Parameter in Clinical Flow Cytometry, Am. J. Clin. Pathol. 88, 447–456 (1987).
[16] R. C. McCarthy, T. J. Fetterhoff, Issues for Quality Assurance in Clinical Flow Cytometry,
      Arch. Pathol. Lab. Med. 113, 658–666 (1989).
[17] J. P. McCoy, J. L. Carey, J. R. Krause, Quality Control in Flow Cytometry for Diagnostic
      Pathology: I. Cell Surface Phenotyping and General Laboratory Procedures, Am. J. Clin.
      Pathol. 93, 27–37, 1990.
[18] A. Landay, Clinical Applications of Flow Cytometry: Quality Assurance and Immunophe-
      notyping of Peripheral Blood Lymphocytes, NCCLS Document H42-P 9, 765–849 (1989).
[19] A. L. Jackson, N. L. Warner, Preparation, Staining, and Analysis by Flow Cytometry of
      Peripheral Blood Leukocytes, in: N. R. Rose, H. Friedman, J. C. Fahey (eds.), Manual of
      Clinical Laboratory Immunology, American Microbiological Association, Washington D.C.
      1986, pp. 226–235.
[20] L. M. Ashmore, G. M. Shopp, B. S. Edwards, Lymphocyte Subset Analysis by Flow
      Cytometry, J. Immunol. Methods 118, 209–215 (1989).
[21] P. K. Horan, K. A. Muirhead, S. E. Slezak, Standards and Controls in Flow Cytometry, in: M.
      R. Melamed, T. Lindmo, M. L. Mendelsohn (eds.), Flow Cytometry and Sorting, Wiley-Liss,
      New York 1990, pp. 397–414.
[22] M. R. Loken, Immunofluorescence Techniques, in: M. R. Melamed, T. Lindmo, M. L.
      Mendelsohn (eds.), Flow Cytometry and Sorting, Wiley-Liss, New York 1990, pp.
      397–414.
[23] M. G. Wing, A. M. P. Montgomery, J. V. Watson, An Improved Method for the Detection of
      Cell Surface Antigens in Samples of Low Viability Using Flow Cytometry, J. Immunol.
      Methods 126, 21–27 (1990).
[24] P. S. Rabinovitch, R. M. Torres, D. Engel, Simultaneous Cell Cycle Analysis and Two-Color
      Surface Immunofluorescence using 7-Aminoactinomycin D and Single Laser Excitation:
      Applications to Study of Cell Activation and the Cell Cycle of Murine LY-1 B-Cells, J.
      Immunol. 136, 2769–2775 (1986).
[25] M. Kubbies, High Resolution Cell Cycle Analysis: The Flow Cytometric Bromodeoxyuridine
      – Hoechst Quenching Technique, in: A. Radbruch (ed.), Flow Cytometry and Cell Sorting,
      Springer Verlag, Berlin 1992, pp. 75–85.
[26] P. S. Rabinovitch, C. H. June, A. Grossmann, J. A. Ledbetter, Heterogeneity of T Cell
      Intracellular Free Calcium Responses After Mitogen Stimulation with PHA or Anti-CD3:
      Use of Indo-1 and Simultaneous Immunofluorescence with Flow Cytometry, J. Immunol. 137,
      952–961 (1986).
[27] M. Kubbies, Indo-1 Ratiometric Analysis of Intracellular Ionized Calcium, in: A. Radbruch
      (ed.), Flow Cytometry and Cell Sorting, Springer Verlag, Berlin 1992, pp. 89–99.
[28] W. Mc Lean Grapen, J. M. Collens, Guide to Flow Cytometric Method, Marcel Libber, New
      York 1990, pp. 138–153.

6 Application of Phenotype Analysis

6.1   Immunological Detection of Membrane-Bound Antigens and Receptors

Philippe Poncelet, Françoise George and Thierry Lavabre-Bertrand

6.1.1   General

A cell phenotype may be defined at the three fundamentally different levels of genetic, immunological and functional organization. Likewise, the genetic information in cellular DNA is transformed into biological phenomena through the use of cell-surface molecules. This emphasizes the crucial role of the cell membrane and its associated receptors as the interface for the interactions of cells with their environment made up of other cells, the extracellular matrix, soluble substances, etc. Methods for immunological detection of surface molecules were initially developed to classify cell types and subtypes but can also enable an explanation of biological phenomena on a molecular basis.

In using immunological methods to detect membrane-bound molecules, the aim, in the first place, is to localize or enumerate a given cell type, possibly its relation to a function; then cell-surface molecules represent differentiation antigens, used as markers to which to attach antibodies. In the second place, these molecules are effectors of biological function whose level of expression may well be related to the intensity of the function.

6.1.2   Technical Considerations

As a consequence of the advent of monoclonal antibody technology [1], numerous immunological methods have been developed for phenotype analysis of cells and tissues. Before considering their applications, it is important to compare their characteristics to optimize the technical choice according to the expected response. Fundamental scientists will look for the most precise and complete information, whereas clinical applications may require time- and cost-effective tests. As can be seen in Table 1, some of these methods are directed to the detection of cell-surface rather

Table 1. Characteristic features of the main technological approaches applied for immunological detection of cell-surface antigens and receptors. Capital letters (S or I) suggest major frequency, small letters (s or i) minor frequency of reactions.

Characteristic features		Surface (S) Intracellular (I)	Quantitative (Yes or No)	Mass (M) Individual cells (I)	Architecture (Yes or No)	Morphology (Yes or No)
Methods	*Detection system*					
RIA	Radioactivity	S + I	Y	M	N	N
Immunoprecipitation	Radioactivity	S + I	N	M	N	N
Histo-autoradiography	Radioactivity	S + I	N/Y	I	N	Y
Complement dependent cytotoxicity	Radioactivity	S	N	M	N	N
Cell mediated cytotoxicity	Radioactivity	S	N	M	N	N
Immunocytology	Fluorescence	S + I	N	I	N	Y
Immunohistology	Fluorescence	S + I	N	I	Y	Y
Imagecytometry	Fluorescence	S + I	Y	I	Y	Y
Flowcytometry	Fluorescence	S + I	Y	I	N	N
Immunocytology	Enzymology	S + I	N	I	N	Y
Immunohistology	Enzymology	S + I	N	I	Y	Y
ELISA	Enzymology	S + I	Y	M	N	N
Immuno-gold/ electron microscopy	Micro/nano particles	S	N	I	Y	Y
Immunomagnetic separation	Micro/nano particles	S	N	I	N	Y
Red cell rosetting	Micro/nano particles	S	N	I	N	Y

than intracellular Ag. This is the case with, for example, cell-mediated reactions (mixed lymphocyte reaction, cytotoxicity) which indirectly reflect the presence of histocompatibility Ags. This is also the case for both analytical and preparative methods using antibody-coated micro-particles. In contrast, when immunocytochemistry deals with sections of tissues, it is thus more concerned with intracellular structures. Some important applications of immunocytochemistry will be illustrated in the subsequent sections.

Methods analysing individual cells can be applied to heterogeneous cell preparations, whereas mass detection methods require purified cell preparations or will provide only crude information on the population at large.

On the one hand, immunohistological methods only may reflect architectural organization between cells, an invaluable parameter for certain applications; on the other hand, morphological features are most often defined without generating quantitative data. Image cytometry, especially using fluorescence, will potentially associate both features, but up to now limited access to such a technology has impaired its applicability.

Several authors [2–6] have stressed that quantitation of membrane-bound Ags and receptors should be emphasized and developed both for fundamental research and clinical applications. In reviewing the main applications of immunological phenotype analysis the feasability and potential interest of the "quantitative immune phenotype" concept will be illustrated. This concept corresponds to the expression of the absolute number of receptors or Ag sites per cell that can also be referred to as "antigen density".

The technological problem of how to determine this absolute number of sites per cell should be considered first. Thermodynamic studies of receptor-ligand interactions using radiolabelled ligands or mAbs offer the classical means of measuring the number of bound molecules per cell or per gram of tissue [7]. This methodology is limited by at least two constraints: first, the use of radioactive compounds and second, the need for purified homogeneous target-cell populations. Radioactivity can be replaced by enzyme-mediated absorbance in a cell ELISA [8, 9]. Both limitations have recently been overcome in a new concept of cell-surface oriented sandwich ELISA [10]. In such a way, a defined cell subset, previously captured on an antibody-coated solid phase, is assayed for the level of expression of a selected membrane Ag. This new type of test responds to the need of more quantitative information (cf. 5.8) by combining biochemistry with cytology.

Fig. 1. Quantitation of cell-surface antigens using the QIFI assay. Calibrated cell lines (CEM) or ▶ bead standards (QIFIKIT^{TM}, *Biocytex,* Marseille) are used to construct an internal standard curve relating the corrected mean fluorescence intensity (M_o, lower histogram) with the mean number of mAb molecules bound per cell. Assuming monovalent binding, this standardization leads to a new abscissa, expressed in number of sites per cell (antigen density, upper histogram). In the present example, the CD4 molecule has been quantitated on positive lymphocytes, with a mean density of 51,000 sites per cell [96].

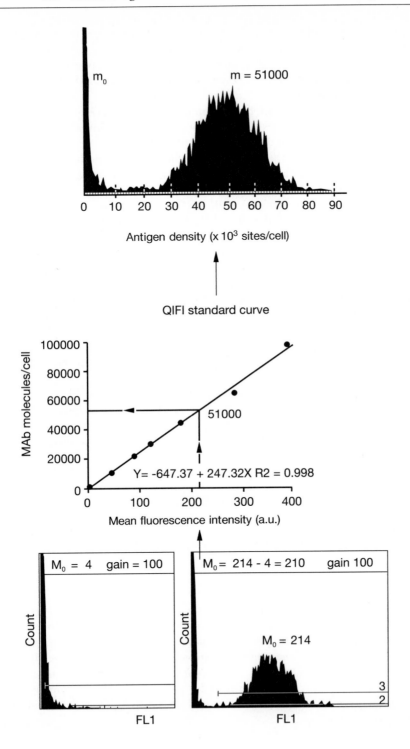

m_0

m = 51000

Antigen density (x 10^3 sites/cell)

QIFI standard curve

MAb molecules/cell

51000

Y= -647.37 + 247.32X R2 = 0.998

Mean fluorescence intensity (a.u.)

$M_0 = 4$ gain = 100

$M_0 = 214 - 4 = 210$ gain 100

$M_0 = 214$

Count

Count

FL1

FL1

Clinically useful information can be obtained by measurement of soluble molecules, originating from cell membranes, such as differentiation Ags, activation Ags or adhesion receptors [11–14]. Ultimately, membrane Ag may be extracted from the cell surfaces and quantitated in the same way as are soluble molecules [8, 15, 16]. However, these are all mass techniques.

More refined information can be obtained by combining measurements of cell-surface density and percent of positive cells using quantitative flow cytometry in which a fluorescent signal from a bound mAb is related to Ag density (Fig. 1).

In the QIFI assay (Quantitative Immuno-Fluorescence Indirect assay), internal standards are used to relate the mean fluorescence intensity calculated from flow cytometry histograms to the mean number of antibody molecules bound per cell. The standards were originally made of cell lines [17, 18], but more recently, a series of micro-bead standards has been developed (QIFIKIT^{TM}, *Biocytex,* Marseille, France). Since, under saturating conditions, mAbs are likely to bind to cell-surface antigens through monovalent interaction, the epitope density or number of antigenic sites per cell can be inferred from the amount of bound mAb. The QIFI assay can be used with any crude source of mAb such as those utilized during workshop studies [18, 19]. Alternatively, if fluorescent mAb conjugate sources are available for use in direct fluorescence protocols, appropriate standards (*Flow Cytometry Standards Corporation,* Research Triangle Park, N. C., USA) and protocols also permit quantitation of binding of mAbs to cell subpopulations [20–25]. Thus the precise definition of cell-surface antigen density on an absolute basis has become an accessible approach which can be applied routinely by flow cytometry.

The field of immunological cell-surface phenotype applications is so wide that it is obviously impossible to cover it comprehensively. Valuable reviews have been published elsewhere [26–33] so here the aim is to illustrate how quantitative approaches may often complement the more classical methods of qualitative phenotype analysis.

6.1.3   Basic Research Applications

Aside from immunology, other domains including haematology, oncology, infection studies, pharmacology, neurology and cell biology in general have gained invaluable information from cell surface phenotype analysis. The appropriate methods were originally developed to answer basic questions about cell and tissue distribution, development and differentiation, genetic origins and regulation, and mechanisms of biological processes, as can be illustrated by the research on human leucocyte differentiation Ags co-ordinated in several successive international workshops [34–39].

6.1.3.1   Cell and Tissue Distribution of Antigens

In this international effort, any new Ag, identified by mAbs, was first defined by its cell and tissue distribution. This was tested on an extended panel of cell lines and samples using flow cytometry as the common method to determine the percentage of positive cells as the main parameter; this served to compare mAbs and assemble them into clusters of differentiation (CDs), which are groups of mAbs with similar binding properties and corresponding to the various human leucocyte Ags [34]. For such computer-assisted clustering analysis, Ag density was found to be a useful parameter [18]. Whereas all of the homogeneous cell samples tested scored 90–100% for all reactive mAbs, quantitative evaluation of binding levels could clearly discriminate between mAbs recognizing a mean of "n" molecules per cell from those reacting with a different Ag expressed at a higher density, say "2.5 × n" molecules per cell. The power of these complementary data has been experienced many times [18, 19, 40, 41] and it also underlines the heterogeneity among established CDs such as CD9 [42].

In addition to flow cytometry (FCM) analysis, immunocytochemistry is important to confirm a precise cluster analysis on the basis of tissue distribution; although this more descriptive method does not currently provide quantitative data, it can reveal functional roles from the architectural organization of cell types in specialized tissues [32, 43].

Although initially cell-lineage or cell-subset specific Ags were preferentially sought [27, 28, 44], differentiation schemes have recently evolved towards a more quantitative analysis, thus obtaining information about molecules as poorly specific as CD45, a pan-leucocyte Ag. In bone marrow, for example, the density of this ubiquitous molecule increases with maturation [45]. Most progenitors display a 5–10 times lower level than mature lymphocytes. On the other hand, some Ags decline with maturation: transferrin receptor, whose maximal level is found on erythroblasts, decreases with reticulocyte maturation, being undetectable on mature red blood cells [46]. Also, the density of CD24 expression distinguishes between pre-B (CD24^{++}) and mature B-cells (CD24^{+}) as shown by *Duperray* et al. [47]. Such information should be refined by defining absolute density values. For normal mature lymphocytes, CD45 levels are around 190000 ± 15000 molecules per cell [48]. For CD24, *Lavabre-Bertrand* [49] recently measured high densities on immature B-cells (240000 molecules per cell) such as fetal liver or fetal bone marrow B-cells and lower densities (40000 molecules per cell) on mature blood B-cells.

Phylogenetic studies may take advantage of phenotype analysis. The first homologies were made between human T1 and murine Lyt 1 molecules, or human T8 (CD8) and the murine Lyt 2,3 complex, according to Ag distribution profiles on blood, splenic and lymph node lymphocytes [50]. Studies of CD4 in various species, and especially monkeys, have provided comparative information on conserved and variable epitopes [51, 52]. NK cell-related molecules have been characterized in species like sea urchins quite distant from mammals [53].

6.1.3.2   Biochemistry of Antigens

Various techniques of immunological detection are involved in the biochemical characterization of cell-surface molecules. Whereas immunoprecipitation and Western-blot methods elucidate antigen size, molecular weight and polymerism, mAb-binding assays are needed to study potential enzymatic cleavages and thus define precisely the nature of the Ag (i.e. protein, glycoprotein, glycolipid, etc.), the type of membrane insertion (transmembrane, phospho-inositol anchor, etc.) [54–56]. They serve to reveal Ag fate through description and kinetic studies of movements such as clustering, patching or capping, and internalization processes such as pinocytosis or endocytosis, as well as later re-expression. Modulation in general is an important aspect of Ag behaviour, with major consequences especially for immunological cell-targeting approaches [57–59].

Defining the precise levels of expression of a newly discovered Ag on the various positive cell types is an important criterion is defining the molecule. As an example, such information was provided to illustrate the high expression on umbilical vein endothelial cells of the Ag recognized by the endothelium-related S-Endo1 mAb [60]. Finally, from co-capping [61, 62] to energy transfer experiments [63], batteries of techniques are used to evaluate molecular linkages and communications [6].

6.1.3.3   Molecular Genetics

The association of molecular biology with immunological detection techniques has lead to major discoveries. Many genes coding for cell-surface receptors have been cloned by virtue of the membrane expression of their products (detected immunologically) obtained after transfection of either whole DNA [64–68] or cDNA libraries [69, 70]. Chromosome localization can be obtained through phenotype analysis of various human x mouse hybrids retaining only a limited number of human chromosomes, resulting in selective maintenance of the corresponding Ags [71]. Gene transcription depends on a series of regulatory events which affect the expression of the resulting products. This underlines the interest of phenotypic analysis in gene regulation studies.

6.1.3.4   Biological Functions

The first step in the evaluation of cell function is the isolation of the subpopulation of interest. This is then either eliminated by cytotoxic or negative selection processes, or positively separated from a heterogeneous mixture by immunophysical methods. Techniques such as cell chromatography, panning, rosetting, magnetic separation and electronic cell-sorting have been extensively used for cell function studies (cf. 2 and 4). Such methods all make use of cell-surface antigens, the density of which influences the

Table 2. Quantitative changes in antigen density induced by various stimuli. Cell-surface Ag density may be modified by various inducers/repressors. Selected examples are shown with final state density data provided either as relative terms (d_0 to $z \times d_0$) or as absolute densities (number of molecules/cell).

Molecule	Function	Cell	Initial state	Final state	Inducer	Ref.
CD 11b	C3bi receptor, CR3	NK, Mono, PMN	d_0	3 to 5 $\times$ d_0	PMA	76
CD 11c	C3bi receptor, CR4	NK, Mono, PMN	d_0	1.5 to 2 $\times$ d_0	PMA	76
CD 11b	C3bi receptor, CR3	PMN	d_0	15 $\times$ d_0	FMLP, LPS	76
CD 11b	C3bi receptor, CR3	PMN	d_0	15–30 $\times$ d_0	Infection	2
CD 48	adhesion	B cells	d_0	10–20 $\times$ d_0	EBV	70
CD 48	adhesion	B lymphoid lines	d_0	> 2 $\times$ d_0	IL-4	70
CD 2	signalling	T cells	25–30,000	300,000	PHA	40
CD 11a	adhesion	T cells	50–60,000 Naive	300,000 Memory	Ag priming	74
CD 5	proliferation	T-CLL	40,000	500,000	IFN γ	77
ICAM-1/ CD 54	adhesion	endothelial cells	100,000	5000,000	TNF, LPS	78
Thrombo-modulin	haemostasis	endothelial cells	50,000	< 5,000	TNF	79
Thrombo-modulin	haemostasis	endothelial cells	d_0	1.3 $\times$ d_0	histamine	80
Thrombo-modulin	haemostasis	endothelial cells	d_0	1.2 $\times$ d_0	dc-AMP	15
Thrombo-modulin	haemostasis	endothelial cells	d_0	1.3 $\times$ d_0	pentoxifyline	9
Thrombo-modulin	haemostasis	endothelial cells	d_0	2.5 $\times$ d_0	retinoic acid	81
EGF receptor	growth	corneal endoth. cells	4800			82
HLA-class II	Ag presentation	ML-3 (myeloid)	10,000	> 100,000	IFN γ	83
CD 64	Fc receptor	PMN	700	10,000	IFN γ	84
Fc receptor	Fc receptor	Human NK	42,000			85

efficacy of the separation process [72]. Alternatively, the cell subset of interest can be traced without separation by delineation of its surface phenotype: as an example, *Rabinovitch* et al. [73] described the calcium influx in subsets of T-lymphocytes using multiparametric FCM analysis.

As a second step, extended batteries of tests have been used to identify the biological functions of cell-membrane molecules functioning as receptors for immunoglobulins, complement or haemostasis factors, growth or differentiation inducers, viruses or adhesive structures which mediate cell-cell and cell-matrix interactions. Obviously, quantitative changes in the expression of such receptors may lead to functional modifications with physiological or physiopathological consequences.

Thus, surface density of adhesion receptors and ligands controls leucocyte adhesiveness, as do other intrinsic properties of receptors such as affinity and diffusivity [74]. For example, the surface expression of leucocyte adhesion molecules such as ICAM-1, VCAM-1 and E-selectin is increased at sites of inflammation [74]. As shown by *Zola* et al. [75], the density of the protrusion-associated molecule, LAM1, is different on thymocytes involved in generative process (high density) from those progressing to intrathymic death (low density). Memory T-cells express higher levels of most adhesion receptors compared to naive T-cells [74]: LFA-1 densities range from 50000 sites on naive T-cells up to 300000 sites on each primed T- or NK-cells. These last figures, as well as some selected examples of quantitative changes in antigen density, are compiled in Table 2.

Such variations in the quantitative immune phenotype of a cell may be induced either physiologically or experimentally or by exposure to various inducers. Studies *in vitro* most often provide the appropriate baseline control and variations can simply be expressed as a percentage of it. Absolute measurements may be important in clinical studies where experimental densities may be compared to either normal values, potentially common to all laboratories, or to a value previously determined for the same patient. Activated or pathological states may be detected by an uncommon level of expression of constitutive markers, rather than only by the appearance of neo-antigens. The use of the quantitative immune phenotype in patient monitoring has already been illustrated in the follow-up of B-CLL patients [18, 86].

6.1.4   Clinical Applications

6.1.4.1   Acquired and Congenital Immunodeficiency Disorders

The diagnosis, prognosis and monitoring of patients with human immunodeficiency virus (HIV) infection has probably been the most widely used application of immunophenotype analysis. The CD4$^+$ T-cell number has important prognostic implications and is utilized for stratification of patients upon entry into various therapeutic protocols as well as for monitoring their response [26, 28, 87, 88]. Following the extensive use of flow cytometry for enumeration of CD4+ cells, alternative methods have arisen which do not need expensive apparatus such as immunomagnetic separations [89, 90] or cell-related CD4 ELISA [16, 91]. On the other hand, flow cytometry capabilities create new applications in the field of HIV investigations.

In the first place, multicolour fluorescence techniques lead to the study of new clinically relevant lymphocyte or leucocyte subsets [28, 87, 88]. For example, CD8+ lymphocyte subsets co-expressing either HLA-DR, CD38, CD57 or gamma-delta phenotypes may have separate roles in HIV diseases [28]. Moreover, some NK cell subsets such as the CD16+/CD56+ cells, which also express CD8 (although at low density) are reduced in number in AIDS patients, together with NK function [28]. The main problem remains to define clearly which of these subset alterations reflects the individual clinical changes associated with AIDS. Some of them may be due to chronic antigenic stimulation either through administration of blood products in patients with congenital coagulation disorders as shown by *Prince* et al. [92], or *via* other viral infections.

Secondly, phenotypic evaluation of the monocyte population separately from other white cells within the peripheral blood clearly illustrates the multi-parametric capability of flow cytometry. *Passlick* et al. [93] have identified a new subset of peripheral blood monocytes which co-express CD14 and the Fc-receptor CD16 and which potentially represent important targets for viral enhancement. Other studies of antigens such as CD4, CD11b and HLA-DR have mainly identified decreased expression of these molecules rather than frequency changes in monocyte subsets.

So far, relatively few studies have addressed the question of quantitative modifications in the expression of membrane antigens during HIV-related disease, and even fewer have dealt with density data expressed in terms of molecules per cell. *Jouvin* et al. [94] measured the expression of the human C3b receptor (CR1/CD35) on erythrocytes of normal and seropositive individuals using radiolabelled anti-CR1 mAb. They reported a significant decrease in the number of CR1 sites on erythrocytes from AIDS patients compared to normal individuals, suggesting that this parameter may represent a marker of the severity and natural history of the disease. This was confirmed using an ultra-sensitive flow cytometric quantitation of CR1 on erythrocytes [95]. On the other hand, CD4 density on CD4+ lymphocytes remained surprisingly stable throughout the progression of the disease, totally independent of the absolute cell count whichever CD4 epitope was studied [96]. This may lead to new ELISA assays quantitating cell-related CD4 molecules [91, 97] rather than directly enumerating cells.

6.1.4.2   Genetically Inherited Immunodeficiency Disorders

Common variable hypogammaglobulinaemia, the most frequent inherited abnormality of the humoral response, has often been associated with defects in Ig+ B-cells, whereas lymphocytes from patients with severe combined immunodeficiency disease (SCID) generally do not express some of the major T-cell differentiation antigens [98]. Genetically inherited defects have been observed in phospholipid-anchored proteins such as DAF/CD55, acetylcholine esterase and LFA-3/CD58 [55, 99–101] as well as CD16 [56] on erythrocytes and/or leucocytes from patients with paroxysmal nocturnal haemoglobinuria (PNH).

Other immunodeficiency disorders may benefit from quantitative immunophenotypic studies. Leu-CAM deficiency is an inherited disorder of leucocytes characterized by recurrent and often fatal bacterial infection [102, 103]. This disease is due to a lack of (or a reduced) surface expression of the beta-2 integrins LFA1, Mac1, p150-95 (CD11a, b, c and CD18) [104, 105]. The definitive diagnosis of Leu-CAM deficiency is made by quantitating the levels of these integrins on the surface of leucocytes [106]. Based on surface expression, two types of clinically significant Leu-CAM deficiency have been delineated [107]. In the group of patients with the "severe" form, less than 2% of the normal expression level is found, whereas a group of "moderate deficiency" is associated with levels between 5% and 15% of normal and with a more benign clinical course and survival into adulthood.

Chediak-Higashi Syndrome (CHS) and chronic granulomatous disease (CGD) are other inherited diseases characterized by defective phagocytic, adhesive and bactericidal functions. Again, quantitative evaluation of functional receptors may be applied to the clinical diagnosis of these diseases [108, 109].

6.1.4.3   Infectious Diseases

Aside from the detection of the microbial or viral antigens themselves, the application of immunophenotype analysis in infectious diseases deals with the detection of neo-antigens induced by the pathogen on the surface of infected cells or with the phenotypic consequences of the infection on the balance of number of the different cells of the immune system. The classical parameter, the CD4/CD8 ratio, is generally reduced in the active phase of viral infections, due to an increase in CD8 cells, and returns to normal values during the recovery phase of the disease. In bacterial infections also, abnormalities in the numbers of T-cells, CD4$^+$ or CD8$^+$ levels have been observed especially in severe forms of diseases, generally returning to normal with response to therapy [31]. Leucocyte sub-typing has been proposed to differentiate between viral and bacterial infections [110], emphasizing the value of granulocyte typing.

Again, quantitative evaluations of surface markers may prove informative in the study of infectious diseases. In conditions in which they should play their bactericidal role, granulocytes express more CR3/CD11b, a C3bi receptor, which binds complement-opsonized particles [2, 110]. Surface expression of CD3, CD4 and CD8 molecules is decreased by *Trypanosoma cruzi* infection, during the acute phase of *Chagas* disease [111]. Pathogen infection may even induce the expression of neo-antigens as seen on reticulocytes infected by *Plasmodium spp.* [112] or on leucocytes in response to *Rubella* vaccine [113].

6.1.4.4   Autoimmune Diseases

Diseases in which immunophenotypic studies of peripheral blood cells have been performed include multiple sclerosis, systemic lupus erythematosus, sarcoidosis, thyroiditis, rheumatoid arthritis, *Sjögren's* syndrome, myasthenia gravis, chronic liver disease, and type I diabetes. The CD4/CD8 ratio has generally been found to be elevated during active phases of autoimmune disease, but such changes are not consistent. With the development of dual and multicolour fluorescence flow cytometry [88], numerous lymphocyte subsets have been tested in such patients [8, 26, 27, 31]. However, definitive conclusions are difficult to draw from so many complex results and several reasons render immunophenotyping partially unreliable for these diseases [31]:

- Changes in lymphocyte subsets may be relevant only in the affected tissue and not in peripheral blood.
- Very few cells may in fact be implicated in the pathogenesis of the disease and appropriate reagents recognizing antigenic determinants associated with the disease are still not available [114].
- Functional rather than numerical alterations in immune cells may be involved in the pathogenesis of the disease.

The analysis of cells in inflammatory lesions may lead to more informative results. For example, in immunophenotypic analysis of synovial tissue lymphocytes from patients with rheumatoid arthritis, significant increases in density of HLA-DR, VLA-1 and LFA-1 associated with decreased expression of CD3, CD4 and mainly CD7 have been noted [115, 116]. Several types of autoimmune diseases have been associated with elevated expression of MHC Class II or adhesion molecules in the target tissues [115, 117–120].

6.1.4.5   Transplantation Immunology

Immunophenotyping is currently applied to determine histocompatibility requirements before transplantation and to monitor immune reactions (rejection episodes) after transplantation.

HLA typing

The determination of MHC antigens is of importance in tissue transplantation, since allograft survival is influenced by the similarity of MHC antigens in the donor and recipient. Micro-cytotoxicity has been the standard technique for HLA typing. This approach is hampered by the cross-reactivity between available antisera and the subjective, complex and time-consuming procedure for performing and reading the assay. Improvements have been introduced recently through the use of immunomagnetic beads which shorten the cell-separation and washing steps [121] and automated microplate readers. The availability of anti-HLA mAbs gives some hope that automation of HLA typing, as proposed for HLA-B27, will be achieved with flow cytometry [122–124]. However, since many problems in raising and applying such mAb reagents remain, molecular biology gene typing techniques may intervene as more widely used alternatives.

HLA cross-match

HLA cross-matching is used to determine the presence of pre-formed antibodies to donor HLA antigens. A positive anti-T-cell cross-match is a contra-indication to transplantation since it is associated with early and irreversible graft rejection. The significance of a positive B-cell cross-match is controversial [31]. Study of both types of antibody involves either micro-cytotoxicity tests or flow cytometric evaluation of binding of recipient antibodies to the donor's lymphocytes [125]. FCM analysis generally offers higher sensitivity, is not limited to the detection of cytotoxic antibodies and discriminates between IgM and IgG antibodies. The use of dual-colour FCM technique or pre-clearing of Fc-receptors from non-T-cells have been proposed as an improvement by *Talbot* et al. [126]. The information gained is particularly useful for transplantation programmes that include donor-specific transfusion before transplantation [127]. Also, preventative immunization of pregnant women with their partner's lymphocytes is a useful strategy in many cases to prevent spontaneous recurrent abortion [128]. The same techniques as those for HLA-cross-matching can be used but the clinical importance of sub-liminal anti-donor T-cell antibodies that are detected only by FCM and not confirmed by other techniques is not certain [31].

Post-transplant monitoring

In the follow-up of transplant recipients, evaluation of peripheral blood lymphocyte subsets has been extensively used [26, 31, 129–134]. The tendency is to study these at the level of the transplanted organ [135, 136] and to evaluate supra-normal levels of transplantation Ags or adhesion molecules induced by local immune responses [137, 138]. The monitoring of the progress of therapeutic immuno-modulation also requires immune phenotyping [139, 140].

6.1.4.6   Platelet Immunology

The major clinical impact of platelet immunology still relates to the transplantation field through the study of specific alloantigen systems [141]. New assays such as MAIPA [142] in which platelet glycoproteins are pre-extracted and purified from membranes by means of specific mAbs bring significant improvements in such serological tests.

Quantitation of platelet surface-bound human IgG is often required for the distinction between immune and non-immune thrombocytopenia [143].

Platelet immunology also deals with genetically inherited diseases: in *Glanzmann's* disease and *Bernard-Soulier* syndrome, almost 30-fold less than normal amounts of gpIIb/IIIa and gpIb may be encountered. Quantitation of these molecules helps discrimination between heterozygous and homozygous forms [144]. Quantitation of platelet glycoproteins and activation markers has been applied using radioimmunoassays or flow cytometry in both fundamental studies [145] and also in clinical studies on the detection of activated platelets in pre-thrombotic states [146–148].

6.1.5   Oncology

The evaluation of cancer makes use of immunological markers for tumour diagnosis, classification, staging and prognosis as well as for monitoring therapy [149].

6.1.5.1   Solid Tumours

In solid tumours, clinically useful information is most often found at the intracellular level. This emphasizes the importance of immuno-cytochemical approaches and the limited value of the detection of surface antigens. Thus, cytokeratin staining shows greater specificity for epithelial cells and is easier to detect than the membrane staining of epithelial membrane antigen. Proliferation markers, like Ki-67 or PCNA, are found inside cells rather than on the outer surface as in the case of the transferrin receptor. Also, the more clinically relevant hormone receptors are located intracellularly.

However, specific domains of oncology take significant advantage of cell-surface immuno-detection. This has become an integral part of the diagnosis and classification of haematopoietic malignancies (see below) and detection as well as grading of bladder cancer cells [150, 151] benefits from the advent of new mAbs. For solid tumours, the study of factors influencing metastasis requires quantitative assays since overexpression or down-regulation processes are more frequent phenomena than complete appearance or disappearance. The expression of proteins involved in cell transport such as drug-resistance gene-encoded products, cell surface lectins or lectin receptors, proteases, ectoenzymes and adhesion molecules may be modulated on tumour cells. The MHC molecules are involved in genetically restricted cytotoxic mechanisms and reduced expression of such molecules on the tumour cells may be responsible for their increased metastatic potential [152]. Adhesion molecules on solid tumours include carcino-embryonic antigen (CEA), an important molecule in colon cancer biology, the

EGF-like transmembrane receptor encoded by the HER2/*neu* oncogene which is amplified in resected breast cancers [153, 154], and N-CAM on neuroblastomas and small cell lung carcinomas [155]. The latter adhesion molecule is down-regulated by N-myc amplification in neuroblastomas, resulting in increased metastatic behaviour [156]. The MDR gene encodes the P-glycoprotein which acts as a pump to remove drugs from the cells [157]. MDR expression correlates with resistance to various drugs and can be modified by many agents [158, 159]. So far, these factors have been investigated only in an experimental context and not as prognostic indicators in routine clinical practice [149].

6.1.5.2   Immune Phenotype in Haemopoietic Malignancies

For a long time it was assumed that a neoplastic cell would carry the same phenotype as its normal counterpart. In many cases, an aberrant phenotype can be observed in the form of an aberrant combination of antigens, an asynchrony in appearance or disappearance of a few immune markers as compared to others, or even an abnormal level of expression of "normal" cell-surface molecules. This could provide new insights for diagnosis, prognosis, pathophysiology and follow-up of haemopoietic malignancies.

Distinction between haemopoietic and nonhaemopoietic malignancies

The leucocyte-common antigen (LCA, CD45) is expressed at the surface of the great majority of haemopoietic cells and is absent from cells of other origins. Its combined use with intracellular markers, such as cytokeratin and vimentin, for example, would in many cases allow the determination of the haemopoietic origin of a given cell [33, 160]. Some restrictions, however, should be noted. First, rare anaplastic malignant lymphomas may display a CD45$^-$ and/or a cytokeratin$^+$ phenotype [161, 162]. Second, acute leukaemia cells can express only very low or undetectable amounts of CD45. This is in agreement with normal haemopoietic differentiation since CD45 expression increases along with maturation [45, 163]. This may also bear prognostic significance since low CD45 expression on ALL cells may be related to a better prognosis [164, 165].

Distinction between benign and malignant proliferations

In the absence of any formal immune marker of malignancy, indirect information can argue for a malignant process. First, monoclonality may be associated with malignancy and sought for through surface immunoglobulin detection [26, 166–168]. However, the rule is not absolute since oligoclonality can be detected in certain specific benign situations such as allogeneic bone marrow engraftment [169–171], while AIDS-related lymphomas are frequently polyclonal [172]. Second, a major B-cell CD5$^+$ phenotype may argue for a neoplastic process [173, 174]. Third, a phenotype considered aberrant or at least unusual in a given site [175–179] can evoke malignancy. Triple colour immuno-flow-cytometry is now proposed for such studies [180, 181] and again unusually over- or underexpression of certain surface antigens may also be beneficial for diagnostics.

Classification of haemopoietic malignancies

Acute leukaemias may be classified in accordance with normal differentiation schemes [44] and today immuno-staining is part of leukaemia typing, together with morphology and cytochemistry. A short series of surface markers most often helps in relating blast cells to T, B or myeloid lineages, but cytoplasmic staining is also of great significance [180]. Special cases of lineage infidelity require the care and extended knowledge of the pathologist. For instance, CD19, a classical B-cell lineage marker has been described at the surface of monocytic blasts [182] and CD7, a T-cell lineage antigen, is found on about 15% of myeloid leukaemias [178].

Among each cell lineage, immune classification allows for sub-groupings that bear prognostic significance. Different levels or stages are proposed for B-lineage ALLs [44, 163, 183–185] and T-ALLs [44, 186]. For myeloid leukaemias, the interpretation of immune phenotype and its correlation with morphological classification (FAB) are more difficult because of heterogeneity [181, 187–190]. Nevertheless, phenotypic features such as the expression of immaturity markers bring diagnostic and prognostic information [191, 192].

Lymphomas may be considered in the same manner as solid tumours with emphasis on immunocytochemical investigations for both intra-cytoplasmic and membrane markers. Immune phenotype is, for example, useful to distinguish between *Hodgkin's* and non-*Hodgkin's* lymphomas [193], to characterize rare groups of lymphomas such as anaplastic Ki1 [161, 162] or the pure mediastinal B-cell type [194] and to distinguish those of centro-follicular origin from mantle zone types according to expression of CD5 and CD10 antigens [195, 196].

Prognostic value of immune phenotype

The prognostic relevance of an immune phenotype has been obtained first by the presence or absence of certain markers: CD34 positivity is related to poor prognosis in AML [197, 198], as well as CD19 in myelo-monocytic leukaemia [182, 199, 200], whereas absence of HLA-DR suggests poor prognosis in NHL [201]. The search for new and informative markers is evolving, with a major interest in adhesion molecules such as CD44 in NHL [202]. Well-known antigens may be of greater value if tested in a quantitative fashion. Thus, a high level of expression of CD10, with a potential cut-off around 20000 molecules per cell (*Brunet C.* et al., unpublished results) of CD 10 is correlated with better prognosis in childhood ALL [203], as is low expression of CD45

[204]. When quantitated on an absolute basis with the QIFI assay, several antigens including CD9, CD10, CD20, CD23, CD24, CD45 and HLA appear to be of diagnostic, pathophysiological and/or prognostic value [165].

Pathophysiological implications of immune phenotype

Immune phenotype is a basis for comparison of neoplastic cells with their putative normal counterparts [44], to define the so-called "hybrid acute leukaemia" [205, 206] and to define precisely the origin of a given cell. It will provide more information as knowledge of the biological role of differentiation antigens grows. Numerous studies now deal with the significance of adhesion molecules for lymphomatous cell diffusion [202, 207]. The local and cell-surface density of such receptors will no doubt be critical to the expression of the function as also seen for the ectoenzyme activity of Calla [208].

Evaluation of minimal residual disease

This long-lasting problem has been approached with immunological methods in three ways. First, detection of clonal excess has been used to detect minor malignant subpopulations [209]. Second, abnormal phenotypes, i. e., those not normally seen in a given localization such as CD1 expression outside of the thymus, or aberrant phenotypes such as TdT/CD13 co-expression [178] have been used to detect contaminations by leukaemic cells as low as 10^{-5}. Third, abnormally high or low expression of a given antigen may also make the basis for distinction, using absolute quantitative immunocytometry.

   In this field, the combination of various immunological and/or non-immunological techniques is mandatory. Strategies associating electronic or magnetic cell-sorting with second-step phenotype or *in situ* hybridization or PCR may succeed in developing very sensitive procedures.

6.1.6   Other Applications

6.1.6.1   Therapy and Monitoring of Therapy

Therapeutic decisions or monitoring make more and more use of cell surface phenotypes [59]. In modern therapy, cell-surface antigens not only serve as markers for monitoring but also as targets for therapy. Cytokine- and monoclonal antibody-based treatments require a follow-up of both the targeted cells and the targeted molecules [139, 210–214]. The optimization of treatment regimens needs preclinical studies involving phenotypic investigation. Bone marrow purging, for instance, has required numerous attempts optimally to eradicate cells which express the target surface antigens [59, 215, 216]. The efficacy of killing or purging is often related to the density of the target antigen(s) [72, 217–221] thus emphasizing the interest in designing cocktails of antibodies with functionally high affinity for the target antigen.

6.1.6.2 Detection of Rare Cells

The high affinity and specificity of monoclonal antibodies has allowed the recognition, staining and separation of rare cells from heterogeneous populations. Again, membrane antigens are used as markers to which antibody molecules can anchor specifically. This is especially true with immunophysical sorting methods such as panning, rosetting and immunomagnetic sorting which are influenced by the cell-surface density of the target antigen [72, 221]. Detection and sorting of rare cells may be clinically applied in ante-natal diagnosis, where extremely rare ($< 10^{-6}$) fetal cells may be isolated from maternal blood and provide material for genetic studies [133, 222, 223] and monitoring of minimal residual disease as seen above. It has been considered for early diagnosis of viral diseases [224] and quality-control of cellular blood products before transfusion [225], and may be involved in new cell-based tests for monitoring pre-thrombotic states [226].

References

[1] G. Köhler, C. Milstein, Continuous Culture of Fused Cells Secreting Antibody of Predefined Specificity, Nature 256, 495–497 (1975).
[2] G. Stelzer, Analysis of Leukocyte Function by Flow Cytometric Techniques, Cytometry 9, 52–59 (1988).
[3] C. W. Caldwell, Fluorescence Intensity of Immunostained Cells as a Diagnostic Aid in Lymphoid Leukemias, Diagn. Clin. Immunol. 5, 371–376 (1988).
[4] H. M. Shapiro, H. M. Shapiro, Putting the -metry into Immunofluorescence Flow Cytometry, Cytometry 12, Supp. 5, 70 (1991).
[5] P. Poncelet, M. Mutin, C. Brunet, F. George, P. Ambrosi, J. Sampol, Quantification of Cell-Membrane Antigenic Sites in Immuno-cytometry with Indirect IF: The QIFI Assay, Cytometry 12, Supp. 5, 417D (1991).
[6] T. Springer, Adhesion Receptors of the Immune System, Nature 346, 425–434 (1990).
[7] D. W. Mason, A. F. Williams, The Kinetics of Antibody Binding to Membrane Antigens in Solution and at the Cell Surface, Biochem. J. 187, 1–20 (1980).
[8] H. Baumgarten, H. Beulshausen, J. Bätzing-Feigenbaum, F. Bieber, R. Zierz, O. Götze, Determination of the T3-3A1 Antigen in PHA-Induced Human T Cells by Standardized Cell ELISA, J. Immunol. Methods 96, 201–209 (1987).

[9]   S. Ohdama, S. Takano, K. Ohashi, S. Miyake, N. Aoki, Pentoxyfylline Prevents Tumor Necrosis Factor-Induced Supression of Endothelial Cell Surface Thrombomodulin, Thrombosis Res. 62, 745–755 (1991).

[10] D. Carriere, Trousse et méthode de dosage immunométrique applicable à des cellules entières, Brevet France, Demande 87.13.537 (1987).

[11] C. M. Ballantyne, E. A. Mainolfi, J. B. Young, N. T. Windsor, E. O. Laurence, R. Rothlein, Prognostic Value of Increased Levels of Circulating Intercellular Adhesion Molecule 1 After Heart Transplantation, Clin. Res. 39, 285a (1991).

[12] D. Maimone, A. T. Reder, Soluble CD8 Levels in the CSF and Serum of Patients with Multiple Sclerosis, Neurology 41, 851–854 (1991).

[13] H. F. Weissman, T. Bartow, M. K. Leppo, H. C. Marsh, G. R. Carson, N. F. Concino, N. P. Boyle, K. H. Roux, M. L. Weisfeldt, D. F. Fearon, Soluble Human Complement Receptor Type 1: in vivo Inhibitor or Complement Suppressing Post-Ischemia Myocardial Inflammation and Necrosis, Science 249, 146 (1990).

[14] S. Sawada, S. Sugai, S. Imima, M. Takei, E. Paredes, T. Hayama, S. Nishinarita, Y. Nosokawa, T. Noric, T. Obara, Increased Soluble CD4 and Decreased Soluble CD8 Molecules in Patients with Sjögren's Syndrome, Am. J. Med. 92, 134 (1992).

[15] K. Hirokawa, N. Aoki, Up-Regulation of Thrombo-Modulin by Activation of Histamine H1 Receptors in Human Umbilical Vein Endothelial Cells in vitro, J. Cell. Physiol. 147, 157–165 (1991).

[16] K. Murphy, S. Kline, H. Paxton, M. Johns, G. Parsons, A New Method for the Enumeration of CD4+ and CD8+ Lymphocytes – Presented at the 8th International Congress of Immunology Budapest, Hungary (August 25, 1992), Abs. 63-30.

[17] P. Poncelet, P. Carayon, Cytofluorometric Quantification of Cell-Surface Antigens by Indirect Immunofluorescence Using Monoclonal Antibodies, J. Immunol. Methods 85, 65–75 (1985).

[18] P. Poncelet, T. Lavabre-Bertrand, P. Carayon, Quantitative Phenotypes of B Chronic Lymphocytic Leukemia B Cells Established with Monoclonal Antibodies from the B Cell Protocol, in: E. L. Reinherz, B. F. Haynes, L. M. Nadler, I. D. Bernstein (eds.), Leukocyte Typing II, Springer-Verlag, New York 1986, pp. 329–343.

[19] P. Poncelet, J. F. Cantaloube, P. Delon, C. Duperray, T. Lavabre-Bertrand, Quantitative Expression of CD37, the New 40–45 kd Cluster, on B and T Cells, in: A. J. McMichael et al. (eds.), Leucocyte Typing III, Oxford University Press, Oxford 1987, pp. 341–345.

[20] P. Le Bouteiller, Z. Mishal, F. A. Lemonnier, F. M. Kourilsky, Quantification by Flow Cytofluorimetry of HLA Class I Molecules at the Surface of Murine Cells Transformed by Cloned HLA Genes, J. Immunol. Methods 61, 301–315 (1983).

[21] T. Oonishi, N. Uyesaka, A New Standard Fluorescence Microsphere for Quantitative Flow Cytometry, J. Immunol. Methods 84, 143–154 (1985).

[22] M. R. Wilson, J. S. Wotherspoon, A New Microsphere-Based Immunofluorescence Assay Using Flow Cytometry, J. Immunol. Methods 107, 225–230 (1988).

[23] R. Vogt, G. Cross, L. Henderson, D. Phillips, Model Systems Evaluating Fluorescein-Labelled Microbeads as Internal Standards to Calibrate Fluorescence Intensity on Flow Cytometers, Cytometry 10, 294–302 (1989).

[24] R. Dux, G. Kindler-Rohrborn, K. Lenmartz, M. F. Rajewsky, Calibration of Fluorescence Intensities to Quantify Antibody Binding Surface Determinants of Cell Subpopulations by Flow Cytometry, Cytometry 12, 422–428 (1991).

[25] C. D. Dawson, J. A. Scheppler, J. K. A. Nicholson, R. C. Holman, Enumeration of Antigen Sites on Cells by Flow Cytometry, Pathobiology 59, 57–61 (1991).

[26] D. H. Ryan, M. A. Fallon, P. K. Horan, Flow Cytometry in the Clinical Laboratory, Clin. Chim. Acta 171, 125–174 (1988).

[27] J. V. Giorgi, A. M. Kesson, C. C. Chou, Immunodeficiency and Infectious Diseases, in: N. R. Rose, E. C. de Macario, J. L. Fahey, H. Freidman, G. M. Penn (eds.), Manual of Clinical Laboratory Immunology, Amer. Soc. for Microbiol., Washington 1992, pp. 174–181.

[28] A. Landay, B. Ohlsson-Wilhelm, J. V. Giorgi, Application of Flow Cytometry to the Study of HIV Infection, AIDS 4, 479–497 (1990).

[29] *C. C. Stewart*, Clinical Applications of Flow Cytometry. Immunologic Methods for Measuring Cell Membrane and Cytoplasmic Antigens, Cancer *69*, 1543–1552 (1992).

[30] *J. V. Giorgi, P. E. Hurtubise, L. S. Cram, J. W. Parker, M. F. La Via*, Clinical Applications of Cytometry: 6th Annual Meeting, Cytometry *13*, 445–447 (1992).

[31] *R. S. Riley, E. J. Mahin, W. Ross* (eds.), Clinical Applications of Flow Cytometry, Ijaku-Shoin, New York 1992.

[32] *D. Mason, K. C. Gatter*, The Role of Immunocytochemistry in Diagnostic Pathology, J. Clin. Pathol. *40*, 1042–1054 (1987).

[33] *K. C. V. Gatter, Z. Abdulaziz, P. C. L. Beverley, J. R. F. Corvalan, C. Ford, E. B. Lane, M. Mota, J. R. G. Nash, K. Pulford, H. Stein, P. J. Taylor, C. Woodhouse, D. Y. Mason*, Use of Monoclonal Antibodies for the Histopathological Diagnosis of Human Malignancy, J. Clin. Pathol. *35*, 1253–1267 (1982).

[34] *A. Bernard, L. Boumsell, J. Dausset, C. Milstein, S. F. Schlossman* (eds.), Leucocyte Typing, Springer-Verlag, Heidelberg 1982.

[35] *E. L. Reinherz, B. F. Haynes, L. M. Nadler, I. D. Bernstein* (eds.), Leucocyte Typing II, Springer-Verlag, New York 1986.

[36] *A. J. McMichael, P. C. L. Beverley, S. Cobbold, M. J. Crumpton, W. Gilks, F. M. Gotch, N. Hogg, M. Horton, N. Ling, I. C. M. McLennan, D. Mason, C. Milstein, D. Spiegelhalter, H. Waldmann* (eds.), Leucocyte Typing III, Oxford University Press, Oxford 1987.

[37] *S. Shaw*, Characterization of Human Leucocyte Differentiation Antigens, Immunology Today *8*, 1–3 (1987).

[38] *W. Knapp, B. Dorken, W. R. Gilks, P. Rieber, R. E. Schmidt, H. Stein, A. E. G. K. Von dem Borne* (eds.), Leucocyte Typing IV, Oxford University Press, Oxford 1989.

[39] *W. Knapp, B. Dorken, P. Rieber, R. E. Schmidt, A. E. G. K. Von dem Borne*, CD Antigens, Blood *74*, 1448–1450 (1989).

[40] *T. Durroux, P. Delon, D. Carriere, P. Carayon, P. Poncelet*, Quantitative Expression of Molecules Defined by the "New-T" Workshop Antibodies on Various T-Cells; Modulation of T-Lymphocytes upon PHA Activation, in: *A. J. McMichael* et. al. (eds.), Leucocyte Typing III, Oxford University Press, Oxford 1987, pp. 242.

[41] *T. Lavabre-Bertrand, D. Delon, B. Klein, P. Poncelet*, Quantitative Expression of Surface Antigens Recognized by the "New B" Monoclonal Antibodies on an Variety of Human B Cells, in: *A. J. McMichael* et al. (eds.), Leucocyte Typing III, Oxford University Press, Oxford 1987, pp. 410.

[42] *A. E. K. G. Von dem Borne, P. V. Moddermann*, Cluster report CD9, in: *W. Knapp, B. Dorken, W. R. Gilks, P. Rieber, R. E. Schmidt, H. Stein, A. E. K. G. Von dem Borne* (eds.), Leucocyte Typing IV, Oxford University Press, Oxford 1989, pp. 989–990.

[43] *K. A. F. Pulford, P. M. Knight, K. C. Gatter, D. Y. Mason*, Immunocytochemical Characterization of Monoclonal Anti-Leucocyte Antibodies, in: *A. Bernard, L. Boumsell, J. Dausset, C. Milstein, S. F. Schlossman* (eds.), Leucocyte Typing, Springer-Verlag, Heidelberg 1984, pp. 453–465.

[44] *K. A. Foon, R. F. Todd*, Immunologic Classification of Leukemia and Lymphoma, Blood *68*, 1–31 (1986).

[45] *V. O. Shah, C. I. Civin, M. R. Loken*, Flow Cytometric Analysis of Human Bone Marrow. IV. Differential Quantitative Expression of T200 Common Leucocyte Antigen During Normal Hemopoiesis, J. Immunol. *140*, 1861–1867 (1988).

[46] *M. R. Loken, V. O. Shah, K. Dattilio, C. Civin*, Flow Cytometric Analysis of Human Bone Marrow. I. Normal Erythroid Development, Blood *69*, 255–263 (1987).

[47] *C. Duperray, J. H. Boiron, J. F. Cantaloube, C. Boucheix, T. Lavabre-Bertrand, M. Attal, J. Brochier, F. Favier, R. Bataille, B. Klein*, The CD24 Antigen Makes the Discrimination of pre-B Cells from B Cells Possible in Human Bone Marrow, J. Immunol. *145*, 3678–3683 (1991).

[48] *P. Poncelet, A. Bikoué, T. Lavabre, G. Poinas, M. Parant, C. Duperray, J. Sampol*, Quantitative Expression of Human Lymphocytes Membrane Antigens: Definition of Normal Densities Measured in Immuno-Cytometry with the QIFI Assay, Cytometry *12*, Supp. 5, 418A (1991).

[49] T. Lavabre-Bertrand, Apport de Techniques Immunologiques à l'Étude des Hémopathies Malignes: Cytométrie Quantitative, Cytométrie en trois Couleurs, Purification Immuno-magnétique, Étude Multi-paramétrique en Microscopie Électronique, PhD Thesis (Université Montpellier I, 1991).

[50] J. A. Ledbetter, R. V. Rouse, H. S. Micklem, L. A. Herzenberg, T Cells Subsets Defined by the Expression of Lyt-1,2,3 and Thy-1 Antigens. Two Parameter IF and Cytotoxicity Analysis with MAbs Modifies Current Views, J. Exp. Med. 152, 280–285 (1980).

[51] M. Jonker, F. J. M. Nooij, The Phylogeny of T Cell Antigens, in: E. L. Reinherz et al. (eds.), Leucocyte Typing II, Springer-Verlag, New York 1986, pp. 373–387.

[52] M. Jonker, W. Slingerland, Reactivity of MAb Specific for Human CD Markers with Rhesus Monkey Leucocytes, in: W. Knapp, B. Dorken, W. R. Gilks, P. Rieber, R. E. Schmidt, H. Stein, A. E. K. G. Von dem Borne (eds.), Leucocyte Typing IV, Oxford University Press, Oxford 1989, pp. 1058–1063.

[53] A. M. C. Koros, M. J. Taylor, J. C. Hiserodt, B. Stephens, R. J. Lakomy, M. Dalbow, R. Raikow, J. Lange, M. Wagner, Sea Urchin Coelomocytes, Human Peripheral Blood NK Cells and Human Small-cell Lung Cancer Lines may Share Evolutionarily Conserved Antigens HNK1 and NKH1, in: A. J. McMichael et al. (eds.), Leucocyte Typing III, Oxford University Press, Oxford 1986, pp. 866–869.

[54] H. Zola, H. A. Moore, I. K. Hunter, J. Bradley, Analysis of Chemical and Biochemical Properties of Membrane Molecules in situ by Analytical Flow Cytometry with Monoclonal Antibodies, J. Immunol. Methods 74, 65–77 (1984).

[55] T. Kinoshita, M. E. Medof, R. Silber, V. Nussensweig, Distribution of Decay-accelerating Factor in the Peripheral Blood of Normal Individuals and Patients with Paroxysmal Nocturnal Hemoglobulinuria, J. Exp. Med. 162, 75–81 (1985).

[56] P. Selvaraj, W. F. Rosse, R. Silber, T. A. Springer, The Major Fc Receptor in Blood has a Phosphatidyl-Inositol Anchor and is Deficient in Paroxysmal Nocturnal Hemoglobulinuria, Nature 333, 565–567 (1988).

[57] J. Ritz, J. M. Pesando, S. E. Sallan, L. A. Clavell, J. Notis-McConarty, P. Rosenthal, S. F. Schlossman, Serotherapy of Acute Lymphoblastic Leukemia with Monoclonal Antibody, Blood 58, 141–152 (1981).

[58] A. B. Cosimi, R. B. Colvin, R. C. Burton, R. H. Rubin, G. Goldstein, P. C. Kung, W. P. Hansen, F. L. Delmonico, R. S. Russel, Monoclonal Antibodies for Immunologic Monitoring and Treatment in Recipients of Renal Allografts, N. Engl. J. Med. 305, 308–313 (1981).

[59] P. Gros, F. K. Jansen, P. Poncelet, R. Roncussi (eds.), Flow Cytometry and Monoclonal Antibodies for the Monitoring of Therapy, Quo Vadis?, Medsi/McGraw-Hill, Paris 1982.

[60] F. George, P. Poncelet, J. C. Laurent, O. Massot, D. Arnoux, N. Lequeux, P. Ambrosi, C. Chicheportiche, J. Sampol, Cytofluorometric Detection of Endothelial Cells in Whole Blood Using S-Endo1 Monoclonal Antibody, J. Immunol. Methods 139, 65–75 (1991).

[61] J. M. Rojo, K. Saizawa, C. A. Janeway, Physical Association of CD4 and the T-Cell Receptor can be Induced by Anti-T-Cell Receptor Antibodies, Proc. Natl. Acad. Sci. USA 86, 3311–3316 (1989).

[62] P. Andersen, M. L. Blue, S. F. Schlossman, Co-Modulation of CD3 and CD4. Evidence for a Specific Association Between CD4 and Approximately 5% of the CD3/T-Cell Receptor Complexes on Helper T Lymphocytes, J. Immunol. 140, 1732–1737 (1988).

[63] R. S. Mittler, S. J. Goldman, G. L. Spitalny, S. J. Burakoff, T-Cell Receptor CD4 Physical Association in a Murine T-Cell Hybridoma: Induction by Antigen Receptor Ligation, Proc. Natl. Acad. Sci. USA 86, 10044–10048 (1989).

[64] P. Kavathas, L. A. Herzenberg, Amplification of a Gene Coding for Human T Cell Differentiation Antigen, Nature 306, 385–387 (1983).

[65] P. Kavathas, L. A. Herzenberg, Stable Transformation of Mouse L Cells for Human Membrane T Cell Differentiation Antigens, HLA and Beta-2 Microglobulin: Selection by Fluorescence-activated Cell Sorting, Proc. Natl. Acad. Sci. USA 80, 524–528 (1983).

[66] P. J. Maddon, A. G. Dalgleish, J. C. McDougal, P. R. Clapham, R. A. Weiss, R. Axel, The T4 Gene Encodes the AIDS Virus Receptor and is Expressed in the Immune System and the Brain, Cell 47, 333–348 (1986).

[67] J. E. Sims, C. J. March, D. Cosman, M. B. Widmer, H. R. McDonald, C. J. McMahan, C. E. Grubin, J. M. Wignall, J. L. Jackson, S. M. Call, D. Friend, A. R. Alpert, S. Gillis, D. L. Urdal, S. K. Dower, cDNA Expression Cloning of the IL-1 Receptor, a Member of the Immunoglobulin Superfamily, Science 241, 585–589 (1988).

[68] J. F. Cantaloube, M. Piechaczyk, A. Calender, G. Lenoir, A. Minty, D. Carrière, E. Fisher, P. Poncelet, Stable Expression and Function of EBV/C3d Receptor Following Genomic Transfection into Murine Fibroblast L Cells, Eur. J. Immunol. 20, 409–416 (1990).

[69] B. Seed, A. Aruffo, Molecular Cloning of the CD2 Antigen, the T-Cell Erythrocyte Receptor, by a Rapid Immunoselection Procedure, Proc. Natl. Acad. Sci. USA 84, 3365–3369 (1987).

[70] S. Yokoyama, D. Staunton, R. Fisher, M. Amiot, J. J. Fortin, D. A: Thorley-Lawson, Expression of the Blast-1 Activation Adhesion Molecule and Its Identification as CD48, J. Immunol. 146, 2192–2200 (1991).

[71] C. Milstein, What next?, in: W. Knapp, B. Dörken, W. R. Gilks, E. P. Rieber, R. E. Schmidt, H. Stein, A. E. G. K. Von dem Borne (eds.), Leucocyte Typing IV, Oxford University Press, Oxford 1989, pp. 1–5.

[72] P. Poncelet, C. Brunet, F. George, A. Bikoué, J. Sampol, Influence of Target-Antigen Density on the Efficacy of Immuno-Magnetic Separation (IMS) of Cells, in: J. Kemshead (ed.), Magnetic Separation Techniques Applied to Cellular and Molecular Biology. Abstracts of the John Ugelstad Conference, Cromwell Press, Broughton, Gifford UK 1991.

[73] P. S. Rabinovitch, C. H. June, A. Grossmann, J. A. Ledbetter, Heterogeneity Among T Cells in Intracellular Free Calcium Responses after Mitogen Stimulation with PHA or Anti-CD3. Simultaneous Use of Indo-1 and Immunofluorescence with Flow Cytometry, J. Immunol. 137, 952–961 (1986).

[74] R. Pardi, L. Inverardi, J. R. Bender, Regulatory Mechanisms in Leucocyte Adhesion: Flexible Receptors for Sophisticated Travelers, Immunology Today 13, 224–230 (1992).

[75] L. M. Pilarski, E. A. Turley, A. R. E. Shaw, W. M. Gallatin, M. P. Laderoute, R. Gillitzer, I. G. R. Beckman, H. Zola, FMC46, a Cell Protrusion-Associated Leucocyte Adhesion Molecule-1 Epitope on Human Lymphocytes and Thymocytes, J. Immunol. 147, 136–141 (1992).

[76] T. Werfel, W. Witter, O. Götze, CD11b and CD11c Antigens are Rapidly Increased on Human Natural Killer Cells upon Activation, J. Immunol. 142, 2423–2427 (1991).

[77] M. Chiron, J. M. Darbon, F. Roubinet, G. Cassar, J. P. Jaffrezou, C. Bordier, G. Laurent, Quantitative Analysis of CD5 Antigen Modulation by TPA in T-Lymphoblastic Leukemia Cells: Individual Response Patterns and Their Relationships with Both Maturation and Protein Kinase C Content, Cell. Immunol. 130, 339–351 (1990).

[78] M. L. Dustin, T. A. Springer, Lymphocyte Function-Associated Antigen-1 (LFA-1) Interaction with Intercellular Adhesion Molecule-1 (ICAM-1) is One of at Least Three Mechanisms for Lymphocyte Adhesion to Cultured Endothelial Cells, J. Cell Biol. 107, 321–331 (1988).

[79] G. A. Soff, R. W. Jackman, R. D. Rosenberg, Expression of Thrombomodulin by Smooth Muscle Cells in Culture: Different Effects of TNF and CAMP on Thrombomodulin Expression by Endothelial Cells and Smooth Muscle Cells in Culture, Blood 77, 515–518 (1991).

[80] K. Hirokawa, N. Aoki, Up-Regulation of Thrombomodulin by Activation of Histamine H1-Receptors in Human Umbilical Vein Endothelial Cells in vitro, Biochem. J. 276, 739–743 (1991).

[81] S. Horie, K. Kizaki, H. Ishii, M. Kazama, Retinoic Acid Stimulates Expression of Thrombomodulin, a Cell Surface Anti-coagulant Glycoprotein, on Human Endothelial Cells, Biochem. J. 281, 149–154 (1992).

[82] J. Lopez, M. Inster, H. Thompson, J. Malter, R. Beuerman, EGF Cell Surface Receptor Densities by an Immunocytochemical Flow Cytometry Technique, Cytometry 12, Suppl. 5, 230 (1991).

[83] M. Chiron, J. P. Jaffrezou, P. Carayon, C. Bordier, F. Roubinet, C. Xavier, M. Brandely, G. Laurent, Induction and Increase of HLA-DR Expression by Immune Interferon on ML-3

Cell Line Enhances the Anti-HLA-DR Immunotoxin Activity, Clin. Exp. Immunol. *82*, 214–220 (1990).

[84] *K. Petroni, L. Shen, P. McGuyre*, Modulation of Human Polymorphonuclear Leucocyte IgG Fc Receptors and Fc Receptor-mediated Functions by Gamma Interferon and Glucocorticoids, J. Immunol. *140*, 3467–3472 (1988).

[85] *J. A. Titus, S. O. Sharrow, J. M. Conolly, D. M. Segal*, Fc(IgG) Receptor Distributions in Homogeneous and Heterogeneous Cell Populations by Flow Microfluorometry, Proc. Natl. Acad. Sci. USA *78*, 519–523 (1981).

[86] *N. Genetet, B. Grosbois, G. Merdrignac, P. Poncelet, Y. Avril, M. Le Carrour, D. Bourel, R. Leblay, B. Genetet*, Quantitative Phenotypes of B-CLL Cells: A Longitudinal Study, in: A. J. McMichael et al. (eds.), Leucocyte Typing III, Oxford University Press, Oxford 1987, pp. 493–495.

[87] *T. Ohno, T. Kanoh, T. Suzuki, T. Masuda, K. Kuribayashi, S. Araya, H. Arai, H. Uchino*, Comparative Analysis of Lymphocyte Phenotypes Between Carriers of Human Immunodeficiency Virus (HIV) and Adult Patients with Primary Immunodeficiency Using Two-Color Immunofluorescence Flow Cytometry, J. Exp. Med. *154*, 157–172 (1988).

[88] *Cheng-Ming Liu, K. A. Muirhead, S. P. George, A. L. Landay*, Flow Cytometric Monitoring in Human Immunodeficiency Virus-infected Patients. Simultaneous Enumeration of Five Lymphocyte Subsets, Am. J. Clin. Pathol. *92*, 721–728 (1989).

[89] *J. E. Brinchmann, F. Vartdal, G. Gaudernack, G. Markussen, S. Funderud, J. Ugelstad, E. Thorsby*, Direct Immunomagnetic Quantification of Lymphocyte Subsets in Blood, Clin. Exp. Immunol. *71*, 182–186 (1988).

[90] *Dynal*, Dynabeads® T4/T8 Quant., Total Cell Count Directly from Whole Blood to Monitor Immune Status, Product Description Sheets, Dynal (Oslo, Norway).

[91] *Sanofi*, Capcellia® CD4-CD8, Product Description Sheets, *Sanofi Diagnostic-Pasteur* (Paris, France).

[92] *H. E. Prince, J. K. Kreiss, C. K. Kasper, S. Kleinman, A. M. Saunders, L. Waldbeser, G. Mandigo, H. S. Kaplan*, Distinctive Lymphocyte Subpopulation Abnormalities in Patients with Congenital Coagulation Disorders who Exhibit Lymph Node Enlargement, Blood *66*, 64–68 (1985).

[93] *B. Passlick, D. Flieger, H. W. Ziegler-Heitbrock*, Identification and Characterization of a Novel Monocyte Subpopulation in Human Peripheral Blood, Blood *74*, 2527–2534 (1989).

[94] *M. H. Jouvin, W. Rozenbaum, R. Russo, M. D. Kazatchkine*, Decreased Expression of the C3b/C4b Complement Receptor (CR1) in AIDS and AIDS-related Syndromes Correlates with Clinical Subpopulations of Patients with HIV Infection, AIDS *1*, 89–94 (1987).

[95] *J. H. M. Cohen, B. Autran, M. H. Jouvin, J. P. Aubry, W. Rozenbaum, J. Bancherau, P. Debré, J. P. Revillard, M. Kazatchkine*, Decreased Expression of the Receptor for the C3b Fragment of Complement on Erythrocytes of Patients with Acquired Immunodeficiency Syndrome, Presse Méd. *17*, 727–730 (1988).

[96] *P. Poncelet, P. Poinas, P. Corbeau, C. Devaux, N. Tubiana, C. Tamalet, J. C. Cherman, F. Kourilsky, J. Sampol*, Surface CD4 Density Remains Constant on Lymphocytes from HIV-infected Patients in the Progression of Disease, Res. Immunol. *142*, 291–298 (1991).

[97] *K. Murphy, S. Kline, H. Paxton, M. Johns, G. Parsons*, A New Method for the Enumeration of CD4+ and CD8+ Lymphocytes, Communisation at the 8th International Congress of Immunology Budapest, Hungary (August 25, 1992), Abs. 63-30.

[98] *E. L. Reinherz*, Abnormalities of T Cell Maturation and Regulation in Human Beings with Immunodeficiency Disorders, J. Clin. Invest. *68*, 699–704 (1981).

[99] *A. Nicholson-Weller, J. P. March, C. E. Rosen, D. B. Spicer, K. F. Austen*, Surface Membrane Expression by Human Blood Leucocytes and Platelets of Decay-accelerating Factor, A Regulatory Protein of the Complement System, Blood *65*, 1237–1244 (1985).

[100] *A. Nicholson-Weller, D. B. Spicer, K. F. Austen*, Deficiency in the Complement Regulatory Protein DAF on Membranes of Granulocytes, Monocytes and Platelets in Paroxysmal Nocturnal Hemoglobulinuria, N. Engl. J. Med. *312*, 1091–1097 (1985).

[101] *E. Ueda, T. Kinoshita, T. Terasawa, T. Shichishima, Y. Yawata, K. Inoue, T. Kitani,* Acetylcholinesterase and Lymphocyte-function-associated Antigen 3 Found on DAF Negative Erythrocytes from Some Patients with PNH are Lost During Erythrocyte Aging, Blood *75,* 762–769 (1990).

[102] *D. C. Anderson, F. C. Schmalsteig, M. J. Finegold, B. Hughes, R. Rothlein, L. J. Miller, S. Kohl, M. F. Tosi, R. L. Jocobs, T. C. Waldrop, A. S. Goldman, W. T. Shearer, T. A. Springer,* Abnormalities in Polymophonuclear Leucocyte Function Associated with a Heritable Deficiency of a High Molecular Weight Surface Glyco-proteins (GP138): Common Relationship to Diminished Cell Adherence, J. Clin. Invest. *74,* 536–551 (1984).

[103] *T. J. Bowen, H. D. Ochs, L. C. Altman, T. H. Price, D. E. Van Epps, D. L Brautigan, R. E. Rosin, W. D. Perkins, B. M. Babior, S. J. Klebanoff, R. J. Wedgwood,* Severe Reccurent Bacterial Infections Associated with Defective Adherence and Chemotaxis in Two Patients with Neutrophils Deficient in a Cell-associated Glycoprotein, J. Pediatrics *101,* 932–940 (1982).

[104] *M. R. Buchanan, C. A. Crowley, R. E. Rosin, M. A. J. Gimbrone, B. M. Babior,* Studies on the Interaction Between GP180-deficient Neutrophils and Vascular Endothelium, Blood *60,* 160–165 (1982).

[105] *D. C. Anderson, T. A. Springer,* Leucocyte Adhesion Deficiency: An Inhereted Defect in the Mac-1, LFA-1 and p150-95 Glycoproteins, Ann. Rev. Med. *38,* 175–194 (1987).

[106] *M. A. Arnaoult, H. Spits, C. Terhorst, J. Pitt, R. F. Todd,* Deficiency of a Leucocyte Surface Glycoprotein (LFA-1) in Two Patients with Mo1 Deficiency: Effects of Cell Activation on Mo1/LFA-1 Surface Expression in Normal and Deficient Leucocytes, J. Clin. Invest. *74,* 1291–1300 (1984).

[107] *D. C. Anderson, F. C. Schmalsteig, M. A. Arnaout, S. Kohl, M. F. Tosi, N. Dana, G. J. Buffone, B. J. Hughes, B. R. Brinkley, W. D. Dickey, J. S. Abramson, T. Springer, L. A. Boer, J. M. Hollers, C. W. Smith,* The Severe and Moderate Phenotypes of Heritable Mac-1, LFA-1 Deficiency: Their Quantitative Definition and Relation to Leucocyte Dysfunction and Clinical Features, J. Infect. Dis. *152,* 668–689 (1985).

[108] *C. A. Crowley, J. T. Curnutte, R. E. Rosin, J. Andre-Schwartz, J. I. Gallin, M. Klempner, R. Snyderman, F. S. Southwick, T. P. Stossel, B. M. Babior,* An Inherited Abnormality of Neutrophil Adhesion: Its Genetic Transmission and Its Association with a Missing Protein, N. Engl. J. Med. *302,* 1163–1168 (1980).

[109] *M. S. Cairo, C. Vandeven, C. Toy, D. Tischler, L. Sender,* Fluorescent, Cytometric Analysis of Polymorphonuclear Leucocytes in *Chediak-Higashi* Syndrome: Diminished C3bi Receptor Expression (OKM1) with Normal Granular Cells Density, Pediatr. Res. *24,* 673–676 (1988).

[110] *S. A. Bentley, N. D. Pegram, D. W. Ross,* Diagnosis of Infective and Inflammatory Disorders by Flow Cytometric Analysis of Blood Neutrophils, Am. J. Clin. Pathol. *88,* 177–181 (1987).

[111] *M. B. Sztein, W. R. Cuna, F. Kierszenbaum, Trypanozoma Cruzi* Inhibits the Expression of CD3, CD4, CD8 and IL2r by Mitogen-activated Helper and Cytotoxic Human Lymphocytes, J. Immunol. *144,* 3558–3562 (1990).

[112] *C. F. Ockenhouse, N. N. Tandon, C. Magowan, G. A. Jamieson, J. D. Chulay,* Identification of a Platelet Membrane Glycoprotein as a Falciparum Malaria Sequestration Receptor, Science *243,* 1469–1471 (1989).

[113] *S. O'Shea, D. Nutton, J. M. Best, In vivo* Expression of Rubella Antigens on Human Leucocytes: Detection by Flow Cytometry, J. Med. Virol. *25,* 297–307 (1988).

[114] *C. G. Drake, B. L. Kotzin,* Superantigens: Biology, Immunology and Potential Role in Disease, J. Clin. Immunol. *12,* 149–162 (1992).

[115] *L. L. Cush, N. N. Lipsky,* Phenotypic Analysis of Synovial Tissue and Peripheral Blood Lymphocytes Isolated from Patients with Rheumatoid Arthritis, Arthritis Rheum. *31,* 1230–1238 (1988).

[116] *A. I. Lazarovits, J. Karsh,* Decreased Expression of CD7 Occurs in Rheumatoid Arthritis, Clin. Exp. Immunol. *72,* 470–475 (1988).

[117] *Y. J. Rosenberg, A. D. Steinberg, T. J. Santoro,* The Basis of Autoimmunity in MRL lpr/lpr Mice: A Role for Self Ia Reactive T Cells, Immunology Today *5,* 64–67 (1981).

[118] *G. Janossy, O. Duke, L. W. Poulter, G. Panayi, M. Bofill, G. Goldstein,* Rheumatoid Arthritis: A Disease of T Lymphocyte/Macrophage Immunoregulation, Lancet *II,* 839–842 (1981).

[119] *I. Todd, M. Londei, R. Pujoll-Borrell, R. Mirakian, M. Feldmann, G. F. Bottazzo,* HLA-DR Expression on Epithelial Cells: The Finger on the Trigger?, Ann. N. Y. Acad. Sci. *475,* 241–250 (1986).

[120] *R. P. A. Wuthrich, M. Jevnikar, F. Takei, L. H. Glimcher, V. E. Kelley,* Intercellular Adhesion Molecule-1 (ICAM-1) Expression is Upregulated in Autoimmune Murine Lupus Nephritis, Am. J. Pathol. *136,* 441–450 (1990).

[121] *T. Hansen, K. Hannestad,* Direct HLA Typing by Rosetting with Immunomagnetic Beads Coated with Specific Antibodies, J. Immunogenetics *16,* 137–140 (1989).

[122] *T. Hansen, K. Hannestad,* Simple Rosette Assay for HLA-B27 Typing of Whole Blood Samples, Tissue Antigens *30,* 198–203 (1987).

[123] *J. Albrecht, H. A. G. Muller,* HLA-B27 Typing by Use of Flow Cytofluorometry, Clin. Chem. *33,* 1619–1623 (1988).

[124] *D. Fizet, C. Hitte, A. M. Ferrer, G. Vezon,* Identification de l'antigène HLA-B27 par cytométrie de flux, Ann. Biol. Clin. *47,* 408–411 (1989).

[125] *D. Talbot,* A Rapid, Objective Method for the Detection of Lymphocytotoxic Antibodies Using Flow Cytometry, J. Immunol. Methods *99,* 137–140 (1987).

[126] *D. D. Talbot, A. L. Givan, B. K. Shenton, A. Stratton, G. Proud, R. M. Taylor,* Rapid Detection of Low Levels of Donor Specific IgG by Flow Cytometry with Single and Dual Colour Fluorescence in Renal Transplantation, J. Immunol. Methods *112,* 279–283 (1988).

[127] *M. R. Garovoy, B. W. Colombe, J. Melzer, N. Feduska, C. Shields, D. Cross, W. Amend, F. Vincenti, S. Hoffer, R. Duca and O. Salvatierra,* Flow Cytometry Cross-matching for Donor-specific Transfuson Recipients and Cadaveric Transplantation, Transplantation Proc. *17,* 693–695 (1985).

[128] *M. F. Reznikoff-Etievant, N. Simmoney, A. Janaud, Y. Darbois, A. Netter,* Treatment of Reccurent Spontaneous Abortions by Immunization whith Paternal Leucocytes, Lancet *I,* 1985–1989 (1985).

[129] *A. Van Es, H. J. Tanke, W. M. Baldurin, P. J. Oljans, J. S. Ploem, L. A. Vanes,* Ratios of T Lymphocyte Subpopulations Predict Survival of Cadaveric Renal Allografts in Adult Patients on Low Dose Cortocosteroid Therapy, Clin. Exp. Immunol. *52,* 13–20 (1983).

[130] *L. Fuller, D. Roth, C. Flaa, V. Esquenazi, J. Miller,* Is Immunologic Monitoring Helpful in Renal Transplantation?, Transplantation Proc. *17,* 553–555 (1985).

[131] *H. G. Herrod, J. Williams, P. J. Dean,* Alterations in Immunologic Measurements in Patients Experiencing Early Hepatic Allograft Rejection, Transplantation *45,* 923–925 (1988).

[132] *S. Roodman, L. W. Miller, C. C. Tsai,* Role of Interleukin-2 Receptors in Immunologic Monitoring Following Cardiac Transplantation, Transplantation *45,* 1050–1056 (1988).

[133] *K. Ault, J. H. Antin, D. Ginsburg, S. H. Orkin, J. M. Rappeport, M. L. Keohan, P. Martin, B. R. Smith,* Phenotype of Recovering Lymphoid Cell Populations after Marrow Transplantation, J. Exp. Med. *161,* 1483–1502 (1985).

[134] *L. G. Lum,* The Kinetics of Immune Reconstitution after Human Marrow Transplantation, Blood *69,* 369–380 (1987).

[135] *R. Mazaheri, C. R. Stiller, P. A. Keown, N. McKenzie, R. Coles, A. Hellstrom, W. Howson, N. R. Sinclair,* Monitoring the Effect of Cyclosporine Immunosuppression on Lymphocyte Subsets by Flow Cytometry and Monoclonal Antibodies, Transplantation Proc. *16,* 1086–1088 (1984).

[136] *U. Gross, P. Cunningham, C. Sash, C. Matthews, J. Thomas, S. Silverman,* Two-color Flow Cytometric Analysis of Mononuclear Cells Infiltrating Human Renal Allografts, Transplantation Proc. *20,* 102–104 (1988).

[137] *J. S. Pober, M. A. J. Gimbrone, R. S. Cotran, C. S. Reiss, S. J. Burakoff, W. Fiers, K. A. Ault,* Ia Expression by Vascular Endothelium is Inducible by Activated T Cells and by Human Gamma Interferon, J. Exp. Med. *157,* 1339–1353 (1983).

[138] *D. M. Briscoe, F. J. Schoen, G. E. Rice, M. P. Bevilacqua, P. Ganz, J. S. Pober,* Induced Expression of Endothelial-leukocyte Adhesion Molecules in Human Cardiac Allografts, Transplantation *51,* 537–547 (1991).

[139] *A. B. Cosimi, R. B. Colvin, R. C. Burton, R. H. Rubin, G. Goldstein, P. C. Kung, W. P. Hansen, F. L. Delmonico, P. S. Russel,* Use of Monoclonal Antibodies to T-Cell Subsets for Immunologic Monitoring and Treatment of in Recipients of Renal Allografts, N. Engl. J. Med. *305,* 308–314 (1981).

[140] *ORTHO multicenter transplant study group,* A Randomized Clinical Trial of OKT3 Monoclonal Antibody for Acute Rejection of Cadaveric Renal Transplants, N. Engl. J. Med. *313,* 337–342 (1985).

[141] *A. K. G. Von dem Borne, R. W. A. M. Kuijpers,* Platelet Antigens, New Aspects, in: *C. Kaplan-Gouet, N. Schlegel, C. Salmon, J. McGregor* (eds.), Platelet Immunology: Fundamental and Clinical Aspects, J. Libbey Eurotext Ltd, Paris, Londres 1991, pp. 219–240.

[142] *S. Santoso, V. Kiefel, E. Skribelka, C. Mueller-Eckhardt,* Human Platelet-specific Antibodies as a Tool to Identify the Glycoprotein Specificity of MAb by MAIPA Assay, in: *W. Knapp, B. Dörken, E. P. Rieber, H. Stein, W. R. Gilks, R. E. Schmidt, A. K. G. Von dem Borne* (eds.), Leucocyte Typing IV, Oxford University Press, Oxford 1989, pp. 971–973.

[143] *W. S. Court, J. M. Bozeman, S. J. Soong, M. N. Saleh, D. R. Shaw, A. F. Lobuglio,* Platelet-surface Bound IgG in Patients with Immune and Non-immune Thrombocytopenia, Blood *69,* 278–283 (1987).

[144] *L. K. Jennings, R. A. Ashmun, W. C. Wang, M. E. Dockter,* Analysis of Human Platelet Glycoprotein IIb-IIIa and Glanzmann's Thrombasthenia in Whole Blood by Flow Cytometry, Blood *68,* 173–179 (1986).

[145] *C. Kaplan-Gouet, N. Schlegel, C. Salmon, J. McGregor* (eds.), Platelet Immunology: Fundamental and Clinical Aspects, Vol. *230,* J. Libbey Eurotext, Paris 1991.

[146] *S. J. Shattil, M. Cunningham, J. A. Hoxie,* Detection of Activated Platelets in Whole Blood Using Activation-Dependent Monoclonal Antibodies and Flow Cytometry, Blood *70,* 307–315 (1987).

[147] *C. S. Abrams, N. Ellison, A. Z. Budzynski, S. J. Shattil,* Direct Detection of Activated Platelets and Platelets-derived Micro-particles in Humans, Blood *75,* 128–138 (1990).

[148] *P. Ambrosi, F. George, P. Poncelet, I. Besson-Faure, C. Chicheportiche, R. Luccioni, J. Sampol,* Effect of Recombinant Tissue-type Plasminogen on Ten Platelet Membrane Glycoproteins, Fibrinolysis *6,* 193–197 (1992).

[149] *C. M. Fenoglio-Preiser,* Selection of Appropriate Cellular and Molecular Biologic Test in the Evaluation of Cancer, Cancer *69,* 1607–1632 (1992).

[150] *C. W. Lin, D. A. Young, S. D. Kirley, A. H. Khaw, G. R. J. Prout,* Detection of Tumor Cells in Bladder Washings by a Monoclonal Antibody to Human Bladder Tumor-Associated Antigen, J. Urol. *140,* 672–677 (1988).

[151] *A. Longin, B. Fontaniere, N. Berger-Dutrieux, M. Devonec, J. C. Laurent,* A Useful Monoclonal Antibody (BL2-10D1) to Identifiy Tumor Cells in Urine Cytology, Cancer *65,* 1412–1417 (1990).

[152] *R. M. Zinkernagel, P. C. Doherty,* MHC Cytotoxic T-Cells: Studies on the Biological Role of Polymorphic Major Histocompatibility Antigens Determining T-Cell Restriction Specificity, Function and Responsiveness, Adv. Immunol. *27,* 151–177 (1979).

[153] *A. L. Schechter, D. F. Stern, L. Vaidyanathan, S. J. Decker, J. A. Drebin, M. I. Greene, R. A. Weinberg,* The Neu Oncogene: An Erb-B Related Gene Encoding a 185 000 Tumor Antigen, Nature *312,* 513–516 (1984).

[154] *C. R. King, M. H. Kraus, S. Aaronson,* Amplification of a Novel v-erbB Related Gene in Human Mammary Carcinoma, Science *229,* 974–976 (1985).

[155] *V. Combaret, B. Kremens, M. C. Favrot, J. C. Laurent, T. Philip,* S-L 11.14: A Monoclonal Antibody Recognizing Neuroectodermal Tumors with Possible Value for Bone Marrow Purging Before Autograft, Bone Marrow Transpl. *3,* 221–227 (1988).

[156] *R. Akeson, R. Bernards,* N-myc Down-regulates Neural-cell Adhesion Molecule Expression in Rat Neuroblastoma, Mol. Cell. Biol. *10,* 2012–2016 (1990).

[157] B. Roninson, Structure and Evolution of P-Glycoproteins, in: B. Roninson (ed.), Molecular and Cellular Biology of Multidrug Resistance in Tumors, Plenum Press, New York 1991, pp. 189–211.

[158] K. L. Deuchars, V. Ling, P-Glycoprotein and Multi-drug Resistance in Cancer Chemotherapy, Semin. Oncol. 16, 159–169 (1989).

[159] P. Musto, N. Cascavilla, N. Renzo, S. Ladogana, A. La Sala, L. Melillo, M. Nobile, R. Matera, G. Lombard, M. Carotenuto, Clinical Relevance of Immunocytochemical Detection of Multidrug-resistance Associated P-Glycoprotein in Hematologic Malignancies, Tumori 76, 353–359 (1990).

[160] R. A. Warnke, K. C. Gatter, B. Falini, P. Hildbreth, R. E. Woolston, K. Pulford, J. L. Cordell, B. Cohen, C. De Woolf-Peeters, D. Y. Mason, Diagnosis of Human Lymphoma with Monoclonal Anti-Leucocyte Antibodies, N. Engl. J. Med. 309, 1275–1281 (1983).

[161] B. Falini, S. Pileri, H. Stein, D. Dieneman, F. Dallenbach, G. Delsol, O. Minelli, S. Poggi, M. F. Martelli, G. Pallesen, G. Pallestro, Variable Expression of Leucocyte Common (CD45) Antigen in CD30 (Ki-1)-positive Anaplastic Large Cell Lymphomas. Implications in the Differential Diagnosis Between Lymphoid and Non-lymphoid Malignancies, Hum. Pathol. 6, 624–629 (1990).

[162] C. Gustmann, M. Altmannsberger, M. Osborn, H. Griesser, A. C. Feller, Cytokeratin Expression and Vimentin Content in Large Anaplastic Lymphomas and Other Non-Hodgkin's Lymphomas, Am. J. Pathol. 138, 1413–1422 (1991).

[163] M. R. Loken, V. O. Shah, Z. Hollander, C. I. Civin, Flow Cytometric Analysis of Normal B Lymphoid Development, Pathol. Immunopathol. Res. 7, 357–370 (1988).

[164] F. G. Behm, S. C. Raimondi, M. J. Schell, A. T. Look, G. K. Rivera, Ching-Hon Pui, Lack of CD45 Antigen on Blast Cells in Childhood Acute Lymphoblastic Leukemia is Associated with Chromosomal Hyperdiploidy and Other Favorable Prognostic Features, Blood 79, 1011–1016 (1992).

[165] T. Lavabre-Bertrand, P. Poncelet, D. Donadio, N. Fegueux, J. Taib, N. Navarro, I. Momas, Quantitative Expression of B Markers, HLA Molecules and Leucocyte Common Antigen During Neoplastic B Cell Differentiation, Blood 76, 1427a (1990).

[166] K. A. Ault, Detection of Small Numbers of Monoclonal B Lymphocytes in the Blood of Patients with Lymphomas, N. Engl. J. Med. 300, 1401–1405 (1979).

[167] D. S. Weinberg, G. S. Pinkus, K. A. Ault, Cytofluorometric Detection of B Cell Clonal Excess: A New Approach to the Diagnosis of B Cell Lymphomas, Blood 63, 1080–1087 (1984).

[168] M. Nakano, S. Kuge, S. Kuvabara, M. Yaguchi, Y. Kawanishi, K. Kodama, T. Akiya, K. Toyama, The Basic Study on Kappa-Lambda Imaging by Delta-curve for the Detection of a Monoclonal B Cell Population in the Peripheral Blood, Blood 72, 1461–1466 (1988).

[169] B. Corront, M. Michallet, J. M. Renversez, Study of Monoclonal Immunoglobulins after Allogeneic Bone Marrow Transplantation: Allotype and Antibody Activity, Bone Marrow Transpl. 2, 296–300 (1987).

[170] M. Palutke, B. Schnitzer, I. Mirchandani, P. M. Tabacza, R. Franklin, L. Eisenberg, K. So, G. Carillo, Increased Number of Lymphocytes with Single Class Surface Immunoglobulins in Reactive Hyperplasia of Lymphoid Tissue, Am. J. Clin. Pathol. 78, 316–323 (1982).

[171] N. Levy, J. Nelson, P. Meyer, R. Lukes, J. Parker, Reactive Lymphoid Hyperplasia with Single Class (Monoclonal) Surface Immunoglobulins, Am. J. Clin. Pathol. 80, 300–308 (1983).

[172] P. G. Pelici, D. M. Knowles, Z. A. Arlin, Multiple Monoclonal B Cell Expansion and c-Myc Oncogene Rearrangements in Acquired Immune Deficiency Syndrome-related Disorders, J. Exp. Med. 164, 2049–2053 (1986).

[173] T. Al Saati, G. Laurent, P. Caverivière, F. Rigal, G. Delsol, Reactivity of Leu-1 and T101 Monoclonal Antibodies with B Cell Lymphomas (Correlation with Other Immunological Markers), Clin. Exp. Immunol. 58, 631–638 (1984).

[174] L. J. Picker, L. M. Weiss, L. J. Medeiros, G. S. Wood, R. A. Warnke, Immunophenotype Criteria for the Diagnosis of Non-Hodgkin's Lymphoma, Am. J. Pathol. 128, 181–201 (1987).

[175] D. Campana, J. S. Thomson, P. Amlot, S. Brown, G. Janossy, The Cytoplasmic Expression of CD3 in Normal and Malignant Cell of the T Lymphoid Lineage, J. Immunol. 138, 648–655 (1987).

[176] A. Chu, J. Patterson, C. Berger, E. Vonderheid, R. Edelson, In Situ Study of T-Cell Subpopulations in Cutaneous T-Cell Lymphoma. Diagnostic Criteria, Cancer, 2414–2422 (1984).

[177] T. Suchi, K. Lennert, L. Y. Tu, M. Kikuchi, E. Sato, A. G. Stansfeld, A. C. Feller, Histopathology and Immunohistochemistry of Peripheral T Cell Lymphomas: A Proposal for Their Classification, J. Clin. Pathol. 40, 995–1015 (1987).

[178] D. Campana, E. Coustan-Smith, G. Janossy, The Immunologic Detection of Minimal Residual Disease in Acute Leukemia, Blood 76, 163–171 (1990).

[179] C. A. Hurwitz, M. R. Loken, M. L. Graham, J. E. Karp, M. J. Borowitz, D. J. Pullen, C. I. Civin, Asynchronous Antigen Expression in B Lineage Acute Lymphoblastic Leukemia, Blood 72, 299–307 (1988).

[180] G. Janossy, D. Campana, Monoclonal Antibodies in the Diagnosis of Acute Leukemia, in: D. Catovsky (ed.), The Leukemic Cell, Churchill and Livingstone, Edimbourg 1989.

[181] L. W. M. M. Terstappen, M. R. Loken, Myeloid Cell Differentiation in Normal Bone Marrow and Acute Myeloid Leukemia Assessed by Multi-dimensional Flow Cytometry, Anal. Cell. Pathol. 2, 229–240 (1990).

[182] L. Campos, D. Guyotat, A. Larese, L. Mazet, J. P. Bourgeot, A. Ehrsam, D. Fiere, Expression of CD19 Antigen on Acute Monoblastic Leukemia Cells at Diagnosis and After TPA-Induced Differentiation, Leuk. Res. 12, 369–372 (1988).

[183] L. M. Nadler, S. J. Korsmeyer, K. C. Anderson, A. W. Boyd, B. Slaugenhoupt, E. Park, J. Jensen, F. Coral, R. J. Mayer, S. E. Sallan, J. Ritz, S. F. Schlossman, B Cell Origin of Non-T-Cell Acute Lymphoblastic Leukemia. A Model for Discrete Stages of Neoplastic and Normal Pre-B Cell Differentiation, J. Clin. Invest. 74, 332–340 (1984).

[184] R. Garand, J. P. Vannier, M. C. Bene, G. C. Faure, A. Bernard, Correlations Between Acute Lymphoid Leukemia (ALL) Immunophenotype and Clinical and Laboratory Data at Presentation. A Study of 350 Patients, Cancer 64, 1437–1446 (1989).

[185] F. M. Uckun, Regulation of Human B Cell Ontogeny, Blood 76, 1908–1923 (1990).

[186] R. Garand, J. P. Vannier, M. C. Bene, G. Faure, M. Favre, A. Bernard, GEIL, Comparison of Outcome and Clinical Laboratory and Immunological Features in 164 Children and Adults with T-ALL, Leukemia 1, 697–705 (1990).

[187] H. G. Drexler, Classification of Acute Myeloid Leukemias. A Comparison of FAB and Immunophenotyping, Leukemia 1, 697–705 (1987).

[188] L. W. M. M. Terstappen, M. Safford, S. Könemann, M. R. Loken, K. Zurlutter, T. Büchner, W. Hiddemann, Flow Cytometric Characterization of Acute Myeloid Leukemias. II. Phenotypic Heterogeneity at Diagnosis, Leukemia 5, 757–767 (1991).

[189] D. C. Linch, C. Allen, P. C. L. Beverley, A. G. Bynoe, C. S. Scott, N. Hogg, Monoclonal Antibodies Differentiating Between Monocytic and Non-monocytic Variants of AML, Blood 63, 566–573 (1984).

[190] H. Merle-Béral, L. Ngyen Cong Duc, V. Leblond, C. Boucheix, A. Michel, C. Chastang, P. Debre, Diagnostic and Prognostic Significance of Myelomonocytic Cell Surface Antigens in Acute Myeloid Leukemia, Br. J. Hematol. 73, 323–330 (1989).

[191] F. Brito-Babapulle, H. Pullon, D. M. Layton, A. Etches, A. Huxtable, M. Mangi, A. J. Bellingham, G. J. Mufti, Clinicipathological Features of Acute Undifferentiated Leukemia with a Stem Cell Phenotype, Br. J. Hematol. 76, 210–214 (1990).

[192] M. J. Borowitz, J. P. Gockerman, J. O. Moore, C. I. Civin, S. O. Page, J. Robertson, S. H. Bigner, Clinipathologic and Cytogenetic Features of CD34 (My10)-positive Acute Non-lymphocytic Leukemia, Am. J. Clin. Pathol. 91, 265–270 (1989).

[193] S. M. Chittal, P. Caverivière, R. Schwarting, J. Gerdes, T. Al Saati, F. Rigal-Huguet, H. Stein, G. Delsol, Monoclonal Antibodies in the Diagnosis of Hodgkin's Disease. The Search for a Rational Panel, Am. J. Surg. Pathol. 12, 9–21 (1988).

[194] T. Lavabre-Bertrand, D. Donadio, N. Fegueux, D. Jessueld, J. Taib, D. Charler, T. Rousset, J. M. Emberger, P. Baldet, M. Navarro, A Study of 15 Cases of Primary Mediastinal Lymphoma of B-Cell Type, Cancer 69, 2561–2566 (1992).

[195] *J. Ritz, L. M. Nadler, A. K. Bhan, J. Notis-McConarty, J. M. Pesando, S. F. Schlossman*, Expression of Common Acute Lymphoblastic Leukemia Antigen (Calla) by Lymphomas of B-Cell and T-Cell Lineage, Blood *58*, 648–652 (1981).

[196] *D. D. Weisenburger*, Mantle-zone Lymphoma. An Immunohistological Study, Cancer *53*, 1073–1080 (1984).

[197] *R. B. Geller, M. Zahurak, C. A. Hurwitz, P. J. Burke, J. E. Karp, S. Piantadosi, C. I. Civin*, Prognostic Importance of Immunophenotyping in Adults with Acute Myelocytic Leukemia: The Significance of the Stem-Cell Glycoprotein CD34 (My10), Br. J. Hematol. *76*, 340–347 (1990).

[198] *E. Solary, R. O. Casasnovas, L. Campos, M. C. Béné, G. Faure, P. Maingon, A. Falkenrodt, B. Lenormand, N. Genetet*, GEIL, Surface Markers in Adult Acute Myeloblastic Leukemia: Correlation of CD19$^+$, CD34$^+$ and CD14$^+$/DR-Phenotypes with Shorter Survival, Leukemia *6*, 393–399 (1992).

[199] *J. D. Griffin, R. Davis, D. A. Nelson, F. R. Davey, R. J. Mayer, C. Schiffer, O. R. McIntyre, C. D. Bloomfield*, Use of Surface Marker Analysis to Predict Outcome of Adult Myeloblastic Leukemia, Blood *68*, 1232–1241 (1986).

[200] *L. Campos, D. Guyotat, E. Archimbaud, Y. Devaux, D. Treille, A. Larese, J. Maupas, O. Gentilhomme, A. Ehrsam, D. Fiere*, Surface Marker Expression in Adult Acute Myeloid Leukemia: Correlations with Initial Characteristics, Morphology and Response to Therapy, Br. J. Hematol. *72*, 161–166 (1989).

[201] *T. P. Miller, S. M. Lippman, C. M. Spier, D. J. Slymen, T. M. Grogan*, HLA-DR (Ia) Immune Phenotype Pedicts Outcome for Patients with Diffuse Large Cell Lymphoma, J. Clin. Invest. *82*, 370–372 (1988).

[202] *S. Jalkanen, H. Joensuu, K. O. Söderström, P. Klemi*, Lymphocyte Homing and Clinical Behavior of Non-Hodgkin's Lymphoma, J. Clin. Invest. *87*, 1835–1840 (1991).

[203] *A. T. Look, S. L. Melvin, L. K. Brown, M. E. Dockter, P. K. Roberson, S. B. Murphy*, Quantitative Variation of the Common Acute Lymphoblastic Leukemia Antigen (gp100) on Leukemic Bone Marrow Blasts, J. Clin. Invest. *73*, 1617–1628 (1984).

[204] *C. W. Caldwell, W. P. Patterson, N. Hakami*, Alterations of HLe-1 (T200) Fluorescence Intensity on Acute Lymphoblastic Leukemia Cells May Relate to Therapeutic Outcome, Leuk. Res. *11*, 103–106 (1987).

[205] *R. P. Gale, I. Ben Bassat*, Hybrid Acute Leukemia, Br. J. Hematol. *65*, 261–264 (1987).

[206] *W. D. Ludwig, C. R. Bartram, J. Ritter, A. Raghavachar, W. Hiddemann, G. Heil, J. Harbott, H. Seibt-Jung, J. V. Teichmann, H. Riehm*, Ambiguous Phenotypes and Genotypes in 16 Children with Acute Leukemia as Characterized by Multiparameter Analysis, Blood *71*, 1518–1828 (1988).

[207] *A. S. Freedman, J. M. Munro, C. Morimoto, B. W. McIntyre, K. Rhynhart, N. Lee, L. M. Nadler*, Follicular *Non-Hodgkin's* Lymphoma Cell Adhesion to Normal Germinal Centers and Neoplastic Follicles Involves very Late Antigen-4 and Vascular Cell Adhesion Molecule-1, Blood *79*, 206–212 (1992).

[208] *R. Tran-Paterson, G. Boileau, V. Giguere, M. Letarte*, Comparative Levels of Calla / Neutral Endopeptidase on Normal Granulocytes, Leukemic Cells and Transfected Cos-1 Cells, Blood *76*, 775–782 (1990).

[209] *B. R. Smith, D. S. Weinberg, N. J. Robert, M. Towle, E. Luther, G. S. Pinkus, K. A. Ault*, Circulating Monoclonal B Lymphocytes in Non-Hodgkin's Lymphomas, N. Engl. J. Med. *311*, 1476–1480 (1984).

[210] *J. H. Phillips, B. T. Gemlo, W. W. Myers, A. A. Rayner, L. L. Lanier*, In vivo and in vitro Activation of Natural Killer Cells in Advanced Cancer Patients Undergoing Combined Recombinant Interleukin-2 and LAK Cell Therapy, J. Clin. Oncol. *5*, 1933–1941 (1987).

[211] *S. Nasr, J. McKolanis, R. Pais, H. Findley, R. Hnath, K. Waldrep, A. H. Ragab*, A Phase I Study of Interleukin-2 in Children with Cancer and Evaluation of Clinical and Immunologic Status During Therapy, Cancer *64*, 783–788 (1989).

[212] *E. L. Hänninen, A. Körfer, M. Hadam, C. Schneekloth, I. Dallmann, T. Menzel, H. Kirchner, H. Poliwoda, J. Atzpodien*, Biological Monitoring of Low-dose Interleukin-2 in

Humans: Soluble Interleukin-2 Receptors, Cytokines and Cell-Surface Phenotypes, Cancer Res. *50*, 6312–6316 (1991).

[213] *G. Laurent, J. Pris, J. P. Farcet, P. Carayon, H. Blythman, P. Casellas, P. Poncelet, F. K. Jansen*, Effects of Therapy with T101 Ricin A-chain Immunotoxin in Two Leukemia Patients, Blood *67*, 1680–1687 (1986).

[214] *D. M. Fishwild, E. A. Saria*, Investigation and Prevention of Artifactual Staining in Flow Cytometric Analyses of Whole Blood Samples from Patients Treated with H65-RTA, an Anti-CD5 Monoclonal Antibody Conjugated to Ricin A-chain, J. Immunol. Methods *144*, 27–34 (1991).

[215] *P. Casellas, X. Canat, A. A. Fauser, O. Gros, G. Laurent, P. Poncelet, F. K. Jansen*, Optimal Elimination of Leukemic T Cells from Human Bone Marrow with T101-ricin-A-chain Immunotoxin, Blood *65*, 289–297 (1985).

[216] *J. M. Derocq, G. Laurent, P. Casellas, H. Vidal, P. Poncelet, A. Fauser, C. Demur, F. Jansen*, Rationale for the Selection of Ricin A Chain Anti-T Immunotoxins for Mature T Cell Depletion, Transplantation *44*, 763–769 (1987).

[217] *G. Laurent, E. Kuhlein, P. Casellas, X. Canat, P. Carayon, P. Poncelet, S. Correll, F. Rigal, F. K. Jansen*, Determination of Sensitivity of Fresh Leukemia Cells to Immunotoxins, Cancer Res. *46*, 2289–2294 (1986).

[218] *M. A. Taupier, J. F. Kearney, P. J. Leibson, M. R. Loken, H. Schreiber*, Non-random Escape of Tumor Cells from Immune Lysis due to Intra-clonal Fluctuations in Antigen Expression, Cancer Res. *43*, 4050–4057 (1987).

[219] *M. D. P. Boyle, A. P. Gee*, Low Antigen Density on Tumor Cells: An Obstacle to Effective Bone Marrow Purging?, Cancer Invest. *5*, 113–118 (1987).

[220] *W. E. Janssen, C. Lee, C. Gross, A. P. Gee*, Low Antigen Density Leukemia Cells: Selection and Comparative Resistance to Antibody-mediated Marrow Purging, Exp. Hematol. *17*, 252–257 (1989).

[221] *A. Gee, V. H. Mansour, M. B. Weiler*, Effects of Target Antigen Density on the Efficacy of Immunomagnetic Cell Separation, J. Immunol. Methods *142*, 127–136 (1991).

[222] *L. A. Herzenberg, D. W. Bianchi, J. Schroder, H. M. Cann, G. M. Iverson*, Fetal Cells in the Blood of Pregnant Women: Detection and Enrichment by Fluorescence Cell Sorter, Proc. Natl. Acad. Sci. USA *76*, 1453–1460 (1979).

[223] *M. Adinolfi*, Detection of Trophoblast Cellular Elements in Maternal Peripheral Blood Using Monoclonal Antibodies and Flow Cytometry, Cytometry Suppl. *3*, 104–105 (1988).

[224] *J. E. Brinchmann, G. Gaudernack, E. Thorsby, T. O. Jonassen, F. Vartdal*, Reliable Isolation of Human Immunodeficiency Virus From Cultures of Naturally Infected CD4$^+$ T Cells, J. Virol. Methods *25*, 293–300 (1989).

[225] *C. Chicheportiche, P. Poncelet, O. Massot, J. C. Laurent, L. Passarelli, L. Morel, J. Sampol*, Quality-control of Leukocyte-depleted Blood Products: A New Simple Assay to Count Very Low Numbers of Residual White Blood Cells, Boletim *14*, 213–214 (1992).

[226] *F. George, C. Brisson, P. Poncelet, J. C. Laurent, O. Massot, D. Arnoux, P. Ambrosi, C. Klein-Soyer, J. P. Cazenave, J. Sampol*, Rapid Isolation of Human Endothelial Cells from Whole Blood Using S-Endo1 Monoclonal Antibody Coupled to Immuno-magnetic Beads: Demonstration of Endothelial Injury after Angioplasty, Thrombosis and Haemostasis *67*, 147–153 (1992).

6.2   Development of the Immune System

Françoise Dieterlen-Lièvre and Josselyne Salaün

6.2.1   General Considerations of Developmental Biology

Immunological methods have become very important for the investigation of developmental problems. A critical asset of these methods in this field has been their applicability to *in-situ* detection of antigens, thereby bypassing the problems due to the small number of embryonic cells available. Furthermore, *in-situ* detection is a particularly appropriate approach for developmental studies, since ontogeny usually involves cell interaction processes. The techniques for detection of antigens in embryonic cells are those applicable generally (cf. 5.1 *et seq.*).

Other important developmental applications derive from hybridoma methodology [1] which, together with molecular biology, has permitted the identification of several classes of molecules that mediate crucial processes of development. The strategy leading to such identification starts with the preparation of an mAb that detects a protein, and provides information about its location, developmental modulation and hence potential importance. In many cases such mAbs have been obtained after immunization of mice with cell populations or membrane preparations. The molecule recognized by the mAb may be purified by means of immunoaffinity chromatography and its sequence determined by one of two approaches: 1. fragments of the polypeptide can be sequenced and used to deduce nucleotide sequences, which in turn will serve as probes for screening a cDNA library; 2. the antibody can be applied directly to the screening of a cDNA expression library. In favourable circumstances the subsequent sequencing of selected cDNA clones will eventually lead to the complete amino acid sequence of the antigen and to the cloning of the gene. Thereafter a host of investigations can be undertaken: search for homologues in a data bank; study of ontogenic expression at the messenger RNA level; gene knockout by homologous recombination in embryonic stem (ES) cells and creation of mutant mice by the integration of these ES cells; analysis of the mutant phenotype. Developmental molecules of prime importance have been thus discovered, such as cell adhesion molecules, and extracellular matrix molecules and their receptors; furthermore, the function of several cell surface or extracellular matrix molecules has been analysed with blocking antibodies directed against them. Such powerful approaches are likely to become increasingly important.

The account that follows will focus on the structural and functional genesis of the immune system, as it has been studied by the combined use of embryological and immunological methods. Applications of the latter methods have made possible both the tracing of movements of cells "marked" by specific surface antigens and the study of the acquisition of differentiated phenotypes. This approach will enable a complete ontogenic process to be described and will illustrate how some of the cellular and molecular mechanisms important in developmental biology have been unravelled by means of immunological methods. The development of the immune system will be considered in higher vertebrates, namely birds and mammals.

Avian embryos yield particularly informative developmental models, because they are suitable to many experimental approaches in the early phases of morphogenesis and organogenesis, so that single components of their immune system can be manipulated, prior to their interaction with cells of other types. Embryos which have undergone experimental manipulations can eventually hatch and their functional capacities can be analysed in the adult state. A further advantage of the avian model is the feasibility of constructing chimaeras from two closely related species such as the chick and quail [2]. Quail cell nuclei possess a prominent heterochromatin mass associated with the nucleolus. This "nucleolar marker" makes it possible to identify quail cells combined with chick cells. In earlier years, the quail and chick nuclei were recognized on tissue sections stained for DNA by the *Feulgen Rossenbeck* reaction. Now, further resolution is accomplished with mAbs that have affinity for a cell lineage or a cell subpopulation derived from only one of the two species.

Knowledge derived from chick-quail chimaeras has often provided leads to investigations of mammalian development. In mice, a limited assortment of chimaeras may be constructed *in utero* or, more simply, immediately after birth. Mutant mice with a deficient immune system (nude or SCID) are often selected as hosts for rudiment transplantation, since these mice will not reject an allogeneic graft even if they are raised until adulthood. The analysis of chimaerism in mice relies on allogeneic markers, a rich variety of which have been obtained from numerous inbred strains selected by genetic studies during the last fifty or so years. It is not possible here to review the exploitation of transgenic mice for the understanding of the role of the MHC in the acquisition of self recognition.

Cell phenotype analysis in normal or experimental embryos and fetuses has laid the basic rules governing the development of the immune system and has shown the sequential appearance of defined cell populations. Some of these populations, such as the $\gamma\delta^+$ T lymphocytes produced uniquely in early ontogeny, may have an important regulatory role in the immune system, in relationship to other cell populations that are produced in a more sustained fashion. These cell populations, rare in the adult, are predominant and mutually interactive early in ontogeny; they probably have a crucial role in the establishment of mature immune repertoires. The combination of immunological and embryological methods has led to the dissection of the role of various populations, and emphasized crucial issues, such as the role of the thymic epithelium in the establishment of tolerance.

6.2.2   Primary Lymphoid Organ Differentiation

Birds have contributed uniquely to the knowledge of the immune system, because they constitute the only class, among vertebrates, which possesses a lymphoid organ devoted to the development of B lymphocytes. The existence of the bursa of *Fabricius* was actually instrumental in the discovery that the immune system is divided into a humoral and a cellular limb [3]. Another original trait of birds in the rearrangement strategy of immunoglobulin genes.

A number of rules that govern the development as well as the steady state operation of the immune system have been worked out in avian chimaeras:

1. The development of thymus and bursa, like that of all haemopoietic organs, involves seeding of the rudiment by stem cells [4, 5]. The rudiments are composed of endoderm (pharyngeal or cloacal) and mesenchyme (of neural crest origin in the case of the thymus), which give rise respectively to the epithelial network and to the connective tissue stroma. The thymic epithelium is responsible, at least in part, for T-cell education while the bursal epithelium provides an environment that promotes B-cell progenitor amplification and eliminates B-cells with unproductive immunoglobulin (Ig) chain rearrangements. The mesenchyme is indispensable for the correct development of the organs (for instance, the *Di George*'s syndrome athymic condition results from a deficiency in the mesectodermal neural crest cells that give rise to the connective tissue of the thymus).

2. The colonization of the rudiments follows very precise patterns. The thymus receives periodic inputs of progenitors [5, 6, 7] (Fig. 1). The bursa of *Fabricius* is colonized during a single period of short duration [8] while around the time of hatching, progenitors capable of colonizing the bursa and undergoing lymphoid differentiation altogether disappear [9].

These basic patterns of development were discovered before the advent of immunological methods. Chimaeric lymphoid organs were first obtained by *Moore & Owen* [4], who parabiosed chick embryos and used the sexual chromosomes as markers. They inferred the extrinsic origin of progenitors from the chimaerism of the lymphoid population in heterosexual pairs of embryos (the chimaerism actually extended to all haemopoietic organs). The precise patterns of colonization were established by grafting thymus and bursa rudiments from the quail embryo into the chick body wall, the quail nucleolus serving as the marker [5, 6, 8]. Cyclic colonization was confirmed for the chick thymus grafted in the quail embryo body wall [7]. In this case, cell migrating from the host into the rudiment were traced by means of mAb MB1 [10] that recognizes the quail haemangioblastic lineage (haemopoietic and endothelial cells).

Colonization of the thymus rudiment has also been studied in the mouse embryo or fetus. The first wave of progenitors enters the thymus rudiment at E11 (day 11 of gestation) [11]. Thus, when the third branchial pouches are retrieved on E10, the presumptive thymic rudiment, present in these pouches, is not yet colonized by blood-borne progenitors; this is an important point in experiments probing the role of cell subpopulations in the establishment of tolerance. The mouse precolonization

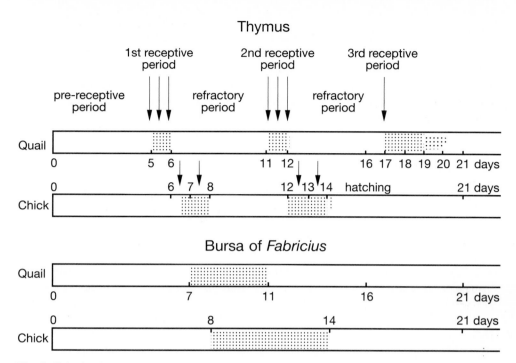

Fig. 1. Colonization patterns of primary lymphoid organs in birds.

rudiments become lymphoid when associated in organ culture with organs capable of contributing lymphoid progenitors, such as the E8 to E10 yolk sac, E12 to E17 liver or spleen, and adult bone marrow [12]; in these instances the origin of the progenitors has been determined through either glucose phosphate isomerase isoenzymes or Thy-1 antigen alleles. Progenitors from the E11 fetal liver colonizing a thymic rudiment acquire the capacity to respond to phytomitogens [13]. The entry of progenitors in the mouse thymus also proceeds in waves, although the waves are much less clear-cut than in birds because of a heavy overlap: a first wave takes place in E11 to E12 thymuses but a second wave begins after E14 while the progeny of the first wave is still multiplying and differentiating [14].

Colonization of the avian bursa of *Fabricius* has also been analysed by similar methods. After its unique wave of colonization, the bursa functions for several weeks producing a large contingent of pre B-cells that settle into the bone marrow, where they undergo their final maturation. The bursa is composed of tightly packed follicles arranged around a central lumen, which is a diverticulum of the cloaca. Each follicle is populated by very few stem cells (1 to 3), as has been shown in embryonic parabionts or cyclophosphamide-treated embryos whose contingents of B precursors were restored with a mixed suspension of precursors bearing one of two alleles of Bu1, a B-cell surface antigen [15].

The rearrangement of immunoglobulin genes during chicken ontogeny has been worked out in detail. It entails the use of a single functional Vλ1 gene from the light chain locus that always becomes joined to the Jλ sequence during the rearrangement event. The other Vλ genes are pseudogenes, from which sequences are used in successive gene conversion events that introduce somatic diversity in the originally rearranged Vλ1 gene [16]. A similar strategy is used for diversification of the heavy chain repertoire [17].

6.2.3   T-Cell Differentiation during Ontogeny Followed through Phenotype Analysis

The fate of the successive progenitor waves entering the thymus was established [18] using a panel of mAbs directed against cell surface molecules present on chicken T-cells [19]. Avian homologues of the CD2, CD3 and CD8 molecules are very similar to their mammalian counterparts. Three distinct TCR isotypes (TCR1, 2 and 3 according to their order of appearance during ontogeny) were identified and found to be expressed by mutually exclusive sublineages of avian T-cells. The TCR1 sublineage appears to be homologous to the mammalian γδ-bearing cells, while the TCR2 cells are homologous to the mammalian TCR αβ cells. The TCR2 and TCR3 sublineages may express distinct TCR β chains but probably share the same TCR α chain. The TCR1 cells preferentially home to the splenic red pulp and to the intestinal epithelium, like their mammalian counterparts (T-cells are rare in the skin of chickens). The TCR2 cells migrate preferentially to the periarteriolar areas of the splenic white pulp and the lamina propria of the intestines.

The differentiation of T-cells begins in the E9 thymus (the first colonization wave occurs at E6.5 to E8, cf. Fig. 1) with the expression of cytoplasmic CD3 molecules, soon followed by cell-surface expression of CD2.

The T-cells first generated express the TCR1/CD3 receptor. The TCR1 cells begin to appear in the thymic cortex on E12, reach the nascent medullary region of the thymus on E13, and begin their migration to peripheral organs where many express CD8 by E15 (spleen) and E16 (intestine).

The second T-cell subpopulation, generated in the thymus and expressing the TCR2/CD3 complex, develop more slowly than TCR1 cells. First recognized at E14–15, they expand rapidly, becoming the major thymocyte subpopulation, and reaching the spleen on E19. As in mammals, most of the immature TCR2 cells in the thymic cortex express both CD4 and CD8, whereas more mature TCR2 cells express either CD4 or CD8. The TCR3/CD3 cells appear last in the thymic cortex around E17. Their pattern of development closely resembles that of TCR2, except that they are fewer in number.

In the avian model, all mAbs recognizing T-cell surface antigens are restricted to the chick species and make good markers in interspecific chimaeras. Each wave of precursors was shown to give rise to TCR1, 2 or 3 T-cells: E9 chicken thymuses containing the first wave of precursors, when transplanted to quail hosts, generated T-cells bearing any of these three isotypes. Similar data concerning the second wave of progenitors were also obtained. The entire intrathymic maturation and seeding process of TCR1, 2 and 3 cells from each wave of precursor cells lasted approximately 3 weeks [20].

These analyses have also uncovered the existence of a novel cell population, the so-called TCR0 cells. These cells lack Ig or TCR/CD3 on their surface but express CD3 in their cytoplasm. They frequently express CD8. TCR0 cells first appear in the spleen at E8 and can be found later in the spleen and intestines. They are thymus-independent in their development and share many characteristics of mammalian natural killer cells. It is speculated that these cells represent a primitive population of lymphocytes that evolved before T- and B-cells but remain important participants in defence mechanisms, even in higher vertebrates.

In the mouse, descendants of thymocytes from the first wave migrate to the peripheral lymphoid organs during the first post-natal week where they constitute a unique subpopulation of lymphocytes characterized by the expression of TCR$\gamma\delta$, in which $\gamma3$ is always the rearranged allele [21, 22]. In adult lymphoid tissues V$\gamma3$ cells are not detectable, except in the skin Thy-1$^+$ dendritic cells. V$\gamma3$ T-cells are the progeny of the first wave of stem cells as shown by the following experiment. Thy-1-1 thymic lobes were grafted into newborn Thy-1-2 recipients: donor-type Thy-1-1 dendritic cells were found in the epidermis of the host when E14 fetal, but not newborn, thymus had been grafted, proving that the ability to generate this particular subpopulation has already disappeared at birth. Furthermore, by exposing embryos to injected anti-V$\gamma3$ antibody, mice without V$\gamma3$ Thy-1$^+$ dendritic epidermal cells were produced [22].

6.2.4   Haemopoietic Stem Cells

Since haemopoietic organs are all seeded by extrinsic stem cells, where do these cells come from? *Moore & Owen,* who had detected this feature, put forward the hypothesis of a unique yolk sac origin of all stem cells [23]. This hypothesis was tested later by means of "yolk sac chimaeras", in which the embryonic area of a quail is grafted onto the extra-embryonic area of a chick blastodisc (Fig. 2) [24]. The extra-embryonic area gives rise to the yolk sac in the next two days. In these chimaeras, the haemopoietic organs were entirely populated by quail cells [25, 26]. The blood was studied in a haemolysis assay using polyclonal antibodies directed against quail or chick erythrocytes. These chimaeras had 95 to 100% chick cells until E5, then quail erythrocytes were released in the blood in increasing proportions [27]. Some chimaeras had up to 80% quail red cells on E13; however, the replacement of chick by quail fluctuated greatly. This experiment

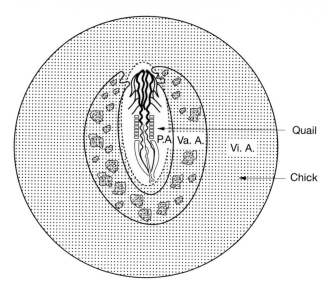

Fig. 2. Construction of quail chick "yolk-sac chimaeras" [24]. The stippled line indicates the site of the suture between the quail body and the chick extraembryonic area. P.A. = pellucid area. Va. A = vascular area. Vi.A = vitelline area.

was repeated using yolk sac chick-chick chimaeras, in which immunoglobulin allotypes and MHC antigens served as markers. Yolk sac stem cells never gave rise to B lymphocytes [28]. In that type of chimaera, erythrocyte replacement was very regular and very swift: on E10 only 20% of the red cells were progeny from yolk sac stem cells and these had disappeared altogether by hatching [29].

Thus, in birds, yolk stem cells give rise to the early erythrocytes of the primitive series; their contribution then tapers off and they become extinct without giving rise to stem cells with life-long renewal capacity. The origin of intra-embryonic stem cells could be traced to the region of the aorta in E3–E4 chick and quail embryos [30–32].

The question of the site of emergence of haemopoietic stem cells in mammals is still open. While several approaches have suggested the existence of distinct populations with differing potentialities, the only stem cells with a well-identified origin are the ones that arise in the yolk sac. The difficulty in working out these problems in the mouse comes from the nonaccessibility of the embryo to experimental manipulations at the stages of morphogenesis or organogenesis; furthermore migrations and interactions involved in the commitment of these cells do not occur *in vitro* in dissociated cells. The long-term potentialities of yolk sac stem cells have been probed some years ago. *Weissman* et al. [33] attempted to obtain chimaeras by injecting yolk sac cells into the yolk sac cavity of E8–E11 fetal mouse recipients *in utero* and found a low degree of chimaerism in a few fetuses' bone marrow and, exceptionally, thymus. *Paige* et al. [34] tried to restore with yolk sac cells the B lymphocyte population of a B-cell-deficient strain of mice (Xid). A long delay was necessary for the development of a low level of B-cell progenitors. Clearly, yolk sac cells were not as efficient as bone marrow or fetal liver cells in these two assays. Yolk sacs, organ cultured for 2–4 days prior to cell collection, provided cells that restored irradiated adults more efficiently [35]. Recently *Liu and Auerbach* [36] obtained the colonization of E14 thymocyte-depleted thymuses by co-culture with E9 yolk sac. The repopulating cells acquired mature T-cell markers (CD3/TCR, CD4, CD8). In contrast, cells from the E9 embryonal body did not reconstitute the thymus. The most thorough investigations, carried out on the erythropoietic capacities of yolk sac cells, have indicated clearly that the yolk sac is capable of producing stem cells that undergo both primitive and definitive erythropoiesis [37].

Some data do indicate that cells with the potential of a stem cell are present in other sites than the yolk sac and at other times in the mouse embryo. The omentum is often considered a possible site for the production of intraembryonic stem cells. This mesothelial structure contains, in the E13.5 mouse embryo, cells that generate $Ly1^+$ B lymphocytes capable of homing to the spleen, peritoneal cavity and lymph glands of SCID mice [38]. Cells from the omentum can also give rise to T-cells, when they are grafted to the anterior chamber of the eye in irradiated adults [39]. Earlier data indicated the presence of T-cell progenitors in the embryo at E9 [40]. Furthermore, on the same day of development, cells capable of giving rise to B-cells, when seeded on an appropriate stromal cell line, are present in the embryo prior to their appearance in the yolk sac [41].

All in all, the evidence shows that the mouse yolk sac is capable of producing a secondary "wave" of stem cells after the primitive wave, the progeny of the first wave being exclusively primitive erythrocytes. The other issues are open to speculation. For instance: 1. "secondary" stem cells produced in the yolk sac may or may not be the daughters of the "primitive" stem cells; 2. these yolk sac "definitive" stem cells may not be endowed with permanent self renewal potential; 3. the emergence of "secondary" stem cells might occur in parallel in the yolk sac and the embryo. While these propositions reflect what occurs in the avian embryo, no experimental evidence is available about them.

Interestingly, however, some indications have been obtained about changing potentialities of stem cells, namely the possible occurrence in mouse fetuses of waves of stem cells. The experiment draws upon a remarkable stem cell enrichment strategy [42], implementing negative sorting out of stem cells using mAbs; all cells bearing one or several of an array of cell surface antigens (B220 on B-cells, Gr-1 on granulocytes, Mac-1 present on myelomonocytic cells, CD4 and CD8 on T-cells) are depleted from a bone marrow cell suspension. The cells selected through this negative procedure (Lin^- for lineage) express a low grade of the Thy-1 marker ($Thy-1^{lo}$) and are submitted to further selection for the expression of the Sca-1 antigen (Stem Cell Antigen 1). As few as 30 $Thy-1^{lo}$ Lin-$Sca-1^+$ cells suffice to rescue one half of lethally irradiated mice. This selection procedure was used and the interactions between stem cells and thymic environment studied [43]. $Thy-1^{lo}$ Lin^-Sca-1^+ haemopoietic stem cells were isolated either from fetal liver or adult bone marrow and used to repopulate fetal or adult thymuses *in vitro*. Donor-derived $V\gamma3$ cells (with the fetus-specific γ chain rearrangement) were detected in fetal thymuses repopulated with fetal liver cells. At limiting dilutions, thymic progeny of a single fetal haemopoietic stem cell included $V\gamma3^+$, other

$g\delta^+$ and $\alpha\beta^+$ T-cells. However donor-derived Vγ3 T-cells were not found in fetal thymuses repopulated with adult bone marrow haemopoietic cells, nor in adult thymuses repopulated with fetal liver cells. Thus, both the fetal cells and the fetal micro-environment are needed to support the differentiation of the fetal specific trait. The developmental potential of haemopoietic stem cells thus changes during ontogeny. Whether this results from a changing developmental clock within the progeny of an embryonic or fetal stem cell or results from waves of stem cells not related to each other in a lineage awaits further examination.

The number of progenitors necessary to populate the thymus has intrigued many investigators. This question was studied in the adult. Irradiated mice were reconstituted with limiting numbers of bone marrow cell mixtures, marked by the Thy-1 alleles. A few cells or even one cell could reconstitute an entire thymic lobe. The pattern of reconstitution indicated that two independent lineages exist in the mouse thymus, one colonizing the cortex plus medulla and the other the medulla alone [44].

In experiments on fetuses, the rudiments usually came from E14, because earlier rudiments do not survive *in vitro*. The lymphoid progenitors already present were depleted either by a 5-day culture in the presence of deoxyguanosine (dGuo) [45] or by incubation at 24°C for 7 days [46]. The number of stem cells necessary to colonize a thymus and the potentialities of a single stem cell were investigated using these dGuo depleted thymuses and E14 dissociated thymuses as sources of immature progenitors [47]. A hanging drop culture system ensured a 2-day contact between thymic stroma and precursors. After this colonization period, the thymuses were placed in organ cultures for 10 days. The number of lobes recolonized was related to the number of cells in the hanging drop, presumably reflecting the colonizing potential of the cells (80% of lobes were colonized with 2000 precursors per well and 10% with 50–75 precursors per well). In a small proportion of cases (2–3% of 300 lobes), recolonization was achieved with one manually seeded cell. Despite this very low success rate, the significance of the results lies in the phenotypic analysis of the progeny of a single cell. Over a 12-day culture period, the single precursor gave rise to a minimum estimate of 2 to 11×10^4 cells bearing three different Lyt phenotypes [47]. Multiple rearrangements of the TCR β chain could be demonstrated in nine thymic lobes repopulated by a single progenitor [48].

Another line of research concerns the existence of a common lymphoid progenitor. It is clear that, in birds around hatching, lymphoid progenitors become restricted to the T lineage, since B progenitors disappear altogether. Do bipotential precursors exist earlier in development? To answer this question, irradiated chick embryos with cells bearing the Bu1 antigen and another genetically polymorphic cell surface antigen were reconstituted. Two classes of progenitors, $Bu1^+$ committed to the B lineage and $Bu1^-$ committed to the T lineage, could be demonstrated in E14 embryos [49], indicating clearly that colonization of the two primary lymphoid organs is accomplished by distinct progenitors.

6.2.5   Tolerance

Neural tube chimaeras (chick embryos in which a segment of the neural tube was replaced by a quail segment), raised for a few months after hatching, display signs of "autoimmune" disease, although the foreign neural tissue has been present since a very early embryonic stage (E2) [50]. In order to study the rejection process in an experimental model that would not kill the animal, the wing was grafted *in situ* in 5-day embryos. Inflammatory signs appeared much earlier than after neural tube grafting and within a few days, the grafted wing became auto-amputated. The rejection in this xenogeneic system is indeed extremely acute. The delayed rejection of grafted neural tissue has been attributed to the blood-brain barrier, which eventually breaks down. Rejection of the wing could be alleviated or prevented altogether by engrafting the chick host embryo with a quail thymic rudiment two days before grafting the quail wing bud [51]. The thymus was grafted *in situ,* in place of the host rudiments that were cauterized. This operation is delicate and often some host thymus remains and/or the foreign tissue does not engraft completely. One third of the total thymic tissue of foreign origin was found sufficient to ensure tolerance. At the time of grafting, the thymus rudiments are purely epithelial, i. e., deprived of cells of the blood lineage. At the time of sacrifice the cell origins of the differentiated thymus were studied by means of mAbs recognizing MHC class II antigens of the chick or the quail [52]: this analysis was consistent with the conclusion that only the quail tissue gave rise to thymic epithelium. Thus, this thymic component is by itself capable of educating lymphocytes for self recognition. This capacity was previously attributed to accessory cells of the thymus (dendritic cells and macrophages) which belong to the blood lineage.

   In the mouse, many investigators have attempted to induce tolerance in allogeneic situations by grafting E14 thymuses depleted of haemopoietic cells under the adult kidney capsule. Colonization of the explants by recipient haemopoietic stem cells was observed in this situation. However, with regard to tolerance induction, the results of these experiments have been controversial. In nude-mice recipients, *Jordan* et al. [53, 54] could induce *in vitro* tolerance (tested by mixed lymphocyte culture) in allogeneic situations, whereas *von Bœhmer* et al. concluded that thymic epithelium induced tolerance only to minor histocompatibility antigens [55, 56].

   Surgery was performed *in utero* to construct early allogeneic chimaeras [57]. E10 BALB/c embryos (*H-2^d* haplotype) were donors of thymic rudiments that were grafted onto E16 C3H fetuses (*H-2^k*). Several weeks after birth, the grafted thymus from the operated animals, submitted to immunocytological analysis, was found to be chimaeric, with epithelial cells expressing MHC class II molecules of donor origin (Ia^d) and haematopoietic cells expressing MHC class II molecules of host origin (Ia^k). Despite the maintenance of the chimaeric thymus, tolerance to donor-type skin was never obtained. The presence of the recipient's own thymus, already colonized when the allogenic thymic rudiment was grafted, was probably responsible for the absence of tolerance. Subsequently a new strategy, involving newborn nude mice, which are genetically deprived of a thymus, was devised. These nude mice were reconstituted at birth by the graft of E10 thymic epithelium [57]. T-cell functions were fully restored by syngeneic epithelium as shown by rejection of allogeneic skin grafts and *in vitro* responses of splenic cells (MLR). When the grafted thymic epithelium was allogeneic, a chimaeric thymus developed. Double staining with donor-specific anti-class II and anti-keratin antibodies identified the epithelial cells in the cortex and medulla as donor type, while accessory cells in the medulla were of host origin. Lymphocytes, identified with anti-Thy-1 antibody, were especially dense in the cortex. Several months after thymus grafting, three kinds of skin grafts were performed: host, donor and third-party haplotypes. All reconstituted mice rejected third-party skin grafts while they accepted host and donor skin grafts. Specific cytolytic activity of splenic lymphocytes against irradiated donor haplotype cells or third-party cells was studied. In this assay some mice appeared tolerized while others retained T-cells reactive against donor haplotype cells. Thus the noncolonized thymic epithelium has the ability to reconstitute allogeneic nude mice, and to induce tolerance *in vivo*. However, in most animals this tolerance is split, not extending to reactivity *in vitro* between lymphocytes [58].

References

[1] *G. Köhler, C. Milstein*, Continuous Cultures of Fused Cells Secreting Antibody of Pre-Defined Specificity, Nature *256*, 495–497 (1975).

[2] *N. M. Le Douarin*, Particularités du noyau interphasique chez la Caille japanaise, Utilisation de ces particularités comme "marquage biologique" dans les recherches sur les interactions tissulaires et les migrations cellulaires au cours de l'ontogénèse, Bull. Biol. Fr. Belg. *103*, 432–452 (1969).

[3] *M. Cooper, R. D. A. Peterson, R. A. Good*, Delineation of the Thymic and Bursal Lymphoid Systems in the Chicken, Nature *4967*, 143–146 (1965).

[4] *M. A. S. Moore, J. J. T. Owen*, Chromosome Marker Studies on the Development of the Haematopoietic System in the Chick Embryo, Nature *208*, 958–989 (1965).

[5] *N. M. Le Douarin, F. Dieterlen-Lièvre, P. D. Oliver*, Ontogeny of Primary Lymphoid Organs and Lymphoid Stem Cells, Am. J. Anat. *170*, 261–299 (1984).

[6] *N. M. Le Douarin, F. Jotereau*, Origin and Renewal of Lymphocytes in Avian Embryo Thymuses Studied in Interspecific Combinations, Nature New Biol. *246*, 25–27 (1973).

[7] *M. Coltey, F. V. Jotereau, N. M. Le Douarin*, Evidence for a Cyclic Renewal of Lymphocyte Precursor Cells in the Embryonic Chick Thymus, Cell Differ. *22*, 71–82 (1987).

[8] *N. M. Le Douarin, E. Houssaint, F. V. Jotereau, M. Belo*, Origin of Haemopoietic Stem Cells in Embryonic Bursa of Fabricius and Bone Marrow Studied through Interspecific Chimaeras, Proc. Natl. Acad. Sci. USA *72*, 2701–2705 (1975).

[9] *A. Toivanen, P. Toivanen*, Stem Cells of the Lymphoid System, in: *A. Toivanen, P. Toivanen* (eds.), Avian Immunology: Basis and Practice, Vol. 1; CRC Press, Boca Raton, Florida 1987, pp. 23–37.

[10] *B. Péault, J. P. Thiery, N. M. Le Douarin*, A Surface Marker for the Haemopoietic and Endothelial Cell Lineages in the Quail Species Defined by a Monoclonal Antibody, Proc. Natl. Acad. Sci. USA *80*, 2976 (1983).

[11] *D. Metcalf, M. A. S. Moore* (eds.) Frontiers of Biology, Vol. 24, Haemopoietic Cells, North-Holland Publishing Company, Amsterdam London 1971, pp. 550.

[12] *J. Fontaine-Pérus. F. M. Calman, C. Kaplan, N. M. Le Douarin*, Seeding of the 10-day Mouse Embryo Thymic Rudiment by Lymphocyte Precursors *in vitro*, J. Immunol. *126*, 2310–2316 (1981).

[13] *K. W. Pyke, P. F. Bartlett, T. E. Mandel*, The *in vitro* Production of Chimaeric Murine Thymus from Nonlymphoid Embryonic Precursors, J. Immunol. Methods *58*, 243–254 (1983).

[14] *F. Jotereau, F. Heuze, V. Salomon-Vie, H. Gascan*, Cell Kinetics in the Fetal Mouse Thymus: Precursor Cell Input, Proliferation and Emigration, J. Immunol. *138*, 1026–1030 (1987).

[15] *J. R. Pink, O. Vainio, A. M. Rijnbeek*, Clones of B Lymphocytes in Individual Follicules of the Bursa of Fabricius, Eur. J. Immunol. *15*, 83–87 (1985).

[16] *J. C. Weill, C. A. Reynaud*, The Chicken B Cell Compartment, Science *238*, 1094–1098 (1987).

[17] *C. A. Reynaud, A. Dahan, V. Anquez, J. C. Weill*, Somatic Hyperconversion Diversifies the Single VH gene of the Chicken with a High Incidence in the D Region, Cell *59*, 171–183 (1989).

[18] *N. M. Le Douarin, F. Dieterlen-Lièvre, J. Smith* (eds.), The Avian Model in Developmental Biology: from Organism to Genes. T Cell Development in Birds, Editions du CNRS, Paris 1990, pp. 239–250.

[19] *C. L. H. Chen, M. D. Cooper*, Identification of Cell Surface Molecules on Chicken Lymphocytes with Monoclonal Antibodies, in: *A. Toivanen, P. Toivanen* (eds.), Avian Immunology: Basis and Practice, Vol. 1; CRC Press, Boca Raton, Florida 1987, pp. 138–154.

[20] *M. Coltey, R. P. Bucy, C. H. Chen, J. Cihak, U. Lösch, D. Char, N. M. Le Douarin, M. D. Cooper*, Analysis of the First Two Waves of Thymus Homing Stem Cells and Their T Cell Progeny in Chick-Quail Chimaeras, J. Exp. Med. *170*, 543–557 (1989).

[21] *W. Havran, S. Grell, G. Duwe, J. Kimura, A. Wilson, A. Kruisbeek, R. O'brien, W. Born, R. Tigelaar, J. Allison*, Limited Diversity of T-cell Receptor γ-chain Expression of Murine Thy-1$^+$ dendritic Epidermal Cells Revealed by Vγ3-specific Monoclonal Antibody, Proc. Natl. Acad. Sci. USA *86*, 4185–4189 (1989).

[22] *W. Havran, J. Allison*, Origin of Thy-1$^+$ Dendritic Epidermal Cells of Adult Mice from Fetal Thymic Precursors, Nature *344*, 68–70 (1990).

[23] *M. A. S. Moore, J. J. T. Owen*, Experimental Studies on the Development of the Thymus, J. Exp. Med. *126*, 715 (1967).

[24] *C. Martin*, Technique d'explantation *in ovo* de blastodermes d'embryons d'oiseaux, C. R. Soc. Biol. *116*, 283–285 (1972).

[25] *F. Dieterlen-Lièvre*, On the Origin of Haemopoietic Stem Cells in the Avian Embryo: an Experimental Approach, J. Embryol. Exp. Morphol. *33*, 607–619 (1975).

[26] *C. Martin, D. Beaupain, F. Dieterlen-Lièvre*, Developmental Relationships Between Vitelline and Intra-embryonic Haemopoiesis Studied in Avian "Yolk Sac Chimaeras", Cell Differ. *7*, 115–130 (1978).

[27] *D. Beaupain, C. Martin, F. Dieterlen-Lièvre*, Are Developmental Hemoglobin Changes Related to the Origin of Stem Cells and Site of Erythropoiesis? Blood *53*, 212–225 (1979).

[28] *O. Lassila, J. Eskola, P. Toivanen, C. Martin, F. Dieterlen-Lièvre*, The Origin of Lymphoid Stem Cells Studied in Chick Yolk Sac-embryo Chimaeras, Nature *272*, 353–354 (1978).

[29] *O. Lassila, C. Martin, P. Toivanen, F. Dieterlen-Lièvre*, Erythropoiesis and Lymphopoiesis in Chick Yolk Sac-embryo Chimaeras: Contribution of Yolk Sac and Intraembryonic Stem Cells, Blood *59*, 377–381 (1982).

[30] *F. Dieterlen-Lièvre*, Emergence of Intraembryonic Blood Stem Cells Studied in Avian Chimaeras by means of Monoclonal Antibodies, Dev. Comp. Immunol. Suppl. *3*, 75–80 (1984).

[31] *F. Cormier, P. De Paz, F. Dieterlen-Lièvre*, In vitro Detection of Cells with Monocytic Potentiality in the Wall of the Chick Embryo Aorta, Dev. Biol. *118*, 167–175 (1986).

[32] *F. Cormier, F. Dieterlen-Lièvre*, The Wall of the Chick Embryo Aorta Harbours M-CFC, G-CFC, GM-CFC and BFU-E, Development *102*, 279–285 (1988).

[33] *I. L. Weissman, V. Papaioannou, R. Gardner*, Fetal Haematopoietic Origins of the Adult Hematolymphoid System, in: Cold Spring Harbor Conference on Cell Proliferation *5*, 33–47 (1978).

[34] *C. J. Paige, M. W. Kincade, M. A. S. Moore, G. Lee*, The Fate of Fetal and Adult B-cell Progenitors Grafted into Immunodeficient CBA/N Mice, J. Exp. Med. *150*, 548–563 (1979).

[35] *G. Perah, M. Feldman, In vitro* Activation of the *in vivo* Colony-forming Units in the Mouse Yolk Sac, J. Cell. Physiol. *91*, 193–199 (1977).

[36] *C. P. Liu, R. Auerbach, In vitro* Development of Murine T Cells from Prethymic and Preliver Embryonic Yolk Sac Haematopoietic Stem Cells, Development *113*, 1315–1324 (1991).

[37] *I. N. Rich* (ed.), Molecular and Cellular Aspects of Erythropoietin and Erythropoiesis; NATO ASI Series, Vol. H8; Respective Roles of Programme and Differentiation Factors During Hemoglobin Switching in the Embryo, Springer Verlag, Berlin Heidelberg 1987, pp. 127–148.

[38] *N. W. Solvason, J. F. Kearney,* Reconstitution of Lymphocyte Subsets in Scid Mice by Transplantation of Fetal Primordia, Curr. Top. Microbiol. Immunol. *152*, 161–168 (1989).

[39] *L. Kubai, R. Auerbach,* A New Source of Embryonic Lymphocytes in the Mouse, Nature *301*, 154–156 (1986).

[40] *M. L. Tyan, L. A. Herzenberg,* Studies on the Ontogeny of the Mouse Immune System. II. Immunoglobulin-producing Cells, J. Immunol. *101*, 446–450 (1968).

[41] *M. Ogawa, S. Nishikawa, K. Ikuta, F. Yamamura, M. Naito, K. Takahashi, S. I. Nishikawa,* B. Cell Ontogeny in Murine Embryo Studied by a Culture System with the Monolayer of a Stromal Cell Clone, ST2: B Cell Progenitor Develops First in the Embryonal Body rather than in the Yolk Sac, EMBO J. *7*, 1337–1343 (1988).

[42] *G. J. Spangrude, S. Heimfeld, I. L. Weissman,* Purification and Characterization of Mouse Haematopoietic Stem Cells, Science *241*, 58–62 (1988).

[43] *K. Ikuta, T. Kina, I. Macneil, N. Uchida, B. Péault, Y. H. Chien, I. L. Weissman,* A Developmental Switch in Thymic Lymphocyte Maturation Potential Occurs at the Level of Haematopoietic Stem Cells, Cell *62*, 863–874 (1990).

[44] *S. Ezine, I. Weissman, R. Rouse,* Bone Marrow Cells Give Rise to Distinct Cell Clones within the Thymus, Nature *309*, 629–631 (1984).

[45] *E. J. Jenkinson, L. L. Franchi, R. Kingston, J. J. Owen,* Effect of Deoxyguanosine on Lymphopoiesis in the Developing Thymus Rudiment *in vitro:* Application in the Production of Chimaeric Thymus Rudiments, Eur. J. Immunol. *12*, 583–587 (1982).

[46] *J. Robinson, R. K. Jordan,* Thymus *in vitro,* Immunol. Today *4*, 41–45 (1983).

[47] *R. Kingston, E. J. Jenkinson, J. J. T. Owen,* A Single Stem Cell can Recolonize an Embryonic Thymus, Producing Phenotypically Distinct T-cell Populations, Nature *317*, 811–813 (1985).

[48] *G. T. Williams, R. Kingston, M. J. Owen, E. J. Jenkinson, J. J. T. Owen,* A Single Micromanipulated Stem Cell Gives Rise to Multiple T-cell Receptor Gene Rearrangements in the Thymus *in vitro,* Nature *324*, 63–64 (1986).

[49] *E. Houssaint, A. Mansikka, O. Vainio,* Early Separation of B and T Lymphocyte Precursors in Chick Embryo, J. Exp. Med. *174*, 397–406 (1991).

[50] *M. Kinutani, M. Coltey, N. M. Le Douarin,* Postnatal Development of a Demyelinating Disease in Avian Spinal Cord Chimaeras, Cell *45*, 307–314 (1986).

[51] *H. Ohki, C. Martin, C. Corbel, M. Coltey, N. M. Le Douarin,* Tolerance Induced by Thymic Epithelial Grafts in Birds, Science *237*, 1032–1035 (1987).

[52] *F. P. Guillemot, P. D. Oliver, B. M. Péault, N. M. Le Douarin,* Cells Expressing Ia Antigens in the Avian Thymus, J. Exp. Med. *160*, 1803–1819 (1984).

[53] *R. K. Jordan, A. L. Bentley, G. A. Perry, D. A. Crouse,* Thymic Epithelium. I. Lymphoid-free Organ Cultures Grafted in Syngeneic Intact Mice, J. Immunol. *134*, 2155–2160 (1985).

[54] *R. K. Jordan, J. H. Robinson, N. A. Hopkinson, K. C. House, A. L. Bentley,* Thymic Epithelium and the Induction of Transplantation Tolerance in Nude Mice, Nature *314*, 454–456 (1985).

[55] *H. von Boehmer, K. Schubiger,* Thymocytes Appear to Ignore Class I Major Histocompatibility Complex Antigens Expressed on Thymus Epithelial Cells, Eur. J. Immunol. *14*, 1048–1052 (1984).

[56] *H. Von Boehmer, K. Hafen,* Minor but not Major Histocompatibility Antigens of Thymus Epithelium Tolerize Precursors of Cytolytic T Cells, Nature *320*, 626–628 (1986).

[57] *J. Salaün, F. Calman, M. Coltey, N. M. Le Douarin,* Construction of Chimaeric Thymuses in the Mouse Fetus by *in utero* Surgery, Eur. J. Immunol. *16*, 523–530 (1986).

[58] *I. Khazaal, J. Salaün, M. Coltey, F. Calman, N. M. Le Douarin*, Restoration of T-cell Function in Nude Mice by Grafting the Epitheliomesenchymal Thymic Rudiment from 10-day-old Euthymic Embryos, Cell Differ. Dev. *26*, 211–220 (1989).

[59] *J. Salaün, A. Bandeira, I. Khazaal, F. Calman, M. Coltey, A. Coutinho, N. M. Le Douarin*, Thymic Epithelium Tolerizes for Histocompatibility Antigens, Science *247*, 1471–1474 (1990).

6.3 Immunological Detection of Intracellular Structures/Antigens

6.3.1 Cytoskeleton, Filaments and Tubules

Kay E. Foster and Keith Gull

The cytoskeleton is the dynamic, complex, intracellular scaffold which enables the cell to adopt a variety of shapes, to move and to divide. There are three major types of proteinaceous networks which comprise the cytoskeleton, namely, microfilaments (MFs), microtubules (MTs) and intermediate filaments (IFs). These three groups are characterized by their different protein monomers, their associated proteins and the structures that they form within the cell [1]. In addition to the characteristic single cytoskeletal elements, these components can also be involved in higher-order specialized complexes or organelles. Examples include MTs in mitotic spindle, centrioles, cilia and flagella, the aggregation of MFs into stress fibres, and the association of IFs with desmosomes.

The component proteins of the cytoskeleton become assembled into particular, recognizable structures and, as such, are extremely amenable to analysis *via* immunological probes. Antibodies have provided information on individual protein species and so facilitated biochemical analyses, and they have also been extremely valuable probes for the analysis of the cellular organization, differentiation and polymerization dynamics of the cytoskeletal filaments.

The cytoskeleton is complex both in the nature of its components and also their organization into varying polymeric structures. Antibodies have proved to be exquisitely sensitive tools in describing this complexity. The approaches taken to providing these immunological probes have been varied. Sometimes the route has been a classical purification of a protein and raising of an antibody. However, many particularly interesting and novel insights into the cytoskeleton have come from use of antibodies with interesting, yet initially cryptic, discriminatory properties and specificities. Immunological analysis of the cytoskeleton illustrates the particular attributes of antibodies as experimental tools. They have aided the identification of rare isotypes of the main structural proteins such as tubulin and the cloning of genes encoding cytoskeletal components by screening of expression libraries, and they have assisted *in-vivo* functional studies by use in microinjection experiments.

There are many approaches to generating antibodies to cytoskeletal components. Use has been made of existing antibodies from patients with autoimmune disorders; of highly complex antigens such as complete organelles; of purified single component antigens, and of highly specific antigens such as peptides corresponding to particular sequences of proteins. In each approach either monoclonal antibodies or polyclonal antisera may be used to particular advantage. Each of the major approaches to the immunological analysis of the cytoskeleton are described below, illustrating the nature of the analysis with examples of successful applications.

6.3.1.1   Autoantibodies Against the Cytoskeleton

Autoantibodies found in the serum of patients have often been important in the analysis of the insoluble components of the cytoskeleton and its associated organelles. Patients suffering from CREST syndrome (calcinosis, *Raynaud's* phenomenon, oesophageal dysmotility, sclerodactyly and telangiectasia) often have antibodies that recognize certain cytoskeletal-associated elements, e.g., kinetochores and centrosomes. The advantage of such sera is that they can be screened easily by immunofluorescence and western blotting and can then often be sub-fractionated by specific protocols of absorption to immobilized, fractionated antigens, so producing more specific sub-probes. Of course, limitations of the approach are its initial randomness and the fact that the antibody specificity may be unique and therefore limited to an individual patient.

Early immunofluorescence studies with sera from scleroderma patients showed a kinetochore staining pattern in mammalian cells [2, 3] and electron microscopical analysis showed that the antibody is located to the inner and outer kinetochore plates [3]. With such sera, as discussed in more detail later (cf. 6.3.3.3), it has been possible to monitor the purification [4] and likely location [5] of the kinetochore-associated proteins. Specific antibodies prepared by affinity purification [6] have been used to screen cDNA expression libraries for the proteins [7] and to use fusion proteins in turn to raise specific antibodies.

Similar analyses have been performed on centrosomes [8] and topoisomerase I [9] and the approach has the particular advantage of facilitating studies of virtually unpurifiable cellular structures of cryptic composition.

6.3.1.2   Organelle Shot-gun Approach to Making Antibodies

The organelle shot-gun approach has been very successful as a technique for the generation of antibodies to those cytoskeletal constituents characterized by their low abundance and high insolubility. Organelles are isolated and then partially or fully extracted prior to use as immunogens in programmes of mAb production. Precise and extensive sceening following the initial fusion can identify the potentially useful mAbs very early in the process. Immunofluorescence is often a most informative screen at this stage as the structures recognized are easily observed in the context of the cytoskeleton. An ELISA or western blot screen may reveal little of the role of the antigen in the cytoskeleton whilst immunofluorescence of a field of cells can give instant and extensive information related to the cytoskeleton component recognized and its possible modulation in relation to cell shape or the cell cycle. Immunofluorescence also has the advantage of enabling the detection of antigens of very low abundance.

Woods et al. [10] used either detergent-extracted cytoskeletons of trypanosome cells or a salt extract thereof to generate a library of mAbs *via* this route. The complex immunogens produced four different anti-tubulin antibodies together with antibodies recognizing the nucleus, basal body, flagellar attachment zone and paraflagellar rod. The latter antibodies detected minor insoluble proteins, previously uncharacterized. This study resulted in a set of probes for each of the major organelles of the trypanosome cell cytoskeleton. The probes also revealed the identity of novel components. For example, the antibody recognizing the paraflagellar rod was not to the previously-characterized major protein doublet of that structure ($M_r = 68000–76000$) [11, 12] but to polypeptides of $M_r = 180000$ and 200000. This antibody was also found to cross-react with human and porcine spectrin and thus confirms other work suggesting that spectrin is present in trypanosomes [13]. The flagellar attachment zone has been defined ultrastructurally [14] and the two mAbs generated in this study should aid biochemical analysis of this structure.

A similar study used the Triton X-100 extracted cytoskeleton of bull sperm as immunogen [15] and produced six mAbs to different regions of the sperm cytoskeleton. These mAbs revealed novel cytoskeletal elements or were found to recognize structures which had already been defined ultrastructurally but not biochemically.

Mitotic cells have also been popular targets for the organelle shot-gun approach. Many modulations of protein metabolism occur at division and cells at this stage of the cell cycle are easy to recognize in screens. Thus, the use of mitotic cells as an inoculum allows mAb probes to either novel mitotic proteins or uniquely modified proteins to be made.

A saline extract (NaCl, 150 mmol/l) of synchronized mitotic HeLa cells was used in one programme of mAb production [16]. Two Abs, MPM 1 and MPM 2, were found to react with many polypeptides in mitotic cells but strongly with only three; these bands corresponded to those labelled with $^{32}PO_4$ and the signal was abolished by alkaline phosphatase treatment. The results indicated that the antibodies recognized an epitope phosphorylated at mitosis and possibly important in the regulation of mitotic events (cf. p. 6.3.3.5). Immunofluorescence showed that the signal increased towards metaphase and further studies indicated that the signal located to the centrosome, kinetochores and mid-body of the mitotic spindle [17]. The epitope has also been demonstrated in other organisms and these mAbs have found widespread use in the study of cytoskeletal modulations associated with mitosis [18]. In a similar study [19], mAbs recognizing the mid-body and centrosomes were generated using isolated mitotic spindles as the antigen.

Neurofilaments are the neuronal IFs and are composed of three major proteins. When the whole filaments have been used as immunogen, many mAbs have been produced to the individual protein subunits [20]. Moreover, other studies have shown that antibodies can be obtained which recognize the differing phosphorylated states of the proteins which may be involved in regulation of neurofilament function [21, 22].

6.3.1.3   Purified and Expressed Proteins as Cytoskeletal Antigens

Monoclonal and polyclonal antibodies can, of course, be raised to purified components of the cytoskeleton. Often it is not practical to purify such proteins to homogeneity by standard biochemical means as very small amounts of protein are needed for antibody production. Thus, it is often sufficient to separate a partially purified protein by SDS-PAGE, excise the band of interest and use this as the antigen. The protein may be electroeluted from the gel, or the polyacrylamide may be homogenized to a fine suspension which may be injected. In other studies the proteins have been electroblotted onto nitrocellulose and the band excised, the nitrocellulose dried, powdered and injected [23].

The antibody raised to the isolated flagellar rootlets of the green alga *Tetraselmis striata* provides an example of this technique. When analysed by SDS-PAGE, a major component of the isolated rootlets was found to be a polypeptide of $M_r = 20\,000$. Thus the band could be readily excised from gels and the protein electroeluted and used as immunogen for pAb production [24]. This antibody has been instrumental in identifying the Ca^{2+}-binding phosphoprotein ($M_r = 20\,000$) largely responsible for the motile behaviour of striated flagellar rootlets [24] and has also been used to identify an analogous protein and its role in the cell cycle in animal cells [25].

This technique was also used to raise Abs to a protein, $M_r = 77\,000$, [26] known to be a major component of isolated taxol-stabilized MTs from mitotic sea urchin eggs [27]. In this case the protein was not separated from the polyacrylamide and was used in a programme of mAb production. Five different mAbs were made and they revealed that, although the protein of $M_r = 77\,000$ was a component of cytoplasmic and mitotic MTs, it was not present in ciliary or flagellar MTs.

Expressed fusion proteins may also be used as antigens for the production of antibodies which can then be used to analyse the original protein of interest. A recent example of this has been the discovery and analysis of γ-tubulin. Investigation of the *mip*A gene of *Aspergillus nidulans* identified a third tubulin sub-type (γ-tubulin) [28] and showed it to be essential for nuclear division and MT function [29]. cDNA encoding

Drosophila melanogaster γ-tubulin was identified using the *A. nidulans* gene probe and the *D. melanogaster* gene was then used in the next phylogenetic step to *H. sapiens*. The *A. nidulans* γ-tubulin fusion protein was expressed in *E. coli* and used to raise pAbs in rabbits. The antiserum was then affinity purified with the aid of purified, expressed human fusion polypeptide. The resulting antibody was highly specific and, when used in immunofluorescence studies of γ-tubulin, revealed centrosomal staining in mitotic cells with staining intensity increasing towards metaphase, so correlating with an increased number of MTs nucleating at the centrosome. The authors propose that the staining is in fact pericentriolar and that γ-tubulin may be a minus end nucleator of MT assembly [30].

A second antibody to γ-tubulin has been raised using a peptide corresponding to a sequence of γ-tubulin found to be conserved in many species [31]. The resulting pAb was affinity-purified with the aid of expressed fusion protein and this produced a highly specific anti-centrosomal antibody with a high degree of species cross-reactivity. γ-tubulin is present at very low levels (less than 1% of αβ-tubulin [31]) and purification of the natural protein would be difficult, especially as it is thought to be complexed in the pericentriolar material. The expression of fusion proteins provides a ready source of the protein under study which may then be used to generate further antibodies.

6.3.1.4   Peptides and Specific Isotype Probes

The genes encoding many cytoskeletal proteins have now been cloned and subjected to sequence analysis. Thus, it is possible to synthesize peptides that conform to a portion of the primary sequence and to use such peptides to generate highly specific antibodies. This methodology has been particularly useful in the study of the tubulin multigene family. In vertebrates there are at least 6–7 functional genes for both α and β tubulin [32, 33]. The precise role of these different isotypes is unknown and has been the subject of much debate. One hypothesis suggests that the different isotypes confer different properties on the MTs whereas others suggest that the isotypes are functionally similar but arise from the need for differential regulatory controls. The multi-tubulin gene families of chick and man have been analysed and patterns of expression defined [32, 33]. However, this does not describe the isotype composition of MTs within a cell in which two or more isotypes might be expressed. To this end, highly specific antibodies to the different isotypes have been produced. One approach was to synthesize peptides corresponding to the 15 carboxy-terminal amino acids of the individual members of the chick β-tubulin family; this region is variable in the different members of the family. pAbs were raised and affinity purified using the peptides [34]. An alternative approach has been to use expressed fusion proteins, purified by excision from SDS gels, to produce pAbs. Tolerance to shared epitopes was induced by initially injecting a mixture of fusion proteins not of interest, followed by an injection of cyclophosphamide. The fusion protein of interest was then used to raise pAbs which were subsequently purified by affinity purification [36].

In both studies the antibodies were then used to analyse the composition of MTs in various cell types, revealing that the MTs were copolymers of the available tubulin isotypes in a particular cell. In addition, when a highly divergent tubulin was transfected into an inappropriate cell type, immunofluorescence studies showed that the isotype was incorporated into all classes of MTs without any effect on the cell [36, 37].

Similar transfection studies with IFs have demonstrated that some members of the IF family form copolymers. When fibroblasts were transfected so that they inappropriately expressed either the low or medium molecular-weight neurofilament proteins, immunofluorescence studies with antibodies to the neurofilament proteins or to vimentin (the endogenous IF constituent protein) showed that the IFs were in fact copolymers formed with no obvious effect on the cell [38].

Post-translational modification of components of the cytoskeleton is thought to be a means of regulating cytoskeletal function and antibodies recognizing the specific protein domain have been important in analysing the role of these modifications. The post-translational phosphorylation of IFs [21, 22] has been discussed; however, other cytoskeletal protein modifications have been revealed through the use of highly selective antibodies. For example, tubulin may be modified by acetylation; an antibody recognizing this acetylated tubulin epitope was made using axonemal tubulin from sea urchin sperm and later was found to detect sub-sets of acetylated MTs in mammalian cells. This and other modifications reviewed in [32, 33] and immunological probes have been of paramount importance in providing descriptions of the distribution of these modified tubulins, in particular MT organelles. However, although the antibodies have proved to be superb probes for revealing the distribution of such modified MTs they have not succeeded in revealing their role.

6.3.1.5   Antibodies and Function of the Cytoskeleton

Most of the successful applications of antibodies to the study of the cytoskeleton described above are the results of analysis performed on fixed cells; the study of many such cells allows proposals to be made regarding the role of various proteins in cytoskeletal functions. A combination of antibodies with microinjection protocols has sometimes allowed a more detailed analysis of the interactions within the cytoskeleton and also measurements of cytoskeletal dynamics.

The injection of anti-MT antibodies into mammalian cells caused the collapse of the IF network, demonstrating the interaction of the two cytoskeletal elements [39]. Similarly, the injection of anti-IF antibodies into cells caused the collapse of the IF network, forming perinuclear caps [40]. In this study cells were chosen which expressed two IF types: injection of antibodies to one of the types caused total collapse of the network, indicating that the IFs in these particular cells were copolymers.

Lysed cell models have also been used to study cytoskeletal function: centrosomal MT nucleating ability was blocked using the MPM2 mAb described above. The antibody recognizes an epitope phosphorylated at mitosis and present in the centrosome; thus, use of this probe demonstrates the importance of this protein modification in centrosomal MT nucleating activity at mitosis [41].

Injection of antibodies into living cells may cause perturbation of the cell and collapse of the cytoskeleton and therefore analysis of cytoskeleton dynamics has used antibodies in a different way. Modified proteins (e. g. biotinylated [42]) or heterologous proteins (e. g. *Physarum* tubulin into PtK2 cells [43]) have been used as markers of MT growth. After injection, the cells are fixed at various time points and the distribution of the injected tubulin probe determined using highly selective antibodies. Measurements of the proportion of the MT labelled by the antibody allow determination of polymer dynamics. Similar technology has now been applied to analysis of the IF network in cells [44].

Antibodies have played a powerful role as highly selective or pan-reactive probes for analysis of the cytoskeleton. When combined with molecular biology and microinjection studies they can facilitate the discovery and provide almost a complete description of the distribution, protein structure and ultimately, function of a cytoskeletal component in the living cell.

References

[1] *B. Alberts, D. Bray, J. Lewis, M. Raff, K. Roberts, J. D. Watson,* Molecular Biology of the Cell, 2nd Edition, Garland Publishing Inc., New York 1989, pp. 629–676.

[2] *Y. Moroi, A. C. Hartman, P. K. Nakane, E. M. Tan,* Distribution of Kinetochore (Centromere) Antigen in Mammalian Cell Nuclei, J. Cell Biol. *90,* 254–259 (1981).

[3] *S. Brenner, D. Pepper, M. W. Berns, E. M. Tan, B. R. Brinkley,* Kinetochore Structure, Duplication, and Distribution in Mammalian Cells: Analysis by Human Autoantibodies, From Scleroderma-Patients, J. Cell Biol. *91,* 95–102 (1981).

[4] *M. M. Valdivia, B. R. Brinkley,* Fractionation and Initial Characterization of the Kinetochore from Mammalian Metaphase Chromosomes, J. Cell Biol. *101,* 1124–1134 (1985).

[5] *D. K. Palmer, K. O'Day, M. H. Wener, B. S. Andrews, R. L. Margolis,* A M-KD Centromere Protein (CENP-A) Copurifies with Nucleosome Core Particles and with Histones, J. Cell Biol. *104,* 805–815 (1984).

[6] *J. B. Olmsted,* Analysis of Cytoskeletal Structure Using Blot-purified Nonspecific Antibodies, Methods Enzymol. *134,* 467–472 (1986).

[7] *W. C. Earnshaw, K. F. Sullivan, P. S. Machlin, C. A. Cooke, D. A. Raiser, T. D. Pollard, N. F. Rothfield, D. W. Cleveland,* Molecular Cloning for cDNA for CENP-B the Major Human Centromere Autoantigen, J. Cell Biol. *104,* 817–829 (1987).

[8] *P. D. Calarco-Gillam, M. C. Siebert, R. Hubble, T. Mitchison, M. Kirschner,* Centrosome Development in Early Mouse Embryos as Defined by an Autoantibody against Pericentriolar Material, Cell *35,* 621–629 (1983).

[9] *J. H. Shero, B. Bordwell, N. F. Rothfield, W. C. Earnshaw,* High Titers of Autoantibodies to Topoisomerase I (Sci-70) in Sera from Scleroderma Patients, Science *231,* 737–740 (1986).

[10] *A. Woods, T. Sherwin, R. Sasse, T. H. MacRae, A. J. Baines, K. Gull,* Definition of Individual Components within the Cytoskeleton of *Trypanosoma brucei* by a Library of Monoclonal Antibodies, J. Cell Sci. *93,* 491–500 (1989).

[11] *D. G. Russell, R. J. Newsam, G. C. N. Palmer, K. Gull,* Structural and Biochemical Characterisation of the Paraflagellar Rod of *Crithidia fasciculata,* Eur. J. Cell Biol. *30,* 137–143 (1983).

[12] *J. M. Gallo, J. Schrevel,* Homologies between Paraflagellar Rod Proteins from Trypanosomes and Euglenoids Revealed by a Monoclonal Antibody, Eur. J. Cell Biol. *36,* 163–168 (1985).

[13] *A. Schneider, H. U. Lutz, R. Margg, P. Gehr, T. Seebeck*, Spectrin like Proteins in the Paraflagellar Rod of *Trypanosoma brucei*, J. Cell Sci. *90*, 307–315 (1988).

[14] *T. Sherwin, K. Gull*, Visualisation of Detyrosination along Single Microtubules Reveals Novel Mechanisms of Assembly during Cytoskeletal Duplication in Trypanosomes, Cell *57*, 211–221 (1989).

[15] *T. H. MacRae, B. M. H. Lange, K. Gull*, Production and Characterization of Monoclonal Antibodies to the Mammalian Sperm Cytoskeleton, Mol. Reprod. Dev. *25*, 384–392 (1990).

[16] *F. M. Davis, T. H. Tsao, S. K. Fowler, P. N. Rao*, Monoclonal Antibodies to Mitotic Cells, Proc. Natl. Acad. Sci. U.S.A. *80*, 2926–2930 (1983).

[17] *D. D. Vandre, F. M. Davis, P. N. Rao, G. G. Borisy*, Phosphoproteins are Components of Mitotic Microtubule Organising Centers, Proc. Natl. Acad. Sci. U.S.A. *81*, 4439–4443 (1984).

[18] *D. D. Vandre, F. M. Davis, P. N. Rao, G. G. Borisy*, Distribution of Cytoskeletal Proteins Sharing a Conserved Phosphorylated Epitope, Eur. J. Cell Biol. *41*, 72–81 (1986).

[19] *C. Sellitto, R. Kuriyama*, Distribution of a Matrix Component of the Midbody during the Cell Cycle in Chinese Hamster Ovary Cells, J. Cell Biol. *106*, 431–440 (1987).

[20] *B. H. Anderton, D. Breinberg, M. J. Downes, P. J. Green, B. E. Tomlinson, J. Ulrich, J. N. Wood, J. Kahn*, Monoclonal Antibodies Show that Neurofibrillary Tangles and Neurofilaments Share Antigenic Determinants, Nature *298*, 84–86 (1982).

[21] *M. J. Carden, W. W. Schlaepfer, V. M. Y. Lee*, The Structure, Biochemical Properties and Immunogenicity of Neurofilament Peripheral Regions are Determined by Phosphorylation State, J. Biol. Chem. *260*, 9805–9817 (1985).

[22] *L. A. Sternberger, N. M. Sternberger*, Monoclonal Antibodies Distinguish Phosphorylated and Non-phosphorylated Forms of Neurofilaments *in Situ*, Proc. Natl. Acad. Sci. U.S.A. *80*, 6126–6130 (1983).

[23] *M. Diano, A. Le Bivic, M. Hirn*, A Method for the Production of Highly Specific Polyclonal Antibodies, Anal. Biochem. *166*, 224–229 (1987).

[24] *J. L. Salisbury, A. Baron, B. Surek, M. Melkonian*, Striated Flagellar Roots: Isolation and Partial Characterization of a Calcium-modulated Contractile Organelle, J. Cell Biol. *99*, 962–970 (1984).

[25] *A. T. Baron, T. M. Greenwood, J. L. Salsbury*, Localisation of the Centrin-Related 165000-M_r Protein of PtK$_2$ Cells during the Cell Cycle, Cell Motil. Cytoskeleton *18*, 1–14 (1991).

[26] *G. S. Bloom, F. C. Luca, C. A. Collins, R. B. Vallee*, Use of Multiple Monoclonal Antibodies to Characterize the Major Microtubule-associated Protein in Sea Urchin Eggs, Cell Motil. Cytoskeleton *5*, 431–446 (1985).

[27] *R. B. Vallee, G. S. Bloom*, Isolation of Sea Urchin Egg Microtubules with Taxol and Identification of Mitotic Spindle Microtubule Associated Proteins with Monoclonal Antibodies, Proc. Natl. Acad. Sci. U.S.A. *80*, 6259–6263 (1983).

[28] *C. E. Oakley, B. R. Oakley*, Identification of Gamma-tubulin, a New Member of the Tubulin Superfamily Encoded by *Mip* A gene of *Aspergillus nidulans*, Nature *338*, 662–664 (1989).

[29] *B. R. Oakley, C. E. Oakley, Y. Yoon, M. K. Jung*, γ-Tubulin is a Component of the Spindle Pole Body that is Essential for Microtubule Function in *Aspergillus nidulans*, Cell *61*, 1289–1301 (1990).

[30] *Y. Zheng, M. K. Jung, B. R. Oakley*, γ-Tubulin is Present in *Drosophila melanogaster* and *Homo sapiens* and is Associated with the Centrosome, Cell *65*, 817–823 (1991).

[31] *T. Stearns, L. Evans, M. Kirschner*, γ-Tubulin is a Highly Conserved Component of the Centrosome, Cell *65*, 825–836 (1991).

[32] *K. F. Sullivan*, Structure and Utilization of Tubulin Isotypes, Ann. Rev. Cell Biol. *4*, 687–716 (1988).

[33] *K. E. Foster*, Tubulin and Microtubule Associated Proteins, Life Chem. Reports *7*, 83–112 (1989).

[34] *M. A. Lopata, D. W. Cleveland*, *In vivo* Microtubules are Co-polymers of Available β-Tubulin Isotypes: Localisation of Each of Six Vertebrate β-tubulin Isotypes Using Polyclonal Antibodies Elicited to Synthetic Peptide Antigens, J. Cell Biol. *105*, 1707–1720 (1987).

[35] *S. A. Lewis, W. Gu, N. J. Cowan*, Free Intermingling of Mammalian β-tubulin Isotypes Among Functionally Distinct Microtubules, Cell *49*, 539–548 (1987).

[36] *H. C. Joshi, T. Y. Yen, D. W. Cleveland*, *In vivo* Co-assembly of a Divergent β-tubulin Subunit (cβ6) into Microtubules of Different Function, J. Cell Biol. *105*, 2179–2190 (1987).

[37] *W. Gu, S. A. Lewis, N. J. Cowan*, Generation of Antisera that Discriminate among Mammalian α-Tubulins: Introduction of Specialised Isotypes into Cultured Cells Results in Their Co-assembly without Disruption of Normal Microtubule Function, J. Cell Biol. *106*, 2011–2022 (1987).

[38] *M. J. Monteiro, D. W. Cleveland*, Expression of NF-L and NF-M in Fibroblasts Reveals Co-assembly of Neurofilament and Vimentin Subunit, J. Cell Biol. *108*, 579–593 (1989).

[39] *S. H. Blose, D. I. Meltzer, J. R. Feramisco*, 10-nm Filaments are Induced to Collapse in Living Cells Microinjected with Monoclonal and Polyclonal Antibodies against Tubulin, J. Cell Biol. *98*, 847–858 (1984).

[40] *H. G. Tolle, K. Weber, M. Osborn*, Microinjections of Monoclonal Antibodies to Vimentin. Desmin and GFA in Cells which Contain more than one IF Type, Exp. Cell Res. *162*, 462–474 (1986).

[41] *V. E. Centonze, G. G. Borisy*, Nucleation of Microtubules from Mitotic Centrosomes is Modulated by a Phosphorylated Epitope, J. Cell Sci. *95*, 405–411 (1990).

[42] *E. Schulze, M. Kirschner*, Microtubule Dynamics in Interphase Cells, J. Cell Biol. *102*, 1020–1031 (1986).

[43] *A. R. Prescott, K. E. Foster, R. M. Warn, K. Gull*, Incorporation of Tubulin from an Evolutionarily Diverse Source, *Physarum polycephalum* into the Microtubules of a Mammalian Cell, J. Cell Sci. *92*, 595–605 (1989).

[44] *K. L. Vikstrom, G. G. Borisy, R. D. Goldman*, Dynamic Aspects of Intermediate Filaments Network in BHK-21 Cells, Proc. Natl. Acad. Sci. U.S.A. *86*, 549–553 (1989).

6.3.2   Chromatin and Chromosomal Proteins

Michael Bustin

The nucleoprotein fibre present in both interphase chromatin and metaphase chromosomes is built from an array of repeating subunits known as the core particle. The core particle is composed of 145 base pairs of DNA wrapped around a histone octamer in which two molecules each of histones H2A, H2B, H3, and H4 are complexed into a precise structure. The DNA between adjacent core particles, the linker DNA, consists of 40–70 base pairs of DNA and is complexed with histone H1. Thus, the genetic information encoded in DNA is packed into a fibre-like structure resembling a beaded string. This structure, composed of histones and DNA, is the backbone of the chromatin fibre. However, during the life-cycle of a cell, many other chromosomal proteins interact with this backbone, modifying its structure and influencing its function [1].

The chromatin fibre is a dynamic structure. Gross structural changes occur during the cell cycle and are easily observed in the light microscope. In addition, the chromatin fibre is a substrate for a variety of complex processes such as transcription, replication and DNA repair. Both the nucleic acid and the protein components of chromatin are subject to modification, degradation and replacement. Furthermore, chromosomal proteins may be associated only temporarily with select regions in chromatin. Studies on the structure and function of such a complex and dynamic structure as the chromatin fibre require analytical techniques capable of recognizing defined components at various stages of chromatin organization. Immunochemical approaches are uniquely suited for such studies.

The use of immunochemical techniques for the study of chromatin, chromosomes and nuclear proteins is complicated by a conflicting situation. The production of sera specific for a defined chromosomal protein requires a purified immunogen. Yet, in chromatin and chromosomes, proteins are complexed with other proteins or nucleic acids, and their purification requires procedures which alter their native structure. Thus, antisera elicited against purified and characterized chromosomal components may not recognize the immunogen complexed in its nucleoprotein conformation. Antisera to "native" chromatin or chromosomes contain antibodies elicited by complex determinants composed of several components. Since purification of chromosomal components often disrupts the antigenic site, the immunogens cannot be identified and the contribution of the individual chromosomal components to the various parameters cannot be identified. In spite of these limitations, serological approaches have been used for a variety of structural and functional studies on chromatin and chromosomal proteins. In fact, due to their versatility, specificity and sensitivity, immunological approaches are the methods of choice for studies which require identification of specific chromosomal components, and the results have provided information which is very difficult to obtain by other methods. Antibodies have been used to estimate homologies between related chromosomal components, to detect structural modifications associated with functional changes in the genome, to visualize the location of a protein or a modified base in metaphase or polytene chromosomes, to study the location of components at the level of resolution of a single nucleosome, to study the role of a specific protein in the transcribing chromatin fibre, and to fractionate chromatin and nucleosomes according to their content of nuclear proteins.

The contribution of immunological approaches to understanding the structure and function of chromosomal proteins, chromatin, and chromosomes is reviewed and evaluated in the following. The focus is on histones, which are the major protein component of chromatin, and on the High Mobility Group (HMG) chromosomal proteins, which are the major nonhistone class of chromosomal proteins. The many elegant studies involving antisera elicited by nucleic acids are not covered. Many methodological aspects are not included. For a more detailed treatment of these subjects, consult published reviews [2–8].

6.3.2.1   Immunogens, Antigens, Antisera and Assays

The dynamic nature of the chromatin fibre and the transient association of some proteins with chromatin must be taken into account when preparing the immunogen. Purified immunogens are required for preparation of specific polyclonal antisera or for reliable assays and characterization of monoclonal antibodies. In the case of histone fractions, the most common contaminants are other histones or nonhistone proteins. Histones are poor immunogens [9, 12]; therefore, even a small amount of cross-contamination, especially with nonhistone chromosomal proteins, may create a situation in which a significant fraction of the antibodies is not specific for the intended immunogen. Serological techniques are more sensitive than most analytical techniques used to detect proteins. Thus, an immunogen which may seem pure by accepted criteria may elicit antibodies against minor components. Careful purification of antigens and examination of their purity on overloaded polyacrylamide gels, or by HPLC, minimize the complications which arise from impure immunogens. The primary sequence of the histones and the major HMG species is evolutionarily conserved; therefore, it is possible to elicit antisera against immunogens prepared from one species in order to test antigens from a heterologous species. This approach minimizes complications due to species-specific contaminants. Histones and HMG proteins from calf thymus are well characterized; therefore, the sera elicited by these proteins have been used as "standard" reagents in many experimental systems.

Accessibility of antigenic sites

The accessibility of an antigenic determinant to antibody binding is of particular relevance in studies of complex macromolecular structures such as chromatin and nucleosomes. For example, less than 10% of the antigenic determinants present in isolated histones are available to antibody binding in native chromatin [9]. The loss of antigenic determinants reflects conformational changes occurring in the molecules upon cross-complexing with other histones and with DNA in their final nucleosomal organization. In addition, some antigenic sites are shielded due to steric hindrance. The accessibility of antigenic determinants is of special relevance in studies on the cellular localization of chromosomal components. An antigenic site present in a protein in the cytoplasm or nucleoplasm may not be accessible in the chromatin-bound state, which may lead to a false conclusion that the component is absent from chromatin. These considerations are of special importance when monoclonal or anti-peptide antibodies are used. However, the ability to measure exposure of antigenic determinants is an additional analytical tool for various studies on chromatin.

It is possible to measure the availability of antigenic sites in chromatin in a precise and semiquantitative way by an immunoadsorption assay [10, 11]. In this assay, incubate antibodies with either chromatin or nucleosomes at low ionic strength under conditions in which these nucleoproteins are relatively soluble. After incubation, raise the ionic strength with NaCl to 150 mmol/l and separate the bound antibody from the free antibody by sedimentation. Test the supernatant containing unabsorbed antibodies by ELISA and compare to a control serum preparation that has been treated identically but not adsorbed on chromatin. This assay allows for the use of high concentrations of chromatin, which often interfere with immunological assay. In a variation of this assay, the amount of labelled, affinity-purified antibodies sedimenting with the chromatin can be measured directly [13].

Preparation of antibodies

Native preparations of chromatin and chromosomes have been used to elicit both polyclonal and monoclonal antibodies. The antibodies have been used as qualitative reagents to detect changes in the nucleoproteins. However, difficulties in identifying the specific antigenic moiety complicated the interpretation of the results. Interestingly, antisera elicited by chromatin do not contain antibodies which react with free histones [9]. Antisera elicited against limited and defined regions of chromosomal proteins are among the most useful specific reagents for studies on chromatin structure and function. Initially, these studies involved histone fragments obtained by proteolytic or chemical cleavage [14–18]. More recently, synthetic peptides have been used to elicit antibodies against defined regions of histones [5] and HMGs [17]. Antibodies to acetylated histone H4, which recognize nucleosomes, have been elicited and used to study functional aspects of histone acetylation [18–21]. Autoimmune sera obtained from human subjects and animals are an additional source of reagents useful for studies of chromatin and chromosomal proteins [22–24]. Some of these sera contain antibodies against components such as native DNA, which usually do not elicit an immune response, or against components that are difficult to isolate.

Monoclonal antibodies against isolated chromatin, chromosomes and chromosomal proteins have been elicited. However, since in most cases the antigenic moiety has not been identified, their use in studies of chromatin has been limited. Definition of the epitopes recognized by the antibodies would significantly enhance their usefulness. *Mendelson* et al. [25] elicited a panel of mAbs against histone H5, identified the epitopes with some degree of accuracy, and described an approach based on steric hindrance measurements to identify overlapping epitopes. The antibodies which bind to chromatin can be used as markers to determine accessible regions of the proteins. Changes in the binding of the mAb to chromatin are indicative of rearrangements in the chromatin structure. Analysis of the antigenic sites for monoclonals elicited by histone H5 and H1^0 [25–27] indicate that the globular domain and the boundaries between the globular domain and the unstructured domain of the proteins are the most immunogenic region of the protein. Monoclonals against H1 have also been used to map accessible regions in chromatin and to define evolutionarily conserved epitopes in this histone family [28]. Immunofluorescence studies with mAbs against an H1 variant from *Chironomus thummi* revealed differences between homologous chromosome sites in the content of H1 variants [29]. Monoclonals to HMG-1 and 2 have been used to study the specificity and chromatin distribution of these proteins [30].

6.3.2.2   The Specificity of Chromosomal Proteins and Chromatin

Histones, HMGs, and many other chromosomal proteins are structural proteins lacking a function which can be readily assayed. Therefore, serological techniques have been used widely to identify and compare chromosomal proteins and chromatin obtained from various sources. Microcomplement fixation has proved to be one of the most sensitive techniques to distinguish related proteins differing by as little as a single amino acid [31]. Although determination of amino acid sequence is, by far, the method of choice for comparing proteins, the microcomplement fixation technique is a reasonable second choice for assessing the degree of similarity among related proteins. This technique has been used widely to assess the specificity of H1 histones from various species. These studies indicate that the range of differences among various H1 subfractions in one tissue is of the same order of magnitude as that among H1 subfractions from various species. This suggests that each H1 subfraction evolved independently [32, 33]. Additional examples where this technique has been used to assess the relationship among various chromosomal proteins and to study protein conformation and modification have been reviewed [3, 4]. The microcomplement fixation technique is relatively cumbersome and has been replaced by ELISA and Immunoblotting, although these are less sensitive to minor differences in the structure or conformation of proteins. They have been used to identify newly isolated proteins from various species or to follow post-translational modifications which may alter the mobility of the protein. Antisera elicited against histones H2A, H2B, H3 and H4 recognize histones from a variety of species, including insects and fish. Likewise, anti-HMG sera react with HMGs isolated from a range of sources, including plants [28, 34].

Antisera elicited by chromatin or a nucleoprotein preparation devoid of histones, and by most (not all) of the nonhistones, exhibit a remarkable specificity for the immunogen [35]. In fact, these serological analyses are the only studies which have detected significant differences among chromatins from various sources. Surprisingly large differences have been reported between normal and malignant tissues, among chromatins obtained from different organs of the same species, among different developmental stages of one organ, and even between a cell and its virally transformed counterpart [36]. Histones and DNA are not immunogenic in native chromatin. The specificity of these sera resides in specific nonhistone-DNA complexes and is lost upon digestion with DNase. The serological specificity is reversible, i.e., upon dissociation and reassociation of the complex [37]. The molecular basis of the immunological specificity is not understood. It may be due to the tissue specificity of the nonhistone proteins, to the tissue-specific structural relation of the proteins with the DNA, or both. Most of the immunological differences among various chromatin preparations have been detected by the microcomplement fixation technique which, as mentioned above, maximizes the differences among antigens. The availability of antibodies elicited in chickens [38], which are reactive at high ionic strength, may allow additional studies on the immunological specificity of chromatin.

6.3.2.3   Localization and Organization of Components in Chromatin and Chromosomes

The intracellular localizations of histones and HMGs in various cells have been studied by immunofluorescence. Purified antihistone antibodies invariably localize to the nucleus [39]. In contrast, antibodies to the HMG-1/-2 class of nonhistones indicate that the proteins are present both in the nucleus and cytoplasm [40]. Most probably, the proteins shuttle between these two cellular compartments in synchrony with the cell cycle. Specific staining of both metaphase and polytene chromosomes with antibodies to either histones or nonhistones has been obtained in many laboratories. Among various experimental parameters involved in immunofluorescence studies, the results are most affected by the method of chromosome preparation and by the concentration of the antisera used to stain the chromosomes [2]. At low serum dilutions the entire axis of the chromosome fluoresces and the band resolution is very poor. At high dilutions only the regions containing a relatively high concentration of antigens can be detected. Thus, the immunofluorescent pattern reflects the *relative availability* of the antigenic determinants rather than the absolute presence of an antigen in a specific region. Controlled treatment of chromosomes with methanol-acetic acid fixative produces a spotty fluorescent pattern with antihistone antibodies [41]. The spotty fluorescent pattern (resulting from differential extraction of histones along the chromatin fibre) differs among the various chromosomes present in a cell. This suggests a potential application for cytological studies.

Polytene chromosomes have features which render them suitable for various studies on the role of chromosomal proteins in maintaining the structure and regulating the functions of chromatin. Antibodies can be used to study the distribution of proteins in bands, interbands, and "puffed" regions of the chromosomes. Antisera to histone H1 preferentially stain the bands while antisera to core histones preferentially stain the interbands [42]. Monoclonal antibodies have been used to demonstrate that homologous chromosome sites differ in their content of H1 variants [29]. Antisera to RNA polymerase localize to interbands, suggesting that active genes are located in these regions [42]. Transcribed regions, which often appear as "puffs" in the phase microscope, stain very intensely with antibodies to RNA polymerase. This indicates that the enzyme is highly concentrated in this region [43]. Antisera to histones stain weakly "puffed" regions of chromosomes fixed with acetic acid [44]. The same regions stain more intensely in formaldehyde-fixed chromosomes, indicating that histones are present in transcribed regions [44]. Apparently, in transcribed regions, histones are easily extracted by the fixative. The banding pattern obtained with anti-HMG-1 is uneven. This suggests variability in the organization of the protein along the chromosome axis [45]. In fact, most nonhistone proteins localize to select regions of the chromosomes [46–48]. Antisera prepared against various nonhistone fractions or purified proteins have been used to demonstrate heterogeneity among various transcribed regions in the polytene chromosomes [49].

The content of proteins at the level of resolution of nucleosome has been investigated by immunoelectron microscopy [49–53] and by immune sedimentation [54]. By electron microscopy, the interaction of a nucleosome with an antibody can be detected by an increase in the diameter of the particle [49]. The diameter of a nucleosome is about 10 nm. When the nucleosome is fully covered with antibodies, which are 11 nm long, the diameter of the particle is about 30 nm. However, if only one or two antibodies are bound to the nucleosome or if the antibodies do not bind to the periphery of the nucleosome, the resulting particle has a smaller diameter. Thus, there is a correlation between the amount of antibody bound and the size of the particle, ranging from 10 nm for the free nucleosome to 30 nm for a particle fully saturated with antibodies. Such an analysis reveals heterogeneity among the nucleosomes with respect to the exposure of histone antigenic determinants [50]. The heterogeneity most probably reflects differences in the content of nonhistone proteins, which sterically hinder histone antigenic determinants, rather than differences in histone content among nucleosomes. Indeed, antisera against nonhistone proteins increase the diameter of all nucleosomes. The multiplicity of the nonhistone chromosomal protein fraction is large; therefore, it is inconceivable that each nucleosome can contain a full set of nonhistones. None of the nonhistone protein molecules is present in sufficient amounts to have one copy per nucleosome. Since all nucleosomes in a preparation react with antibodies, it can be concluded that the nucleosomes differ in their content of nonhistones. Support for this conclusion comes from immune sedimentation experiments in which ^{32}P end-labelled nucleosomes have been incubated with affinity purified antibodies to a histone fraction. The reaction mixtures were sedimented under conditions where free nucleosomes with an SW_{20} of 11 separated from free IgG (SW_{20} of 7) and from the nucleosome-antibody complex. At high antibody-to-nucleosome ratios, all nucleosomes migrated as a complex. Analysis of the complex revealed that each nucleosome contained two molecules of the core histones. This provided, for the first time, direct experimental evidence that each nucleosome contains a full set of core histones [54].

Antibodies against synthetic peptides or proteolytic fragments and mAbs against defined regions of a protein have been used to gain insight into the organization of protein in the chromatin fibre. Exposed regions will bind antibodies while sterically hindered regions will not. A recent example is a study on the organization of chromosomal proteins HMG-14 and HMG-17 in nucleosomes [17]. Antibodies were elicited against synthetic peptides corresponding to distinct protein domains. Immunoadsorption experiments (see above) revealed that the *N*-terminal and C-terminal region of the protein were relatively exposed and available to interact with other molecules, while the central regions were tightly bound to the core particles and did not bind antibodies. These results are relevant to understanding the function of these proteins.

6.3.2.4   Immunofractionation of Chromatin and Nucleosomes

The ability to isolate biologically meaningful fractions is a longstanding goal in chromatin research. Chromatin fractions may yield information about the association of specific chromosomal proteins with unique DNA sequences, the distribution of modified nucleotides in the genome, and the compositional rearrangement occurring during transcription, replication, or DNA repair. The availability of antisera against defined chromosomal components allows fractionation of chromatin and nucleosomes according to their content of antigenic determinants.

It is important to realize that results obtained from nucleoprotein immunofractionation are affected by considerations unique to this system. In particular, the methods of chromatin and nucleosome preparation and the size of the oligonucleosome fractions are relevant to such basic considerations as to whether the nucleosome preparation faithfully represents the entire nucleosome population in the nucleus and to whether protein rearrangement and migration occur during the preparation of the nucleosomes [55]. Cross-linking by ultraviolet irradiation [56, 57] or formaldehyde [58] and the use of low ionic strength buffers [55] avoid potential problems of protein rearrangement during chromatin and nucleosome fractionation. Preferential loss of a specific subset of nucleosomes can be minimized by preparing nucleosomes from chromatin rather than nuclei. *Landsman* et al. [55] described a sensitive test for protein rearrangement in which chromatin or nucleosomes prepared from one species are mixed with a salt-stripped preparation of chromatin or nucleosomes from another species. The mixture is immunofractionated and analysed with probes which can distinguish between the DNA of the two species. Immunoaffinity chromatography on columns containing antibodies to HMG-17 reveals that fractions of chromatin enriched in HMG-17 are also enriched in acetylated histones [59]. The DNA bound to such columns is 2 to 3-fold enriched in coding sequences as compared to total cellular DNA [60]. A similar enrichment has been observed by analysis of the chicken β-globin gene in cross-linked chromatin [61]. An enrichment of HMG-17 in active genes in chicken tissue has also been observed by immunoprecipitation with mAbs [62]. Further analysis indicates that the transition from HMG-17-free to HMG-17-containing chromatin occurs at the start of transcription [63]. In contrast, the proteins known to associate with the linker DNA between nucleosomes, namely histones H1 and H1^0, HMG-1, chicken HMG-E, and the trout HMG-T, seem to be somewhat depleted in chromatin regions containing active genes [56, 61, 64]. The results obtained with H1 and H1^0 support the results obtained by immunofluorescence with polytene chromosomes (see above).

6.3.2.5   Functional Analysis

The involvement of a protein in a cellular function is frequently inferred from its cellular location. The association of histones and HMG proteins with transcriptionally active regions has been investigated in many laboratories. Thus, the presence of histone H1 in interbands of polytene chromosomes suggests that the protein may be involved in inactivation of transcription [43]. However, recent immunoelectron microscopy studies on active *Balbiani* ring genes in salivary glands indicate that transcribed regions contain histone H1 [52]. In fact, the signal is stronger in active genes compared with the same region in the repressed state. The stronger signal reflects an increased accessibility of H1 antigenic determinant in the extended, transcriptionally active state. This example clearly illustrates one of the pitfalls in the use of antibody techniques to determine the presence of an antigen. As already elaborated, only a small proportion of the antibodies elicited by free histones bind to "native" chromatin. Immunofractionation experiments also indicate that histones H1 and $H1^0$ are present in transcribed regions, including enhancer-promoter DNA, albeit at a reduced concentration [61, 64]. Early immunoelectron microscopy studies demonstrating that the core histones remain associated with the transcriptionally active regions [65] have been verified by a variety of techniques.

The presence of select nonhistones in defined regions of the genome usually is taken as an indication that the protein directly affects the function of the region or the expression of a local gene. It is desirable to verify this by additional experiments. Antibodies to RNA polymerase localize to active regions in chromosomes [42]. Likewise, the presence of HMG-14 in transcriptionally active loci of polytene chromosomes [66] is consistent with a role in active chromatin. Immunofractionation experiments indicate that active genes are somewhat enriched in HMG-14/-17 proteins (for references see above). A few studies have examined the presence of the major chromosomal proteins in the regions of replicating DNA. The results indicate that histones are present near the replicating fork [65]. The use of antibodies to bromodeoxyuridine to map the pattern of DNA replication may serve as an example of the application of serological techniques to study replication of DNA in chromatin [67]. The role of histone modification. especially acetylation of histone H4 in transcription, has been studied by several groups [18–21, 24].

A more direct approach to studying the involvement of a chromosomal protein in chromatin function is antibody microinjection. Microinjection into amphibian oocytes and examination of lampbrush chromosomes and the amplified nucleoli present in the oocytes has been used in several studies of gene expression in living cells [68]. With this system, it has been demonstrated that appropriate antibodies interfere with the activity of RNA polymerases [69] and that histones [70] and HMGs [71] are present in transcriptionally active regions. Similar conclusions have been reached by injecting antibodies into tissue culture cells [72]. In these studies, the location of the antibody was visualized with antibodies labelled with a fluorescent tag. The ability of the microinjected cells to transcribe was monitored by autoradiography after brief incubations with radioactive precursors.

Immunodepletion experiments may also provide insights into the possible involvement of chromosomal proteins in gene expression. In a study with HMG-1 and HMG-2 proteins, *Singh* and *Dixon* [73] found that affinity-purified, fluorescent-labelled antibodies inhibited run-off transcription of several genes. Additional studies suggest that HMG-1/-2 may, in fact, be transcription factor TFIIB.

Serological approaches are uniquely suited to studies on the function and structure of complex and dynamic macromolecular structures such as chromatin and chromosomes. The examples presented illustrate the wide applicability of antibodies to a variety of studies. Immunological approaches will find an increasingly important role in functional studies on complex processes such as transcription and replication, especially as factors involved in these processes are identified and specific antisera or mAbs are elicited.

Likewise, advances in electron (cf. 5.7) and light microscopy (cf. 5.10) techniques, as well as in antibody labelling and 3-dimensional reconstitution techniques, will merge to yield information on the organization of chromosomal proteins *in situ*. Some of the pitfalls and limitations inherent in various experiments have been mentioned. The information obtainable by immunological approaches complements that obtained by other biophysical and biochemical techniques and can provide insights which presently cannot be obtained by other methods.

References

[1] *K. E. van Holde*, Chromatin, Springer-Verlag, New York 1988l
[2] *M. Bustin*, Immunological Probes for Nucleosomes, Methods Enzymol. *170*, 214–251 (1989).
[3] *M. Bustin*, Immunological Studies on the Structure and Function of HMG Proteins, in: *I. Beckhor* (ed.), Progress in Nonhistone Protein Research, CRC Press, Boca Raton 1985, pp. 75–90.
[4] *M. Bustin*, Immunological Approaches to Chromatin and Chromosome Structure and Function, Curr. Top. Microbiol. Immunol. *88*, 105–137 (1979).
[5] *S. Muller, M. H. Van Regenmortel*, Antihistone Antibodies, Methods Enzymol. *170*, 251–263 (1989).
[6] *B. D. Stollar*, Antibodies to DNA, CRC Crit. Rev. Biochem. *20*, 1–36 (1986).
[7] *J. S. Zlatanova*, Immunochemical Approaches to the Study of Histone H1 and HMG Chromatin Proteins, Mol. Cell. Biochem. *92*, 1–22 (1990).
[8] *E. A. Nigg*, Nuclear Function and Organization: the Potential for Immunochemical Approaches, Int. Rev. Cytol. *110*, 27–92 (1988).
[9] *D. Goldblatt, M. Bustin*, Exposure of Histone Antigenic Determinants in Chromatin, Biochemistry *14*, 1689–1695 (1975).
[10] *M. Bustin*, Arrangement of Histones in Chromatin, Nature *245*, 207–209 (1973).
[11] *M. Bustin*, Histone Antibodies and Chromatin Structure, in: *R. S. Sparkes, D. E. Comings, C. F. Fox* (eds.), Molecular Human Cytogenetics, Academic Press, New York 1977, pp. 25–40.
[12] *B. D. Stollar, M. Ward*, Rabbit Antibodies to Histone Fractions as Specific Reagents for Preparative and Comparative Studies, J. Biol. Chem. *245*, 1261–1266 (1970).
[13] *Y. Zick, D. Goldblatt, M. Bustin*, Exposure of Histone F1 Subfractions in Chromatin, Biochem. Biophys. Res. Commun. *65*, 637–643 (1975).
[14] *M. Bustin, B. D. Stollar*, Antigenic Determinants in Lysine Rich Histones, Biochemistry *12*, 1124–1129 (1973).
[15] *G. Sapeika, D. Absalom, M. H. V. Regenmortel*, Three Antigenic Determinants in Histone F3 from Chicken Erythrocytes, Immunochemistry *13*, 1–3 (1976).
[16] *D. Mathiew, C. V. Mura, L. Y. Frado, C. L. Woodcock, B. D. Stollar*, Differing Accessibility in Chromatin of the Antigenic Sites of Regions 1–58 and 63–125 of Histone H2B, J. Cell Biol. *91*, 135–141 (1981).
[17] *M. Bustin, M. P. Crippa, J. M. Pash*, Immunochemical Analysis of the Exposure of High Mobility Group Protein 14 and 17 Surfaces in Chromatin, J. Biol. Chem. *265*, 20077–20080 (1990).
[18] *U. Pfeffer, N. Ferrari, G. Vidali*, Availabity of Hyperacetylated H4 Histone in Intact Nucleosomes to Specific Antibodies, J. Biol. Chem. *261*, 2496–2498 (1986).
[19] *U. Pfeffer, N. Ferrari, F. Tosethi, G. Vidali*, Histone Acetylation in Conjugating *Tetrahymena thermophilia*, J. Cell Biol. *109*, 1007–1014 (1989).
[20] *B. M. Turner, L. Franchi, H. Wallace*, Islands of Acetylated H4 in Polytene Chromosomes and

Their Relationship to Chromatin Packaging and Transcriptional Activity, J. Cell Sci. *96*, 335–346 (1990).

[21] *R. Lin, J. W. Leone, R. G. Cook, C. D. Allis*, Antibodies Specific to Acetylated Histones Document the Consistence of Deposition and Transcription-related Histone Acetylation in Tetrahymena, J. Cell Biol. *108*, 1577–1588 (1989).

[22] *M. Monestier, T. M. Fasy, L. Bohn*, Monoclonal Antihistone H1 Autoantibodies from MRL lpr/lpr mice, Mol. Immunol. *26*, 749–758 (1989).

[23] *R. Laskov, S. Muller, M. Hochberg, H. Gieoh, M. H. V. Regenmortel, D. Eilat*, Monoclonal Autoantibodies to Histones from Autoimmune NZB/NZW F1 Mice, Eur. J. Immunol. *14*, 76–81 (1984).

[24] *S. Muller, D. Bonnier, M.Thiry, M. H. V. van Regenmortel*, Reactivity of Autoantibodies in SLE with Synthetic Core Histone Peptides, Int. Arch. Allergy Appl. Immunol. *89*, 288–296 (1989).

[25] *E. Mendelson, B. J. Smith, M. Bustin*, Mapping the Binding of Monoclonal Antibodies to Histone H5, Biochemistry *23*, 3466–3471 (1984).

[26] *M. Rozalshi, L. Lafleur, A. Rueiz-Carrillo*, Monoclonal Antibodies against Histone H5, J. Biol. Chem. *260*, 14379–14385 (1985).

[27] *S. Doussow, C. Gorka, C. Gilly, J. J. Lawrence*, Histone H1 Mapping Using Monoclonal Antibodies, J. Immunol. *19*, 1123–1129 (1989).

[28] *L. Mazzolini, M.Valk, M.V. Montagu*, Conserved Epitopes on Plant H1 Histones Recognized by Monoclonal Antibodies, Eur. J. Biochem. *178*, 779–787 (1989).

[29] *E. Mohr, L. Trieschmann, U. Grossbach*, Histone H1 in two Subspecies of *Chironomus thummi* with Different Genome Sizes: Homologous Chromosome Sites Differ Largely in Their Content of H1, Proc. Nat. Sci. U.S.A. *86*, 9308–9312 (1989).

[30] *J. N. Vanderbilt, J. N. Anderson*, Monoclonal Antibodies as Probes for the Complexity, Phylogeny and Chromatin Distribution of HMG-1 and 2, J. Biol. Chem. *260*, 9336–9345 (1985).

[31] *L. A. Blankstein, B. D. Stollar, S. G. Franklin, A. Zweidler, S. B. Lay*, Biochemical and Immunological Characterization of two Distinct Variants of Histone H2A in *Friend Leukemia*, Biochemistry *16*, 4556–4562 (1977).

[32] *M. Sluyser, M. Bustin*, Immunological Specificities of Lysine-rich Histones from Tumors, J. Biol. Chem. *248*, 2507–2511 (1974).

[33] *M. Bustin, B. D. Stollar*, Immunological Relatedness of Thymus and Liver F1 Subfractions, J. Biol. Chem. *248*, 3506–3510 (1973).

[34] *S. Spiker, K. M. Everett*, Blotting Index of Dissimilarity: Use to Study Immunological Relatedness of Plant and Animal HMG Chromosomal Proteins, Plant Mol. Biol. *9*, 431–442 (1987).

[35] *L. S. Hnilica* (ed.), Chromosomal Nonhistone Proteins, CRC Press.

[36] *R. C. Briggs, W. F. Glenn*, in: *L. S. Hnilica* (ed.), Chromosomal Nonhistone Proteins, CRC Press, Boca Raton 1983, pp. 103–113.

[37] *K. Wakabayashi, S. Wang, L. S. Hnilica*, Immunospecificity of Nonhistone Proteins in Chromatin, Biochemistry *13*, 1027–1032 (1974).

[38] *L. Zardi*, Chicken Antichromatin Antibody, Eur. J. Biochem. *55*, 231–238 (1975).

[39] *E. Mendelson, M. Bustin*, Monoclonal Antibodies against Distinct Determinants of Histone H5 Bind to Chromatin, Biochemistry *23*, 3459–3466 (1984).

[40] *M. Bustin, N. K. Neihart*, Antibodies against Chromosomal HMG Proteins Stain the Cytoplasm of Mammalian Cells, Cell *16*, 181–190 (1979).

[41] *M. Bustin, H. Yamasaki, D. Goldblatt, M. Shani, E. Huberman, L. Sachs*, Histone Distribution in Chromosomes revealed by Anti-histone Antibodies, Exp. Cell Res. *97*, 440–444 (1976).

[42] *M. Jamrich, A. L. Greenleaf, E. K. F. Bautz*, Localization of RNA Polymerase in Polytene Chromosomes of *Drosophila melanogaster*, Proc. Nat. Acad. Sci. U.S.A. *74*, 2079–2083 (1977).

[43] *M. Jamrich, A. L. Greenleaf, F. A. Bautz, E. K. Bautz*, Functional Organization of Polytene Chromosomes, Cold Spring Harbor Symp. Quant. Biol. *XLII*, 389–396 (1977).

[44] *P. D. Kurth, E. N. Moudrianakis, M. Bustin,* Histone Localization in Polytene Chromosomes by Immunofluorescence, J. Cell Biol. *78,* 910–918 (1978).

[45] *P. D. Kurth, M. Bustin,* Localization of Chromosomal Protein HMG-1 in Polytene Chromosomes of *Chironomus thummi,* J. Cell Biol. *89,* 70–77 (1981).

[46] *L. M. Silver, S. C. R. Elgin,* Immunological Analysis of Protein Distributions in Drosophila Polytene Chromosomes, in: *H. Busch* (ed.), The Cell Nucleus, Academic Press, New York 1978, Vol. 4, pp. 216–262.

[47] *T. C. James, J. C. Eisenberg, C. Craig, V. Dietrich, A. Hobson, S. C. Elgin,* Distribution of HP1 a Heterochromatin-Associated Nonhistone Chromosomal Protein in Drosophila, Eur. J. Cell Biol. *50,* 170–180 (1989).

[48] *G. C. Howard, L. A. Abmayr, L. A. Shinefeld, V. L. Sato, S. C. Elgin,* Monoclonal Antibodies against a Specific Nonhistone Chromosomal Protein of Drosophila Associated with Acitve Genes, J. Cell Biol. *88,* 219–225 (1981).

[49] *M. Bustin, D. Goldblatt, R. Sperling,* Chromatin Structure Visualization by Immuno Electron Microscopy, Cell 7, 297–304 (1976).

[50] *D. Goldblatt, M. Bustin, R. Sperling,* Heterogeneity in the Interaction of Chromatin Subunits with Anti-histone Sera Visualized by Immunoelectron Microscopy, Exp. Cell Res. *112,* 1–14 (1978).

[51] *C. Woodcock,* Immunoelectron Microscopy of Nucleosomes, Methods Enzymol. *170,* 180–192 (1989).

[52] *C. Ericsson, V. Grossbach, B. Bjorhroth, B. Daneholt,* Presence of Histone H1 on an Active *Balbiani* Ring Gene, Cell *60,* 73–83 (1990).

[53] *L. Frado, C. V. Mura, B. D. Stollar, C. L. F. Woodcock,* Mapping of Histone H5 Sites on Nucleosomes Using Immunoelectron Microscopy, J. Biol. Chem. *258,* 11984–11990 (1983).

[54] *M. Bustin, R. Simpson, R. Sperling, D. Goldblatt,* Molecular Homogeneity of Histone Content of HeLa Chromatin Subunits, Biochemistry *16,* 5381–5385 (1977).

[55] *D. Landsman, E. Mendelson, S. Druckmann, M. Bustin,* Exchange of Proteins during Immunofractionation of Chromatin, Exp. Cell Res. *163,* 95–102 (1986).

[56] *J. Blanco, J. C. States, G. H. Dixon,* General Method for Isolation of DNA Sequences that Interact with Specific Nuclear Proteins in Chromosomes, Biochemistry *24,* 8021–8028 (1985).

[57] *D. S. Gilmour, T. J. Lis,* Detecting Protein-DNA Interactions *in vivo*; Distribution of RNA Polymerase on Specific Bacterial Genes, Proc. Nat. Acad. Sci. U.S.A. *81,* 4275–4279 (1984).

[58] *P. C. Dedon, J. A. Soults, D. C. Allis, M. A. Gorowsky,* Formaldehyde Cross-linking and Immunoprecipitation Demonstrate Developmental Changes in H1 Association with Active Genes, Mol. Cell Biol. *11,* 1729–1733 (1991).

[59] *N. Malik, M. Smulson, M. Bustin,* Enrichment in Acetylated Histones in Polynucleosomes Containing HMG-17 Revealed by Immunoaffinity Chromatography, J. Biol. Chem. *259,* 699–702 (1984).

[60] *S. Druckmann, E. Mendelson, D. Landsman, M. Bustin,* Immunofractionation of DNA Sequences Associated with HMG-17 in Chromatin, Exp. Cell Res. *166,* 486–496 (1986).

[61] *Y. V. Postnikov, V. V. Shick, A. V. Belyavsky, K. R. Khrapko, K. L. Brodolin, T. A. Nikolskaya, A. D. Mirzabekov,* Distribution of High Mobility Group Proteins 1/2, E and HMG-14/-17 and Linker Histones H1 and H5 on Transcribed and Non-transcribed Regions of Chicken Erythrocyte Chromatin, Nucleic Acids Res. *19,* 717–725 (1991).

[62] *T. Dorbic, B. Wittig,* Isolation of Oligonucleosomes from Chromatin Using HMG-17 Specific Monoclonal Antibodies, Nucleic Acids Res. *14,* 3363–3376 (1986).

[63] *T. Dorbic, B. Wittig,* Chromatin from Transcribed Genes Contains HMG-17 only Downstream from the Starting Point of Transcription, EMBO J. *6,* 2393–2399 (1987).

[64] *E. Mendelson, D. Landsman, S. Druckmann, M. Bustin,* Immunofractionation of Chromatin Region Associated with Histone H1^0, Eur. J. Biochem. *160,* 253–260 (1986).

[65] *S. L. McKnight, M. Bustin, O. L. Miller,* Electron Microscopic Analysis of Chromosome Metabolism in the Drosophila Melanogaster Embryo, Cold Spring Harbor Symp. Quant. Biol. *XLII,* 741–754 (1977).

[66] *R. Westermann, U. Grossbach*, Localisation of Nuclear Proteins Related to High Mobility Group Protein 14 (HMG-14) in Polytene Chromosomes, Chromosoma *90*, 355–365 (1984).

[67] *L. Allison, D. J. Arndt-Jovin, H. Gratzner, T. Ternyck, M. Robert-Nicoud*, Mapping the Pattern of DNA Replication in Polytene Chromosomes from *Chironomus thummi* Using Monoclonal Anti-bromodeoxyuridine Antibodies, Cytometry 6, 584–590 (1985).

[68] *U. Scheer*, Injection of Antibodies into the Nucleus of Amphibian Oocytes: An Experimental Means of Interfering with Gene Expression in the Living Cell, J. Embryol. Exp. Morphol. Suppl. 97, 223–242 (1986).

[69] *M. Bona, U. Scheer, E. K. F. Bautz*, Antibodies to RNA Polymerase II Inhibit Transcription after Microinjection into Living Amphibian Oocytes, J. Mol. Biol. *151*, 81–99 (1981).

[70] *U. Scheer, J. Sommerville, M. Bustin*, Injected Histone Antibodies Interfere with Transcription of Lampbrush Chromosome Loops in Oocytes of Pleurodeles, J. Cell Sci. *40*, 1–20 (1979).

[71] *J. A. Kleinschmidt, U. Scheer, M. C. Dabauvalle, M. Bustin, W. W. Franke*, High Mobility Group Proteins of Amphibian Oocytes: A Large Pool of Soluble HMG-1 Like Proteins and Involvement in Transcriptional Events, J. Cell Biol. 97, 838–848 (1983).

[72] *L. Einck, M. Bustin*, Inhibition of Transcription in Somatic Cells by Micro Injection of Antibodies to Chromosomal Proteins, Proc. Nat. Acad. Sci. U.S.A. *80*, 6735–6739 (1983).

[73] *J. Singh, G. H. Dixon*, High Mobility Group Proteins 1 and 2 Function as General Class II Transcription Factors, Biochemistry 29, 6295–6302 (1990).

6.3.3   The Mitotic Apparatus and Chromosomes

Claudio E. Sunkel

The application of a variety of immunological techniques to the structural and functional analysis of the mitotic apparatus and chromosomes in eukaryotes has made a significant contribution to the study of mitosis. It has become apparent that mitotic chromosomes are embedded in a very complex and dynamic protein matrix, the scaffold. This structure contains elements required for chromosome condensation, as well as those which form the interphase between spindle microtubules and the DNA fibre. A number of immunological studies on this structure have indicated that, independently of the DNA, it has a large degree of autonomy during mitosis. The structure of the spindle and its interactions with other components of the mitotic apparatus, the kinetochore and the centrosome, have also been studied through very elegant immunological techniques. The picture that is emerging is that spindle microtubules are nucleated by the centrosome as they migrate to the poles during late prometaphase. During these early stages, chromosomes are organized in a metaphase plate as plus-ends microtubules are captured by the kinetochores. Immunological evidence indicates that motor proteins such as dynein are located in the kinetochore, supporting the hypothesis that, during anaphase, chromosomes move to the poles along spindle microtubules by chemical energy produced at the kinetochore.

Immunological techniques have also been applied to the characterization of molecules which seem to regulate mitosis, thus providing clues to the general mechanisms of mitotic control. The localization of cdc2, a protein kinase which forms an integral part of maturation promoting factor, to the kinetochore and the centrosome, and its involvement with histone H1 and lamins, suggests that phosphorylation might play a significant role during the assembly or disassembly of macromolecular structures of the mitotic apparatus and chromosomes.

6.3.3.1   Organization of the Chromosome Scaffold

The genome of eukaryotic cells is organized at two levels: first, by the binding of histones to form nucleosomes and, second, by interaction with other non-histone proteins that appear to define and maintain looped domains ranging in size from $M_r = 10000$ to 100000. During metaphase, the chromosomes assume a highly condensed organization, associated with a proteinaceous structure which can be isolated after DNA and histone extraction. This structure has been called the chromosome scaffold [1].

The use of purified scaffold for immunization protocols has not been generally successful. It will be seen later that this approach has produced monoclonal antibodies to a limited subset of scaffold associated proteins. However, most of them are antigens related to specific components of the mitotic apparatus and do not meet the criteria for an epitope that correlates with the expected distribution of a structurally important scaffold component. So far, the only protein which partially fulfills this expected distribution and abundance is topoisomerase II. Antibodies raised against whole scaffold recognized a single protein ($M_r = 170000$) in mitotic chromosomes [2]. Immunolocalization within mitotic chromosomes showed this protein to concentrate at the base of what might be the DNA fibre loops along the length of the chromosome [3].

Chromosome condensation

Chromosome condensation can be envisaged as a two-step process. The first is a reduction in nuclear volume, independent of topoisomerase II levels, which might be related to histone H1 phosphorylation [4]. A second step is the resolution of individual chromosomes and for this, scaffold-bound topoisomerase II seems to be essential [5].

Chromosome organization at prometaphase

The whole nuclear arrangement of chromosomes during mitosis has been studied in detail using immunofluorescence techniques. In *Drosophila*, the prometaphase transition was analysed with the aid of various antibodies against tubulin, centrosomes and lamins. At this stage of mitosis, chromosomes are attached to the apical nuclear envelope by their centromeres and, after condensation is completed, the telomers locate basally. Nuclear envelope breakdown starts apically, concomitantly with the mitotic spindle formation and, probably, attachment of the spindle microtubules to the centromeres, and continues as an apical-basal wave which can be correlated with congression of chromosomes to the metaphase plate [6]. In mammalian cells in culture the prometaphase configuration is slightly different. By the use of CREST sera which recognize centromere antigens (cf. 6.3.3.3, Kinetochore) and anti-tubulin antibodies it has been shown that centromeres appear to be located towards the inside of the nucleus while the telomeres remain attached to the nuclear envelope. The centrosomes seem to push their way into the nucleus as they migrate to the poles, organizing the metaphase plate and the spindle [7].

6.3.3.2   Centromeric DNA

The centromere domain of eukaryotic mitotic chromosomes is structurally defined as the primary constriction at which the kinetochore, the attachment site of mitotic spindles, is located. Although the ultrastructure of the centromere has been extensively studied, the molecular basis for its structure and function have only recently begun to be elucidated. The kinetochore of metaphase chromosomes is in close contact with centromeric chromatin. In higher eukaryotes, these regions are known to be composed of heterochromatic DNA, a fact that has hindered their molecular analysis. Early reports indicated that mouse α-satellite DNA was a major component of centromeric regions [8]. More recently, some elegant experiments resulted in the isolation of human centromeric DNA. By performing limited endonuclease digestion of isolated chromatin and monitoring the gel filtration fraction which contained centromere antigens, it was possible to build a mini-library of DNA enriched for centromeric DNA. Subsequent *in-situ* hybridization revealed that one clone contained a series of short 150 bp repeats which hybridized to the centromere of some human chromosomes. These repeats show strong homology to known α-satellite DNA [9].

6.3.3.3   The Kinetochore

Kinetochore – associated antigens

The kinetochore is a multiprotein complex formed at the centromere in close contact with the DNA fibre. Since this chromosomal structure is the site of spindle microtubule attachment, we can consider it to be both part of the chromosome and also part of the mitotic apparatus. Electron-microscopy studies of metaphase mammalian kinetochores indicate that it consists of a trilaminar disk composed of outer, middle and inner layers [10, 11] and a fibrous corona [12]. The inner layer may be involved in holding sister chromatids together. Indeed, a set of proteins has been identified and named the Inner Centromere Proteins (INCENPs) which concentrate next to the centromere of chromosomes during metaphase to anaphase transition [13]. The INCENPs were identified after immunization of mice with isolated scaffolds, to which the proteins remain attached during sequential extraction. Another set of antigens showing similar distribution was defined using autoimmune sera. The Chromatin Linking Proteins (CLIPs) localize to a filamentous structure that transects the central centromeric domain and also to discreet sites along the pairing surface of the chromatids [14].

Kinetochore antigens

The molecular characterization of the major kinetochore antigens started after the discovery that some human patients suffering from CREST or other autoimmune diseases had high titres of anti-kinetochore antibodies [16]. Using their sera it was possible to map the autoantigens directly onto chromosome spreads by an immunoperoxidase technique [17]. Further studies showed that the antibodies recognized three immunologically related protein species in western blots [18] designated CENP-A, CENP-B and CENP-C. Partial cDNAs for CENP-B were isolated from a human endothelial cDNA expression library, and the β-gal fusion protein was used to produce both monoclonal and polyclonal antibodies [19]. Neither CENP-A or CENP-C have been cloned or specific antibodies obtained. However, sequential extraction of proteins from the nucleus and immunological monitoring with CREST sera have indicated that CENP-A is released from the scaffold with histones [20] while CENP-B remains attached [21]. The original CREST sera and the polyclonal antibodies against CENP-B have been used in ultra-thin sections to map the location of these antigens. CENP-B specific antibodies localized thoughout the centromeric heterochromatin beneath the kinetochore [22] and CENP-B recognized *in vitro* a 17 bp motif present in human α-satellite DNA [23]. However, when whole CREST serum was used a "collar" of label, presumably bound to CENP-A and/or CENP-C surrounded the kinetochore plates [24].

Another well-characterized protein was recently identified as a component of mammalian kinetochores. Monoclonal antibodies directed against cytoplasmic dynein recognized a similar molecular species in mitotic spindles and kinetochores [24, 25]. These results are the first direct evidence that a molecular motor protein is localized to the kinetochore, thus providing support for the hypothesis that the mechanochemical energy responsible for chromosome translocation is associated with the kinetochore (cf. 6.3.3.5, below).

Further insights into the dynamics of this crucial chromosomal structure were obtained by studying its behaviour *in vivo* after being detached from mitotic chromosomes. By forcing CHO cells to enter mitosis prematurely after treatment with cafeine during G_1/S arrest, the mitotic spindle begins to assemble and chromosomes partially condense into fragments which become disperse. The kinetochores labelled with CREST sera can be seen to detach from chromosomes and aggregate near the center of the nucleous as in normal congression. To follow the fate of the kinetochores, synchronized populations of cells were released from the microtubule depolymerizing block and observed at various stages of cell cycle progression. After aggregating near the centre of the nucleus, the kinetochores "split" and move to opposite poles and cytokinesis takes place leaving the chromatin randomly distributed among daughter cells [26]. Since no DNA was detected in the detached kinetochores it seems that, in its absence, kinetochores can still retain the capacity to interact with spindle microtubules and undergo all anaphase movements. These results show that the mitotic chromosome scaffold is highly structured and very dynamic and that, even in the absence of the DNA fibre, it can interact normally with the other components of the mitotic apparatus and perform complex behaviour.

In-vivo functional tests for the major kinetochore antigens have also been performed. Injection of immunopurified antibodies from CREST sera against CENP-A, CENP-B or CENP-C into living cells at different stages of the cell cycle causes arrest at two points in interphase. These events might involve centromere assembly in coordination with α-satellite DNA replication and maturation of the kinetochore at prophase [27, 28].

6.3.3.4   The Centrosome

Structure of the centrosome

The centrosome can act as the site for microtubule polymerization-depolymerization [29] and it also plays a crucial role in the temporal and spatial organization of the cellular matrix [30]. In most higher eukaryotes, this structure is the anchoring site for microtubules throughout the cell cycle. It is composed of a pair of centrioles and associated electron-dense pericentriolar material. The centrosome is a complex structure capable of duplication and there are indications that it might contain DNA [31]. Microinjection of biotinylated tubulin into LLC-Pk culture cells followed by indirect immunofluorescence has been used to analyse the mode of centriole duplication and distribution. After mitosis each cell receives a centrosome containing a new and an old centriole, indicating that incorporation of tubulin into centrioles is conservative and distribution is semiconservative [32].

Studies on the molecular composition of centrosomes were initiated after the discovery that the sera from patients with progressive systemic sclerosis have antibodies to the eukaryotic centrosome [33]. Ultrastructural localization of these antigens using immunoperoxidase methods indicated that they are not the tubulin component [34] but are located either in the matrix or the centriolar rim which surrounds the blade microtubules [35]. Human CREST sera which recognize centrosomes have been used successfully for the screening of *S. cerevisiae* gt11 expression libraries. Thus it was possible to identify and clone the Spindle Pole Antigen 1 (SPA1), a protein of

$M_r = 59\,000$, which has been shown genetically to be directly involved with chromosome segregation [36].

Centrosomal antigens

Although many attempts have been made to produce monoclonal antibodies against centrosomal antigens by immunization with highly enriched centrosomal fractions, they have encountered limited success. The poor results obtained with this strategy suggest some basic biochemical constraints in the use of these protein preparations as immunogens. However, it is most interesting that in autoimmune related diseases these antigens can induce high antibody titres. To date, only one mAb has been obtained by immunization with a crude centrosomal fraction from PtK cells. It recognized a $M_r = 35\,000$ component of the murine centrosome [37], and was used to isolate from an expression library full length cDNAs which code for a lamin-related protein called centrosomin A [38]. Other centrosome-related proteins have been cloned through the fortuitous identification of antibodies which were not specifically sought. For example, in *Drosophila*, cDNAs coding for a $M_r = 185\,000$ protein were isolated by screening a gt11 expression library with the mAb BX63 [39]. This antibody had been recovered after immunization of mice with embryonic nuclear fractions and it recognizes only centrosomes in this species [40]. Another mAb against centrosomal components is MPM13, raised originally against extracts from mitotic cells, which recognizes a $M_r = 13\,000$ protein [41]. Recently, a kinesin-related antigen of $M_r = 120\,000$ has been identified by polyclonal antibodies raised against purified kinesin [42].

There are no data on the ultrastructural localization of any of the antigens so far described. However, molecular characterization and localization of a pericentriolar material antigen has been achieved. Centrin is a $M_r = 165\,000$ protein of which little is known about its function but it has been localized to the pericentriolar material of PtK cells [43].

Cell cycle-related post-translational modifications of centromeric antigens have also been studied using antibodies. MPM-2 is a mAb, raised against mammalian mitotic antigens [44], which recognizes a specific subset of centrosomally-associated phospho-proteins [45]. Immunofluorescence shows that these centrosomal antigens attain maximum phosphorylation just prior to anaphase onset [46]. These results might be related to the localization of the p34^{cdc2} serine/threonine protein kinase to the centrosome, kinetochore microtubules and kinetochore of Hela and Indian muntjac cells during late G^2_M[47]. This protein is now believed to be a major mitotic regulator for many different species (cf. 6.3.3.6, Control of Mitosis).

6.3.3.5   The Mitotic Spindle

Microtubules are protein filaments, made up of α- and β-tubulin subunits, about 20–25 nm in diameter which form part of the cytoskeleton of eukaryotic cells. More specifically, what concerns us here are the spindle microtubules which become organized into a bipolar structure during the first stages of mitosis and function primarily for the separation of sister chromatids. There is now a wealth of data indicating that higher eukaryotes contain multiple genes for α- and β-tubulin [48]. However, there is still some discussion of whether different tubulin isotypes serve different functions. While this question remains essentially unanswered, some elegant experiments which combine molecular genetics and immunological techniques suggest that both α and β isotypes are interchangeable, allowing functional co-polymerization *in vivo* [49, 50].

Both α- and β-tubulin subunits have been shown to be modified after translation. α-Tubulins are synthesized with a carboxyl terminal tyrosine which can be removed by a carboxypeptidase and added back by a ligase. Specific antibodies which can differentiate between tyrosinylated and detyrosinylated tubulin show that young microtubules tend to contain more tyrosinylated subunits than older ones, permitting stable microtubules to be distinguished from those turning over rapidly [51]. α-Tubulin can also be acetylated on lysine 40 [52] and specific antibodies show that old microtubules tend to be more highly acetylated than younger ones. Therefore, while the *in-vivo* role of these post-translational modifications remains unclear, stable microtubules are often both acetylated and detyrosinylated [53]. It is intriguing, however, that none of these modifications seems to affect microtubule polymerization *in vitro*. β-Tubulins are also modified. They can be phosphorylated on a serine residue near the carboxyl terminus. The same serine has been found to be phosphorylated *in vivo* [54].

The first stages of spindle organization require microtubule assembly which is a two-step process involving nucleation and elongation. For elongation to occur, GTP must be bound to tubulin subunits giving rise to a polarized microtubule, so that addition of subunits takes place at the plus ends and loss at the minus ends [55]. Overall, microtubules display rather unusual properties both *in vitro* and *in vivo,* alternating between growing and shrinking states, a phenomenon which has been called dynamic instability and which reflects the inherent instability of the polymer unless stabilized by continuous subunit addition [56].

Microtubule nucleation *in vivo* is thought to occur essentially by the centrosome. Specific proteins which might be involved in microtubule nucleation have been identified. A distinct microtubule assembly-promoting factor was isolated from *Xenopus* eggs. This is a $M_r = 215000$ protein which preferentially promotes microtubule assembly at the plus ends [57]. Also, a $M_r = 145000$ protein termed STOP has been isolated which binds microtubules and makes them super-stable under a variety of conditions [58].

During prometaphase, spindle microtubules are nucleated by the centrosome and captured by the kinetochore of condensed chromosomes. In a series of elegant experiments, biotinylated tubulin was incorporated *in vitro* into microtubules and their interaction with isolated kinetochores was studied by antibiotin antibodies. The results suggest that plus-ends microtubules are preferentially stabilized at the kinetochore [59]. By extensive use of this experimental approach it was possible to show that chromosomes move polewards during anaphase along stationary microtubules, while depolymerization takes place coordinately at the kinetochore end [60]. Similar experiments *in vivo* confirmed these results and suggested that the energy for chromosome translocation could be solely derived from microtubule depolymerization at the kinetochore [61].

Other major components of the mitotic spindle are the microtubule-associated proteins (MAPs). A highly successful approach to isolating these components was developed recently. Soluble cytoplasmic extracts made from *Drosophila* embryos were subjected to microtubule affinity chromatography. Taxol-stabilized microtubules were bound to an agarose-Sepharose matrix through which whole cell extracts were passed. Release of bound proteins from the columns yielded more than 50 proteins. Mouse polyclonal antibodies were raised to 24 of these and at least 20 of them stained microtubule-associated structures [62]. Other well-characterized MAPs such as tau and MAP2 have been shown to induce linkage between microtubules to produce bundles and to stabilize the polymers [63].

6.3.3.6 The Control of Mitosis

Even though the biochemical pathways that control cell-cycle progression had been the focus of much research, they remained poorly understood. Only recently have biochemical, genetic and immunological analysis been combined systematically, with unprecedented success. Biochemical studies showed that when the Maturation Promoting Factor (MPF) of early *Xenopus* eggs was isolated from the appropriate stage and injected into pre-mitotic eggs it could induce maturation and entry into mitosis [64]. Subsequently, it has become clear that MPF plays a general role in mitotic induction in somatic cells ranging from yeast to human cells [65].

The development of cell free systems to analyse the activity of particular components of MPF has greatly facilitated molecular analysis. It has been possible to reconstruct interphase extracts which re-assemble chromatin [66], replicate their DNA [67] and perform other functions efficiently. It is possible to induce an interphase-free system to undergo early mitotic events by addition of active MPF [68].

From a very different standpoint, genetics had begun to dissect the yeast cell cycle by isolating conditional lethals that affect cell cycle progression in some way [69]. Two of these loci proved later to be crucial components of mitotic control, the *S. cerevisiae* (CDC28) and its homologue in *S. pombi* (cdc2). Molecular cloning of these genes proved them to encode a protein kinase [70, 71]; later, immunological analysis showed the *Xenopus* homologue of cdc2 and CDC28 to co-purify with MPF activity [72].

The general nature of MPF activity as a mitotic regulator across most species was shown by mAbs prepared against highly conserved amino acid domains of these protein kinases. The use of these antibodies for immunoprecipitation after *in-vitro* phosphorylation studies in human cells indicated that p34^{cdc2} showed cell cycle-dependent phosphorylation, and MPF, significant subunit rearrangement [73]. p34^{cdc2} was highly phosphorylated during G_2/M transition, declining during G_1 and S phases. *In vitro*, p34^{cdc2} and its various homologues have been shown to phosphorylate a number of proteins including histone H1 and lamins [74]. However, none has been shown conclusively to be an *in-vivo* substrate. Nevertheless, both of these *in-vitro* substrates are known to be phosphorylated during M phase. Histone H1 phosphorylation had been shown to be essential for chromosome condensation [4] and lamin phosphorylation occurs concomitantly with nuclear envelope breakdown [75, 76].

Two other proteins have been shown to be essential components of MPF. The mitotic cyclins were first identified in embryos of marine invertebrates. They accumulate during interphase but undergo abrupt selective degradation at the end of each mitosis [77]. Cyclins A and B can be immunoprecipitated with anti-p34^{cdc2} antibody, and there is a clear correlation between inactivation of the p34^{cdc2} kinase and cyclin degradation [78]. Indeed, intact cells or extracts which contain a proteolysis-resistant cyclin can not exit from mitosis [79]. Finally, the addition of exogenous p34^{cdc2} kinase to a cell-free extract of interphase *Xenopus* eggs induces precocious cyclin degradation [80], suggesting that in this way cdc2 provides a negative feedback loop thereby terminating mitosis.

References

[1] *K. W. Adolph, S. M. Cheng, J. R. Paulson, U. K. Laemmli,* Isolation of a Protein Scaffold from Mitotic Hela Cell Chromosomes, Proc. Natl. Acad. Sci. U.S.A. *11,* 4937–4941 (1977).

[2] *W. C. Earnshaw, B. Halligam, C. A. Cooke, M. M. S. Heck, L. F. Lin,* Topoisomerase II is a Structural Component of Mitotic Chromosomes Scaffolds, J. Cell Biol. *100,* 1706–1715 (1985).

[3] *W. C. Earnshaw, M. M. S. Heck,* Localization of Topoisomerase II in Mitotic Chromosomes, J. Cell Biol. *100,* 1716–1725 (1985).

[4] *Y. Matsumoto, H. Yasuda, S. Mita, T. Marunochi, M. Yamada,* Evidence for the Involvement of H1 Histone Phosphorylation in Chromosome Condensation, Nature *284,* 181–183 (1980).

[5] *E. R. Wood, W. C. Earnshaw,* Mitotic Chromatin Condensation *in vitro* Using Somatic Cell Extracts and Nuclei with Variable Levels of Endogenous Topoisomerase II, J. Cell Biol. *111,* 2839–2850 (1990).

[6] *Y. Hiraoka, D. A. Agard, J. W. Sedat,* Temporal and Spacial Coordination of Chromosome Movement, Spindle Formation, and Nuclear Envelope Breakdown during Prometaphase in Drosophila melanogaster Embryos, J. Cell Biol. *111,* 2815–2828 (1990).

[7] *N. Chaly, D. Brown,* The Prometaphase Configuration and Chromosome Order in Early Mitosis, J. Cell Sci. *91,* 325–335 (1988).

[8] *A. Wong, J. B. Rattner,* Sequence Organization and Cytological Localization of the Minor Satellite of Mouse, Nucleic Acids Res. *16,* 11645–11661 (1988).

[9] *H. Masumoto, K. Sugimoto, T. Okazaki,* Alphiod Satellite DNA is Tightly Associated with Centromere Antigens in Human Chromosomes throughout the Cell Cycle, Exp. Cell Res. *181,* 181–196 (1989).

[10] *P. T. Jokelainen,* The Ultrastructure and Spatial Organization of the Metaphase Kinetochore in Mitotic Rat Cells, J. Ultrastruct. Res. *16,* 19–44 (1967).

[11] *J. B. Rattner, D. P. Bazett-Jones,* Kinetochore Structure: Electron Spectroscopic Imaging of the Kinetochore, J. Cell Biol. *108,* 1209–1219 (1989).

[12] *A. F. Pluta, C. A. Cooke, W. C. Earnshaw,* Structure of the Human Centromere at Metaphase, TIBS *15,* 181–185 (1990).

[13] *C. A. Cooke, M. M. S. Heck, W. C. Earnshaw,* The Inner Centromere Protein (INCENP) Antigens: Movement from Inner Centromere to Midbody during Mitosis, J. Cell Biol. *105,* 2053–2067 (1987).

[14] *J. B. Rattner, B. G. Kingwell, M. J. Tritzler,* Detection of Distinct Structural Domains within the Primary Constriction Using Autoantibodies, Chromosoma *96,* 360–367 (1988).

[15] *C. L. Reider,* The Formation, Structure and Composition of the Mammalian Kinetochore and Kinetochore Fiber, Int. Rev. Cytol. *79,* 1–58 (1982).

[16] *Y. Moroi, C. Peebles, M. J. Fritzler, J. Stergerwarld, E. M. Tan*, Autoantibodies to Centromere (Kinetochore) in Scleroderma Sera, Proc. Natl. Acad. Sci. U.S.A. *77*, 1627–1631 (1980).

[17] *S. Brenner, D. Pepper, M. W. Bernz, E. M. Tan, B. R. Brinkley*, Kinetochore Structure, Duplication and Distribution in Mammalian Cells: Analysis by Human Autoantibodies from Scleroderma Patients, J. Cell Biol. *91*, 95–102 (1981).

[18] *W. C. Earnshaw, N. Rothfield*, Identification of a Family of Human Centromere Related Proteins Using Autoimmune Sera from Patients with Scleroderma, Chromosoma *91*, 313–321 (1985).

[19] *W. C. Earnshaw, K. F. Sullivan, P. S. Machlin, C. A. Cooke, D. A. Kaiser, T. D. Pollard, N. F. Rothfield, D. W. Cleveland*, Molecular Cloning of cDNA for CENP-B, The Major Human Centromere Autoantigen, J. Cell Biol. *104*, 817–829 (1987).

[20] *D. K. Palmer, K. O'Day, M. H. Wener, B. S. Andrews, R. L. Margolis*, A 17 kD Centromere Protein (CENP-A) Copurifies with Nucleosome Core Particles and with Histones, J. Cell Biol. *104*, 805–815 (1987).

[21] *M. Valdivia, B. R. Brinkley*, Fractionation and Initial Characterization of the Kinetochore From Mammalian Metaphase Chromosomes, J. Cell Biol. *101*, 1124–1134 (1985).

[22] *C. A. Cooke, R. L. Bernat, W. C. Earnshaw*, CENP-B: A Major Human Centromere Protein Located Beneath the Kinetochore, J. Cell Biol. *110*, 1475–1488 (1990).

[23] *H. Masumoto, H. Masukata, Y. Muro, N. Nozaki, T. Okazaki*, A Human Centromere Antigen (CENP-B) Interacts with Short Specific Sequence in Alphoid DNA, a Human Centromeric Satellite, J. Cell Biol. *109*, 1963–1973 (1989).

[24] *E. R. Steuer, L. Wordemann, T. A. Schroer, M. P. Sheetz*, Localization of Cytoplasmic Dynein to Mitotic Spindles and Kinetochores, Nature *345*, 266–268 (1990).

[25] *C. M. Pfarr, M. Coue, P. M. Garrison, T. S. Hays, M. E. Porter, J. R. McIntosh*, Cytoplasmic Dynein is Localized to the Kinetochores during Mitosis, Nature *345*, 263–265 (1990).

[26] *B. R. Brinkley, R. P. Zinkowski, W. L. Mollon, F. M. Davis, M. A. Pisegna, M. Pershouse, P. N. Rao*, Movement and Segregation of Kinetochores Experimentally Detached from Mammalian Chromosomes, Nature *336*, 251–254 (1988).

[27] *C. Simerly, R. Balczon, B. R. Brinkley, G. Schatten*, Microinjected Kinetochore Antibodies Interfere with Chromosome Movement in Meiotic and Mitotic Mouse Oocytes, J. Cell Biol. *111*, 1491–1504 (1990).

[28] *R. L. Bernat, G. G. Borisy, N. F. Rothfield, W. C. Earnshaw*, Injection of Anticentromere Antibodies in Interphase Disrupts Events Required for Chromosome Movement at Mitosis, J. Cell. Biol. *111*, 1519–1533 (1990).

[29] *L. Evans, T. Mitchison, M. Kirschner*, Influence of the Centromere on the Structure of Nucleated Microtubules, J. Cell Biol. *100*, 1185–1191 (1985).

[30] *J. W. Raff, D. M. Glover*, Centrosomes and not Nuclei, Initiate Pole Cell Formation in the Drosophila Embryo, Cell *57*, 611–619 (1989).

[31] *J. L. Hall, Z. Ramanis, D. J. Luck*, Basal Body/Centriolar DNA: Molecular Genetic studies in *Chlamydomonas*, Cell *59*, 121–132 (1989).

[32] *R. S. Kochanski, G. G. Borisy*, Mode of Centriole Duplication and Distribution, J. Cell Biol. *110*, 1599–1605 (1990).

[33] *Y. Moroi, I. Murata, A. Tackeuchi, N. Kamatani, K. Tamimoto, R. Yokohari*, Human Anticentriole Autoantibodies in Patients with Scleroderma and *Reynaud's* Phenomenon, Clin. Immunol. Immunopathol. *29*, 381–390 (1980).

[34] *T. G. Osborn, J. S. Ryerse, N. E. Bauer, J. M. Urhahim, D. Blair, T. L. Moore*, Anticentriole Antibody in a Patient with Progressive Systemic Sclerosis, Arthritis Rheum. *29*, 142–146 (1986).

[35] *D. A. Fais, E. S. Nadezhdina, Y. S. Chentsov*, The Centriolar Rim, Exp. Cell Res. *164*, 27–34 (1986).

[36] *M. Snyder, R. W. Davis*, SPA1: A Gene Important for Chromosome Segregation and Other Mitotic functions in *S. cerevisiae*, Cell *54*, 743–754 (1988).

[37] *G. Joswig, C. Petzelt*, The Centrosomal Cycle. Its Visualization in PtK Cells by a Monoclonal Antibody to a 32 kD Protein, Cell Motil. Cytoskeleton *15*, 181–192 (1990).

[38] *G. Joswig, C. Petzelt, D. Werner,* Murine cDNAs Coding for the Centrosomal Antigen Centrosomin A, J. Cell Sci. *98,* 37–43 (1991).

[39] *W. G. Whitfield, S. E. Millar, H. Saumweber, M. Frasch, D. M. Glover,* Cloning of a Gene Encoding an Antigen Associated with the Centrosome in Drosophila, J. Cell Sci. *89,* 467–480 (1988).

[40] *M. Frasch, D. M. Glover, H. Saumweber,* Nuclear Antigens Follow Different Pathways into Daughter Nuclei During Mitosis in Early Drosophila Embryos, J. Cell Sci. *82,* 155–172 (1986).

[41] *P. N. Rao, J. Zhao, R. K. Ganju, C. L. Ashorn,* Monoclonal Antibody against the Centrosome, J. Cell Sci *93,* 63–69 (1989).

[42] *B. W. Neighbors, R. C. Williams, J. R. McIntosh,* Localization of Kinesin in Cultured Cells, J. Cell Biol. *106,* 1193–1204 (1988).

[43] *A. T. Baron, J. L. Salisbury,* Identification and Localization of a Novel, Cytoskelethal, Centrosome-associated Protein in PtK$_2$ Cells, J. Cell Biol. *107,* 2669–2678 (1988).

[44] *F. M. Davis, T. Y. Tsao, S. K. Fowler, P. N. Rao,* Monoclonal Antibodies to Mitotic Cells, Proc. Natl. Acad. Sci. U.S.A. *80,* 2926–2930 (1983).

[45] *F. M. Davis, P. N. Rao,* Antibodies to Mitosis-specific Phosphoproteins. In Molecular Regulation of Nuclear Events in Mitosis and Meiosis, in: *R. A. Schlegel, M. S. Halleck, P. N. Rao* (eds.), Academic Press, New York 1987, pp. 259–293.

[46] *D. D. Vandre, G. G. Borisy,* Anaphase Onset and Dephosphorylation of Mitotic Phosphoproteins Occur Concomitantly, J. Cell Sci. *94,* 245–258 (1989).

[47] *J. B. Rattner, J. Lew, J. H. Wang,* p34[cdc2] Kinase is Present at Several Distinct Domains within the Mitotic Apparatus, Cell Motil. Cytoskeleton *17,* 227–236 (1990).

[48] *D. Cleveland,* The Multitubulin Hypothesis Revisited, What Have we Learned? J. Cell Biol. *104,* 381–383 (1987).

[49] *M. A. Lopata, D. W. Cleveland, In vivo* Microtubules Are Copolymers of Available β-tubulin Isotypes: Localyzation of Each of Six Vertebrate β-Tubulin Isotypes Using Polyclonal Antibodies Elicited by Synthetic Peptide Antigens, J. Cell Biol. *105,* 1707–1720 (1987).

[50] *W. Gu, S. A. Lewis, N. J. Cowan,* Generation of Antisera That Discriminate Among Mammalian α-Tubulin: Introduction of Specialized Isotypes into Cultured Cells Results in Their Coassembly without Disruption of Normal Microtubule Function, J. Cell Biol. *106,* 2011–2022 (1988).

[51] *D. R. Webster, G. G. Gundersen, C. Bulinski, G. G. Borisy,* Differential Turnover of Tyrosinated and Detyrosinated Microtubules, Proc. Natl. Acad. Sci. U.S.A. *84,* 9040–9044 (1987).

[52] *M. LeDizet, G. Pipermo,* Identification of an Acetylation Site of Chlamydomonas α-Tubulin, Proc. Natl. Acad. Sci. U.S.A. *84,* 5720–5724 (1987).

[53] *J. C. Bulinski, J. E. Richards, G. Pipene,* Posttranslational Modifications of α-Tubulin: Detyrosination and Acetylation Different Populations of Interphase Microtubules in Cultures Cells, J. Cell Biol. *106,* 1213–1220 (1988).

[54] *L. Serrano, J. Diaz-Nido, F. Wandosell, J. Avila,* Tubulin Phosphorylation by Casein II is Similar to that Found *in vivo,* J. Cell Biol. *105,* 1731–1740 (1987).

[55] *R. L. W. Margolis, L. Wilson,* Microtubule Theadmillspossible Molecular Machinery, Nature *293,* 705–711 (1981).

[56] *T. Mitchison, M. Kirschner,* Dynamic Instability of Microtubule Growth, Nature *312,* 237–242 (1984).

[57] *D. L. Gard, M. Kirschner,* A Microtubule-associated Protein from Xenopus Eggs that Specifically Promotes Assembly at the Plus-ends, J. Cell Biol. *105,* 2203–2216 (1987).

[58] *D. Job, C. T. Raugh, R. L. Margolis,* High Concentrations of STOP Protein Induce a Microtubule Super-stable State, Biochem. Biophys. Res. Commun. *148,* 429–434 (1987).

[59] *P. Huitorel, M. Kirschner,* The Polarity and Stability of Microtubule Capture by the Kinetochore, J. Cell Biol. *106,* 151–159 (1988).

[60] *G. J. Gorbsky, P. J. Sammak, G. G. Borisy,* Chromosomes Move Polewards in Anaphase along Stationary Microtubules that Coordinately Dissassemble from Their Kinetochore Ends, J. Cell Biol. *104,* 9–18 (1987).

[61] *J. E. Koshland, T. Mitchison, M. Kirschner,* Polewards Chromosome Movement Driven by Microtubule Depolymerization *in vitro,* Nature *331,* 499–504 (1988).

[62] *D. R. Kellogg, C. M. Field, B. M. Alberts,* Identification of Microtubule-associated Proteins in the Centrosome, Spindle, and Kinetochore of the Early *Drosophila* Embryo, J. Cell Biol. *109,* 2977–2991 (1989).

[63] *Y. Kanai, R. Takemura, T. Oshima, H. Mori, Y. Ihara, M. Yanagisawa, T. Masaki, N. Hirokawa,* Expression of Multiple Tau Isoforms and Microtubule Bundle Formation in Fibroblasts Transfected with a Single Tau cDNA, J. Cell Biol. *109,* 1173–1184 (1989).

[64] *Y. Masui, C. L. Markert,* Cytoplasmic Control of Nuclear Behaviour during Meiotic Maturation of Frog Oocytes, J. Exp. Zool. *177,* 129–146 (1971).

[65] *T. Kishimoto, R. Kuriyama, H. Kondo, H. Kanatani,* Generality of the Action of Various Maturation Promoting Factors, Exp. Cell Res. *137,* 121–126 (1982).

[66] *J. Newport,* Nuclear Reconstruction *in vitro:* Stages of Assembly around Protein-free DNA, Cell *48,* 205–217 (1987).

[67] *J. J. Blow, R. A. Laskey,* Initiation of DNA Replication in Nuclei and Purified DNA by a Cell-free Extract of *Xenopus* Eggs, Cell *47,* 577–587 (1986).

[68] *R. Miake-lye, M. W. Kirschner,* Induction of early Mitotic Events in a Cell-free System, Cell *41,* 165–175 (1985).

[69] *L. H. Hartwell, Saccharomyces cerevisiae* Cell Cycle, Bacteriol. Rev. *38,* 164–198 (1974).

[70] *V. Simanis, P. Nurse,* The Cell Cycle Control Gene cdc2+ of Yeast Encode a Protein Kinase Potentially Regulated by Phosphorylation, Cell *45,* 261–268 (1986).

[71] *S. I. Reed, J. A. Hadwiger, A. Lorincz,* Protein Kinase Activity Associated with the Product of the Yeast Cell Cycle Gene CDC28, Proc. Natl. Acad. Sci. U.S.A. *82,* 4055–4059 (1985).

[72] *J. Gautier, C. Norbury, M. Lohka, P. Nurse, J. Maller,* Purified Maturation-Promoting Factor Contains the Product of a *Xenopus* Homolog of the Fission Yeast Cell Cycle Control Gene cdc2+, Cell *54,* 433–439 (1988).

[73] *G. Draetta, D. Beach,* Activation of cdc2 Protein Kinase during Mitosis in Human Cells; Cell Cycle-dependent Phosphorylation and Subunit rearrangement, Cell *54,* 17–26 (1988).

[74] *L. Moreno, P. Nurse,* Substrates for p34^{cdc2}, *in vivo* Veritas? Cell *61,* 549–551 (1990).

[75] *G. E. Ward, M. W. Kirschner,* Identification of Cell-Cycle Regulated Phosphorylation Sites on Nuclear Lamin C, Cell *61,* 561–577 (1990).

[76] *R. Heald, F. McKeon,* Mutations of Phosphorylation Sites in Lamin A that Prevent Nuclear Lamina Disassembly in Mitosis, Cell *61,* 579–589 (1990).

[77] *T. Evans, E. T. Rosenthal, J. Youngbloom, D. Distel, T. Hunt,* Cyclins: A Protein Specified by Maternal mRNA in Sea Urchin Eggs that is Destroyed at Each Cleavage Division, Cell *33,* 389–396 (1983).

[78] *G. Draetta, F. Luca, J. Westendorf, L. Brizuela, J. Rudeiman, D. Beach,* cdc2 Protein Kinase Is Complexed with Both Cyclins A and B. Evidence for Proteolytic Inactivation of MPF, Cell *56,* 829–838 (1989).

[79] *A. W. Murray, M. J. Solomon, M. W. Kirschner,* The Role of Cyclin Synthesis and Degradation in the Control of Maturation Promoting Factor Activity, Nature *339,* 280–286 (1989).

[80] *M. A. Felix, J. C. Labbé, M. Dorée, T. Hunt, E. Karsenti,* Triggering of Cyclin Degradation in Interphase Extracts of Amphibian Eggs by cdc2 Kinase, Nature *346,* 379–382 (1990).

6.3.4   Mitochondria

Timothy M. Lever, Sanya J. Sanderson, Anne E. Taylor
and J. Gordon Lindsay

In recent years there have been considerable advances in our understanding of the mechanisms of mitochondrial biogenesis and the nature of the interactions of this organelle with other cellular compartments. As in all areas of scientific endeavour, significant progress has only been made feasible by a number of crucial technological breakthroughs which have provided the impetus for a period of intense research activity on biologically important problems of current interest.

Historically, of course, the isolation of intact, functional mitochondria in the late 1940s was a major stimulus of this type, leading to a period of rapid advancement which contributed greatly to our knowledge of the electron transport chain and the mechanism of ATP production over the next two decades [1, 2]. More recently, a new phase of significant developments in mitochondrial research has been engendered a) by the introduction of routine and reliable techniques of DNA sequence analysis which has resulted in elucidation of the entire mitochondrial genome from several mammalian species [3–5]; b) by gradual improvements in the methodologies and range of detergents available for studying membrane proteins and monitoring their functional reconstitution into artificial membranes [6, 7] and c) in the development of interest in new fields of mitochondrial research, particularly in the area of intracellular protein traffic, with the realization that the vast majority of mitochondrial polypeptides are nuclear-encoded and must be delivered efficiently to the organelle from their site of synthesis in the cytoplasm [8–10].

A key contributory factor to successful progress across this broad front in mitochondrial research has been the increased availability of monoclonal and high-titre monospecific antisera coupled to the appearance of a variety of specific and sensitive immunological techniques for the identification, molecular characterization and intra-organellar localization of individual mitochondrial proteins. This section provides information on the major immunologically-based methods which are in most frequent usage for the analysis of individual mitochondrial proteins, discusses their possible applications including the advantages and limitations of each and provides a source of references.

6.3.4.1   Production of Polyclonal Antiserum and Assessment of Quality

Many standard protocols are reported in the literature and immunological textbooks for the production of polyclonal antibodies (cf. [11, 12] for examples) and the procedures employed in the authors' laboratory have also been published previously [13, 14]. For further details on this important topic, consult Volume 2, 4. However, the key to success, as in all immunological studies, is to obtain high-titre monospecific antiserum, a process which is highly dependent on the purity of the original antigen.

An additional consideration is whether to employ the antigen in its native or denatured state [15]. In practice, with polyclonal sera, a high degree of cross-reaction is normally observed with both native and denatured forms of the protein regardless of the state of the primary antigen although negative results should be treated with caution. For example, in the detection of cytoplasmically-synthesized mitochondrial precursors by immunoprecipitation, it is generally presumed that antibodies to the mature, native protein will recognize the cytoplasmic precursor which is now known to be maintained in an open, "loosely-folded" conformation prior to import. In the case of the dihydrolipoamide succinyltransferase (EC 2.3.1.61), E2, component of the mammalian 2-oxoglutarate dehydrogenase (EC 1.2.4.2) complex (OGDC), however, only antibodies to the denatured enzyme were able to recognize the precursor, indicating major conformational differences in this species with respect to the mature form [16]. Similar effects have been noted when antibodies to holo- or apo-cytochrome c were employed [17]. Where the pure antigen is not readily available, antibodies can be produced to a specific band resolved on, or eluted from, an SDS/polyacrylamide gel [18, 19] or to chemically-synthesized peptides corresponding to a particular region of the protein of interest [20–22].

An alternative approach, yielding small amounts of affinity-purified, subunit-specific IgG, is to recover the fraction of the antibody population directed against an individual subunit from the final immunoblot [23] employing IgG produced against a partially-purified extract or multimeric complex.

6.3.4.2   Immune Electron Microscopy

Colloidal gold is a negatively charged hydrophobic sol, formed by electron-dense metallic particles which under appropriate conditions of pH and concentration bind to macromolecules by non-covalent electrostatic adsorption. This interaction is stable and apparently does not affect the biological activity of the modified macromolecules [24].

In immune electron microscopy, immune-complex formation is detected by employing a second antibody, e. g., goat anti-rabbit IgG or protein A conjugated to colloidal gold particles, which can be purchased in a range of sizes from 5–40 nm for multiple marking of intracellular antigens (cf. 5.7). This specific labelling technique in combination with transmission or scanning EM is proving an increasingly popular strategy for defining the intra-organellar sub-location of important mitochondrial antigens (for methodological details cf. [24]). For example, it has been demonstrated that the mitochondrial pyruvate dehydrogenase (EC 1.2.4.1) multienzyme complex (PDC), normally considered to be a soluble entity, is closely associated with the matrix surface of the mitochondrial inner membrane [25]. Recently, this technique has been employed extensively to examine the distribution of mitochondrial import receptors on the outer surface of the organelle to determine whether these proteins are enriched at contact sites, regions of close proximity between the inner and outer membranes which are believed to contain the translocation apparatus for promoting the import of nuclear-encoded mitochondrial proteins [26, 27]. In addition, it has proved feasible to visualize contact sites directly *via* trapping precursors as membrane-spanning translocation intermediates at low temperature prior to antibody treatment and immunogold labelling, which permits assessment of the number of sites per mitochondrion [28].

Many import receptors were first detected by the simple expedient of producing polyclonal IgG to individual outer membrane proteins resolved on SDS-polyacrylamide gels, and testing for specific inhibitory effects of these immunoglobulins or derived Fab fragments on the *in-vitro* uptake of a range of mitochondrial precursors destined for various locations within the organelle. An alternative strategy involves the production of anti-idiotype antibodies to a mitochondrial targeting sequence with the rationale that a subpopulation of these antibodies will mimic the targeting sequence, thereby producing a specific high affinity interaction with the receptor. A putative receptor was isolated by this approach which has been found to be identical to the mitochondrial phosphate transporter, raising serious concerns as to the validity of this method for identifying functional receptors [29, 30]. Interestingly, immunogold analysis indicates that this protein is also enriched at contact sites between inner and outer membranes, so the possibility remains that it may have a dual function.

An elegant use of subunit-specific mAbs in combination with immunogold studies has resolved the controversy over the subunit stoichiometry of the mitochondrial F1-ATPase (EC 3.6.1.34). Since monoclonals recognise only a single determinant per polypeptide chain, it was possible to establish that the 5 major subunits (α, β, γ, δ, ε) were present in the ratio 3:3:3:1:1 and not 2:2:2:2:2.

6.3.4.3   Immunological Detection and Characterization of Mitochondrial Antigens: the Versatility of Immunoblotting (Western Blotting)

Immunoblotting, otherwise known as Western blotting or immune replica analysis, has become the preferred method for routine detection and analysis of cellular antigens. This reflects the sensitivity and specificity of this approach, its ease and convenience of operation, relative inexpensiveness and great versatility. Several examples illustrating the numerous applications of the basic immunoblotting technique in mitochondrial research are outlined in the following. For information on detailed protocols and the advantages and limitations of the various approaches to detecting the formation of immune complexes cf. Vol. 1, 4.3.4 and [31–33].

Immune monitoring during the purification of mitochondrial antigens

It is now recognized that difficulties in the isolation of mitochondrial enzymes or transporters in high yield often relates to the proteolytically-sensitive nature of the polypeptides in question, rather than to their general susceptibility to denaturation during purification. Immunological monitoring of the proteins at each stage in the process permits the detection of the appearance of degradation products and is particularly applicable to studies of multimeric complexes where specific problems of this type may be confined to an individual subunit. After defining the nature of the problems, it is often possible to develop more focused strategies for their solution; e. g., the inclusion of appropriate protease inhibitors or cofactors to maintain the integrity of

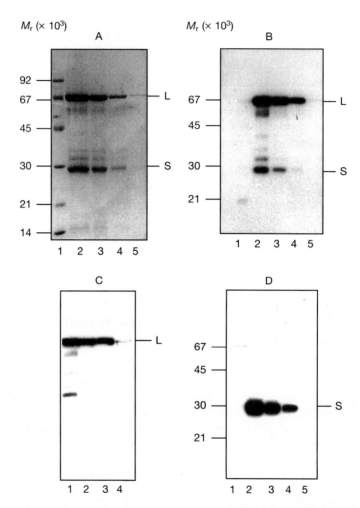

Fig. 1. Immunoblotting analysis of the large and small subunits of succinate dehydrogenase from bovine heart. Panel A. Coomassie blue-stained 10% (w/v) SDS-polyacrylamide gel of purified SDH; Lanes 2–5, 20, 10, 5 and 2 µg, respectively; Lane 1 M_r standards. Panels B, C and D, replicate immunoblots of (A) probed with antibodies to the intact enzyme (B), and the gel-purified large (C) and small (D) subunits. Immune complexes were detected with ^{125}I-labelled protein A.

the protein subunit in question. In the experience of the authors, such procedures have been most useful in devising improved purification protocols for the isolation of the pyruvate dehydrogenase (PDC) and 2-oxoglutarate dehydrogenase (OGDC) multienzyme complexes, especially as these assemblies are difficult to assay routinely during the early stages in the purification owing to the presence of interfering enzyme activities. In the case of PDC, it was observed that there was a tendency for the E1 enzyme (pyruvate dehydrogenase, an $\alpha_2\beta_2$ tetramer) to dissociate into its individual subunits, and that E1 could also be protected from the action of proteases by its cofactors Mg^{2+} and thiamine pyrophosphate which act presumably by stabilizing the enzyme in its native compact tertiary or quaternary state [34]. For OGDC, the sensitivity of the dihydrosuccinyl acyltransferase (E2) core enzyme to proteolysis led to major losses in activity which were not readily overcome by the inclusion of standard protease inhibitors such as PMSF, benzamidine and leupeptin. In pilot immunological analyses on crude extracts, the presence of 0.5% (v/v) rat serum, known to contain a number of protease inhibitors [35], at an early stage in the purification was the most effective in preserving the integrity on the E2 polypeptide. A further example is shown in Fig. 1 where minor contaminants in purified bovine heart succinate dehydrogenase are identified as degradation products of the large 70000 M_r subunit by employing antibody raised to the gel-purified polypeptide.

Immune identification of functionally-equivalent mitochondrial antigens in various species

An extension of the approach outlined above is extremely useful in detecting the presence of the equivalent proteins across a variety of species. The success of this procedure relies on the ability to detect a significant and specific cross-reaction between antibodies raised against a mitochondrial antigen from one species and its counterparts in mitochondrial or cellular extracts from other species. Normally, cross-reactivity is observed only when there are considerable similarities between the two proteins in question with a requirement for a minimum of 50–60% sequence identity at the amino acid level [36, 37]. Fortunately, a high level of homology is normally observed across most equivalent polypeptides from mammalian sources and also extends to other eukaryotes, such as yeast or plants, in some instances.

Specific examples of this approach:

1. Anti-IgG raised against the 34000 M_r polypeptide of the rat liver mitochondrial phosphate transporter was employed in the detection of the carrier in *S. cerevisiae* mitochondria where it exhibits an increased mobility with apparent M_r value of 30000. Subsequently, it was found that the yeast PTP proved amenable to purification by the same regime as employed for the mammalian transporter [38]. As a corollary to these studies a related carrier was identified in human microsomal membranes which forms part of the system for transporting glucose-6-phosphate into the lumen of the endoplasmic reticulum for hydrolysis by the luminal enzyme, glucose-6-phosphatase (EC 3.1.3.9) prior to re-exporting the products, glucose and P_i, *via* specific carriers to the cytoplasm [39].

2. A valuable aspect of immunological screening is the ability to define the intracellular distribution and molecular composition of proteins and multimeric complexes in plant tissues by employing antibodies to the mammalian proteins. Basic biochemical analysis by conventional techniques involving protein purification is often extremely difficult in view of the low abundance of most of the major metabolic enzymes in plants, and the lack of availability of large amounts of tissue in most cases. However, it has been possible to confirm the existence of two separate forms of PDC in plant mitochondria and chloroplasts, to define the subunit composition of their constituent enzymes for the first time and to detect striking differences in the subunit M_r values of some of the individual polypeptides in the two organelles [40].

Immune mapping

A third adaptation of these immunological techniques, termed "immune mapping" can be applied to the characterization of related proteins. This is based on the widely-employed *Cleveland* one-dimensional "mapping" technique in which unique, reproducible patterns of peptide fragments (fingerprints) for specific proteins can be compared by Coomassie-blue staining of SDS-polyacrylamide gels [41]. A major advantage of this procedure is that it can be applied to protein bands, excised as a gel slice from a previous, usually lower-percentage gel, which is then subjected to proteolysis in low-concentration SDS in the well of a second gel prior to electrophoretic resolution of the fragments. More recently, the sensitivity of the method has been greatly enhanced by the use of silver stain [42] or radiolabelled proteins [43].

In immune "mapping" the immunologically-reactive peptides generated from a single protein by various protease treatments can be visualized specifically with high sensitivity without the necessity for purifying the proteins under study. Thus this procedure can be applied to comparison of the proteolytic "fingerprints" of equivalent proteins in crude mitochondrial or chloroplast extracts from different sources. For example, this technique was employed initially to demonstrate that the recently-discovered protein X subunit of mammalian PDC was a distinct polypeptide and not a minor degradation product of the dihydrolipoamide dehydrogenase (E2) component as assumed previously [15]. In a recent study on the related OGDC, it was discovered that domains related to the protein X subunit of PDC form an integral part of the E1 enzyme in a clear case of domain "shuffling", initially suggested by the unexpected observation that anti-X IgG cross-reacted weakly with the E1 enzyme.

Immunoblotting and cross-linking

Cross-linking with homo- or hetero-bifunctional chemical or photo-activatable reagents has been a traditional technique for examining the subunit organization (nearest neighbour associations of constituent proteins) of multimeric complexes; or to identify transient associations between proteins, e.g., mitochondrial translocation intermediates in contact with components of the import apparatus. A major limitation of this approach is that cross-linked aggregates are often formed in low yield, resulting in problems of detection. Moreover, their exact compositions can only be deduced indirectly from analysis of their M_r values relative to those of the unmodified subunits, although these problems were alleviated to some extent by the introduction of cleavable cross-linking reagents. The availability of high-titre, monospecific antibodies against individual subunits has added a new dimension to this area of study and greatly increased both the sensitivity of the detection of cross-linked species and the accuracy of analysis of their compositions.

Elegant studies employing membrane-impermeant cross-linkers and subunit-specific antisera have been employed by *Ragan* and co-workers to probe the topography and subunit contacts in the bovine heart NADH dehydrogenase complex (Complex I), a multimeric, integral membrane assembly comprising approximately 26 distinct subunits [44, 45]. Studies of this type have led to the development of a general model for the organization of Complex I within the inner membrane.

In the case of PDC, interactions between the E2 and X subunits and the number of lipoyl domains per polypeptide chain have been deduced from cross-linking studies with phenylene-2-bis-maleimide in conjunction with immunoblotting utilizing the substrate-generated dihydrolipoamide thiols on these polypeptides [46].

Immunological detection of genetic defects

Standard immune replica analysis of mitochondrial extracts prepared from biopsy samples or cultured fibroblasts derived from patients with putative defects in specific mitochondrial enzymes can provide important additional insights into the precise nature of the lesion. Such analyses are particularly advantageous in the absence of a convenient enzymatic assay in crude extracts, or in multimeric complexes where one is attempting to ascribe the loss of activity to an abnormality in a particular subunit. Such an approach is clearly incapable of detecting point mutations which result in production of a non-functional polypeptide that is still immunologically-reactive; however, regulatory or structural mutations or deletions which alter the level of expression of the protein, its subsequent turnover or apparent M_r value are clearly observed by this technique. In the case of the mitochondrial branched-chain 2-oxoacid dehydrogenase complex which catalyses the committed step in the metabolism of isoleucine, leucine and valine, it has been shown that the E2 subunit is totally absent in one patient exhibiting the symptoms of maple syrup urine disease [47]. Several patients have been described in whom there are abnormally low levels of the E1 component of the PDC [48, 49]. Interestingly, in all cases, levels of both α- and β-subunits are affected similarly, indicating that decreased production of one subunit may lead to enhanced instability of its companion component. Analyses of this type have proved important diagnostic tools in determining the nature of the molecular defect more precisely in a number of inherited diseases associated with defects in mitochondrial function [50].

Detection of mitochondrial precursors in mutants of *S. cerevisiae*

Nuclear-encoded mitochondrial precursors are normally transported rapidly into the organelle and processed to their mature forms from their site of synthesis in the cytoplasm, hence presenting problems in detection. In mitochondrially-defective (*rho*⁻) mutants, however, large amounts of precursors can accumulate in the cytoplasm under appropriate conditions, such that they can be detected directly by immunoblotting [51]. As shown in Fig. 2, heterologous antibodies can often be employed for this purpose. In this example, antibodies to bovine heart PDC cross-react sufficiently strongly with two of the yeast PDC subunits, E2 and E1β, enabling detection of the mature and accumulated precursor states in cellular extracts. As this approach relies on the stability of the unprocessed precursor, it is not always successful. In this instance, there is considerable accumulation of the E2 precursor whereas little or no pre-E1β can be observed.

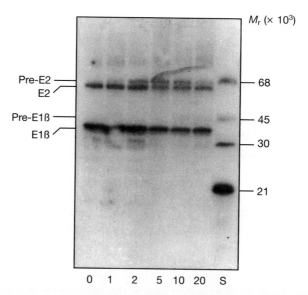

Fig. 2. Accumulation of E2 and E1β precursors of PDC in a mutant of *S. cerevisiae*. A mitochondrially-defective yeast strain was grown in the presence of increasing levels of the uncoupler, carbonyl cyanide 3-chlorophenylhydrazone as indicated in [52]. Cellular extracts were prepared and 100 μg amounts probed with anti-(bovine heart) PDC, prior to detection with ¹²⁵I-labelled protein A.

6.3.4.4   Peptide Antibodies

Detection of mitochondrial gene products

With the sequencing of mitochondrial DNA from several sources, it became clear that 60% of the mammalian mitochondrial genome coded for 8 polypeptides of unknown function, i.e., unidentified reading frames (URFs), although the equivalent sequences were not found in yeast mitochondrial DNA. One of the URFs was eventually identified as the mammalian equivalent of subunit 8 of the yeast ATP synthase complex.

Anti-peptide antibodies raised against predicted amino acid sequences of the remaining URFs were instrumental in establishing their identities as components of the NADH dehydrogenase, an integral inner membrane complex composed of 26 or more distinct polypeptides. Initially, these proteins were found to be expressed as ^{35}S-labelled products on *in-vitro* translation of human mitochondrial DNA. Thereafter, as these radiolabelled species could now be detected on SDS-polyacrylamide gels, immunoprecipitation analysis of the various respiratory chain complexes employing specific antiserum to the NADH dehydrogenase complex (Complex I) confirmed that 6 of the URF products were subunits of this complex [52]. Subsequent studies of this type revealed that the remaining unidentified species was also associated with Complex I [53]. It is likely that this type of analysis will have a general application in facilitating studies on the intracellular compartmentation and possible function of unidentified mitochondrial or chloroplast-encoded gene products in lower eukaryotes or plants which tend to have more complex organelle-based genomes.

Topographical organization of mitochondrial membrane proteins

With improvements in procedures for the routine handling, assay and structural analysis of membrane proteins by biophysical techniques, there has been increased interest in developing refined procedures for mapping the transmembrane organization of mitochondrial transporters and the multi-subunit proton-pumping respiratory chain complexes involved in oxidative phosphorylation. Since the genes for many mitochondrial integral membrane polypeptides have now been cloned and sequenced, a prediction of their possible (two-dimensional) transmembrane organization can be made from hydropathy plots. In eukaryotes, however, it has not yet been feasible to obtain independent biochemical evidence to describe the precise transmembrane/intramembrane arrangement of any integral membrane protein. Most studies have utilized non-permeant chemical reagents, usually radioactive, which react with specific amino acids located on accessible regions of polypeptide chain exposed beyond the confines of the lipid bilayer, on either the cytoplasmic surface or matrix surface of the mitochondrial inner membrane. Identification of the modified residue(s) necessitates purification of the protein, isolation of the radiolabelled peptide(s) and subsequent sequence analysis to identify the appropriate region.

The use of antibodies as specific non-permeant probes can provide important information on the general membrane organization of individual proteins. By the use of populations of mitochondrial inner membrane vesicles which can be sealed in opposite orientations, i.e., right-side out or inside out, it is possible to determine whether the antibody either has an inhibitory effect on a particular mitochondrial function or reacts with the exposed surface in one population of vesicles only. A refinement of this approach is to generate peptide antibodies directed against short stretches of amino acid sequence to test the accessibility of specific regions of the polypeptide. For subunit 8 of the mitochondrial ATP synthase, antibodies to a peptide corresponding to its N-terminal sequence were employed to determine its exposure on the cytoplasmic surface [54]. This approach has general application to the investigation of the topographical arrangement of integral membrane proteins, often to monitor the accessibility of their N- and C-termini on particular faces of the membrane and the exposure of hydrophilic domains as suggested from hydropathy profiles. Two important carriers of the inner membrane, the adenine nucleotide translocase and the phosphate transporter, which are jointly responsible for supplying ADP and P_i for ATP synthesis within the organelle, have been examined in this fashion. In a recent study, for example, the exposure of the C-terminus of the mitochondrial phosphate transporter on the cytoplasmic side of the inner membrane has been demonstrated by competitive radioimmunoassay using antibodies directed against a synthetic peptide corresponding to the eleven C-terminal residues. Moreover, the modification of the reactive cysteine situated near the N-terminus with N-ethylmaleimide reduces the accessibility of the C-terminus to removal by trypsin, suggesting that this modification has induced a conformational change in the entire protein [19]. For the adenine nucleotide translocase, conformational differences in the presence of two specific inhibitors, carboxyatractyloside and bongkrekic acid, are also revealed by alterations in the exposure of the N-terminus on the cytoplasmic surface of the membrane as judged by reactivity with peptide-specific antibodies [18].

Intramembrane organization of mitochondrial membrane proteins

A combination of surface-specific proteolysis using a variety of specific and nonspecific proteinases in combination with immunoblotting with anti-peptide or anti-intact polypeptide IgG has also provided important additional information on the general topography of membrane-associated proteins. For example, in the case of succinate dehydrogenase which has a large FAD-containing subunit, $M_r = 70000$, and a small Fe-S subunit, $M_r = 30000$, it can be shown that this enzyme is only susceptible to proteolytic attack from the matrix side of the inner membrane. Moreover, trypsin treatment generates an immunologically-reactive 27000 M_r soluble fragment of the small subunit, indicating that the vast bulk of this subunit is not intimately associated with the lipid bilayer. This is consistent with the hydropathy profile of this polypeptide, which also predicts that it may be bound to the membrane by a small hydrophobic stretch at its N-terminus. In the case of the large subunit, incubation with a number of proteases of varying specificities yields a protease-resistant, immunoreactive fragment of

32000–34000 M_r which is protected by the presence of an intact bilayer. Some specific proteases generate an additional, stable 27000 M_r membrane-associated peptide which can be degraded to low M_r peptides by suitable proteases. These data would indicate that the large subunit is associated in two separate regions of the molecule with the lipid bilayer, with a large intervening hydrophilic domain and that a substantial proportion of the molecule is located within the confines of the lipid bilayer [55].

6.3.4.5   Immunological Detection of Mitochondrial Proteins Synthesized *in vivo* or *in vitro*

In the past decade, with the realization that the mitochondrial genome has the potential to code for only a limited subset of its own proteins, attention has focused on understanding the complex sequence of molecular events by which the vast majority of mitochondrial proteins (> 95%) which are nuclear-encoded are directed to the mitochondrial surface from their sites of synthesis in the cytoplasm, then translocated across one or more mitochondrial membranes prior to their functional assembly in the correct mitochondrial subcompartment.

Monitoring the intracellular movements of individual mitochondrial precursors has relied heavily on the availability of high-titre, monospecific antibodies to effect the specific detection by immunoprecipitation of (^{35}S) methionine-labelled polypeptides from complex mixtures of radiolabelled proteins synthesized using *in-vivo* or *in-vitro* translation systems primed with poly A$^+$-mRNA. Thereafter, the immunoprecipitates are resolved by SDS-polyacrylamide gel electrophoresis and the cytosolic or mitochondrial forms of specific mitochondrial polypeptides are visualized by fluorography.

Analyses of this type have led to the discovery that cytoplasmic precursor states of mitochondrial proteins generally contain a cleavable pre-sequence located at their *N*-termini, serving as a targeting signal which is removed on entry into the organelle, a process which can also be demonstrated with isolated mitochondria.

General considerations

Protocols for monitoring of nascent mitochondrial proteins *in vivo* differ significantly depending on the organism under study. Much of the original research was conducted in *Saccharomyces cerevisiae* and *Neurospora crassa* and procedures are widely cited in the literature (see [12] for a review), as are protocols for immunoprecipitation of mitochondrial proteins in mammalian cells. Interestingly, mammalian antisera often cross-react with equivalent yeast polypeptides. The procedures described below relate to the accumulation of nuclear-encoded cytoplasmic precursors and analysis of their uptake, processing and mitochondrial assembly in cultured mammalian cells.

To achieve optimal sensitivity in the detection of newly-synthesized proteins, the main aim is to maximize levels of incorporation of radioactive amino acids at high specific activity, since in the case of low-abundance proteins, the immunoprecipitated product may constitute as little as 1:10000 of total cellular protein. Generally (^{35}S) methionine has been the isotope of choice in view of the favourable energy characteristics of sulphur decay for autoradiographic or fluorographic detection. One limitation of this approach concerns the low amounts of methionine present in many proteins, so current practice often involves labelling with a mixture of (^{35}S) methionine and cysteine which is available commercially. Incubation with (^{35}S)-labelled amino acids is also performed in media or buffers containing less than 10% of the normal concentrations of non-radioactive methionine and cysteine.

As mitochondrial polypeptides are normally translocated to the organelle and processed to their mature forms within 2–5 min, *in-vivo* detection of precursors is difficult, particularly in mammalian cells where rates of cell growth are relatively slow. Normally, this problem is circumvented by incubating cultures for 3–4 h in the presence of radioactive amino acids and uncouplers of oxidative phosphorylation e. g. 2,4-dinitrophenol (1–2 mmol/l) or 4-trifluoromethoxyphenylhydrazone (10–20 µmol/l) which dissipate the mitochondrial membrane potential with minimal effects on rates of protein synthesis, leading to the accumulation of precursors in the cytoplasm, provided these are relatively stable. This problem is circumvented in translation studies *in-vitro* where the precursors are formed initally and their import can be followed at a later stage on addition of mitochondria. With the increased availability of cloned genes and coupled *in-vitro* transcription/translation systems, enabling the production of a single (^{35}S) methionine-labelled product, there may be a diminished requirement for specific antibodies in this area in future.

There are several potential problems in achieving high-quality immunoprecipitates with the required degree of specificity: a) the quality of the antiserum or derived IgG fraction is crucial, i. e., it should be of high-titre and monospecific as judged by ELISA and immunoblotting criteria; b) proteolysis of the small amounts of radiolabelled antigen in cellular extracts or reticulocyte lysates is minimized by use of sterile buffers and the inclusion of a range of protease inhibitors during the preparation of cell extracts and the formation of immune complexes, and c) stringent washing conditions are required, usually involving high salt concentration and a combination of 2 or 3 detergents including SDS to ensure the removal of contaminating polypeptides from the final immunoprecipitate.

Principles

Many schemes for the isolation of clean immunoprecipitates are reported (cf. [16, 56, 57] for examples). In mammalian cells, after incorporation of (^{35}S)-methionine, cells are normally lysed in buffers containing 1% (v/v) Triton X-100 to preserve the integrity of nuclei which can be removed rapidly by centrifugation. The presence of lysed nuclei (nuclear DNA) in cellular extracts adversely affects the production of clean immuno-precipitates.

At this stage, SDS in the range of 0.1–0.5% (w/v) is usually added to the cellular extract and occasionally other detergents, e.g., 1% (w/v) sodium deoxycholate or Nonidet P40. These conditions are designed to achieve maximal removal of contaminating proteins bound nonspecifically to the immunoprecipitate while preserving the specific interaction between antibody and antigen. Immune complexes are adsorbed onto commercially-available preparations of formalinized *Staphylococcus aureus* cells, *Cowan I* strain which contain protein A on their surface, or alternatively protein A-agarose beads. Both beads and formalinized cells can be pelleted at low speeds and this permits rapid and extensive washing of the absorbed immune complexes which are finally released by treatment with *Laemmli* sample buffer prior to SDS-polyacrylamide gel electrophoresis.

One advantage in preserving protein-protein interactions during this procedure is that specific, high-affinity associations of the antigen under study with other cellular components can also be monitored. For example, although anti-PDC IgG contains no significant titre to the dihydrolipoamide dehydrogenase (E3) component, this subunit is present in the final immunoprecipitate by virtue of its tight and specific interaction with the intact complex [58]. As expected, this subunit is absent from immune complexes of accumulated precursors as these do not assemble prior to their uptake into the organelle; therefore, appearance of E3 in immune complexes can be used to monitor the *in-vivo* maturation of PDC. In recent studies, similar approaches have identified specific interactions between a trapped membrane-spanning translocation intermediate and 1) a component of the import apparatus, ISP42 [59], 2) two mitochondrial receptors MOM 19 [27] and MOM 72 [26] and 3) a mitochondrial stress protein, hsp 70, providing important new information on the molecular details of the import process [60]. If unknown antigens are obtained in immunoprecipitates, their possible identities can be confirmed by immuno-competition analysis by addition of excess (5–20 µg) of the purified non-radiolabelled protein to the original extract prior to formation of the immune complex. This leads to effective exclusion of the small amounts of radiolabelled antigen from the final immunoprecipitate [58].

Finally, if observations of specific associations with other proteins are not required, these can be disrupted initially by precipitation of polypeptides in the original Triton X-100 extract with 4 volumes of ice-cold acetone and re-solubilization in SDS-based buffer. After re-addition of Triton X-100, isolation of immune complexes can be performed as described previously.

6.3.4.6   Concluding Remarks

All the immunological applications discussed here are variations on one basic theme, in that they rely completely on the ability of antibody to recognize its parent or a related antigen with a high degree of specificity and with high affinity. In immunoglobulins, therefore, nature has provided the scientist with a powerful tool for monitoring the intracellular movements, location, structure, organization and function of specific mitochondrial proteins. It is likely that the capacity of the investigator to exploit the natural advantages of antigen-antibody interactions has not yet been exhausted and that we can look forward to more refined and ingenious applications of this basic phenomenon in the future, particularly in the field of mitochondrial biogenesis.

References

[1] *D. G. Nicholls*, Bioenergetics: An Introduction to the Chemiosmotic Theory, Academic Press, London 1982.

[2] *J. N. Prebble*, Mitochondria, Chloroplasts and Bacterial Membranes, Longman Press, London 1981.

[3] *S. Anderson, A. T. Bankier, B. G. Barrell, M. H. L. de Bruijn, A. R. Coulson, J. Drouin, I. C. Eperon, D. P. Nielich, B. A. Roe, F. Sanger, P. H. Schreier, A. J. H. Smith, R. Staden, I. G. Young*, Sequence and Organisation of the Human Mitochondrial Genome, Nature London *290*, 457–465 (1981).

[4] *M. J. Bibb, R. A. Van Etten, C. T. Wright, M. W. Walberg, D. A. Clayton*, Sequence and Gene Organisation of Mouse Mitochondrial DNA, Cell *26*, 167–180 (1981).

[5] *S. Anderson, M. H. L. de Bruijn, A. R. Coulson, I. C. Eperon, F. Sanger, I. G. Young*, Complete Sequence of Bovine Mitochondrial DNA. Conserved Features of the Mitochondrial Genome, J. Mol. Biol. *156*, 683–717 (1982).

[6] *R. P. Casey*, Membrane Reconstitution of the Energy Conserving Enzymes of Oxidative Phosphorylation, Biochim. Biophys. Acta *768*, 319–347 (1984).

[7] *R. B. Gennis*, Biomembranes: Molecular Structure and Function, Springer-Verlag, New York 1989, pp. 85–103.

[8] *F.-U. Hartl, N. Pfanner, D. W. Nicholson, W. Neupert*, Mitochondrial Protein Import, Biochim. Biophys. Acta *988*, 1–45 (1989).

[9] *F.-U. Hartl, W. Neupert*, Protein Sorting to Mitochondria: Evolutionary Conservations of Folding and Assembly, Science *247*, 930–938 (1990).

[10] *K. P. Baker, G. Schatz*, Mitochondrial Proteins Essential for Viability Mediate Protein Import into Yeast Mitochondria, Nature London *349*, 205–208 (1991).

[11] *A. Johnston, R. Thorpe*, Immunochemistry in Practice, 2nd ed., Blackwell Scientific Publications, Oxford 1987, pp. 30–34.

[12] *S. Werner, W. Sebald*, Immunological Techniques for the Study of the Biogenesis of Mitochondrial Membrane Proteins, Methods Biochem. Anal. *27*, 109–170 (1981).

[13] *O. G. L. De Marcucci, A. Hunter, J. G. Lindsay*, Low Immunogenicity of the Common Lipoamide Dehydrogenase Subunit (E3) of Mammalian Pyruvate Dehydrogenase and 2-Oxoglutarate Dehydrogenase Multienzyme Complexes, Biochem. J. *226*, 509–517 (1985).

[14] *O. G. L. De Marcucci, J. G. Lindsay*, Component X: An Immunologically Distinct Polypeptide Associated with Mammalian Pyruvate Dehydrogenase Multienzyme Complex, Eur. J. Biochem. *149*, 641–648 (1985).

[15] *E. Westhof, D. Altschuch, D. Moras, A. C. Bloomer, A. Mondragon, A. Klug, M. H. V. Van Regenmortel*, Correlation between Segmental Mobility and the Location of Antigenic Determinants in Proteins, Nature London *311*, 123–126 (1984).

[16] *A. Hunter, J. G. Lindsay*, Immunological and Biosynthetic Studies on the Mammalian 2-Oxoglutarate Dehydrogenase Multienzyme Complex, Eur. J. Biochem. *155*, 103–109 (1986).

[17] *B. Hennig, W. Neupert*, Assembly of Cytochrome c: Apocytochrome c is Bound to Specific Sites on Mitochondria before Its Conversion to Holocytochrome c, Eur. J. Biochem. *121*, 203–212 (1981).

[18] *G. Brandolin, F. Boulay, P. Dalbon, P.V. Vignais*, Orientation of the *N*-Terminal Region of the Membrane Bound ADP/ATP Carrier Protein Explored by Anti-Peptide Antibodies and an Arginine Specific Endoprotease. Evidence that the Accessibility of the *N*-Terminal Residue Depends on the Conformational State of the Carrier, Biochemistry *28*, 1093–1100 (1990).

[19] *G. C. Ferraira, R. D. Pratt, P. L. Pedersen*, Mitochondrial Proton/Phosphate Transporter. An Antibody Directed against the COOH Terminus and Proteolytic Cleavage Experiments Provide New Insights about Its Membrane Topology, J. Biol. Chem. *265*, 21202–21206 (1989).

[20] *L. Capobianco, G. Brandolin, F. Palmieri*, Transmembrane Topography of the Mitochondrial Phosphate Carrier Explored by Peptide Specific Antibodies, Biochemistry *30*, 4963–4969 (1991).

[21] *O. G. L. De Marcucci, J. A. Hodgson, J. G. Lindsay,* The M_r 50000 Polypeptide of Mammalian Pyruvate Dehydrogenase Complex Participates in the Acetylation Reactions, Eur. J. Biochem. *158*, 587–594 (1986).

[22] *B. S. Parekh, H. B. Metah, M. D. West, R. C. Montelaro,* Preparative Elution of Proteins from Nitrocellulose Membranes after Separation by SDS-PAGE, Anal. Biochem. *148*, 87–92 (1985).

[23] *R. Bisson, G. Schiavo,* Two Different Forms of Cytochrome c Oxidase Can Be Purified from Slime Mould *Dictostelium discoideum,* J. Biol. Chem. *261*, 4373–4376 (1986).

[24] *M. Bendayan,* The Enzyme-Gold Technique: a New Cytochemical Approach to the Ultrastructural Localization of Macromolecules, in: Techniques in Immunocytochemistry, Volume 3, *G. R. Bullock and P. Petrusy* (eds.), Academic Press, London 1985, pp. 179–201.

[25] *B. Sumegi, Z. Liposits, L. Inman, W. T. Paul, P. A. Srere,* Electron Microscopic Study on the Size of Pyruvate Dehydrogenase Complex *In Situ,* Eur. J. Biochem. *169*, 223–230 (1987).

[26] *T. Sollner, G. Griffiths, R. Pfaller, N. Pfanner, W. Neupert,* MOM19, An Import Receptor for Mitochondrial Precursor Proteins, Cell *59*, 1061–1070 (1989).

[27] *T. Sollner, R. Pfaller, G. Griffiths, N. Pfanner, W. Neupert,* A Mitochondrial Import Receptor for the ADP/ATP Carrier, Cell *62*, 107–115 (1990).

[28] *M. Kiebler, R. Pfaller, T. Sollner, G. Griffiths, T. Horstmann, W. Pfanner, W. Neupert,* Identification of a Mitochondrial Import Receptor Complex Required for Recognition and Membrane Insertion of Precursor Proteins, Nature London *348*, 610–616 (1990).

[29] *D. Pain, H. Murakami, G. Blobel,* Identification of a Receptor for Protein Import into Mitochondria, Nature London *347*, 444–449 (1990).

[30] *H. Murakami, G. Blobel, D. Pain,* Isolation and Characterisation of the Gene for a Yeast Mitochondrial Import Receptor, Nature London *347*, 488–491 (1990).

[31] *J. M. Gershoni,* Protein Blotting: A Manual, Methods Biochem. Anal. *33*, 1–58 (1988).

[32] *J. J. Langone,* ^{125}I-Labelled Protein A: Reactivity with IgG and Use as a Tracer in Radioimmunoassay, Methods Enzymol. *70*, 356–375 (1980).

[33] *R. E. Mandrell, W. D. Zollinger,* Use of a Zwitterionic Detergent for the Restoration of the Antibody-Binding Capacity of Electroblotted Meningococcal Outer Membrane Proteins, J. Immunol. Methods *67*, 1–11 (1984).

[34] *J. C. Neagle, J. G. Lindsay,* Selective Proteolysis of the Protein X Subunit of the Bovine Heart Pyruvate Dehydrogenase Complex, Biochem. J. *278*, 423–427 (1991).

[35] *O. H. Weiland,* On the Mechanism of Irreversible Pyruvate Dehydrogenase Inactivation in Liver Mitochondrial Extracts, FEBS Lett. *52*, 44–47 (1975).

[36] *E. M. Prager, A. C. Wilson,* The Dependence of Immunological Cross-Reactivity upon Sequence Resemblence among Lysozymes I: Microcomplement Fixation Studies, J. Biol. Chem. *246*, 5978–5989 (1971).

[37] *E. M. Prager, E. C. Wilson,* The Dependence of Immunological Cross-Reactivity upon Sequence Resemblence among Lysozymes II: Comparison of Precipitation and Microcomplement Fixation Results, J. Biol. Chem. *246*, 7010–7017 (1971).

[38] *J. A. Hodgson, A. G. James, N. Batayneh, J. G. Lindsay,* Biosynthesis of Precursor Forms of the Pyruvate Dehydrogenase Complex and the Phosphate Transporter in *Saccharomyces cerevisiae,* Biochem. Soc. Trans. *16*, 776–777 (1988).

[39] *I. D. Waddell, J. G. Lindsay, A. Burchell,* The Identification of T2; the Phosphate/Pyrophosphate Transport Protein of the Hepatic Microsomal Glucose-6-Phosphatase System, FEBS Lett. *229*, 179–182 (1988).

[40] *A. Taylor, R. J. Cogdell, J. G. Lindsay,* Immunological Comparison of the Pyruvate Dehydrogenase Complexes from Pea Mitochondria and Chloroplasts, Planta *188*, 225–231 (1992).

[41] *D. W. Cleveland, S. G. Fischer, M. W. Kirschner, U. K. Laemmli,* Peptide Mapping by Limited Proteolysis in Sodium Dodecyl Sulphate and Analysis by Gel Electrophoresis, J. Biol. Chem. *252*, 1102–1106 (1977).

[42] *M. Eschenbruck, R. R. Burk,* Experimentally Improved Reliability of Ultrasensitive Silver Staining of Proteins in Polyacrylamide Gels, Anal. Biochem. *125*, 96–99 (1982).

[43] *M. L. Bryant, R. P. Nalewaik, V. L. Tibbs, G. J. Todaro,* Comparison of Two Techniques for Protein Isolation and Radioiodination by Tryptic Peptide Mapping, Anal. Biochem. *96,* 84–89 (1979).

[44] *S. D. Patel, C. I. Ragan,* Structural Studies on Mitochondrial NADH Dehydrogenase Using Chemical Crosslinking, Biochem. J. *256,* 521–528 (1988).

[45] *S. D. Patel, M. W. J. Cleeter, C. I. Ragan,* Transmembrane Organisation of Mitochondrial NADH Dehydrogenase as Revealed by Radiochemical Labelling and Crosslinking, Biochem. J. *256,* 529–535 (1988).

[46] *J. A. Hodgson, O. G. L. De Marcucci, J. G. Lindsay,* Structure Function Studies on the Lipoate Acyltransferase – Component X Core Assembly of the Ox Heart Pyruvate Dehydrogenase Complex, Eur. J. Biochem. *171,* 609–614 (1988).

[47] *D. J. Danner, N. Armstrong, S. C. Heffelfinger, E. T. Sewell, J. H. Priest, L. J. Elsas,* Absence of the Branch Chain Acyltransferase as a Cause of Maple Syrup Urine Disease, J. Clin. Invest. *75,* 858–860 (1985).

[48] *M. A. Birch-Machin, I. M. Shepherd, M. Solomon, S. J. Yeaman, D. Gardner-Medwin, H. S. A. Sherratt, J. G. Lindsay, A. Aynsley-Green, D. M. Turnbull,* Fatal Lactic Acidosis due to deficiency of E1 Component of the Pyruvate Dehydrogenase Complex, J. Inherited Metab. Dis. *11,* 207–217 (1988).

[49] *L. A. Bindoff, M. A. Birch-Machin, L. Farnsworth, D. Gardner-Medwin, J. G. Lindsay, D. M. Turnbull,* Familial Intermittent Ataxia due to a Defect in the E1 Component of the Pyruvate Dehydrogenase Complex, J. Neurol. Sci. *93,* 311–318 (1989).

[50] *B. H. Robinson,* Cell Culture Studies on Patients with Mitochondrial Diseases: Molecular Defects in the Pyruvate Dehydrogenase Complex, J. Bioenerg. Biomembr. *20,* 313–323 (1988).

[51] *G. A. Reid, G. Schatz,* Import of Proteins into Mitochondria: Yeast Cells Grown in the Presence of Carbonyl Cyanide *m*-Chlorophenylhydrazone Accumulate Massive Amounts of Some Mitochondrial Precursor Polypeptides, J. Biol. Chem. *257,* 13056–13061 (1982).

[52] *A. Chomyn, P. Mariottini, M. W. J. Cleeter, C. I. Ragan, M. Riley, R. F. Doolittle, G. Attardi,* Six Unidentified Reading Frames of Human Mitochondrial DNA Encode Components of the Respiratory NADH Dehydrogenase Complex, Nature London *314,* 592–597 (1986).

[53] *A. Chomyn, M. W. J. Cleeter, C. I. Ragan, M. Riley, R. F. Doolittle, G. Attardi,* URF6 the Last Unidentified Reading Frame of Human Mt. DNA, Codes for an NADH Dehydrogenase Subunit, Science *234,* 614–618 (1986).

[54] *T. Oda, S. Futaki, K. Kitagawa, Y. Yoshihara, I. Tani, T. Higuti,* Orientation of Chargerin II (AL6) in the ATP Synthase of Rat Liver Mitochondria Determined with Antibodies against Peptides of the Protein, Biochem. Biophys. Res. Commun. *165,* 449–456 (1989).

[55] *G. H. D. Clarkson, J. C. Neagle, J. G. Lindsay,* Topography of Succinate Dehydrogenase in the Mitochondrial Inner Membrane – a Study Using Limited Proteolysis and Immunoblotting, Biochem. J. *273,* 719–724 (1991).

[56] *T. R. Mosmann, R. Baumal, A. R. Williamson,* Mutations Affecting Immunoglobulin Light Chain Secretion by Myeloma Cells: Functional Analysis by Cell Fusion, Eur, J. Immunol. *9,* 511–516 (1979).

[57] *L. N. Y. Wu, I. M. Lubin, R. R. Fisher,* Biosynthesis of Rat Liver Transhydrogenase *in vivo* and *in vitro*, J. Biol. Chem. *260,* 6361–6366 (1985).

[58] *O. G. L. De Marcucci, G. M. Gibb, J. Dick, J. G. Lindsay,* Biosynthesis, Import and Processing of Precursor Polypeptides of Mammalian Mitochondrial Pyruvate Dehydrogenase Complex, Biochem. J. *251,* 817–823 (1988).

[59] *D. Vestweber, J. Brunner, A. Baker, G. Schatz,* A 42K Outer Membrane Protein is a Component of the Yeast Mitochondrial Pyruvate Dehydrogenase Complex, Nature London *341,* 205–209 (1988).

[60] *P.-J. Kang, J. Ostermann, J. Shilling, W. Neupert, E. A. Craig, N. Pfanner,* Requirement for Hsp 70 in the Mitochondrial Matrix for Translocation and Folding of Precursor Proteins, Nature London *348,* 137–142 (1990).

6.4   Immunological Detection of Extracellular Matrix Antigens

Robert G. Price and Sarah A. Taylor

The extracellular matrix (ECM) has many differing and highly specialized roles and as a consequence its composition varies with location. However, a common feature is the presence of a characteristic group of macromolecules which are synthesized by specialized cells located in the tissues. These macromolecules are members of several large families of proteins. The strength and rigidity of the ECM is conferred by collagen [1], while flexibility and elasticity arises from the presence of the proteoglycans [2]. Laminin is an abundant glycoprotein found in all basement membranes which binds to type IV collagen, HS-PG, nidogen and the cell surface [3]. Fibronectin is a multi-domain glycoprotein which is also a normal constituent of serum [4].

Various immunocytochemical methods can be used, following standard protocols (cf. 5) to detect ECM components *in situ*. Problems may arise from the nature of the molecular associations in the ECM that limit the effectiveness of antibody-based methods to study the intact matrix. For example, antibodies do not generally penetrate the matrix of connective tissue or cartilage very effectively and some macromolecules are so tightly bound to their neighbours that their epitopes are not naturally accessible to antibodies. Thus, the distribution and variation in amounts of macromolecules in the ECM are usually visualized immunocytochemically by light or electron microscopy in tissue sections or in biopsy material [5]. This section, however, will concentrate upon the detection and analysis of the break-down products of the ECM which is an area of considerable contemporary interest. Many chronic diseases affect the ECM and more quantitative methods are required to monitor the metabolism of the ECM in these diseases since isotopic procedures are unsuitable for use with patients. Breakdown products of the macromolecules of the ECM are found in trace amounts in serum and body fluids [6], with the exception of fibronectin which is present naturally in larger concentrations in serum; as a result, a number of less sensitive assays have been available for many years to quantitate fibronectin concentrations in body fluids. The low quantities of the breakdown products of the other macromolecules present in body fluids required the development of immunoassays, and mainly RIA procedures have been reported [6], several of which are now available as commercial kits. Here the current status of this field will be discussed with emphasis on recent progress in the assessment of chronic disorders involving ECM pathology. The assays can be used to monitor ECM macromolecule synthesis by cells in tissue culture and as a means of determining the efficacy of drugs using experimental animals. Essentially, the assays have been developed against whole molecules or breakdown products which are present in the macromolecule as distinctive domains (Fig. 1 and 2). Only recent studies will be described and further information can be obtained from earlier reviews [7–9]. Discussion of the assay procedures and their applications to each group of macromolecules are presented in sequence.

6.4.1   Collagens

6.4.1.1   Type I Collagen

Although assays have been available for type I collagen and some of its domains for over a decade, only recently have sound assay procedures been established. Initially, solid phase RIA incorporating ^{125}I-labelled IgG were used to detect class-specific antibodies to collagen [10], but since at least three major antigenic sites were present and the preparation of the antigens was imprecise, these procedures were not widely used. *Hartmann* et al. [11] screened patients with a variety of liver diseases with a RIA based on antibodies raised against acid-soluble type I collagen isolated from human skin specimens. These antibodies reacted to two components in serum which could be separated by gel filtration: a high M_r minor peak which proved to be a mixture of undegraded type I collagen and procollagen molecules, and a major peak containing low M_r degradation products of type I collagen. A standard inhibition assay (sequential saturation type) using ^{125}I-labelled collagen was employed in which suitably diluted antiserum was initially incubated with unlabelled human type I collagen (as standard) or with human serum, then twenty-four hours later the ^{125}I-labelled collagen was added. Elevated levels of type I collagen products were found in the serum of patients with cirrhosis and in alcoholic patients without cirrhosis, but not in those with hepatitis. This newly developed assay for serum type I collagen components has been compared with PIIINP (this is the amino-terminal peptide of the type III procollagen molecule – the nomenclature of collagen fragments is described in Fig. 1) as a marker for histological change in chronic hepatitis [12]. Serum type I collagen levels correlated more strongly with liver fibrosis than did PIIINP, while serum PIIINP proved to be a better marker of disease activity than serum alanine aminopeptidase activity or γ-globulin. This suggests that the monitoring of more than one parameter of ECM antigens provides additional information on the differential development of the disease and may also provide an alternative to liver biopsies.

Liver disease is complex, and so the measurement of type I collagen in conjunction with its C-terminal propeptide (PICP, $M_r = 100\,000$) could provide valuable additional information on the progress of the disease. The PICP antigen is a trimeric, globular protein isolated after collagenase digestion of the type I procollagen molecule isolated from cultures of human skin fibroblasts followed by further purification using lectin affinity and column chromatography. Rabbit polyclonal antibodies were prepared [13, 14] and incorporated into a radioimmunoinhibition assay for PICP which could be used to assay 40 samples in 3 h with intra- and inter-assay coefficients of variation between 3 and 5%. Reference intervals for serum PICP are relatively wide (Table 1). There is an inverse correlation between age and serum concentration in men but no similar relationship has been found in women. Only one form of the antigen is present in serum and it is stable during storage at -20 °C with no loss of antigenicity upon repeated freeze-thawing. The amount of PICP is directly proportional to the number of original

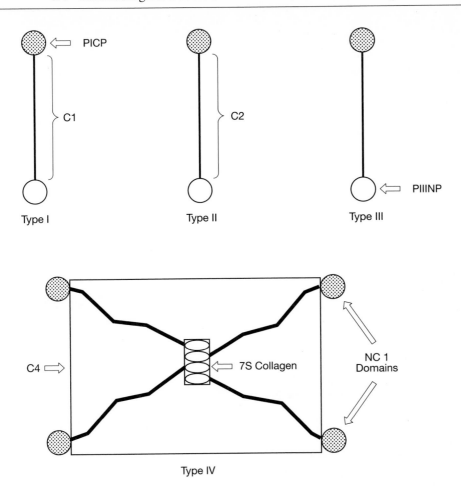

Fig. 1. Schematic representation of the molecular location of antigenic determinants present in collagens which are important in immunological assays. Carboxy-terminal ⊗, amino-terminal ○, triple-helical — regions. The procollagens are designated PI, PII, PIII etc., and their carboxy-terminal and amino-terminal telopeptides CP and NP respectively. The helical degradation products are here referred to as C1, C2, C3 etc.

collagen chains and its concentration in body fluids would be expected to change during periods of rapid growth and with tissue damage. Circulating PICP is cleared from the serum *via* the mannose receptor in liver endothelial cells [15]. The value of this assay for the monitoring of metabolic bone disease is currently being assessed. PICP has also been assayed in inflammatory bowel disease in children [16] and is, together with PIIINP, a useful indicator of growth activity following therapeutic intervention [17].

Table 1. Reported reference ranges for antigens related to ECM macromolecules in serum and urine

Antigen*	Type of Assay	Serum reference range for adults (μg/l or I.U./l**)	Sources
C1	pAb RIA	110–197	11, 12
PICP	pAb RIA	40–200	13
C2	pAb RIA	Not reported	20
PIIINP	pAb RIA	0.0–12.0	41
		3.7–11.7	90
		0.0–12.0	12
	pAb RIA *Behringwerke-Hoechst* Kit	2.0–12.0	39
		4.9–10.3	44
		0.0–12.0	29
		2.9–13.3	30
		2.6–18.2	73
		4.7–9.5	37
		5.0–12.0	74
	Trimeric[+] Specific pAb RIA	1.7–4.2	8, 43
	Rapid Equilibrium Trimeric[+] Specific pAb RIA *Farmos* Kit	1.7–4.2	24
	Rapid Equilibrium Trimeric[+] Specific pAb RIA *Farmos* Kit	1.7–4.2	42, 45
		1.5–4.6	46
		2.1–4.3	35, 36
	pAb Fab RIA *Behringwerke-Hoechst* Kit	29–79	44
		25–72	73
		39–76	30
		10–67	75
		15–63	74
	mAb RIA (coated tubes) *Behringwerke-Hoechst* Kit[++]	6.1–12.3	26
7S	pAb RIA	3.0–10.6	90
		2.5–4.9	37
		0.0–10.0	74
		4.9–10.3	44

Table 1. (Continued)

Antigen*	Type of Assay	Serum reference range for adults (µg/l or I.U./l**)	Sources
NC1	pAb RIA	0.0–12.0	63
	mAb ELISA	93–106	60
		37–84	91
		Urine range:	
		12.0–18.0	60
		1.0–12.0	91
Whole Type IV Collagen	mAb ELISA	70–78	62
C4	One Step Sandwich mAb ELISA	Not reported	66
P1	pAb RIA	14–38	90
		15–37	74
	One Step Sandwich mAb ELISA	73–133	71
	pAb RIA *Behringwerke-Hoechst* Kit	810–1430**	38, 70
		880–1440**	69
		630–1230**	72
		1090–1440**	29
		1260–1460**	77
		640–1600**	73
		760–1360**	92, 93
		860–1820**	37
		1000–1800**	75
		970–1730**	78
HSPG	pAb RIA	Not reported	81
		112–160	82

++   These highly specific assays only recognize the trimeric form of PIIINP, while other assays cross-react with monomeric forms of the antigen.

++   This very recently developed third generation of *Behringwerke-Hoechst* kits have replaced both the pAb and pAb Fab RIA Kits which are now no longer available from this company.

*   For nomenclature of antigens, and their fragments, see Figs. 1 and 2.

**   Concentrations in arbitrary units/l.

6.4.1.2   Type II Collagen

Although anti-type II collagen antibodies occur naturally in joint disease [18], great difficulty has been encountered in the preparation of an antibody for the detection of type II collagen. *Chichester* et al. [19] have attempted to solve this problem by producing a panel of mAbs against type II collagen but even the best monospecific antibodies had multiple activities towards non-collagenous antigens. *Henrotin* et al. [20] have developed what is probably the first sequential saturation RIA for human type II collagen using a polyclonal antibody. They report very good specificity, sensitivity, precision and reproducibility, but have only attempted to quantify native type II collagen in culture media under different culturing conditions. The application of this assay to serum from patients with arthritic conditions will be of great interest.

6.4.1.3   Type III Collagen

The assay of type III collagen and PIIINP [21] are the most widely used methods at present. Since PIIINP arises as a split product of the synthesis of type III collagen, its measurement in serum reflects variations in collagen metabolism in a variety of conditions in which the synthesis of collagen is either stimulated or perturbed. PIIINP is often measured in conjunction with other ECM antigens or other, more commonly measured, clinical chemistry parameters. Circulating intact PIIINP is metabolized in the liver [22], although further studies are needed to determine whether or not hepatic extraction influences the serum concentration of PIIINP. PIIINP ($M_r = 42000$) can be readily isolated from human ascites fluid [23], and a rapid (3 h) equilibrium-type RIA has been developed which overcomes the non-parallelism between standard and human serum samples that was a problem with earlier assays [24]. The intra- and inter-assay CVs were both < 5%. The PIIINP concentration in sera from normal adults determined with this procedure was a third of that obtained with a commercial kit because in previous methods there may have been inhibition by the monomers of PIIINP. To prepare a suitable standard, known amounts of the purified propeptide were added to human serum that had first been treated with DEAE-cellulose for 1 h at room temperature to remove high M_r propeptide antigens. Following the addition of NaN_3 the standards were stable for at least two months. Further improvements in the assay for PIIINP and other antigenic regions of type III collagen may come from the availability of mAbs [25]. *Gressner* [26] has described a RIA which incorporates a monoclonal antibody which does not recognize the monomeric form of PIIINP.

The possibility that the assay of PIIINP would provide valuable diagnostic information about the metabolism of the ECM in the development of fibrosis in liver diseases was suggested over a decade ago [27]. Subsequently, *Niemela* et al. [28] used the assay to study, in particular, alcoholic liver diseases. More recently, assays for both PIIINP and LP1 (the central peptide fragment of laminin – see Fig. 2) in serum have been used to distinguish between patients with cirrhosis and alcoholics with and without cirrhosis [29]. Significantly raised levels of both PIIINP and LP1 were demonstrated in alcoholic cirrhosis and in primary biliary cirrhosis, but only LP1 was significantly elevated in alcoholic patients without cirrhosis, again suggesting the potential of these assays in differential diagnosis.

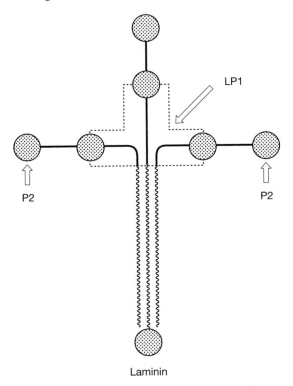

Fig. 2. Schematic representation of the molecular location of antigenic determinants present in laminin which are important in immunological assays. Heavily cross-linked globular domains ☻, α-helical coils ∿, cysteine-rich α-chains ▬.

Similar findings have been reported by *Annoni* et al. [30] who divided patients into 4 groups according to liver histology; namely, those with steatofibrosis, alcoholic hepatitis alone, cirrhosis alone and cirrhosis combined with alcoholic hepatitis. They concluded that PIIINP and LP1 were most significantly elevated in alcoholics with both hepatitis and cirrhosis. Indeed, when they used a PIIINP-Fab assay, only patients with this combined condition showed significant elevation. The LP1 assay proved particularly useful for discriminating between patients with cirrhosis and/or alcoholic hepatitis and those with steatofibrosis – with only the steatofibrotic patients maintaining normal levels of LP1. This assay was 96% specific and highly sensitive (92%). The assays for serum antigens correlated well with each other and with liver histology. Other standard biochemical tests (aspartate aminotransferase, EC 2.6.1.1; alanine aminotransferase, EC 2.6.1.2 and γ-glutamyltranspeptidase, EC 2.3.2.2) showed no significant correlations with LP1 or PIIINP, strongly suggesting that these conventional biochemical assays may fail to detect some cases of hepatitis.

Alcoholic hepatitis has always been particularity difficult to establish by conventional clinical and laboratory methods and definitive diagnosis relies on liver biopsy. However, monitoring patients by means of repeated liver biopsies raises obvious problems, and monitoring by LP1 and PIIINP measurements in alcoholics with cirrhosis could prove useful in detecting bouts of alcoholic hepatitis which would be accompanied by unexpected increases in these antigens. If the potential of serum assay for PIIINP is to be evaluated, correlation with specific changes in the liver demonstrated by histochemical staining of biopsy samples is essential and *Schneider* et al. [31] concluded that serum analyses cannot at present replace diagnostic histological procedures. Their data agreed with that of *Annoni* et al. [30] and indicated that the combined measurement of PIIINP, PIIINP-Fab [32] and LP1 yields better information than any individual parameter in judging the clinical course of liver fibrosis and the efficacy of antifibrotic treatment.

In patients with primary biliary cirrhosis the basement membrane surrounding the bile ducts is disrupted and *Niemela* et al. [33], in an attempt to monitor this process, correlated immunohistochemical staining of ECM antigens with measurements of 7S collagen (cf. Fig. 1), LP1 and PIIINP. LP1 correlated with PIIINP but the increase in the concentration of 7S collagen was a late change. Only PIIINP proved to be significant as a predictor for survival and was a better indicator of prognosis than basement membrane antigens. They and others have suggested that the number of liver biopsies carried out on patients with psoriasis being treated with methotrexate could be reduced so long as they have normal levels of serum PIIINP [34, 35]. PIIINP may also have prognostic value in the management of progressive systemic sclerosis [36]. *Misaki* et al. [37] found that while 7S-collagen and LP1 levels in serum correlated with the grade of fibrosis in chronic viral liver disease, PIIINP only correlated weakly and they accordingly recommended the use of 7S-collagen as a marker. It is apparent that a variety of profiles of ECM antigens may occur in the serum during the course of different connective tissue disorders, suggesting that these tests, if used in parallel, have potential in differential diagnosis. *Gressner* et al. [38] had previously demonstrated that PIIINP was a useful indicator of activity and degree of the fibrotic process in patients with fibrotic liver diseases. In the same report they also demonstrated that LP1, rather than PIIINP, was a potentially important parameter of haemodynamic distortion during fibrotic tissue changes which resulted in portal hypertension. Later, *Gressner* et al. [39] showed that the assay of PIIINP was not useful in the diagnosis of portal hypertension or for monitoring portal vein pressure. *Mutimer* et al. [40] concluded that PIIINP did not give independent prognostic information and conferred no benefit over existing conventional measurements in the routine management of primary biliary cirrhosis.

PIIINP has also been used as a marker in a variety of other situations in which the ECM is changing [41]. Indeed, pregnancy has been shown to affect serum PIIINP and so this condition should be taken into account when evaluating results [41]. *Puistola* et al. [42] measured PIIINP in serum of patients with ovarian carcinomas and found it to be a relatively nonspecific indicator, but they did report that the combined measurement of PIIINP and the tumour maker CA 125 provided more useful information on the clinical behaviour of endometrial carcinoma.

Table 2. Reported reference ranges for antigens related to ECM macromolecules in the serum of children

Antigen*	Type of Assay	Serum reference range for children ($\mu g/l$ or I.U./l*)	Age in years or months**	Sources
PICP	pAb RIA	250–600	4–16	49
		1500–2900	0–3**	17
		280–3120	3–6**	17
		80–2000	6–12**	17
		330–1010	1–2	17
		70–710	2–4	17
		70–690	4–16	17
PIIINP	pAb RIA *Behringwerke-Hoechst* Kit	52–172	1–6**	94
		15–63	6–12**	94
		17–45	1–3	94
		9–29	3–9	94
		5–44	9–16	94
		15–40	4–16	49
	Trimeric+ Specific pAb RIA	Girls		
		3.7–12.2	2–10	47
		4.9–17.2	11–13	47
		2.0–10.0	14–17	47
		Boys		
		3.6–11.8	2–10	47
		3.1–13.3	11–13	47
		5.8–21.5	14–17	47
P1	pAb RIA *Behringwerke-Hoechst* Kit	860–3030*	0–4	48
7S	pAbRIA	<13	0–4	48

+ This assay only recognizes the trimeric form of the PIIINP propeptide, while other assays cross-react with monomeric forms of the antigen.

* For nomenclature of antigens, and their fragments, see Fig. 1 and 2.

If PIIINP is to be a useful parameter of ECM metabolism it should correlate with tissue changes in type III collagen. Such changes occur in wound healing and during this process PIIINP levels can be elevated 1000-fold above the normal serum level in an unaffected fluid such as peritoneal fluid collected through an abdominal drain [43]. The concentration of PIIINP present varied at different stages of the healing process and so represented a quantitative tool for monitoring wound healing. In a further study, *Bentsen* et al. [44] demonstrated a sequential and transitional increase in the serum PIIINP, LP1 and 7S collagen. The changes occurred in parallel with the deposition of type III collagen and basement membrane components in the granulation tissue of wounds, and interestingly serum PIIINP levels reached very high levels when wounds became infected [45]. The ECM rapidly changes during growth and the assay of serum PIIINP may be useful in monitoring prepubertal children receiving growth hormone, since height velocity is reflected by increases in this antigen and early increases may have a predictive value [46, 47] (Table 2). The increase in PIIINP levels in serum of Indian children with cirrhosis has been shown to reflect the very rapid hepatic synthesis of type III collagen which occurs in this condition [48]. Serum concentrations of both PICP and PIIINP were found to reflect growth activity in children with inflammatory bowel disease, but measurement of PIIINP did not have any advantage over PICP [49]. Serum PIIINP is also a sensitive marker for atherosclerosis in coronary heart disease [50] in which there is a known shift in collagen synthesis from type I to type III [51].

6.4.1.4   Type IV Collagen

Type IV collagen is the main collagenous component of basement membranes and is composed of three α-chains of which there are five types [52]. These chains are approximately 350 nm in length and are divided into three distinct domains – the central triple helical region, a non-helical globular region at carboxy-terminal end and a cross-linked region (7S) at the amino-terminal end [53] (Figure 1). The carboxy-terminal globular extensions of two molecules are combined to build a hexameric domain termed NC1. The assay of antibodies in serum against the *Goodpasture* antigen which has been tentatively located in the NC1 region of the α_3-chain of type IV collagen [54] has been widely used in the detection and monitoring of anti-glomerular basement-membranes (GBM) disease [55–57].

Assays for type IV collagen antigens in serum have been used when basement membranes are known to be affected. Competitive RIA for both the 7S collagen [58] and NC1 [59] regions using polyclonal antisera have been used to study liver fibrosis and diabetic microangiopathy.

The concentration of NC1 in serum has been related to the turnover of type IV collagen in the GBM in diabetes. *Torffvit* et al. [60] have developed a sensitive ELISA for NC1 in serum and urine, using a mouse mAb against NC1 prepared from bovine kidneys, and have used the assay on samples from diabetic patients and healthy controls. No difference was found between the serum concentration in the two groups but there was a higher concentration of NC1 in the urine of the diabetic group compared to the controls. If the albumin excretion rate (AER) was normal, NC1 was also normal; if the AER increased so did NC1; however, NC1 values returned to normal when clinical diabetic nephropathy was reached. These findings strongly suggest that NC1 may be an early marker of incipient diabetic nephropathy. Earlier studies had demonstrated that the serum levels of 7S collagen in diabetic rats could be normalized by insulin treatment [61]. Monoclonal antibodies against purified human placental type IV collagen have been used [62] to study diabetic patients with or without clinical signs of retinopathy, nephropathy and/or neuropathy. The concentration of serum type IV collagen increased with the worsening of the disease. The most pronounced effect was found in nephropathy and the increase in type IV collagen correlated with glomerular, rather than tubular, dysfunction. This assay may provide a reproducible marker for the assessment of the activity or progression of diabetic nephropathy. However, the precise nature of the epitope against which the mAb was raised is unclear.

In contrast, the NC1 region of type IV collagen was found to increase in both serum and urine of patients with glomerulonephritis [63] while an increase in NC1 in pre-eclampsia supports the hypothesis that basement membranes are involved in the pathogenesis of this disease [64]. *Gerstmeier* et al. [65] found elevated levels of both LP1 and NC1 in the serum of patients with progressive systemic sclerosis, demonstrating the involvement of basement membranes in this disorder; however, it is doubtful whether assays of these parameters are useful diagnostic or prognostic tools. More encouraging data have been presented [66] on a one-step enzyme immunoassay which utilizes type IV collagen solubilized from placenta by pepsin (EC 2.4.23.1). No cross-reactivity was observed against types I, III,V, acid-extracted type IV collagen, long form 7S and NC1 domains or LP1 fragments. However 7% of cross-reactivity of the anti-pepsin-solubilized type IV collagen antibody was observed with type VI collagen. The pepsin-solubilized collagen used to raise the mAbs consisted mainly of 4 triple-helical strands of type IV collagen connected *via* the 7S region but lacking the NC1 domain [53] and the antigenic specificity of the selected mAbs was dependent on the newly exposed triple-helical conformation after degradation by pepsin. The presence of type IV collagen triple helices in increased amounts in serum is therefore an additional marker for conditions in which basement membranes are degraded, and increased serum concentrations in liver cirrhosis and hepatocellular carcinoma have been demonstrated [66].

6.4.2   Laminin

The presence of antibodies against nidogen and laminin has been shown in sera from streptococcal-related diseases and rheumatoid arthritis [67]. Laminin is a major glycoprotein which is a structurally and biologically active component of basement membranes [3]. The laminin molecule isolated from tumours has a M_r of 850000 and is a cross-shaped structure (Fig. 2). Laminin binds to type IV collagen, heparan sulphate proteoglycan (HS-PG) and nidogen creating an integral structure within the basement membrane [3]. The most immunogenic part of laminin is the heavily disulphide-linked central domain 1 (Fig. 2; [68]), further determinants are located at the globular ends which have been isolated as fragments 2 (P2) and 4.

The most widely used marker for monitoring laminin metabolism in humans is the LP1 fragment. Serum concentration of LP1 has been monitored in patients with a variety of malignancies [69] and can be used to follow the course of malignancies, particularly those of epithelial tumours. *Gressner* et al. [70] measured the laminin concentration in the hepatic and cubital veins of patients with chronic liver diseases by competition RIA and found that levels of LP1 increased with the degree of fibrosis, reaching the highest concentrations in cirrhosis. Fibrotic liver changes are characterized by the development of new basement membranes around the sinusoid, resulting in a narrowing of the lumina and an increase in haemodynamic resistance and portal vein pressure [70]. A cut-off laminin concentration (critical value) above which the result was considered pathological was established in this study.

Recently, a rapid one-step sandwich ELISA has been developed using two mouse mAbs [71] both raised against the laminin P1 fragment ($M_r = 200000$) prepared from human placenta [53]. Essentially, LP1 fragment (as standard) or serum was mixed with the Fab fragment from one of the antibodies, which had been conjugated to POD. This solution was then added to wells coated with the other mAb and incubated for 1 h at room temperature, after which time the wells were washed and the bound POD activity estimated using o-phenylenediamine as substrate in a 15 min assay at room temperature. When this assay was used, the levels of LP1 in the serum of normal individuals was 103 ± 15 µg/l which is 4 times higher than that reported elsewhere [23]. *Iwata* [71] suggested that this high value is due to the fact that this assay is much more specific than the radioimmunoinhibition assay. When patients with liver cirrhosis or primary biliary cirrhosis were studied, they were found to have approximately double normal levels while those with hepatocellular carcinoma had approximately 3.5 times the level of LP1 in their sera.

Essential cryoglobulinaemia is an immune complex-mediated disease with active phases and the monitoring of the course of this disease is therefore difficult. *Gabrielli* et al. [72] measured LP1 in the sera of a group of these patients to determine whether or not it is a sensitive parameter of active vasculitis. A significant increase in LP1 concentration was found with increase in disease activity and LP1 proved to be a better parameter than complement factor assays. In systemic lupus erythematosus, basement membranes are the target for immune complexes and the concentration of LP1 increased in serum with the clinical score for the activity of the disease [73]. Although follow-up studies are required, these authors suggest that an increase of more than 0.5 U/ml in LP1 content within three months will be followed by major organ manifestation.

Two markers for basement membrane, 7S collagen and LP1, have been compared to the activity of galactosylhydroxylysine glucosyltransferase (EC 2.4.1.66) [74], an enzyme participating in the biosynthesis of collagen. The clinical course of progressive systemic sclerosis – acute, subacute and chronic – affected the serum concentrations of both PIIINP and LP1 although there was a considerable overlap between the groups. These findings suggest that such assays have prognostic value but further studies are required. Unfortunately, the laminin assay used had an inter-assay variation of 15–20% which limits its usefulness for detecting small changes. To understand fully the nature of the progression of the disease it would be necessary to have assays which monitored either synthesis or degradation. PIIINP and LP1 were elevated in systemic scleroderma-like disease but not in the sera of patients with silicosis alone, suggesting a certain disease specificity [75]. The isolation and characterization of a novel calcium-binding glycoprotein has been reported [76] and will be worthy of consideration as a potential marker antigen for basement membranes in the future as it is found in large amounts in the serum.

A feature of diabetic microangiopathy is the thickening of basement membranes and changes are most pronounced in the kidney, eye and peripheral nerves. *Pietschmann* et al. [77] reported that LP1 levels correlated with nephropathy but not retinopathy. However, these authors stated that the serum LP1 was not elevated in patients with microalbuminuria, suggesting that it is not a sensitive parameter for incipient renal damage but may be useful for studying the clinical course or the efficacy of therapy. Serum LP1 was found to be elevated in a number of immune-based renal disorders in the nephrotic stage when primarily the GBM was involved [78], but not in IgA nephropathy which affects the mesangium.

The assay of serum components in general does not provide sensitive indicators of early renal damage [79]. Since the large M_r of laminin and LP1 preclude their passage through the glomerulus, it may not be useful to monitor these parameters in urine (*H. Stolte,* personal communication). The value of monitoring the presence of low M_r markers for specific regional or cellular damage has been investigated. A range of laminin fragments of differing M_r have been isolated from human placenta by the procedure of *Dixit* [80] on the basis that lower M_r breakdown products may be excreted into the urine. Three fragments in the M_r range from 50 000 to 150 000 were selected and used for the production of pAbs in rabbits. These antibodies did not cross-react with whole laminin, type IV collagen, human IgG or albumin and so were incorporated into inhibition ELISA procedures for serum and urine. One of these antibodies (NSU3) detected the presence of laminin fragments in the urine of diabetics (1 494 ± 565 µg/l), in contrast nondiabetic controls had low or undetectable levels (170 ± 48 µg/l). This antibody was also able to select components of laminin in serum and may reflect organ damage since workers exposed to cadmium had elevated levels (1 984 ± 216 µg/l) compared to non-exposed control groups (1 097 ± 157 µg/l).

6.4.3 Proteoglycans

The composition of the GBM alters during the development of diabetes in a way which ultimately impairs its function [81]. Using a RIA it has been demonstrated that lower amounts of HS-PG and laminin are present in the GBM of diabetic patients when compared to non-diabetic controls, and little change is observed in the fibronectin content. However, an increase in proteoglycan content has been reported in the serum of diabetic rats [82]. LP1 level in serum was found to be a poor marker of diabetes whereas fibronectin determined by ELISA was increased in urine. It was considered to be of renal origin [83] and was, in fact, increased earlier than the albumin excretion rate which is a recognized marker of early renal damage.

HA is an unusual glycosaminoglycan in that it is never found associated with core proteins which are characteristic of the proteoglycans and as a result it is poorly immunogenic. This problem has recently been overcome by the use of affino-immunoenzymatic methods using a glycoprotein hyaluronectin which has been isolated either from brain [84] or cartilage [85]. Hyaluronectin has a strong affinity for HA and when it is deposited into the wells of a plate coated with HA, the fixation of hyaluronectin on HA can be demonstrated by an inhibition ELISA technique using anti-hyaluronectin antibodies coupled to AP. *Kropt* et al. [86] followed up their studies on portal hypertension by assaying HA as well as LP1 in serum to determine whether or not the diagnostic efficiency was improved. Both analytes are equally useful for the detection of raised portal venous pressure in groups in which liver disease is strongly suspected. *Levesque* et al. [87] found a significant increase in HA and a positive correlation between it and the severity of progressive systemic sclerosis, which may reflect visceral involvement in this disease as well as being an overall indicator of its severity. Serum HA could be an indicator of the degree of systemic involvement in progressive systemic sclerosis [87], but its prognostic value needs to be clarified. *Ramadori* et al. [88] concluded that serum HA concentrations help to differentiate chronic active hepatitis from active cirrhosis. While elevated PIIINP serum concentration mainly correlates with inflammatory activity, the elevation of serum HA appears to result from reduced functional clearance capacity of the liver in chronic liver disease. Thus serum HA determinations are of greater diagnostic value than PIIINP, particularly when inflammatory activity is low [88].

The measurement of the serum concentration of PIIINP and the polysaccharide HA has made it possible to monitor changes in the metabolism of ECM constituents in acute and fibrotic disease. *Horsley-Petersen* et al. [89] compared the serum and synovial fluid levels of PIIINP and HA in patients with arthritis with clinical signs and serological parameters of inflammation. There is an increase of type III collagen around inflammatory cell infiltrates and the correlation between PIIINP and the clinical signs of synovitis supported the assumption that the inflamed synovium is the primary source of serum PIIINP in rheumatoid arthritis [89, 90]. However, serum HA only correlated with serum PIIINP in the initial active phase of synovitis. HA synthesis is dominant during the first stage of formation of granulation tissue which is then followed by the deposition of type III collagen, suggesting that circulating ECM elements reflect the development of disease.

6.4.4   General Considerations

A striking feature of the data presented in Tables 1 and 2 is the variation in the reference ranges for the commonly determined parameters. The normal values quoted for LP1 and PIIINP by different groups vary even when they are using the same procedure. In addition, when the type of antibody used in the assay is changed, wide variation is seen in the reference range. This variation can partly be explained by the difference in the specificity of the antibodies used. An example of this problem is the fall in the reference range for PIIINP when a trimer-specific pAb was incorporated into an RIA compared with the original pAb [41]. However, a mAb for the same analyte which also claimed to be trimer-specific did not result in a lowering of the reference ranges [26]. In this case the difference may be explained by differences in the calibrant or standard antigen. A surprising elevation of the reference range for PIIINP has been reported when a commercial kit (Behringwerke – Hoechst) utilizing the Fab fragment of a pAb was used (Table 1). The reference range increased sixfold and, since this is unlikely to be due to the Fab fragment alone, the difference must be explained by the incoporation of a less specific antibody or again by the standards used. It is therefore critical for each laboratory to set up its own reference range whenever a modification of the assay is introduced. This situation can be expected to improve with the availability of improved commercial kits and standards. The introduction of mAb and ELISA procedures should also contribute to the improved standardization and promote a more widespread use of assays for ECM antigens.

At present the field is not sufficiently standardized to measure absolute values of any particular analyte, but assays can be used to measure trends or changes in levels. A further difficulty is that, at present, it is not certain how much *in-vivo* degradation of many of these analytes occurs, and so more attention needs to be paid to the characterization of the naturally occurring degradation products. The preferred antibody would be one raised against a well-defined, stable, natural breakdown product. Such an approach would be particularly important in the assay of ECM antigens in body fluids other than serum, such as urine and synovial fluid. To date, the serum ECM antigen assays have had limited success when applied to urine. However, it is encouraging that earlier studies [60] have been confirmed [91] to show that the elevation of urinary NC1 may be a sensitive early marker for the development of diabetic nephropathy. Indeed it has been demonstrated that urinary NC1 levels are also elevated in patients with another, unrelated condition: membraneous glomerulonephritis [91].

Despite the problems encountered with the assays for ECM antigens described above, they have considerable promise for the monitoring of a number of chronic diseases. Since they reflect the modification of the composition of tissues in disease they can help reduce, or perhaps eventually remove, the necessity for biopsy samples. They appear to be particularly valuable in fibrotic conditions and those involving basement membranes associated with the microvascular system. It is therefore important to carry out sequential studies to establish the relationship between the changes in the

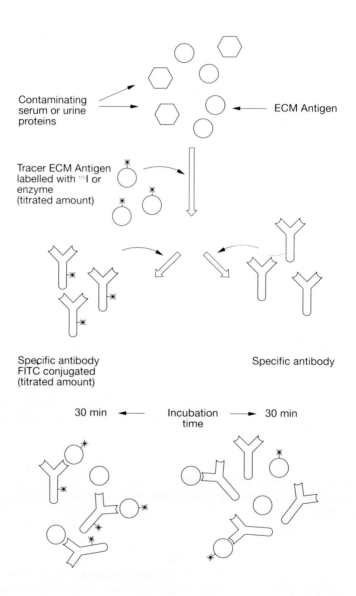

Contaminating serum or urine proteins

ECM Antigen

Tracer ECM Antigen labelled with ¹²⁵I or enzyme (titrated amount)

Specific antibody FITC conjugated (titrated amount)

Specific antibody

30 min ← Incubation time → 30 min

Fig. 3. Schematic representation of a preferred immunological assay for breakdown products of ECM. Further information can be obtained from [95, 96]. Other applications of magnetic bead assays are described in this chapter.

Fig. 3. (continued)

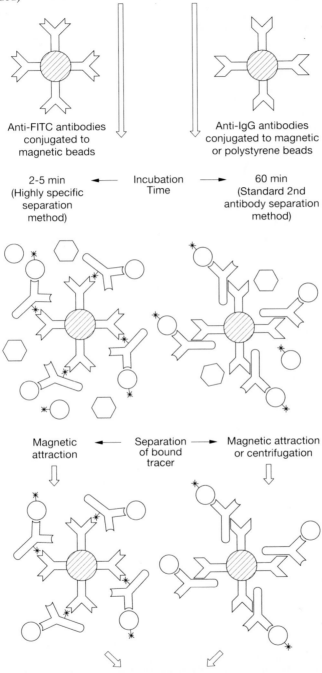

Anti-FITC antibodies
conjugated to
magnetic beads

Anti-IgG antibodies
conjugated to magnetic
or polystyrene beads

2-5 min   ◄── Incubation ──►   60 min
(Highly specific   Time   (Standard 2nd
separation   antibody separation
method)   method)

Magnetic   ◄── Separation ──►   Magnetic attraction
attraction   of bound   or centrifugation
                      tracer

Assay of bound tracer

concentration of ECM antigens and the development of disease. There is still room for the development of assays for additional analytes which might be valuable in other chronic conditions such as rheumatoid arthritis and osteoarthritis, and as markers for renal disease. General acceptance and use of these assays will depend on their ease of use, reliability, specificity and, if they are to be used as early markers, their sensitivity. The requirements for immunological assays for connective tissue antigens are as follows:

1. Good standard or calibrator required.
2. High specificity required: this can be achieved with competitive assays which are therefore preferred.
3. Highly purified and well-characterized antigens are essential for antibody production and standardization.
4. Sensitivity must be sufficient to measure the low concentrations of analytes found in body fluids and the small changes in concentration which are characteristic of pathological processes.
5. Since most of the disorders studied with these techniques are chronic in nature, the rapidity of the assay is not as important as achieving a high degree of sensitivity and specificity.
6. Both RIA and ELISA procedures can be used.

A schematic representation of a preferred procedure which best satisfies these conditions for immunological assay of ECM antigens in body fluids is illustrated in Fig. 3. The more common procedure involves the use of a standard second antibody separation procedure (right hand side). However, a rapid, highly specific separation method has been developed involving the reaction of anti-FITC with FITC. These procedures are equally applicable to ELISA or RIA and can be used for any appropriate antigen.

References

[1] R. Mayne, Collagenous Proteins of Blood Vessels. Arteriosclerosis 6, 585–593 (1986).
[2] L. Kjellen, U. Lindahl, Proteogycans: Structure and Interactions, Annu. Rev. Biochem. 60, 443–475 (1991).
[3] G. R. Martin, R. Timpl, Laminin and Other Basement Membrane Components, Annu. Rev. Cell Biol. 3, 57–85 (1987).
[4] E. Ruoslahti, Fibronectin and Its Receptors, Annu. Rev. Biochem. 57, 375–413 (1988).
[5] A. Martinez-Hernandez, Electron Immunohistochemistry of the Extracellular Matrix: An Overview, Methods Enzymol. 145, 78–102 (1987).
[6] L. Risteli, J. Risteli, Analysis of Extracellular Matrix Proteins in Biological Fluids, Methods Enzymol. 145, 391–411 (1987).
[7] E. G. Hahn, Blood Analysis for Liver Fibrosis [Review], J. Hepatol. 1, 67–73 (1984).
[8] L. Risteli, J. Risteli, Radioimmunoassay for Monitoring Connective Tissue Metabolism [Review], Rheumatology 10, 216–245 (1986).
[9] A. M. Gressner, Measurement of Connective Tissue Parameters in Serum for Diagnosis and Follow-up of Liver Fibrosis [Review], Ann. Clin. Biochem. 24, 283–292 (1987).

[10] *R. B. Clague, R. A. Brown, J. B. Weiss, P. J. Lennox-Holt, J.*, Solid-Phase Radioimmunoassay for the Detection of Antibodies to Collagen, J. Immunol. Methods *27*, 31–41 (1979).
[11] *D. J. Hartmann, J.-C. Trinchet, S. Ricard-Blum, M. Beaugrand, P. Callard, G. Ville*, Radioimmunoassay of Type I Collagen That Mainly Detects Degradation Products in Serum: Application to Patients with Liver Diseases, Clin. Chem. *36*, 421–426 (1990).
[12] *J.-P. Trinchet, D. J. Hartmann, D. Pateron, M. Laarif, P. Callard, G. Ville, M. Beaugrand*, Serum Type I and N-terminal Peptide of Type III Procollagen in Chronic Hepatitis, J. Hepatol. *12*, 139–144 (1991).
[13] *L. Risteli*, The Carboxyterminal Propeptide of Procollagen Type I (PICP) in Serum and Biological Fluids, Scand. J. Clin. Lab. Invest. *50*, 143–146 (1990).
[14] *J. Melkko, S. Niemi, L. Risteli, J. Risteli*, Radioimmunoassay of the Carboxyterminal Propeptide of Human Type I Procollagen, Clin. Chem. *36*, 1328–1332 (1990).
[15] *B. Smedsro, J. Melkko, L. Risteli, J. Risteli*, Circulating C-terminal Propeptide of Type I Procollagen Is Cleared Mainly *via* the Mannose Receptor in Liver Endothelial Cells, Biochem. J. *271*, 345–350 (1990).
[16] *J. S. Hyams, W. R. Treem, D. E. Carey, N. Wyzga, E. Eddy. B. D. Goldberg, R. E. Moore*, Comparison of Collagen Propeptides as Growth Markers in Children with Inflammatory Bowel Disease, Gastroenterol. *100*, 971–975 (1991).
[17] *P. Trivedi, J. Risteli, L. Risteli, P. Hindmarsh, C. G. D. Brook, A. Mowat*, Serum Concentrations of the Type I and III Procollagen Propeptides as Biochemical Markers of Growth Velocity in Healthy Infants and Children, and in Children with Growth Disorders, Pediatr. Res. *30* (31), 276–280 (1991).
[18] *A. S. M. Bari, S. D. Carter, S. C. Bell, K. Morgan, D. Bennett*, Anti-Type II Collagen Antibody in Naturally Occurring Canine Joint Diseases, Brit. J. Rheumatol. *28*, 480–486 (1989).
[19] *C. Chichester, H.-J. Barrach, A. Chichester, A. Matoney, G. R. Srinivas*, Evidence for Polyreactivity Seen with Monoclonal Antibodies Produced against Type II Collagen, J. Immunol. Methods *140*, 259–267 (1991).
[20] *Y. Henrotin, C. Bassleer, J. Collette, B. Nusgens, P. Franchimont*, Radioimmunoassay for Type II Collagen, J. Immunoassay *11*, 555–578 (1990).
[21] *R. Timpl, R. W. Glanville*, The Aminopropeptide of Collagen, Clin. Orthop. *158*, 224–242 (1981).
[22] *K. D. Bentsen, J. H. Henriksen, S. Boesby, K. Horsley-Peterson, I. Lorenzen*, Hepatic and Renal Extraction of Circulating Type III Procollagen Amino-Terminal Propeptide and Hyaluronan in Pig, J. Hepatol *9*, 177–183 (1989).
[23] *O. Niemela, L. Risteli, J. Parkkinen, J. Risteli*, Purification and Characterisation of the N-Terminal Propeptide of Human Type III Procollagen, Biochem. J. *232*, 145–150 (1985).
[24] *J. Risteli, S. Niemi, P. Trivedi, O. Maentiausta, A. T. Mowat, L. Risteli*, Rapid Equilibrium Radioimmunoassay for the Aminoterminal Propeptides of Type III Procollagen, Clin. Chem. *34*, 715–718 (1988).
[25] *J. A. Werkmeister, J. A. Ramshaw*, Multiple Antigenic Determinants on Type III Collagen, Biochem. J. *274*, 895–898 (1991).
[26] *A. M. Gressner*, An Evaluation of a Monoclonal Antibody Based Sandwich Radioimmunoassay for the Col 1–3 Aminoterminal Propeptide of Type III Procollagen in Serum, Clin. Chem. *36*, 1110 (1990).
[27] *H. L. Rohde, L. Vargas, E. Hahn, H. Kalbfleisch, M. Brugguera, R. Timpl*, Radioimmunoassay for Type III Collagen Peptide and Its Application to Human Liver Disease, Eur. J. Clin. Invest. *9*, 451–459 (1979).
[28] *O. Niemela, L. Risteli, E. A. Sotaniemi, J. Risteli*, Aminoterminal Propeptide of Type III Procollagen in Serum in Alcoholic Liver Disease, Gastroenterology *85*, 254–259 (1983).
[29] *R. A. A. van Zanten, R. E. van Leeuwen, J. H. P. Wilson*, Serum Procollagen III N-terminal Peptide and Laminin P1 Fragment Concentrations in Alcoholic Liver Disease and Primary Biliary Cirrhosis, Clin. Chim. Acta. *177*, 141–146 (1988).
[30] *G. Annoni, M. Colombo, M. C. Cantaluppi, B. Khlat, P. Lampertico, M. Rojkind*, Serum Type III Procollagen Peptide and Laminin (Lam-P1) Detect Alcoholic Hepatitis in Chronic Alcohol Abusers, Hepatology *9*, 693–697 (1989).

[31] *M. Schneider, K. Hengst, M. Waldendorf, B. Hogemenn, U. Gerlach,* The Value of Serum Laminin P1 in Monitoring Disease Activity in Patients with Systematic Lupus Erythematosus, Scand. J. Rheumatol. *17,* 417–422 (1988).

[32] *H. L. Rohde, I. Langer, Th. Kreig, R. Timpl,* Serum and Urine Analysis of the Aminoterminal Procollagen Peptide Type III by Radioimmunoassay with Antibody Fab Fragments, Coll. Rel. Res. *3,* 371–379 (1983).

[33] *O. Niemela, L. Risteli, E. A. Sotaniemi, F. Stenback, J. Risteli,* Serum Basement Membrane and Type III Procollagen-Related Antigens in Primary Biliary Cirrhosis, J. Hepatol. *6,* 307–314 (1988).

[34] *J. Risteli, H. Sogaard, A. Oikarinen, L. Risteli, J. Karvoen, H. Zachariae,* Aminoterminal Propeptide of Type III Procollagen in Methotrexate-Induced Liver Fibrosis and Cirrhosis, Br. J. Dermatol. *119,* 321–325 (1988).

[35] *H. Zachariae, H. Sogaard, L. Heickendorff,* Serum Aminoterminal Propeptide of Type III Procollagen, Acta Derm. Venereol. *69,* 241–244 (1989).

[36] *H. Zachariae, L. Halkier-Sorensen, L. Heickendorff,* Serum Aminoterminal Propeptide of Type III Procollagen in Progressive Systemic Sclerosis *69,* 66–70 (1989).

[37] *M. Misaki, T. Shima, Y. Yano, Y. Sumita, U. Kano, T. Murata, S. Watanabe, S. Suzuki,* Basement Membrane Related and Type III Procollagen Related Antigens in Serum of Patients with Chronic Viral Liver Disease, Clin. Chem. *36,* 522–524 (1990).

[38] *A. M. Gressner, W. Tittor, A. Negwer, K.-H. Pick-Kober,* Serum Concentrations of Laminin and Aminoterminal Propeptide of Type III Procollagen in Relation to the Portal Veinous Pressure of Fibrotic Liver Disease, Clin. Chim. Acta. *161,* 249–258 (1986).

[39] *A. M. Gressner, W. Tittor, J. Kropf,* Evaluation of Serum Aminoterminal Procollagen Type III Propeptide as an Index of Portal Hypertension and Oesophageal Varices in Chronic Liver Diseases, Clin. Chim. Acta. *174,* 163–170 (1988).

[40] *D. J. Mutimer, M. F. Bassendine, P. Kelly, O. F. W. James,* Is Measurement of Type III Procollagen Aminopropeptide Useful in Primary Biliary Cirrhosis? J. Hepatal. *9,* 184–189 (1989).

[41] *L. Risteli, U. Puistola, H. Hohtari, A. Kauppila, J. Risteli,* Collagen Metabolism in Normal and Complicated Pregnancy: Changes in the Aminoterminal Propeptide of Type III Procollagen in Serum, Eur. J. Clin. Invest. *17,* 81–86 (1987).

[42] *U. Puistola, L. Risteli, J. Risteli, A. Kauppila,* Collagen Metabolism in Gynaecologic Patients: Changes in the Concentration of the Aminoterminal Propeptide of Type III Procollagen in Serum, Am. J. Obstet. Gynecol. *163,* 1276–1281 (1990).

[43] *K. Haukipuo, L. Risteli, M. I. Kairaluoma, J. Risteli,* Aminoterminal Propeptide of Type III Procollagen in Healing Wound in Humans, Ann. Surg. *206,* 752–756 (1987).

[44] *K. D. Bentsen, C. Lanng, K. Horsley-Petersen, J. Risteli,* The Aminoterminal Propeptide of Type III Procollagen and Basement Membrane Components in Serum during Wound Healing in Man, Acta Chir. Scand. *154,* 97–101 (1988).

[45] *K. Haukipuro, L. Risteli, M. I. Kairaluoma, J. Risteli,* Aminoterminal Propeptide of Type III Procollagen in Serum during Wound Healing in Human Beings, Surgery *107,* 381–388 (1990).

[46] *P. Trivedi, P. Hindsmarsh, J. Risteli, L. Risteli, A. P. Mowat, C. G. D. Brook,* Growth Velocity, Growth Hormone Therapy, and Serum Concentrations of the Amino-Terminal Propeptide of Type III Procollagen, J. Pediatr. *114,* 225–230 (1989).

[47] *P. Tapanainen, L. Risteli, M. Knip, M.-L. Kaar, J. Risteli,* Serum Aminoterminal Propeptide of Type III Procollagen: A Potential Predictor of the Response to Growth Hormone Therapy, J. Clin. Endocrinol. Metab. *67,* 1244–1249 (1988).

[48] *P. Trivedi, J. Risteli, L. Risteli, M. S. Tanner, S. Ghave, A. N. Pandit, A. P. Mowat,* Serum Type III Procollagen and Basement Membrane Proteins as Noninvasive Markers of Hepatic Pathology in Indian Childhood Cirrhosis, Hepatology *7,* 1249–1253 (1987).

[49] *J. S. Hyams, W. R. Treem, D. E. Carey, N. Wyzga, E. Eddy, B. D. Goldberg, R. E. Moore,* Comparison of Collagen Propeptides as Growth Markers in Children with Inflammatory Bowel Disease, Gastroenterology *100,* 971–975 (1991).

[50] *J. Bonnet, P. E. Garderes, M. Aumailley, C. Moreau, G. Gouverneur, D. Benchimol, R. Crockett, L. Larrue, H. Bricaud,* Serum Type III Procollagen Peptide Levels in Coronary Artery Disease (a Marker of Atherosclerosis), Eur. J. Clin. Invest. *18,* 18–21 (1988).

[51] *L. F. Morton, M. J. Barnes,* Collagen Polymorphism in the Normal and Diseased Blood Vessel Wall, Atherosclerosis *42,* 41–51 (1982).

[52] *R. J. Butkowski, G.-Q. Shen, J. Wieslander, A. F. Michael, A. J. Fish,* Characterisation of Type IV Collagen NC1 Monomers and Goodpasture Antigen in Human Renal Basement Membranes, J. Lab. Clin. Med. *115,* 365–373 (1990).

[53] *L. Risteli, J. Risteli,* Assessment of Type IV Collagen and Laminin Metabolism by Radioimmunoassays. In: *R. G. Price, B. G. Hudson* (eds.), Renal Basement Membranes in Health and Disease, Academic Press, London 1987, pp. 219–227.

[54] *J. A. Savige, M. Gallicchio,* The Non-collagenous Domains of the Alpha 3 and 4 Chains of Type IV Collagen and Their Relationship to the *Goodpasture* Antigen, Clin. Exp. Immunol. *84,* 454–458 (1991).

[55] *M. M. Kleppel, C. Kashtan, P. A. Santi, J. Wieslander, A. F. Michael,* Distribution of Familial Nephritis Antigen in Normal Tissue and Renal Basement Membranes of Patients with Homozygous and Heterozygous *Alport* Familial Nephritis, Lab. Invest. *61,* 278–289 (1989).

[56] *R. Saxena, B. Isaksson, P. Bygren, J. Wieslander,* A Rapid Assay for Circulating Anti-glomerular Basement Membrane Antibodies in *Goodpasture* Syndrome, J. Immunol. Methods *118,* 73–78 (1989).

[57] *J. Wheeler, J. Simpson, A. R. Morley,* Routine and Rapid Enzyme Linked Immunosorbent Assays for Circulating Anti-Glomerular Basement Membrane Antibodies, J. Clin. Pathol. *41,* 163–170 (1988).

[58] *B. Hogemann, B. Voss, G. Pott, J. Rauterberg, V. Gerlach,* 7S Collagen: A Method for the Measurement of Serum Concentrations in Man, Clin. Chim. Acta *144,* 1–10 (1984).

[59] *D. Schuppan, M. Besser, R. Schwarting, E. G. Hahn,* Radioimmunoassay for the Carboxy-terminal Cross-linking Domain of Type IV (Basement Membrane) Procollagen in Body Fluids. Characterisation and Application to Collagen Type IV Metabolism in Fibrotic Liver Disease, J. Clin. Invest. *78,* 241–248 (1986).

[60] *O. Torffvit, C.-D. Agardh, B. Cederholm, J. Weislander,* A New Enzyme-Linked Immunosorbent Assay for Urine and Serum Concentration of the Carboxyterminal Domain (NC1) of Collagen IV. Application in Type I (Insulin-Dependent) Diabetes, Scand. J. Clin. Lab. Invest. *49,* 431–439 (1989).

[61] *D. G. Brocks, H. P. Neubauer, H. Strecker,* Type IV Collagen Antigens in Serum of Diabetic Rats: A Marker for Basement Membrane Collagen Biosynthesis, Diabetologia *28,* 928–932 (1985).

[62] *E. Matsumoto, G. Matsumoto, A. Ooshima, H. Kikuoka, H. Bessho, K. Miyamura, K. Nanjo,* Serum Type IV Collagen Concentrations in Diabetic Patients with Microangiopathy as Determined by Enzyme Immunoassay with Monoclonal Antibodies, Diabetes, *39,* 885–890 (1990).

[63] *F. Keller, Y. L. Ser, D. Schuppan,* Increased Type IV Collagen in Serum and Urine of Patients with Glomerulonephritis, Kidney Int. *37,* 258 (1990).

[64] *Ch. Bieglmayer, G. Hofer,* Radioimmunoassay for Immunoreactive Non-Collagenous Domain of Type IV Collagen (NC1) in Serum, J. Clin. Chem. Clin. Biochem. *27,* 163–167 (1989).

[65] *J. Gerstmeier, A. Gabrielli, D. Brocks, M. Meurer, Th. Krieg,* Levels of Basement Membrane Proteins in Sera from Patients with Progressive Systemic Scleroderma, J. Invest. Dermatol. *89,* 437 (1987).

[66] *K. Obata, K. Iwata, T. Ichida, K. Inoue, E. Matsumoto, Y. Muragaki, A. Ooshima,* One Step Sandwich Enzyme Immunoassay for Human Type IV Collagen Using Monoclonal Antibodies, Clin. Chim. Acta *181,* 293–304 (1989).

[67] *J. L. Avila, M. Rojas, G. Velazquez-Avila, M. Rieber,* Antibodies to Basement Membrane Proteins Nidogen and Laminin in Sera from Streptococcal-Related Diseases and Juvenile Rheumatoid Arthritis Patients, Clin. Exp. Immunol. *70,* 555–561 (1987).

[68] *L. Risteli, J. Risteli*, Assessment of Type IV Collagen and Laminin Metabolism by Radioimmunoassays, in: *R. G. Price, B. G. Hudson* (eds.), Renal Basement Membranes in Health and Disease, Academic Press, London 1987, pp. 219–227.

[69] *Ch. Rochliz, Ch. Hasslacher, D. G. Brocks, R. Herrmann*, Serum Concentration of Laminin, and Course of the Disease in Patients with Various Malignancies, J. Clin. Oncol. *5*, 1424–1429 (1987).

[70] *A. M. Gressner, W. Tittor, J. Kropf*, The Predictive Value of Serum Laminin for Portal Hypertension in Chronic Liver Diseases, Hepato-Gastroenterology *35*, 95–100 (1988).

[71] *K. Iwata*, One-Step Sandwich Enzyme Immunoassay for Human Laminin Using Monoclonal Antibodies, Clin. Chim. Acta *191*, 211–220 (1990).

[72] *A. Gabrielli, G. Marchegiani, S. Rupoli, G. Ansuini, D. G. Brocks, G. Danieli, R. Timpl*, Assessment of Disease Activity in Essential Cryoglobinemia by Serum Levels of a Basement Membrane Antigen, Laminin, Arthritis Rheum. *31*, 1558–1562 (1988).

[73] *M. Schneider, B. Voss, B. Hogemann, G. Eberhardt, U. Gerlach*, Evaluation of Serum Laminin P1, Procollagen-III Peptides and N-acetyl-β-glucosaminidase for Monitoring the Activity of Liver Fibrosis, Hepato-Gastroenterology *36*, 506–510 (1989).

[74] *N. G. Guseva, N. V. Anikina, R. Myllyla, L. Risteli, J. Risteli, J. V. Chochlova, K. I. Kivirikko, V. A. Nassonova*, Markers of Collagen and Basement Membrane Metabolism in Sera from Patients with Progressive Systemic Sclerosis, Rheum. Dis. *50*, 481–486 (1991).

[75] *K. Herrmann, E. Schulze, M. Heckmann, I. Schubert, M. Meurer, V. Ziegler, U. F. Haustein, J. Mehlhorn, T. H. Krieg*, Type III Collagen Aminopropeptide and Laminin P1 Levels on Serum of Patients with Silicosis-Associated and Iodiopathic Systemic Scleroderma, Br. J. Dermatol. *123*, 1–7 (1990).

[76] *M. Kluge, K. Mann, M. Dziadek, R. Timpl*, Characterization of a Novel Calcium-Binding 90-kDa Glycoprotein (BM-90) Shared by Basement Membranes and Serum. Eur. J. Biochem. *193*, 651–659 (1990).

[77] *P. Pietschmann, G. Schernthaner, C. H. Schnack, S. Gaube*, Serum Concentrations of Laminin P1 in Diabetics with Advanced Nephropathy, J. Clin. Pathol. *41*, 929–932 (1988).

[78] *S. Horikoshi, H. Koide*, Serum Laminin P1 Fragment Concentration in Renal Diseases, Clin. Chim. Acta *196*, 185–192 (1991).

[79] *R. G. Price*, Urinary Enzymes, Nephrotoxicity and Renal Disease, Toxicology *23*, 99–134 (1982).

[80] *S. N. Dixit*, Isolation, Purification and Characterisation of Intact and Pepsin Derived Fragments of Laminin from Human Placenta, Connect. Tissue Res. *14*, 31–40 (1985).

[81] *H. Shimomura, R. G. Spiro*, Studies on Macromolecular Components of Human Glomerular Basement Membrane and Alteration in Diabetes: Decreased Levels of Heparan Sulphate Proteoglycan and Laminin, Diabetes *36*, 374–381 (1987).

[82] *M. Paulsson, R. Timpl, D. Brock, H. Neubauer*, Increased Basement Membrane Heparan Sulphate Proteoglycan in the Serum of Diabetic Rats, Scand. J. Clin. Lab. Invest. *48*, 379–380 (1988).

[83] *I. Jackle-Meyer, V. Metze, B. Szukics, R. Petzoldt, H. Stolte*, Urinary Excretion of Extracellular Matrix Proteins, Laminin and Fibronectin, and *Tamm-Horsfall* Protein in Diabetes Mellitus (DM), Kidney Int. *37*, 1169 (1990).

[84] *B. Delpech, P. Bertrand, C. Maingonnat*, Immunoenzymo-Assay of Hyaluronic Acid-Hyaluronectin Interaction: Application to the Detection of Hyaluronic Acid in Serum of Normal Subjects and Cancer Patients, Anal. Biochem. *149*, 555–565 (1985).

[85] *A. Engstrom-Laurent, U. B. G. Lilja, T. C. Laurent*, Concentration of Sodium Hyaluronate in Serum, Scand. J. Clin. Lab. Invest. *45*, 497–504 (1985).

[86] *J. Kropf, A. M. Gressner, W. Tittor*, Logistic-Regression Model for Assessing Portal Hypertension by Measuring Hyaluronic Acid (Hyaluronan) and Laminin in Serum, Clin. Chem. *37*, 30–35 (1991).

[87] *H. Levesque, N. Baudot, B. Delpech, M. Vayssairat, A. Gancel, Ph. Lauret, H. Courtois*, Clinical Correlations and Prognosis Based on Hyaluronic Acid Serum Levels in Patients with Progressive Systemic Sclerosis, Br. J. Dermat. *124*, 423–428 (1991).

[88] *G. Ramadori, G. Zohrens, M. Manns, H. Rieder, H. P. Dienes, G. Hess, K.-H. Meyer zum Buschenfelde,* Serum Hyaluronate and Type III Procollagen Aminoterminal Propeptide Concentration in Chronic Liver Disease. Relationship to Cirrhosis and Disease Activity, Eur. J. Clin. Invest. *21,* 323–330 (1991).

[89] *K. Horsley-Petersen, T. Saxne, D. Haar, B. S. Thomsen, K. D. Bentsen, P. Junker, I. Lorenzen,* The Aminoterminal-Type-III Procollagen Peptide and Proteoglycans in Serum and Synovial Fluid of Patients with Rheumatoid Arthritis or Reactive Arthritis, Rheumatol. Int. *8,* 1–9 (1988).

[90] *O. Niemela, L. Risteli, E. A. Sotaniemi, F. Stenback, J. Risteli,* Serum Basement Membrane and Type III Procollagen-Related Antigens in Primary Biliary Cirrhosis, J. Hepatol. *6,* 307–314 (1988).

[91] *O. Torffvit, C.-D. Agardi, P. Alm, J. Wieslander,* Urine and Serum Levels of the Carboxyterminal Domain (NC1) of Collagen IV in Membranous Glomerulonephritis and Diabetic Nephropathy, Nephron *59,* 15–20 (1991).

[92] *J. Kropf, A. M. Gressner, K. Joseph,* Increased Laminin Concentrations in Serum Hyperthyroidism, Clin. Chem. *35,* 1540 (1989).

[93] *J. Kropf, M. Lammers, A. M. Gressner,* Monoclonal Gammopathies as a Cause of High Serum Laminin Concentrations, Clin. Chem. *36,* 390 (1990).

[94] *P. Trivedi, P. Cheesman, B. Portman, J. Hegarty, A. P. Mowat,* Variation is Serum Type III Procollagen Peptide with Age in Healthy Subjects and Its Comparative Value in the Assessment of Disease Activity in Children and Adults with Chronic Active Hepatitis, Eur. J. Clin. Invest. *15,* 69–74 (1985).

[95] *S. J. Rattle, D. R. Purnell, P. I. N. Williams, K. Siddle, G. C. Forrest,* New Separation Method for Monoclonal Immunoradiometric Assay and Its Application to Assays for Thyrotropin and Human Chorionic Gonadotrophin, Clin. Chem. *30,* 1457–1461 (1984).

[96] *B. Mattiasson, C. Borrebaeck,* Novel Approaches to Enzyme-Immunoassay, in: *E. G. Maggio* (ed.), Enzyme-immunoassay, CRC Press, Boca Raton 1980, pp. 213–248.

7 Immunoanalysis of Cell Function

7.1   Enzyme-Linked Immunospot (ELISPOT) Assays for Detection of Specific Antibody-Secreting Cells

Cecil Czerkinsky and Jonathon Sedgwick

7.1.1   General Considerations

7.1.1.1   The Choice of Method

The presence of specific antibodies in body fluids may have considerable biological and pathological significance and can be documented by a variety of techniques. These include conventional seroimmunological techniques and modern solid phase immunoassays which have gained increasing importance in the armamentarium of serologists.

The quantification of antibodies accumulated in various fluids has, however, limited value for analysing the dynamic aspects of immune responses. For instance, the precision of their analysis is influenced by the half-life and the catabolism of antibody molecules, which vary considerably among the different classes and subclasses of immunoglobulins. In addition, the suitability of these approaches for quantitative estimations of autoantibody repertoires is particularly questionable since *in vivo* absorption of self-reactive antibodies by circulating or tissue-bound autoantigens is likely to interfere with their detection. Perhaps the most obvious limitation of these analyses rests in their inability to yield information concerning the precise anatomical location(s) of antibody formation.

The analysis of antibody formation at the cellular level is considerably more informative in this respect. Immunocytochemical methods based on cytoplasmic staining of antibody-containing cells, that use antigens labelled with either a fluorochrome [1], an enzyme [2] or an isotope (autoradiography) [3], have been employed. However, such approaches are cumbersome and, more importantly, make it difficult to distinguish antibody-secreting cells (ASC) from cells that are synthesizing antibody without secreting it, or even from cells that might have internalized antibody and hence also labelled antigen.

For three decades, the haemolytic plaque-forming cell (PFC) assay [4] has been the most widely used indicator system to study antibody secretion and to analyse the regulatory mechanisms that control the expansion of ASC populations. The original technique and its numerous modifications [5–8] have been fundamental tools for the clonal analysis of antibody formation. The method offers the unique possibility of detecting individual ASC even in situations where only a few clones are activated, such as during the early period of a primary immune response or after the induction of antibody production *in vitro*. However, the applicability of the procedure has met with technical and theoretical problems, mainly inherent in the use of the haemolysis reaction as the indicator system of localized antigen-antibody reactions. The difficulties encountered in coupling many antigens to erythrocytes in order to provide lysable targets with an appropriate density of antigenic epitopes are well documented [8–11]. Moreover, the reliability of PFC assays for isotype- [5, 7, 11], allotype- [9, 12], or idiotype-specific [13, 14] determinations is largely based on theoretical predictions [5] and has been questioned in certain circumstances [10, 11, 15–18]. Further, the method does not permit quantification of antibody molecules secreted. Such information might be particularly useful when estimating the metabolic state of the cell population under study.

The limitations of traditional PFC assays have prompted a number of investigators to develop alternative approaches for studying antibody secretion at the cellular level. One such approach consists of quantifying antibodies produced and accumulated in supernatants of short-term cultures of lymphoid cells. The popularity of this approach is largely due to the availability of simple and relatively sensitive methods for the detection of antibodies such as solid phase radio-, enzyme-, or fluoro-immunoassays. However, one should be aware of the pitfalls of these types of solid phase immunoassays in the study of antibody formation at the cellular level. In particular, hybridoma technology has enabled critical evaluation and careful interpretation of solid phase immunoassay data obtained on complex biological fluids such as tissue culture supernatants. It is now apparent that the accuracy of these assays for class- and subclass-specific determinations is critically influenced by phenomena of competition between antibody populations belonging to distinct isotypes and/or expressing different affinities for binding to solid phase antigen. In addition, the threshold of sensitivity of these assays, although rather low, limits their use in situations where relatively few cells are producing antibodies. Most importantly, these procedures do not enable an estimation of the frequency of the corresponding ASC, and thus do not permit analyses of antibody production to be performed at the clonal level.

More recently, an alternative strategy based also on solid phase immunoassay technology has been developed for enumerating specific ASC [19, 20]. The method, termed enzyme-linked immunospot (ELISPOT) assay, is a modification of the classical ELISA [21] that allows localized antigen-antibody reactions to be visualized in the immediate vicinity of individual ASC. *In situ* ELISA quantification of secreted antibodies can be performed in parallel with the detection of ASC [22, 23].

7.1.1.2   Application

The ELISPOT technique is, in principle, applicable to the detection of cells secreting antibodies against any antigen, soluble or particulate, that can be adsorbed (directly or indirectly) onto a solid surface. The method can be employed to detect ASC in cell suspensions prepared from a variety of animal species and from different anatomic compartments. The cells can be tested either directly following collection or after exposure *in vitro* to a mitogen or to an antigen. Since its original description, the ELISPOT assay has been used to detect both animal and human cells secreting antibodies against a variety of soluble as well as particulate antigens.

Soluble antigens

Proteins: a variety of soluble protein antigens have been successfully used in the ELISPOT test to detect corresponding ASC in animal systems. These include prototype antigens such as chicken and bovine albumins [19, 20]. Purified bacterial protein antigens such as tetanus toxoid [24, 25], cholera toxin [26], and *Streptococcus mutans* surface protein antigen I/II [27] have been used to enumerate corresponding ASC in rodents and in humans.

The technique is particularly valuable for the study of autoantibody repertoires and has been used to evaluate the size and organ distribution of cell populations secreting autoantibodies against a variety of soluble protein autoantigens such as the Fc portion of immunoglobulin G (for detection of rheumatoid factor-secreting cells) [28, 29], thyroglobulin [30], and collagen [31].

Polysaccharides: several carbohydrate antigens have been used as solid phase antigens in the ELISPOT assay. For example, specific ASC against bacterial polysac-charides have been detected by the ELISPOT technique [27, 32, 33].

Nucleic acids: specific ASC to single stranded or double stranded DNA have been detected in high numbers in the spleens of certain autoimmune mouse strains by the ELISPOT method [34].

Haptens: chemically defined haptens covalently coupled to a hydrophobic carrier protein, e.g. albumin, have been employed as solid phase antigens in the ELISPOT assay to detect corresponding ASC in mice and rats [30, 35].

Complex antigenic preparations: soluble extracts consisting of multiple antigenic compounds have been used in the ELISPOT technique. Thus, crude parasite extracts from *Ascaris suum* [30], *Schistosoma mansoni* [36], whole lymphocytic choriomeningitis virus [37] and vesicular stomatitis virus [38] have been employed as coats for enumerating corresponding ASC in rodents and in humans.

Particulate antigens

The ELISPOT method can be adapted to enumerate cells secreting specific antibodies to particulate antigens. The use of hydrophilic glass surfaces in combination with polyaldehyde fixatives and/or poly-L-lysine has been described to adsorb sheep erythrocytes and *Escherichia coli* whole bacteria, providing suitable solid phases for detection of corresponding ASC [33]. Others [39] have reported successful detection of human peripheral blood ASC using direct adsorption of *Salmonella typhimurium* whole bacteria to polystyrene wells.

The above examples attest to the versatility of the method. It should be mentioned that "reverse" modifications of the ELISPOT technique using surfaces coated with antibodies [40, 41] or other ligands can be used to detect virtually any cell, eukaryotic or prokaryotic, secreting a given metabolite provided (a) the product is antigenic, (b) that it is secreted in sufficient quantities, and (c) the corresponding antibodies are available. Examples of antigen-secreting cells detected by this modification include lymphocytes secreting immunoglobulins irrespective of antigenic specificity [40, 41], fibronectin-secreting cells [42] and toxin-producing bacteria [43]. More recently, reverse modifications of the ELISPOT assay have been developed to enumerate lymphokine-producing cells [44, 45] (cf. 7.2).

7.1.1.3 Advantages of Enzyme Assays for Enumerating ASC

Using the appropriate enzyme-labelled antiglobulin conjugate, the assay allows for detection of cells secreting antibodies of a given isotype, allotype, or even idiotype [46, 47]. The sensitivity of this method is at least equal to that of conventional PFC assays [19, 20] and permits the detection of extremely small numbers of ASC such as IgE ASC in immunized rodents [48], or specific ASC in cultures of human peripheral blood lymphocytes stimulated *in vitro* with antigen [24].

The ELISPOT assay is an example of a methodological principle in which indicator enzymes cannot be replaced advantageously by radioactive isotopes. It is based on the reaction of antibody secreted by individual lymphoid cells with solid phase antigen. The antibody itself is detected by its reactivity with antiimmunoglobulin antibodies. Therefore, as in the classical indirect immunofluorescence reaction, the method makes use of the antigen-binding capacity of the antibody and its antigenic properties.

The ELISPOT method is designed for the enumeration of individual cells secreting antibodies. It is proposed as an advantageous alternative to the well-known haemolytic plaque-forming cell assay [4]. The latter method is the only comparable technique, as discussed above.

7.1.2 ELISPOT Assays

7.1.2.1 Method Design

The technique described here (Fig. 7) is a typical enzyme-linked immunospot (ELISPOT) assay.

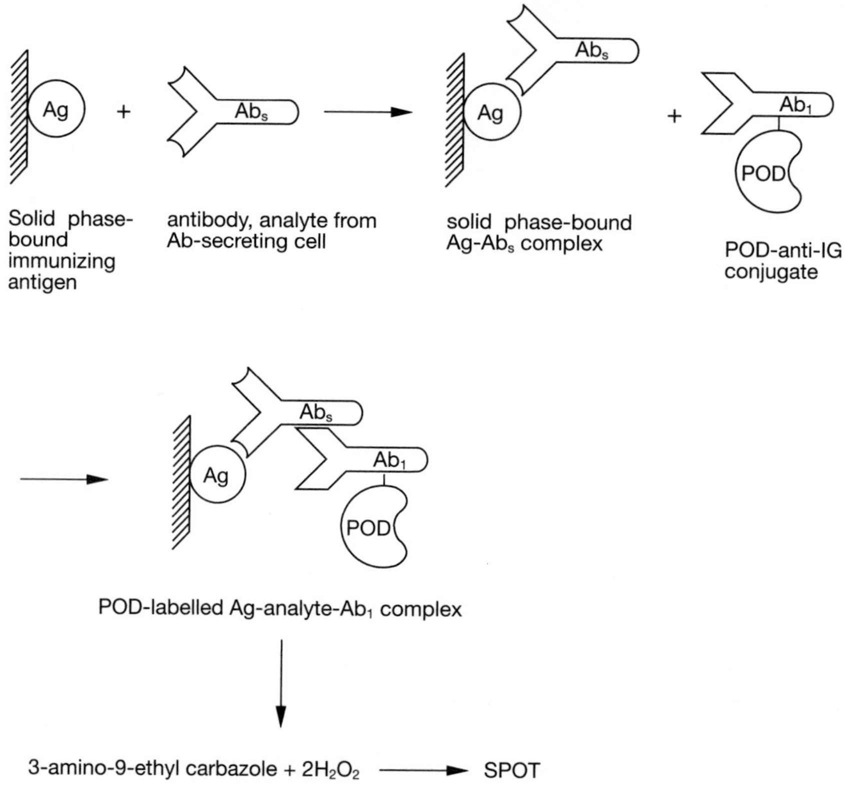

Solid phase-bound immunizing antigen

antibody, analyte from Ab-secreting cell

solid phase-bound Ag-Ab$_s$ complex

POD-anti-IG conjugate

POD-labelled Ag-analyte-Ab$_1$ complex

3-amino-9-ethyl carbazole + 2H$_2$O$_2$ ⟶ SPOT

Fig. 1. Principle of the ELISPOT assay; reaction scheme. Alkaline phosphatase (AP) together with appropriate substrate can be used in place of peroxidase (POD).

A single cell suspension containing putative ASC, e.g., spleen cells from an immunized mouse, is incubated for a few hours at 37 °C in nitrocellulose- or plastic-based vessels whose inner surface has previously been coated with the appropriate antigen. Following removal of the cells, zones of secreted antibodies bound to the solid phase are revealed by stepwise addition of enzyme-labelled antiglobulin conjugate and a suitable enzyme substrate yielding an insoluble coloured product. Coloured foci or spots that can be seen by the naked eye appear at the former location of specific ASC and are accurately enumerated under low magnification (Fig. 2). The indicator enzymes used in the assay are horseradish peroxidase (POD) (EC 1.11.1.7) or alkaline phosphatase (AP) (EC 3.1.3.1) which can be conjugated with antibodies. The conjugated antibodies are used in direct or in indirect techniques that are identical to those described for conventional solid phase ELISA. The indicator reaction depends on the interaction of numerous molecules of substrate with a limited number of enzyme molecules bound to the solid phase. The enzyme-substrate complexes formed react with a chromogenic electron donor to yield a visible coloured product that precipitates onto the solid phase.

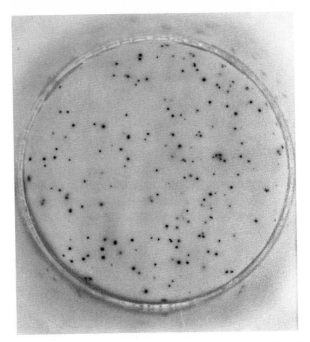

Fig. 2. Typical appearance of ASC spots on a nitrocellulose-bottomed well developed by the ELISPOT technique ($\times$ 40). Spots on plastic surfaces are similar in appearance but somewhat larger and more diffuse.

The original assays employed POD and the substrate 1,4-benzenediamine (*p*-phenylenediamine) /H_2O_2 [19] or AP together with the substrate 5-bromo-4-chloro-3-indolyl phosphate (BCIP) [20] as the detection systems. Both forms of the ELISPOT assay were conducted in plastic-based vessels and the substrate was incorporated into agarose. More recently, 3-amino-9-ethylcarbazole (AEC)/H_2O_2 has been used as the indicator system of POD-based ELISPOT assays in conjunction with nitrocellulose membranes [44]. On such nitrocellulose supports, the sensitivity of the AEC/H_2O_2 substrate system has proved to be far superior to that of other POD-chromogen substrates such as 3,3'-diaminobenzidine, 3,3',5,5'-tetramethylbenzidine and 4-chloro-1-naphthol. In addition, and at variance with 1,4-benzenediamine (the chromogen of choice in POD-based ELISPOT assays performed on plastic surfaces), the AEC/H_2O_2 substrate system does not need to be added as a gel overlay. Note that the BCIP substrate when used in conjunction with a nitrocellulose support can be added without incorporation into agarose [49]. Furthermore, incorporation of nitroblue tetrazolium (NBT) into the BCIP substrate has been shown to increase the sensitivity of AP-based ELISPOT assays [33].

A micromodified two-colour ELISPOT technique that utilizes AEC/H_2O_2 and BCIP as indicator systems of POD and AP, respectively, has been developed [49]. This bichromatic variation makes use of appropriate combinations of POD- and AP-conjugated antiglobulins with distinct specificities and permits the simultaneous detection of distinct types, e. g. isotypes, of ASC (cf. 7.1.3.3).

In the following, a detailed description is given of the standard ELISPOT technique for enumerating mouse spleen cells secreting specific antibodies to a prototype protein antigen, keyhole limpet haemocyanin (KLH). The description concentrates on the use of nitrocellulose-based vessels. Important aspects and specific features of ELISPOT assays employing plastic-based vessels (which are considerably less expensive) are considered in another section (cf. 7.1.3.1).

7.1.2.2   Selection and Adaptation of Assay Conditions

Coating

The adsorption of most macromolecules in solution onto solid surfaces involves random hydrophobic interactions between solid phase and solute. The statistical representation of a given antigenic epitope in the vicinity of a secreting cell can limit the number of specific binding sites geographically accessible to the corresponding secreted antibodies. Thus, a high epitope density would tend to concentrate greater numbers of specific antibody molecules, resulting in stronger reactions. Conversely, a lower epitope density would tend to reduce the surface concentration of the corresponding antibodies, giving rise to comparatively fainter reactions which are then more difficult to detect. In addition, the binding, and more importantly, the retention of antibodies with low affinity can be affected at low epitope density [35] (cf. also Inhibition, 7.1.4.3). Bearing this in mind, it will be clear that accurate determination of the antigen concentration required to achieve appropriate coating of the assay vessel is of paramount importance. In general, antigen concentrations required to achieve appropriate coating in the ELISPOT assay are higher than those required in a corresponding ELISA. The following general points are relevant to most antigens when optimal conditions for coating of the assay vessels are to be determined.

1. The assay dish must be hydrophobic. The more hydrophobic, the lower the antigen concentration required to achieve suitable coating. Nitrocellulose membranes are recommended as the solid phase carrier system since they display a higher binding capacity for most proteins as compared to plastic surfaces [50, see also 7.1.3].
2. The optimal coating concentration may differ from one type of antigen to another and therefore should be determined by experimentation. Concentrations ranging from 1 µg/ml to 20 µg/ml are suitable for most protein antigens.
3. Complex antigenic preparations are generally less suitable than purified antigens. Indeed, nitrocellulose-adsorbable molecules might compete with each other for binding to the solid surface, decreasing the representation of relatively less hydrophobic molecules or even preventing their binding without necessarily being more relevant biologically.
4. Poorly hydrophobic antigens, e. g. haptens, carbohydrates, lipids and nucleic acids, can be covalently coupled to a hydrophobic carrier, e. g., protein or poly-L-lysine,

prior to being used for coating. A variation on this latter theme is to coat the solid phase with low amounts of avidin and use this to capture biotinylated antigen [51, 52].

5. The coating material should not react with the enzyme-labelled conjugate employed and *vice versa*. Such an eventuality will result in complete darkening of the developed dish and will require appropriate absorption of the conjugate.

Cell incubation

1. Culture medium: the use of solid media, e.g. agar or agarose, or of a semisolid medium, e.g. carboxymethylcellulose, is not necessary if the cells are cultured in small volumes, i.e. 50 to 100 μl per assay vessel of about 70, mm² of surface area. Larger volumes are generally associated with decreased definition and poorer distribution of the reactions. A suitable standard assay culture medium consists of Hepes- and carbonate-buffered *Iscove's* medium supplemented with 10% (v/v) serum. Other commonly used media such as *Eagle's* minimal essential medium, *Hank's* balanced salt solution, *Dulbecco's* medium or RPMI 1640 are also suitable.

2. Cell density: should be determined by experimentation and adjusted so that the cells form a non-confluent monolayer. Too many ASC might give rise to partial confluence of the reactions generated, which are then impossible to enumerate with accuracy. Thus, care should be taken when choosing optimal cell densities since considerable variations may be observed among individual animals or subjects. It is convenient to assay most lymphoid cell suspensions at 3 to 4 different densities (serial 4-fold dilutions above and below the expected optimum density) to provide a margin of safety if there are unexpectedly high or low numbers of spot-forming cells.

3. Incubation time: culture periods of 3 to 4 hours are suitable for most mouse and human lymphoid cells. Prolonging the incubation time does not substantially affect the number of detectable spots but may increase their diameter.

4. Plating conditions: the assay-culture vessels must be left absolutely undisturbed throughout the cell incubation period in order to prevent cell movement. The plates should be incubated at 37 °C on a horizontal surface in a cell incubator free from vibrations. The atmosphere should be supplied with 5–10% CO_2 if a bicarbonate-buffered medium is employed.

Enzymatic indicator reaction

1. Specificity of anti-immunoglobulin preparations: the immunological reactivity of unconjugated and/or enzyme-conjugated antiglobulins to be used in the ELISPOT test should first be evaluated by block titrations against purified immunoglobulin preparations, preferably myeloma proteins. Conventional solid-phase ELISA and immuno-dot techniques are adequate for this purpose. The specificity of the antiglobulin preparations should further be documented in the ELISPOT test by

inhibition experiments (cf. 7.1.4). Where necessary, the preparations can be rendered monospecific by absorption against the appropriate insolubilized proteins.

2. Working dilutions: the optimal dilution of any reagent to be used during the immunoenzyme procedure must be determined by chess-board titrations. Dilutions of the reagents yielding the strongest reactions while still producing no or low background are selected for use in the ELISPOT test.

3. Enzyme: protein ratio of the conjugates: several commercial preparations have proved to be unsatisfactory for use in the ELISPOT test because of inadequate conjugation. The molar ratio of enzyme to immunoglobulin appears to be critical, particularly when using direct techniques, and varies according to the method employed for conjugating enzymes with immunoglobulins. For instance, POD conjugates obtained by the two-step glutaraldehyde method [53] exhibit a uniform 1:1 ratio of POD to immunoglobulin whereas conjugates prepared by the sodium periodate method [54] retain higher antibody and enzyme activities and exhibit a higher POD to immunoglobulin molar ratio (1:1 up to 4:1). Thus, whenever possible, the latter conjugates should be preferred for use in the ELISPOT test.

7.1.2.3   Equipment

Vibration-free incubator set at 37 °C (the atmosphere should be saturated with water); if a bicarbonate-buffered medium is used, the atmosphere should be supplied with 5–10% CO_2 in air.

Level platform.

Nitrocellulose bottomed (0.22 µm pore size) 96-well microplates (HA type; *Millipore,* Bedford, MA) or cellulose acetate bottomed (pore size 0.2 µm or 0.8µm) 8-well filter strips (*Costar,* Cambridge, MA).

Stereomicroscope connected with a white light source.

Scissors, forceps, syringes and nylon nets to prepare lymphoid cells from animal organs.

Balances to weigh animal organs (if required).

7.1.2.4   Reagents and Solutions

Purity of reagents: chemicals should be of analytical grade. 3-Amino-9-ethylcarbazole (*Sigma Chemical Company,* St. Louis, MO, or *Aldrich Chemical Company,* Milwaukee, WI) should be stored dry in the dark; 5-bromo-4-chloro-3-indolyl phosphate (toluidine salt) (BCIP) (*Bio-Rad Laboratories,* Richmond, CA) and p-nitroblue tetrazolium chloride (NBT) (e.g. from *Bio-Rad*) must be stored desiccated at -20 °C. Hydrogen peroxide (H_2O_2), 30% (w/v) stock solution, is stored at 4 °C in the dark.

Preparations of solutions: use only repurified water.

1. Fetal bovine serum (FBS):

   available from several commercial sources e.g. *Gibco Europe,* Paisley, U.K. Heat-inactivate at 56 °C for 45 min, aliquot and store at or below −20 °C.

2. Assay culture medium (Hepes, 25 mmol/l; NaHCO$_3$, 36 mmol/l; FBS, 5% (v/v); pH 7.43):

   prepare under sterile conditions; to 90 ml *Iscove's* medium (e.g. from *Gibco*) containing Hepes 25 mmol/l and NaHCO$_3$ 3.024 g/l, add 5 ml FBS (1).

3. Phosphate-buffered saline (PBS); phosphates, 10 mmol/l; NaCl, 0.15 mol/l; pH 7.2):

   dissolve 13.8 g Na$_2$HPO$_4$ · 2 H$_2$O, 3.6 g NaH$_2$PO$_4$ · 2 H$_2$O and 90 g NaCl in 10 l water.

4. Coating solution (phosphates, 10 mmol/l; NaCl, 0.15 mol/l; keyhole limpet haemocyanin, 10 mg/l):

   dissolve 0.1 mg keyhole limpet haemocyanin (e.g. from *Calbiochem-Behring,* San Diego, CA) in 10 ml PBS (3). Aliquot and store at or below −20 °C.

5. PBS/Tween (phosphates, 10 mmol/l; NaCl, 0.15 mol/l; Thimerosal, 0.1 g/l; Tween 20, 0.5 ml/l; pH 7.2):

   add 5 ml Tween 20 to 10 l PBS (3); add 1 g Thimerosal.

6. PBS/Tween/FBS (phosphate, 10 mmol/l; NaCl, 0.15 mol/l; Thimerosal, 0.1 g/l; Tween 20, 0.5 ml/l; FBS, 1%; pH 7.2):

   add 1 ml FBS (1) to 100 ml PBS/Tween (5).

7. PBS/EDTA (phosphate, 10 mmol/l; NaCl, 0.15 mol/l; EDTA, 50 mmol/l; pH 7.2):

   dissolve 18.61 g EDTA-Na$_2$H$_2$ · 2 H$_2$O in 1 l PBS (3); adjust pH to 7.4 with NaOH 0.1 mol/l.

8. Citrate-phosphate buffer (C$_6$H$_8$O$_7$, 0.1 mol/l; Na$_2$HPO$_4$, 0.2 mol/l; pH 5.0):

   dissolve 10.19 g C$_6$H$_8$O$_7$ · H$_2$O and 18.06 g Na$_2$HPO$_4$ · 2 H$_2$O in about 800 ml of water; if necessary, adjust pH to 5.0 by adding citric acid or sodium phosphate and bring to 1 l with water.

9. Carbonate buffer (NaHCO$_3$, 0.1 mol/l; MgCl$_2$, 5 mmol/l; pH 9.8):

   dissolve 8.40 g of NaHCO$_3$ and 1.05 g MgCl$_2$ · 6H$_2$O in 600 ml water. Adjust pH to 9.8 with NaOH 0.1 mol/l and bring final volume to 1 l with water.

10. POD chromogen/substrate solution (citrate, 0.1 mol/l; phosphate, 0.2 mol/l; 3-amino-9-ethylcarbazole, 1.5 mmol/l; H$_2$O$_2$, 4.5 mmol/l; pH 5.0):

    dissolve 30 mg 3-amino-9-ethylcarbazole (AEC) in a minimum volume of dimethylformamide (approx. 500 µl); add 90 ml citrate-phosphate buffer (8) and filter (0.45 µm) the solution to remove particulate matter (the solution becomes colourless). Add 15 µl of 30% H$_2$O$_2$ and use immediately.

11. AP chromogen substrate/solution (NaHCO$_3$, 0.1 mol/l; MgCl$_2$, 5 mmol/l; 5-bromo-4-chloro-3-indolyl phosphate, 0.35 mmol/l; p-nitroblue tetrazolium chloride, 0.35 mmol/l; pH 9.8):

    dissolve separately 15 mg 5-bromo-4-chloro-3-indolyl phosphate (BCIP) and 30 mg p-nitroblue tetrazolium chloride (NBT) in a small volume of dimethylformamide (ca. 0.5 ml for each reagent); mix both reagents and add to 99 ml of carbonate buffer (9). Filter (0.45 µm) the solution to remove particulate matter (the solution remains pale yellow).

12. Enzyme-labelled reagents (> 1 mg/l; POD, > 50 kU/l; AP, ca. 1.5 kU/l):

    unconjugated, POD-, and AP-conjugated rabbit anti-mouse immunoglobulin reagents can be purchased commercially, e.g. from *Dakopatts* (Copenhagen, Denmark); affinity purified goat anti-mouse IgG (Fc fragment specific) and goat anti-mouse IgM (Fc fragment specific) conjugated with either POD or AP can be purchased from, e.g. from *Southern Biotechnology Associates,* Birmingham, AL, USA.

13. Rabbit POD-anti-POD (PAP) and AP-anti-AP (APAAP) immune complexes:

    use commercial preparations, e.g. from *Dakopatts.*

14. Unconjugated, POD-, and AP-anti-rabbit immunoglobulin conjugates:

    use commercial preparations, e.g. swine anti-rabbit immunoglobulins from *Dakopatts.*

15. POD- and AP-avidin conjugates:

    use commercial preparations, e.g. streptavidin from *Dakopatts* or from *Vector Laboratories, Inc.,* Burlingame, CA, or Extravidin© from *Sigma;* avidin/biotinylated POD complexes (ABC complexes) can be purchased from the same commercial sources.

16. Biotinylated antibodies (IgG, ca. 1 mg/l):

    biotinylated goat anti-mouse immunoglobulins are prepared according to the procedure described in Appendix 5 (cf. 7.1.5.5) or can be purchased, e.g. from *Southern Biotechnology,* Goat anti-POD antibodies can be purchased from, e.g. *Dakopatts,* and should be biotinylated (see Appendix 5).

    Dilute reagents (12) to (16) before use in PBS/Tween/FBS (6) to a previously determined concentration (cf. 7.1.2.2).

17. Tris-buffered ammonium chloride (NH₄Cl, 0.14 mol/l; Tris, 17 mmol/l; pH 7.45):

    dissolve 7.47 g NH₄Cl and 2.06 g Tris in 800 ml water; adjust pH to 7.45 with 0.1 mol/l HCl and bring volume to 1 l with water.

18. Tris buffer (Tris base, 0.05 mol/l; NaCl 0.15 mol/l; pH 8.0):

    dissolve 61 g Tris base and 90 g NaCl in 950 ml water; adjust pH to 8.0 with HCl 1 mol/l; make up with water to 10 l.

19. Coated plates: prepare according to Appendix (cf. 7.1.5.2).

Stability of reagents and solutions: 3-amino-9-ethylcarbazole is stable for several years at room temperature, if kept in the dark. FBS (1) can be kept frozen (−70 °C) for several years. Assay culture medium (2) can be kept for several weeks at 4 °C if prepared under sterile conditions and kept protected from light. Solutions (3 to 9, and 18) are stable for several weeks unless contaminated. POD chromogen-substrate solution (10) must be prepared immediately before use. AP chromogen substrate solution (11) is stable for one week if kept at 4 °C protected from light. Immunochemicals (12 to 15) can be stored at 4 °C in the dark for several months. Biotinylated antiimmunoglobulins (16) and unconjugated avidin can be stored at −70 °C for several years. Tris-buffered ammonium chloride solution (17) is stable for several weeks when kept in the dark at 4 °C. Coated plates (19) can be stored for up to three weeks at 4 °C providing a bacteriostatic agent, e.g. Thimerosal (0.1 g/l) has been added to the coating solution (4). Alternatively, coated plates can be stored frozen at −20 °C for several months.

7.1.2.5 Procedure

Collection and treatment of specimen: for immunization and preparation of spleen single cell suspensions, use standard inbred mice, e.g. C57BL/6, CBA, Balb/c, C3H/He, 10–20 weeks old, which are primed with an intraperitoneal injection of KLH (100 µg) emulsified in *Freund's* complete adjuvant (which can be purchased from e.g. *Difco,* Detroit, MI, USA or *Sigma*). One to three weeks later, challenge the animals with a similar injection and sacrifice 4–5 days later. Single cell suspensions are prepared from the spleens (cf. Appendix 7.1.5.1) and assayed for numbers of KLH-specific ASC by the ELISPOT test.

Stability of the analyte in the sample: cells should be processed immediately or cryopreserved.

Assay conditions: prepare 3 to 4 sets of duplicate wells for 1 sample, each set corresponding to 1 cell density.

Cell incubation: for 3 to 4 h at 37 °C.

Immunoreaction: incubation for 2 h at room temperature (or overnight at 4 °C).

Enzymatic indicator reaction: incubate for 3 to 20 min.

Measurement

The assay consists of five stages: first, the preparation of a solid phase immunoadsorbent, then the cell incubation stage, followed by the immunoenzyme reaction stage. The fourth stage consists of adding a chromogenic enzyme substrate which will eventually yield an insoluble coloured product. The corresponding spots are enumerated in the final stage.

Preparation of the antigen-coated dishes

1. Prepare nitrocellulose-bottomed dishes coated with KLH (19) as described in Appendix 2 (cf. 7.1.5.2).
2. To prevent the solid phase from drying and to saturate remaining binding sites on the solid phase, expose the wells for 1 h at 37 °C to 50 µl of assay culture medium (2).

Cell incubation

1. Disperse in each set of antigen-coated wells 50 µl of assay-culture medium (2) containing an appropriate number of cells (e.g. $2 \cdot 10^5$, $5 \cdot 10^4$, $1.25 \cdot 10^4$).
2. Incubate the dishes for 3 to 4 h at 37 °C on a level surface in a 10% CO_2 humified atmosphere.
3. At the completion of the culture period, recover the cells for other purposes or discard them.
4. Rinse the plates three times with PBS (3) by flicking.
5. If necessary elute remaining adherent cells from the solid phase by immersing the plates in a container filled with chilled PBS/EDTA solution (7) for 10 min under continuous shaking.

6. Wash the plates 4 additional times with PBS/Tween (5) by flicking and keep the plates immersed in this solution for 5 min.
7. Empty the wells of wash buffer and carefully dry the outer surface of the nitrocellulose membrane with absorbent paper towels. Fill the wells immediately with 50 μl of PBS/Tween/FBS (6), in order to prevent the membranes from drying.

Immunoreaction

1. After the cell incubation, pipette into individual wells 50 μl of POD-conjugated rabbit anti-mouse immunoglobulin conjugate (12) diluted (usually 1:100–1:300) in PBS/Tween/FBS (6).
2. Incubate for 2 h at room temperature or overnight at 4 °C (whichever is more convenient).
3. Wash 5 times with PBS/Tween (5) to remove unbound POD-antiglobulins and 3 times with PBS (3).
4. Immerse plates in PBS (3) for 5 min.
5. Empty the wells of wash buffer by flicking and carefully blot-dry the outer surface of the nitrocellulose membranes with clean absorbent towel.

Enzymatic indicator reaction

1. Pipette into each well, 0.1 ml of POD chromogen substrate solution (10). After 1–3 min, reddish spots, recognizable by the naked eye begin to appear. These reactions correspond to the former position of individual ASC (Fig. 2).
2. Plates are allowed to incubate for a variable time and up to 10 min.. Note: as excessive background staining may result from over-long incubation, it is important during this time to monitor control wells, i.e., coated wells treated exactly as above but not exposed previously to cells.
3. Wash thoroughly with running tap water and dry plates as above.

Note: developed plates can be stored for several days at ambient temperature before being counted. However, the characteristic appearance of the spots may alter with time, rendering their enumeration more difficult. Alternatively, freshly developed dishes can be kept immersed in tap water allowing the count to be performed whenever convenient.

Enumeration procedure

Although spots begin to appear within minutes after addition of POD chromogen substrate, their number and their intensity are maximal by approximately 5–10 min. They can then be enumerated under low magnification.

Counting: count spots under low magnification ($\times$ 40 to $\times$ 200) under direct illumination. A stereomicroscope equipped with a bifocal white light source is ideal for this purpose.

Appearance of spots: macroscopically, spots are defined as circular, homogeneous and well-individualized red foci. The colour intensity of these reactions varies from orange to dark red. Their diameter also varies, ranging from 0.01 mm to 0.1 mm, rarely larger. There is no relationship between a given isotype of immunoglobulin secreted and a particular pattern of spots. However, differences in the appearance of spots may reflect heterogeneity in the secretion rate of individual cells and/or differences in the affinity of antibody populations secreted [19, 30]. Under low magnification ($\times$ 100 to $\times$ 200), spots exhibit a typical granular appearance. These reactions appear in continuity with the background. The latter feature is the most useful criterion to distinguish true spots from falsely positive reactions that might occasionally be observed. Such artefacts appear as non-circular and non-homogeneously pigmented reactions or as dark granules consisting of precipitates or crystals of enzyme-substrate reaction products which emerge above the background stain (cf. 7.1.4).

Note: computer assisted image-analysing devices can also be employed to allow semi- or fully automated counting (cf. 5.9).

Expression of results: from the total number of spots counted in a well or on a set of replicate wells, relate the results to an arbitrary number of nucleated or mononuclear cells, e. g. 10^6 or 10^7 cells and express data as spot-forming cell (SFC) numbers per 10^6 or 10^7 cells, respectively. Alternatively, estimate the total number of SFC for a given lymphoid organ. Background values, i. e. SFC numbers counted in control wells (cf. 7.1.4), should be substracted from the total number of SFC estimated in test wells.

7.1.3   Alternative Techniques

7.1.3.1   ELISPOT Assays Employing Plastic-based Vessels

As mentioned above, plastic supports for the ELISPOT were first used [19, 20]. The principle advantage of plastic over nitrocellulose is the considerably lower cost. There are a number of technical aspects which distinguish the two forms of the ELISPOT assay and these are considered below.

Principle and method design

Essentially as described above but with a solid phase of plastic as opposed to nitrocellulose membrane.

Assay conditions

Identical to those of nitrocellulose-based ELISPOT assays, including cell incubation conditions, immunoreaction and enumeration procedure (cf. 7.1.2.5). Two important specific features should, however, be considered.

1. Coating: a successful outcome of an ELISPOT procedure is dependent on the attainment of a sufficiently high concentration of antigen on the solid phase and, compared with nitrocellulose, plastic surfaces are relatively poor in their absorptive characteristics. Generally speaking, low molecular weight molecules (ovalbumin for example) coat poorly and high concentrations are required, whereas high molecular-weight complex molecules such as thyroglobulin or KLH can be effectively coated at lower concentrations. Thus for KLH, coating concentrations for plastic surfaces are in the order of 50 to 200 µg/ml [30]. Clearly, most of this will not be adsorbed and it is likely that it is the aggregates of antigen present in this concentrated solution that are of particular importance [30].

   Immunoglobulins can be adsorbed at concentrations around 10 µg/ml even on plastic surfaces [44, 48] so the use of capture antibody, for example to bind a specific antigen and to use this as the solid phase to which cells are added, may be of value.

2. Enzymatic indicator reaction: the localization of spots of insoluble substrate product on nitrocellulose supports is clearly evident when the substrate is added in solution without agarose. This is the case for both the AEC/H_2O_2 and BCIP/NBT systems. *With a plastic solid phase, several POD substrates including AEC/H_2O_2 and 4-chloro-1-naphthol cannot be employed* as the reactions generated are too faint to be visualized. The use of 1,4-benzenediamine /H_2O_2 is recommended in POD-based ELISPOT assays performed on plastic surfaces. The chromogenic substrate 1,4-benzenediamine/H_2O_2 must always be incorporated in agarose. While the substrate BCIP/NBT can be employed in AP-based ELISPOT assays performed on plastic surfaces and can be visualized even without an agarose support, definition is poor and it is advisable to incorporate agarose to aid in product localization.

Equipment

Incubators and viewing apparatus as above. 24-well (16 mm inner diameter) polystyrene plates, preferably *non-tissue culture grade* (e.g. from *Sterilin*, United Kingdom or *Nunc*, Denmark) can be used; a useful alternative is to use the shallow rings of the lid of 24-well polystyrene plates as assay culture vessels. Smaller formats are not recommended. Water bath set at around 40 °C.

Procedure

Preparation of the assay-dishes

1. Prepare polystyrene dishes coated with KLH (19) as described in 7.1.5.3.
2. To prevent the solid phase from drying and to saturate remaining binding sites on the solid phase, expose the wells for 1 h at 37 °C to 0.1 ml of assay culture medium (2).

Cell incubation

1. Decant the wells carefully, e.g. by aspiration with a *Pasteur* pipette.
2. Add immediately to each set of antigen-coated wells 0.1 ml assay-culture medium (2) containing an appropriate number of cells (e.g., $2 \cdot 10^5$, $5 \cdot 10^4$, $1.25 \cdot 10^4$).
3. Incubate the dishes *undisturbed* for 3 to 4 h at 37 °C on a level surface in a 10% CO_2 humidified atmosphere.
4. At the completion of the culture period, recover the cells for other purposes or discard them.
5. Rinse the plates three times with PBS (3) by flicking.
6. If necessary elute the remaining adherent cells from the solid phase by immersing the plates in a container filled with chilled PBS/EDTA solution (7) for 10 min under continuous shaking.
7. Wash the plates 4 additional times with PBS/Tween (5) by flicking.
8. Keep the plates immersed in this solution for 5 min.

Immunoreaction

1. Empty carefully the wells of wash buffer with a *Pasteur* pipette. Fill the wells immediately with 0.1 ml of PBS/Tween/FBS (6) containing appropriately diluted (usually 1:100–1:500) POD- or AP-conjugated rabbit anti-mouse immunoglobulin conjugate (12).
2. Incubate for 2 h at room temperature or overnight at 4 °C (whichever is more convenient).
3. Wash 5 times with PBS/Tween (5) to remove unbound enzyme-labelled antiglobulins and 3 times with PBS (3).
4. Immerse plates in PBS (3) for 5 min.
5. Empty the wells of wash buffer by flicking.

Enzymatic indicator reaction

1. Place the plates to be developed on a stable level surface.
2. Pipette into each well, 0.1 ml of agarose substrate solution which is prepared according to the Appendix (cf. 7.1.5.4).
3. Remove excess agarose substrate immediately by aspirating the content of the wells; this will leave an ultra thin layer of gel which will prevent spontaneous darkening of the substrate.

4. When employing *p*-phenylenediamine/H_2O_2/agarose as indicator substrate of POD-based ELISPOT assays, spots recognizable by the naked eye begin to appear within less than 1 min; these reactions appear as dark brown to almost black foci, ranging from 0.1 mm to 0.5 mm in diameter. They correspond to the former position of individual ASC. Their number and their intensity are maximal by approximately 30 min.

5. When employing BCIP/NBT/agarose as indicator substrate of AP-based ELISPOT assays, dark blue spots, ranging from 0.05 to 0.2 mm in diameter, can appear within 5–10 min but generally 30 min to 1 h is required. As the enzyme substrate reaction does not self-inhibit, increased sensitivity may be achieved by extended incubation (up to 16 h).

Enumeration

1. It is best to enumerate spots within 1–3 h after development.
2. Invert the plates over a light source (e.g. an X-ray viewing box) and count spots without further visual aid.
3. Confirm the positivity of the reactions under low magnification ($\times$ 10 to $\times$ 40). Spots exhibit a typical granular appearance. These granules consist of precipitates of enzyme-substrate reaction products which are *homogeneously* distributed within each spot. The latter feature is the most useful criterion to distinguish true spots from falsely positive reactions that might occasionally be observed. These artefacts appear as non-circular and non-homogeneously pigmented reactions or as dark granules consisting of precipitates or crystals of enzyme-substrate reaction products which emerge above the background.

7.1.3.2 Immunoenzyme Amplification Techniques for Use in ELISPOT Assays

Since the enzyme substrate used in the assay is in excess, the sensitivity of the ELISPOT assay largely depends on the surface concentration of enzyme molecules bound to the solid phase and can be increased by relatively simple modifications of the immunoenzymatic procedure described above. A description of amplification procedures for use in POD-based ELISPOT assays employing nitrocellulose-bottomed vessels is presented below. These amplification techniques can easily be adapted for ELISPOT assays employing other indicator enzymes, e.g. AP, and/or other types of solid supports, e.g. plastic.

Indirect technique

Procedure

1. Add 50 µl unconjugated rabbit anti-mouse immunoglobulins (12) diluted 1:50–1:100 in PBS/Tween/FBS (6) to individual assay wells pre-filled with 50 µl PBS/Tween/FBS (6).
2. Incubate overnight at 4 °C.
3. Remove unbound antiglobulins by washing the plate 4 times with PBS/Tween (5).
4. Add 0.1 ml POD-swine anti-rabbit immunoglobulins conjugate (14) diluted to 1:100–1:200 in PBS/Tween/FBS (6) to wells pre-filled with 0.05 ml of diluent.
5. Incubate for 2 h at room temperature, wash the plate 4 times with PBS (3) and develop.

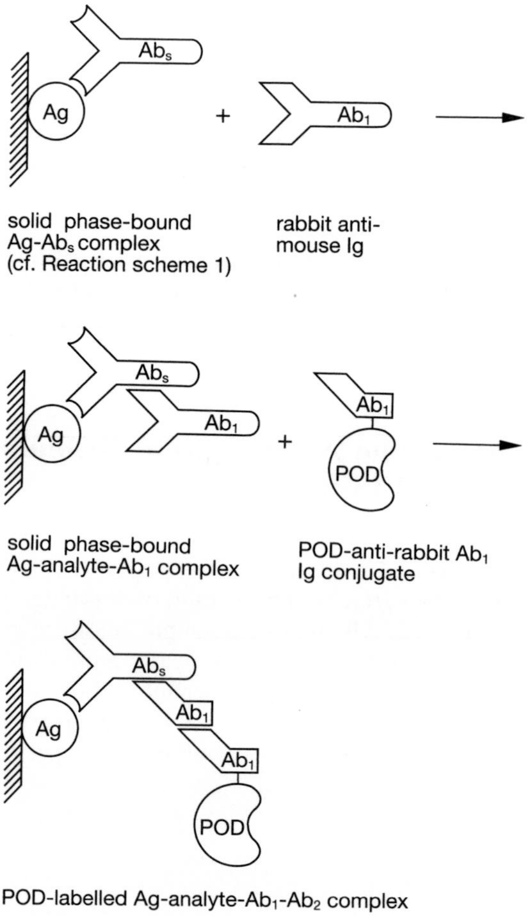

Fig. 3. Indirect technique; reaction scheme.

Remark: the indirect technique is more sensitive and more versatile than the direct technique. Only one conjugated antiglobulin is required for use with a variety of unconjugated first antibodies raised in the same animal species. If increased sensitivity is desired, other immunoperoxidase techniques can be used.

"Reinforced" indirect technique

This technique (Fig. 4) uses the same reaction scheme as the indirect technique but first and second antibodies are both labelled with POD. This approach increases the surface concentration of POD molecules compared to the indirect technique and the reactions (spots) observed are stronger. Despite its sensitivity, this technique has the same practical limitation as that already mentioned for the direct technique in that it requires the use of many POD-conjugated antibodies.

Procedure

The assay wells are treated as described for the indirect technique except that unconjugated first antibodies are substituted for POD-conjugated anti-immunoglobulins (12). Optimal dilutions of both POD-antiglobulins should be determined by chess-board titrations.

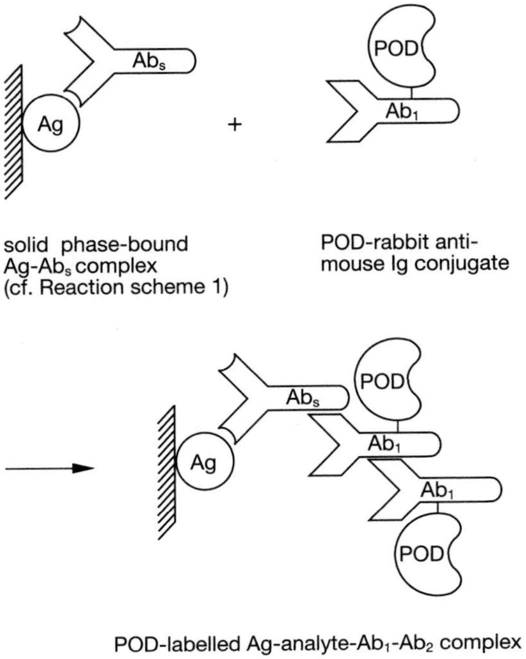
Abs
Ag
+
POD
Ab1
+
Ab2
POD
solid phase-bound Ag-Abs complex (cf. Reaction scheme 1)
POD-rabbit anti-mouse Ig conjugate
POD-anti- rabbit Ig conjugate
Abs
POD
Ab1
Ag
Ab1
POD
POD-labelled Ag-analyte-Ab1-Ab2 complex

Fig. 4. "Reinforced" indirect technique; reaction scheme.

Peroxidase-anti-peroxidase ("PAP") technique

Originally introduced for immunocytological purposes [55] (cf. 5.4.3.1), this elegant technique (Fig. 5) can be used in the ELISPOT test when high sensitivity is desired. The technique uses both first and second unconjugated antiglobulins and POD-anti-POD reagent. The latter consists of complexes of POD and anti-POD antibodies raised in the same animal species as that of the first antibodies which are directed against the immunoglobulin product to be detected, e.g., rabbit anti-mouse immunoglobulins. The second antibodies, e.g., swine anti-rabbit immunoglobulins, when used in excess (so that only one antibody binding site binds to the first antibody) can "bridge" both first antibody and complexed anti-POD antibody. The POD-anti-POD technique is at least as sensitive as the "reinforced" indirect technique but is more versatile since a variety of first and second antiglobulins can be used in unconjugated form. In addition, the preparation of POD-anti-POD reagent obviates the need for chemical conjugation procedures which are known to alter antibody activity. However, POD-anti-POD complexes are expensive and cumbersome to prepare, and the procedure is somewhat time-consuming.

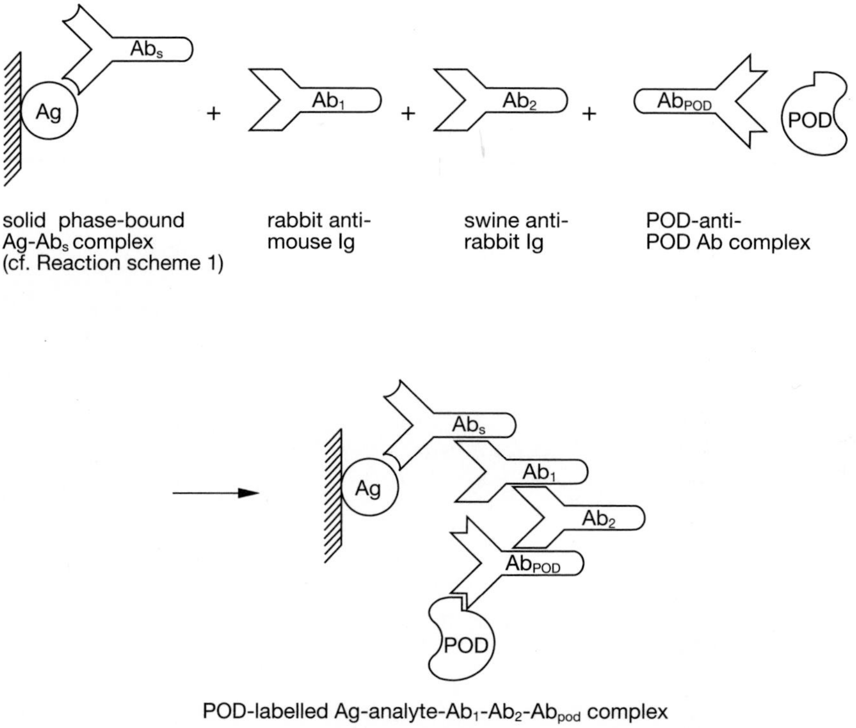
Abs
Ag
+
Ab1
+
Ab2
+
AbPOD
POD
solid phase-bound
Ag-Abs complex
(cf. Reaction scheme 1)
rabbit anti-
mouse Ig
swine anti-
rabbit Ig
POD-anti-
POD Ab complex
Abs
Ag
Ab1
Ab2
AbPOD
POD
POD-labelled Ag-analyte-Ab1-Ab2-Abpod complex

Fig. 5. Peroxidase-anti-peroxidase (PAP) technique; reaction scheme.

Procedure

Perform primary and secondary immunoreactions as described for the indirect technique with the following modifications: use second antibodies (e.g., swine anti-rabbit immunoglobulins (14) in unconjugated form and in excess (1:25 to 1:50). Then add 0.05 ml POD-anti-POD immune complexes (13), appropriately diluted (1:25 to 1:100) in PBS/Tween/FBS (6) and incubate for 3 h at room temperature. Wash 4 times with PBS (3); develop the plate.

Note: when used without first and second antibodies and with dishes coated with anti-immunoglobulin antibodies instead of antigen, the POD-anti-POD technique provides a very useful tool for detecting cells secreting autoanti-IgG antibodies, i.e. rheumatoid factor [28]. In this situation, advantage is taken of the reactivity of rheumatoid antibodies for complexed IgG present in the POD-anti-POD reagent.

Avidin-biotin techniques

These techniques are among the most sensitive immunoenzyme procedures for use in the ELISPOT test. Advantage is taken of the high affinity of avidin, a glycoprotein present in egg white, for the vitamin, biotin. Antibodies can easily be conjugated with biotin (cf. 7.1.5.5). The conjugation procedure is mild and yields conjugated antibodies that have retained virtually all their original activity [56]. Biotinylated antiglobulins can then be used both in direct and indirect techniques. POD-avidin conjugate is then applied to localize the binding of biotinylated antiglobulins (Fig. 6a). Alternatively, a complex made of unconjugated avidin and biotinylated POD ("ABC" complex) can be used for the same purpose (Fig. 6b). Since one molecule of avidin is capable of binding four molecules of biotin, the use of ABC complexes increases the surface concentration of POD molecules giving the method even greater sensitivity.

Procedure

1. Add 0.05 ml biotinylated anti-mouse immunoglobulins (16) to the assay well pre-filled with 0.05 ml of PBS/Tween/FBS (6), replacing the conjugate used in the standard procedure.
2. Incubate for 2 h at room temperature (or overnight at 4 °C).
3. Wash the dish 4 times with PBS/Tween (5) and expose for 1 h at room temperature to either POD-avidin conjugate (15) (0.25 to 1 µg/ml) diluted in PBS/Tween/FBS (6), or to pre-formed complexes of avidin and POD-biotin conjugate (15). In the latter instance, mix equal concentrations (0.1 to 0.5 µg/ml) of avidin and POD-biotin 30 min before adding to the wells.
4. Wash the plate 4 times with PBS (3) and develop.

(A)

solid phase-bound
Ag-Ab$_s$ complex
(cf. Reaction scheme 1)

biotinylated anti-
mouse Ig

solid phase-bound Ag-analyte
biotinylated Ab$_1$ complex

POD-avidin
conjugate

POD-labelled Ag-analyte-biotinylated Ab$_1$-avidin complex

Avidin-biotin-anti-peroxidase ("ABAP") technique

This novel immunoenzyme amplification procedure was recently introduced for use in the ELISPOT assay [45] when extreme sensitivity is desired. The procedure involves the use of a biotinylated anti-POD antibody reagent to enhance the signal provided by antibody- or avidin-POD conjugate used as primary or secondary reagents. Following addition of POD-conjugated avidin (or of POD-biotin-avidin complexes), ELISPOT assay wells are developed (Fig. 7). The procedure can thus be employed to amplify any of the immunoenzyme techniques described above (but cf. 5.4.3.2 for comment on avidinbiotin methods).

(B)

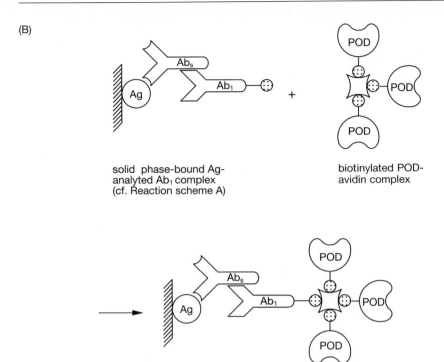

solid phase-bound Ag-
analyted Ab$_1$ complex
(cf. Reaction scheme A)

biotinylated POD-
avidin complex

POD-labelled Ag-analyte-biotinylated Ab$_1$-avidin-
biotinylated POD complex

Fig. 6. Avidin-biotin techniques; reaction schemes. Direct avidin-biotin technique (A) and avidin-biotin complex ("ABC") technique (B).

Procedure

1. Add 0.05 ml of appropriately diluted biotinylated anti-POD (16) to wells that have been treated according to any of the immunoenzyme techniques described above.
2. Incubate for 2 h at ambient temperature.
3. Wash the wells three times with PBS/Tween (6).
4. Expose the wells for 1 h at room temperature to either POD-avidin conjugate (15) (0.25 to 1 µg/ml) diluted in PBS/Tween/FBS (6), or to pre-formed complexes of avidin and POD-biotin conjugate (15).
5. Wash four times with PBS (3) and develop.

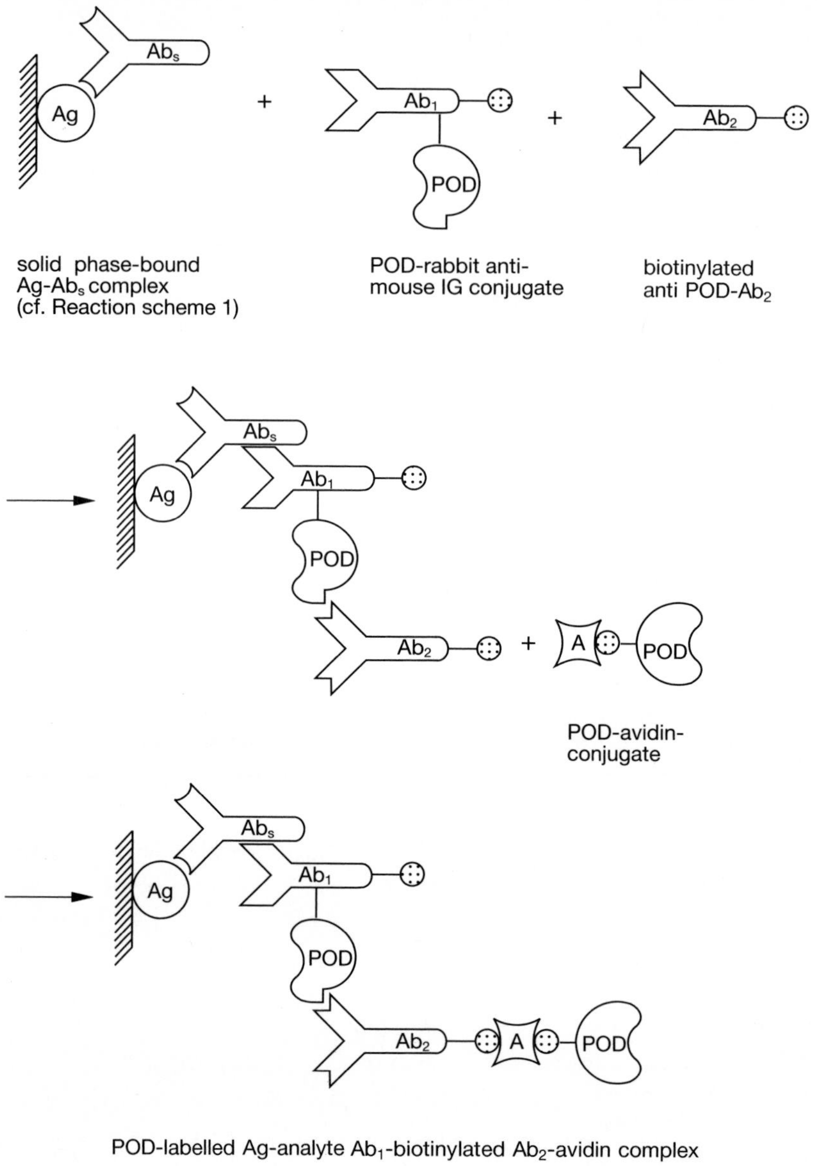
Abs
Ag
+
Ab1
POD
+
Ab2
solid phase-bound
Ag-Abs complex
(cf. Reaction scheme 1)
POD-rabbit anti-
mouse IG conjugate
biotinylated
anti POD-Ab2
Abs
Ag
Ab1
POD
Ab2
+
A
POD
POD-avidin-
conjugate
Abs
Ag
Ab1
POD
Ab2
A
POD
POD-labelled Ag-analyte Ab1-biotinylated Ab2-avidin complex

Fig. 7. Avidin-biotin-anti-peroxidase (ABAP) technique; reaction scheme.

7.1.3.3 Two-Colour Technique (Bichromatic ELISPOT Test)

This variation of the ELISPOT technique has been developed to allow simultaneous detection of distinct isotypes of antibodies [49]. This modification makes use of two antiglobulin conjugates, one labelled with POD, the other with AP, having distinct immunological specificities (Fig. 8). The procedure is particularly useful as it yields twice as much information as the regular monochromatic ELISPOT technique while

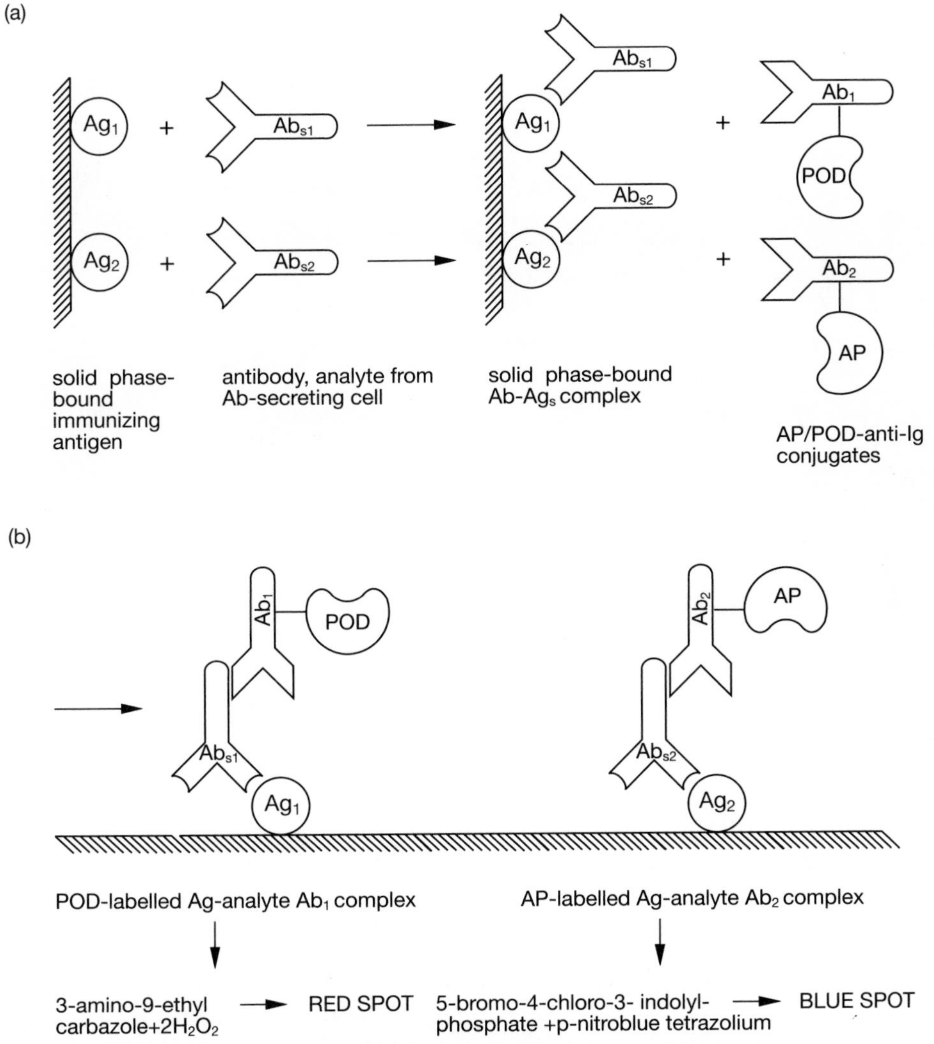

(a)

(b)

Fig. 8. Two-colour ELISPOT technique; reaction scheme.

requiring the same sample and assay vessel sizes. As an example, a bichromatic technique for concurrent detection of KLH specific IgG-secreting cells and KLH specific IgM-secreting cells is described (Figure 9).

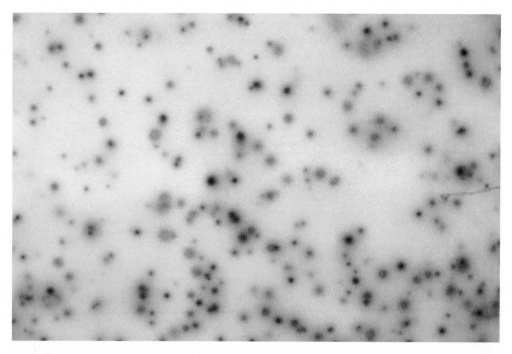

Fig. 9. Typical appearance of a nitrocellulose-bottomed well developed by means of the two-colour ELISPOT technique for simultaneous detection of murine splenocytes secreting KLH specific IgM (blue spots) and IgG (red spots) antibodies (× 60).

Procedure

1. At the completion of the cell incubation stage performed in KLH coated wells, wash the wells as described in the standard technique.
2. To wells pre-filled with 0.05 ml of PBS/Tween/FBS (6), add 0.05 ml of a cocktail of AP-conjugated anti-mouse IgM (12) and POD-conjugated anti-mouse IgG (12) (or *vice versa*) appropriately diluted in PBS/Tween (FBS (6) (optimal dilutions of AP- and POD-conjugates must be determined by chess-board titrations).
3. Incubate for 2 h at room temperature or overnight at 4 °C.
4. Wash the plates 3 times with PBS/Tween (5), twice with PBS, and finally 3 times with Tris buffer (18). Keep the plates immersed in the latter buffer for 5 min.
5. Develop the plates sequentially with AP chromogen substrate and POD chromogen substrate. Add 0.1 ml of BCIP/NBT solution (11) and incubate for 5–20 min at

ambient temperature; examine the wells for appearance of blue spots. These reactions usually appear within 5–10 min. Plates are allowed to develop for an additional period of up to 10 min, provided background staining is not excessive.

6. Rinse the plates with PBS by 3 manual washes and 1 immersion in this buffer.
7. Blot-dry the membranes.
8. Add 0.1 ml of AEC/H_2O_2 solution (10).
9. Examine wells for appearance of red spots.
10. Incubate, wash, and dry the plates exactly as described in the standard ELISPOT technique.

7.1.4 Validation and Performance of Method

7.1.4.1 Precision, Accuracy, Sensitivity and Detection Limit

The percentage of variation between replicate dishes generally does not exceed 10%. However, considerably higher variations can be observed between replicate dishes that have been exposed to suspensions containing small numbers of ASC (< 10 detectable ASC per well). No data are available regarding accuracy. Under optimal conditions the ELISPOT assay described here is 3 to 5 times as sensitive as the PFC assay for enumeration of KLH-specific ASC. Moreover, and as already been indicated, the sensitivity of the ELISPOT assay can be substantially increased by using relatively simple amplification procedures (cf. Alternative techniques 7.1.3).

7.1.4.2 Sources of Error

Artefacts due to the presence of cell debris on the solid phase and/or of aggregates in the enzyme/substrate solution can frequently be observed. Often, these reactions appear as small non-granular dots. Granular spots with a clear centre can also be observed, though less frequently. The use of an appropriate magnifying device is then required to distinguish these false spots from true homogeneously granulated spots.

Another source of error may be encountered when using the ELISPOT test for isotype-specific determinations so it is essential that conjugates of sufficient specificity are used (cf. also Specificity).

7.1.4.3   Specificity

Antigen specificity

Since secreted immunoglobulin may bind nonspecifically to the surface of antigen-coated dishes, the following controls should be included in each experiment:

– wells coated with the immunizing antigen, hereafter referred to as target antigen, but exposed to a cell suspension prepared from either non-immunized animals or animals immunized with an irrelevant antigen preparation, i.e., noncross-reactive with the target antigen.
– "Uncoated" wells, i.e., blocked only with assay culture medium (2), or wells coated with an irrelevant antigen and exposed to cell suspensions prepared from the test animal(s) and from control animal(s) (non-immunized or immunized with an irrelevant antigen).

Cells from animals immunized with the target antigen should generate spots when assayed in wells coated with this antigen but should not produce significant numbers of reactions in the control wells. Conversely, cells from animals immunized with an irrelevant antigen should not form spots when assayed in wells coated with the target antigen or in uncoated wells but should generate reactions when assayed in wells coated with the immunizing antigen. Cells from non-immunized animals should not generate spots when assayed in coated as well as in uncoated wells. An example of results obtained by such experiments is given in Table 1.

Table 1. Specificity of the ELISPOT assay for enumeration of KLH-specific murine ASC

Animals immunized with		$SFC/10^6$ splenocytes assayed in wells coated with		
		OVA (ovalbumin)	KLH	nil
OVA		256*	8	0
KLH		12	540	6
nil		4	0	0
Inhibitor	Antigen µg/well			
OVA	100	18	550	
OVA	10	45		
OVA	1	190		
KLH	100	270	30	
KLH	10		170	
KLH	1		320	
Cycloheximide	25	15	20	

* Results are expressed as mean spot-forming cell (SFC) numbers determined on triplicate wells.

Spots generated by normal cells: in certain situations, cells of animals that have not been actively immunized can generate spots when assayed in dishes coated with a variety of antigens. In general, the frequency of these reactions is negligible and the corresponding spot-forming cells are thought to arise spontaneously or following previous exposure to a cross-reacting antigen. However, in certain situations, the frequency of these reactions can be considerably higher, such as with certain strains of animals that are known to be "polyclonally activated", i.e., whose immune system undergoes B-cell hyperactivity resulting in the expansion of numerous clones of ASC. In these situations, spot formation might be specific as far as the antigen-binding property of the corresponding immunoglobulin secreted is concerned, but this can only be documented by inhibition and/or elution experiments.

Inhibition: spot formation can be inhibited during the cell incubation period by addition of soluble antigen of the same specificity as that of the target Ag used for coating. In contrast, addition of an immunologically irrelevant antigen should not affect spot formation, confirming the specificity of the assay.

In general, the degree of inhibition increases with increasing concentration of free antigen. However, experimental systems using hapten-conjugated proteins for coating, with different hapten substitution ratios of the conjugate, have indicated that the degree of inhibition of spot formation is influenced by the affinity of the different antibody populations secreted and by the density of the corresponding antigenic epitope (hapten substitution ratio of the coating conjugate) immobilized on the solid phase [35]. Thus, a low epitope density preferentially allows monovalent antibody binding [57] and spot formation is mainly due to cells secreting antibodies of relatively high affinity. In that situation, addition of free antigen during the cell incubation period inhibits spot formation in a dose-dependent manner and the lower the amount of free antigen required to inhibit spot formation to an arbitrary degree, the higher is the average affinity of the antibody populations secreted. At high epitope density, which allows binding of both high- and low-affinity antibodies [57], considerably larger amounts of free antigen might be required to inhibit spot formation. Thus, spot formation by cells secreting antibodies of relatively low affinity is more difficult to inhibit than spot formation due to cells secreting antibodies of high affinity.

The specificity of spot formation by cells secreting antibodies of low affinity is thus more difficult to establish by inhibition experiments since large amounts of antigens might be required and are not always available. Elution studies are then more suited for this purpose.

Elution: advantage can be taken of the reversible nature of antigen-antibody reactions and of the relatively weak association between solid-phase antigen and secreted antibodies of low affinity. Addition of free soluble antigen immediately *after* the cell incubation period, and for 2 h at 37 °C, just prior to the immunoenzyme reaction, can dissociate secreted antibodies from solid-phase antigen and thus inhibit subsequent development of the corresponding spots. In that situation added free antigen and solid-phase antigen compete for binding of secreted antibodies. The lower the amount of free antigen required to inhibit spot formation to an arbitrary level, the lower is the average affinity of antibodies secreted and eluted from the solid phase.

Thus, the combination of inhibition and elution experiments not only can document the specificity of spot formation but can also yield information concerning the average affinity of antibodies secreted by individual ASC.

Specificity for immunoglobulin markers

The suitability of the ELISPOT test for detection of cells secreting antibodies of a given marker, e.g., isotype, subclass, or allotype, relies entirely on the immunological specificity of the antiglobulin preparations used during the immunoperoxidase stage. The specificity of such reagents can be evaluated by inhibition experiments. For instance, a preparation which is intended for use as the developing antiglobulin for a given immunoglobulin isotype should inhibit spot formation due to cells secreting antibodies of the corresponding isotype when added during the cell incubation period. In contrast, spot formation due to cells secreting antibodies of other isotypes should not be affected.

The antiglobulin preparations used in such inhibition experiments should be assayed at least at the same dilutions (in culture medium) or in excess of those selected for use in the ELISPOT test.

7.1.4.4   Assessment for *de novo* Protein Synthesis

Antibody formation is a dynamic metabolic process and methodology must provide evidence of active synthesis of antibody by a cell population rather than merely reveal its association with a cell. Indeed, certain antibodies, termed cytophilic antibodies, bind to lymphoid cells which are themselves incapable of synthesizing antibodies. It is important therefore to confirm that spot formation is not merely the result of release of pre-formed antibodies but rather that antibody synthesis by spot-forming cells is taking place during the *in vitro* incubation period. This can be accomplished in a variety of ways, including the use of an inhibitor of protein synthesis.

Procedure

1. Dissolve cycloheximide, e.g. from *Sigma,* in assay-culture medium (2) at a final concentration of 25 µg/ml.
2. Resuspend cells to be assayed in the above medium at a density of 10^6 to 10^7 cells/ml and dispense 1 ml volumes in plastic tissue culture tubes.
3. Incubate the tubes for 3 to 4 h at 37 °C in a humid atmosphere containing 10% CO_2 in air.
4. Subsequently, wash the cells twice with cycloheximide-containing medium by centrifugation at $200 \times g$ for 10 min.

5. Then, resuspend the pelleted cells in the above medium at the appropriate density and assay for SFC numbers by the ELISPOT test. Spot formation should be inhibited by 80%–90% after exposure of the cells to cycloheximide as compared to untreated cells, providing evidence for active metabolism of spot-forming cells (see also Table 1).

7.1.5   Appendix

7.1.5.1   Preparation of Single Cell Suspensions from Mouse Spleen (see also 2.5)

1. Anesthetize animals with ether and/or sacrifice by cervical dislocation.
2. Place individual or pooled spleens in chilled PBS (3).
3. Gently disrupt the organs by scraping them against a nylon sieve with the piston of a syringe.
4. Rinse the sieve with a small volume of cold PBS (3) and filter the resulting suspension through a layer of fine-meshed nylon cloth.
5. Allow clumps to settle for 10 min on ice and transfer the supernatant suspension to a clean tube.
6. Centrifuge at $200 \times g$ for 10 min, gently resuspend the pelleted cells with a small volume of PBS (3) (approximately 1–2 ml per spleen) and expose for 5 min at room temperature to Tris-buffered ammonium chloride (17) (40 ml per spleen) to lyse red blood cells.
7. Underlay the suspension with (FBS) (1) (1 ml per spleen) and centrifuge at $350 \times g$ for 5 min.
8. Count the mononuclear cells, adjust to the desired density with culture medium (2) and keep on ice until use (within 2 h). The viability of the cells can be assayed by a trypan blue exclusion test [58]. More than 98% of the cells prepared by this procedure should be viable (cf. 2.1.1).

7.1.5.2   Preparation of KLH-coated Nitrocellulose-bottomed Dishes

1. Fill individual 9 mm diameter wells of nitrocellulose bottomed plates or strips with 75 to 100 µl coating solution (4) and allow the vessels to stand in humid chambers for 2 h at 37 °C, 4 h at room temperature or overnight at 4 °C, whichever is more convenient.

2. Wash the wells three times with PBS (3) by flicking and further wash by immersing the plates for 5 min in a container containing clean PBS (3).
3. Empty the wells of wash buffer by flicking the plates and carefully blot-dry the outer surface of the nitrocellulose membrane with clean absorbent paper towels.
4. Fill the wells immediately with 50 μl of assay culture medium (2).

7.1.5.3   Preparation of KLH-coated Plastic Dishes

1. Fill individual wells of polystyrene 24-well tissue plates with 100 to 150 μl of coating solution, consisting of KLH diluted to 200 μg/ml in PBS (3). Alternatively, one may use the shallow rings of the lid of a polystyrene 24-well tissue culture plate as assay culture wells which is more hydrophobic and thus displays higher protein absorptive capacity than tissue culture-grade wells of the same plate.
2. Allow the plates (or the lids) to stand in humid chambers for 2 h at 37 °C, 4 h at room temperature or overnight at 4 °C.
3. Wash the plates four times with PBS (3) by flicking.
4. Empty the wells of wash buffer by flicking the plates (or the lids if one uses their rings as assay wells) and fill the wells immediately with 100 μl of assay culture medium (2).

7.1.5.4   Preparation of Agarose Substrate Solutions for Plastic-based ELISPOT Assays

1. Preparation of agarose: a 3% (w/v) solution of type I agarose (e. g. from *Sigma*) is prepared by boiling 3 g agarose in 100 ml sterile filtered distilled water until the agarose is melted. Prepare 10 ml aliquots of agarose in clean glass bottles and store at 4 °C. Before use, melt agarose aliquot by boiling the glass bottle (or by microwave) and place in a water-bath set at about 40 °C to maintain agarose liquidity.
2. 1,4-benzenediamine/H_2O_2/agarose substrate solution: dissolve 5 mg 1,4-benzene-diamine base (e. g. from *Sigma*) in a minimum volume of methanol (0.1 to 0.2 ml). Agitate in water-bath (40 °C) until completely dissolved. Add 5 μl 30% (w/v) H_2O_2 and bring up volume to 8 ml with prewarmed (40 °C) PBS (3). Mix with 2 ml of 40 °C molten agarose solution. If the solution contains aggregates, filter through a clean hot sintered glass filter. Use immediately or within 10 min.
3. BCIP/NBT/agarose solution: dissolve separately 1.5 mg BCIP and 3 mg *p*-nitroblue tetrazolium chloride in a minimum volume of dimethylformamide (0.2 ml for each reagent). Agitate in a water-bath (40 °C) until completely dissolved. Mix the 2 reagents and adjust volume to 8 ml with carbonate buffer (9). Warm to 40 °C. Add 2 ml of 40 °C molten agarose solution. If the solution contains aggregates, filter through a clean hot sintered glass filter.

7.1.5.5   **Biotinylation of Antibodies** (modified from [56])

1. Dialyse the antibody preparation, e.g. affinity purified antibodies, IgG fraction or whole immunoglobulin fraction (obtained by ammonium salt precipitation or by caprilic acid precipitation) extensively against PBS (3) to remove any azide (or other preservatives) and/or ammonium sulphate.
2. Dialyse the preparations against $NaHCO_3$, 0.1 mol/l (42 g $NaHCO_3$ in 5 l water), pH 8.3 ± 0.2.
3. Adjust protein concentration to 1 mg/ml in $NaHCO_3$, 0.1 mol/l; pH 8.3.
4. Dissolve D-biotinyl-ε-aminocaproic acid *N*-hydroxy succinimide ester, e.g. from *Boehringer* (Mannheim, Germany) or from *Biosearch* (San Rafael, CA) in dimethylformamide to a final concentration of 1 mg/ml.
5. Add immediately 150 µl biotin solution per ml protein solution and mix.
6. Incubate for 4 h at room temperature in the dark.
7. Separate conjugated immunoglobulins from unreacted biotin by filtration through a column of Sephadex G25 equilibrated with PBS (3), or alternatively dialyze extensively against PBS (3) containing NaN_3, 0.2 g/l.

References

[1] *A. H. Coons, M. H. Kaplan,* Localization of Antigen in Tissue Cells, II. Improvements in a Method for the Detection of Antigens, J. Exp. Med. *91,* 1–18 (1950).
[2] *C. Bosman, J. D. Feldman, E. Pick,* Heterogeneity of Antibody-forming Cells. An Electron Microscopic Analysis, J. Exp. Med. *129,* 1029–1040 (1969).
[3] *E. Pick, J. D. Feldman,* Autoradiographic Plaques for the Detection of Antibody Formation to Soluble Proteins by Single Cells, Science, *156,* 964–970 (1967).
[4] *N. K. Jerne, A. A. Nordin,* Plaque Formation in Agar by Single Antibody-Producing Cells, Science *140,* 405–406 (1963).
[5] *N. K. Jerne, C. Henry, A. Nordin, H. Fuji, A. M. C. Koros, I. Lefkovits,* Plaque-Forming Cells, Methodology and Theory, Transplant. Rev. *18,* 130–191 (1974).
[6] *J. S. Ingraham, A. Bussard,* Application of a Localized Hemolysin Reaction for Specific Detection of Individual Antibody-Forming Cells, J. Exp. Med. *11,* 667–672 (1964).
[7] *J. Sterzl, I. Riha,* Detection of Cells Producing 7S Antibodies by the Plaque Technique, Nature *208,* 857–858 (1965).
[8] *E. S. Golub, R. I. Mishell, W. O. Weigle, R. W. Dutton,* Modification of the Haemolytic Plaque Assay for Use with Protein Antigens, J. Immunol. *100,* 133–138 (1968).
[9] *G. A. Molinaro, E. Maron, S. Dray,* Antigen-Secreting Cells: Enumeration of Immunoglobulin-Allotype Secreting Cells in Non-Immunized Rabbits by Means of Hybrid Antibody Coated Erythrocytes in a Reverse Hemolytic Plaque Assay, Proc. Natl. Acad. Sci. USA *71,* 1229–1233 (1974).
[10] *B. Merchant, J. K. Inman,* Hapten-Specific Hemolytic Plaque Assays Fail to Detect Most of the Diversity in the Anti-Hapten Response, J. Immunol. Methods *41,* 269–277 (1981).
[11] *N. J. Pasanen, O. Makela,* Effect of the Number of Haptens Coupled to Each Erythrocyte on Haemolytic Plaque Formation, Immunology *16,* 399–407 (1969).
[12] *P. Truffa-Bachi, G. R. Bordenave,* A Reverse Hemolytic Plaque Assay for the Detection and the Enumeration of Immunoglobulin Allotype-secreting Cells, Cell. Immunol. *50,* 261–270 (1980).

[13] *B. Anderson*, Studies on Antibody Affinity at the Cellular Level, J. Exp. Med. *135*, 312–321 (1974).

[14] *E. A. Goidl, A. F. Schrater, G. Siskind, G. J. Thorbecke*, Production of Auto-Antiidiotypic Antibody during Normal Immune Response to TNP-Ficoll. II. Hapten-Reversible Inhibition of Anti-TNP Plaque-Forming Cells by Immune Serum as Assay for Auto-Anti-Idiotypic Antibody, J. Exp. Med. *150*, 154–163 (1979).

[15] *P. H. Plotz, N. Talal, R. Asofsky*, Assignment of Direct and Facilitated Haemolytic Plaques in Mice to Specific Immunoglobulin Classes, J. Immunol. *100*, 744–751 (1968).

[16] *P. J. Baker, P. W. Stahak*, Quantitative and Qualitative Studies on the Primary Antibody Responses to Pneumococcal Polysaccharides at the Cellular Level, J. Immunol. *103*, 1342–1348 (1969).

[17] *B. S. Shepart, G. L. Mayers, R. B. Bankert*, Failure of PFC Inhibition Assays to Distinguish Idiotypically between Clonotypes that are Distinguishable by RIA Analysis, J. Immunol. *135*, 1683–1691 (1985).

[18] *C. DeLisi*, Hemolytic Plaque Inhibition: Physical Chemical Limits on Use as Affinity Assay, J. Immunol. *117*, 2249–2258 (1976).

[19] *C. Czerkinsky, L.-A. Nilsson, H. Nygren, Ö. Ouchterlony, A. Tarkowski*, A Solid-Phase Enzyme-Linked Immunospot (ELISPOT) Assay for Enumeration of Specific Antibody-Secreting Cells, J. Immunol. Methods *65*, 109–121 (1983).

[20] *J. D. Sedgwick, P. G. Holt*, A Solid-Phase Immunoenzymatic Technique for the Enumeration of Specific Antibody-Secreting Cells, J. Immunol. Methods *57*, 301–308 (1983).

[21] *E. Engvall, P. Perlman*, Enzyme-Linked Immunosorbent Assay, ELISA III. Quantification of Specific Antibodies by Enzyme-Labelled Anti-Immunoglobulin in Antigen-Coated Tubes, J. Immunol. *109*, 29–36 (1972).

[22] *B. S. Kelly, J. G. Levy, L. Sikora*, The Use of the Enzyme-linked Immunosorbent Assay (ELISA) for the Detection and Quantification of Specific Antibody from Cell Cultures, Immunology *37*, 45–52 (1979).

[23] *G. H. Boerrigter, A. Vos, R. J. Sheper*, Direct Measurement of *in vitro* Antibody Production Using an Enzyme-Linked Immunosorbent Assay, J. Immunol. Methods *61*, 377–386 (1983).

[24] *C. Czerkinsky, L.-A. Nilsson, Ö. Ouchterlony, A. Tarkowski, C. Gretzer*, Detection of Single Antibody-Secreting Cells Generated after *in vitro* Antigen-Induced Stimulation of Human Peripheral Blood Lymphocytes, Scand. J. Immunol. *19*, 575–579 (1984).

[25] *A. Tarkowski, C. Czerkinsky, L.-A. Nilsson*, Simultaneous Induction of Rheumatoid Factor- and Antigen Specific Antibody-Secreting Cells During the Secondary Immune Response in Man, Clin. Exp. Immunol. *61*, 379–387 (1985).

[26] *N. Lycke, L. Lindholm, J. Holmgren*, Cholera Antibody Production *in vitro* by Peripheral Blood Lymphocytes Following Oral Immunisation of Humans and Mice. Clin. Exp. Immunol. *62*, 39–45 (1985).

[27] *C. Czerkinsky, S. J. Prince, S. M. Michalek, S. Jackson, M. W. Russell, J. R. McGhee, J. Mestecky*, IgA Antibody-Producing Cells in Peripheral Blood after Antigen Ingestion: Evidence for a Common Mucosal Immune System in Humans, Proc. Natl. Acad. Sci. USA *84*, 2449–2454 (1987).

[28] *A. Tarkowski, C. Czerkinsky, L.-A. Nilsson, H. Nygren, Ö. Ouchterlony*, Solid-Phase Enzyme-Linked Immunospot Assay (ELISPOT) for Enumeration of IgG Rheumatoid Factor-Secreting Cells, J. Immunol. Methods *68*, 302–312 (1984).

[29] *A. Tarkowski, C. Czerkinsky, L.-Å. Nilsson*, Detection of IgG-Rheumatoid Factor-Secreting Cells in Autoimmune MRL/lpr Mice: A Kinetic Study, Clin. Exp. Immunol. *58*, 7–12 (1984).

[30] *P. G. Holt, J. D. Sedgwick, G. A. Stewart, C. O'Leary, K. Krska*, ELISA Plaque Assay for the Detection of Antibody-Secreting Cells: Observations on the Nature of the Solid Phase and on Variations in Plaque Diameter, J. Immunol. Methods *74*, 1–8 (1984).

[31] *A. Tarkowski, R. Holmdahl, K. Rubin, L. Klareskog, L.-Å. Nilsson, K. Gunnarsson*, Patterns of Autoreactivity to Collagen Type II in Autoimmune MRL/l Mice, Clin. Exp. Immunol. *63*, 441–447 (1986).

[32] *M. W. Russell, C. Czerkinsky, Z. Moldoveanu,* Detection and Specificity of Antibodies Secreted by Spleen Cells in Mice Immunized with *Streptococcus mutans,* Infect. Immun. *53,* 317–323 (1987).

[33] *C. Franci, J. Ingles, R. Castro, J. Vidal,* Further Studies on the ELISA-Spot Technique. Its Application to Particulate Antigens and Potential Improvement in Sensitivity, J. Immunol. Methods *88,* 225–231 (1986).

[34] *D. G. Ando, F. M. Ebling, B. H. Hahn,* Detection of Native and Denatured DNA Antibody-Forming Cells by the ELISPOT Assay: A Clinical Study of NZB/W F1 Mice, Arthritis Rheum. *29,* 1139–1145 (1985).

[35] *H. Nygren, C. Czerkinsky, M. Stenberg,* Dissociation of Antibodies Bound to Surface-Immobilized Antigen, J. Immunol. Methods *85,* 87–94 (1985).

[36] *C. Czerkinsky, L.-Å. Nilsson, Ö. Ouchterlony,* Kinetics and Isotype Distribution of Parasite Specific Antibody Responses in the Spleen of Mice during Experimental Infection with *Schistosoma mansoni,* Intl. Arch. Allergy. Appl. Immunol. *88,* 280–287 (1989).

[37] *D. Moskophidis, F. Lehmann-Grube,* The Immune Response of the Mouse to Lymphocytic Choriomeningitis Virus. IV. Enumeration of Antibody-Producing Cells in Spleens During Acute and Persistent Infection, J. Immunol. *133,* 3366–3371 (1984).

[38] *D. Moskophidis, J. Lohler, F. Lehmann-Grube,* Antiviral Antibody-Producing Cells in Parenchymatous Organs during Persistent Virus Infection, J. Exp. Med. *165,* 705–712 (1987).

[39] *A. Kantele, H. Arvilommi, I. Jokinen,* Specific Immunoglobulin-Secreting Human Blood Cells After Peroral Vaccination Against *Salmonella typhi,* J. Infect. Dis. *153,* 1126–1132 (1986).

[40] *P. G. Holt, K. J. Cameron, G. A. Stewart, J. D. Sedgwick, K. J. Turner,* Enumeration of Human Immunoglobulin-Secreting Cells by the ELISA-Plaque Method: IgE and IgG Isotypes, Clin. Immunol. Immunopathol. *30,* 159–164 (1984).

[41] *C. Czerkinsky, A. Tarkowski, L.-Å. Nilsson, Ö. Ouchterlony, H. Nygren, C. Gretzer,* Reverse Enzyme-Linked Immunospot (RELISPOT) Assay for Detection of Cells Secreting Immu-noreactive Substances, J. Immunol. Methods *72,* 489–496 (1984).

[42] *C. Czerkinsky, L.-Å. Nilsson, A. Tarkowski, Ö. Ouchterlony, S. Jeansson, C. Gretzer,* An Immunoenzyme Procedure for Enumerating Fibronectin-Secreting cells, J. Immunoassay *5,* 291–298 (1984).

[43] *C. Czerkinsky, A.-M. Svennerholm,* Ganglioside GM1 Enzyme-Linked Immunospot (GM1-ELISPOT) Assay for Simple Identification of Heat-Labile Enterotoxin-Producing *Escherichia coli,* J. Clin. Microbiol. *17,* 965–970 (1983).

[44] *C. Czerkinsky, G. Andersson, L.-Å. Nilsson, H.-P. Eckre, L. Klareskog, Ö. Ouchterlony,* Reverse ELISPOT Assay for Clonal Analysis of Cytokine Production. I. Detection of Gamma Interferon-Secreting Cells, J. Immunol. Methods *110,* 29–37 (1988).

[45] *C. Czerkinsky, G. Anderson, B. Ferrua, I. Nordström, M. Quiding, K. Eriksson, L. Larsson, K. Hellstrand, H.-P. Ekre,* Detection of Human Cytokine-Secreting Cells in Distinct Anatomical Compartments, in: *G. Möller* (ed.), Immunological Reviews, Vol. 119, Munks-gaard, Copenhagen 1991, pp. 1–18.

[46] *J. D. Sedgwick, P. G. Holt,* The ELISA Plaque Assay for Enumerating Specific Antibody-Secreting Cells, in: *D. M. Kemeny, S. J. Challacombe* (eds.), ELISA and Other Solid Phase Immunoassays, John Wiley & Sons Ltd., New York 1988, pp. 241–263.

[47] *C. Czerkinsky, L.-Å. Nilsson, A. Tarkowski, W. J. Koopman, J. Mestecky, Ö. Ouchterlony,* The Solid Phase Enzyme-Linked Immunospot Assay (ELISPOT) for Enumerating Antibody-Secreting Cells: Methodology and Applications, in: *D. M. Kemeny, S. J. Challacombe* (eds.), ELISA and Other Solid Phase Immunoassays, John Wiley & Sons Ltd., New York 1988, pp. 217–239.

[48] *J. D. Sedgwick, P. G. Holt,* Kinetics and Distribution of Antigen-Specific IgE-Secreting Cells During the Primary Antibody Response in the Rat, J. Exp. Med. *157,* 2178–2182 (1983).

[49] *C. Czerkinsky, Z. Moldoveanu, J. Mestecky, L.-Å. Nilsson, Ö. Ouchterlony,* A Novel Two-Colour ELISPOT Assay. I. Simultaneous Detection of Distinct Types of Antibody-Secreting Cells, J. Immunol. Methods *115,* 31 (1988).

[50] *S. A. Möller, C. A. K. Borrebaeck,* A Filter Immuno-Plaque Assay for the Detection of Antibody-Secreting Cells *in vitro,* J. Immunol. Methods *79,* 195–201 (1985).

[51] *A. F. Verheul, A. A. Versteeg, N. A. Westerdaal, G. J. van Dam, M. Jansze, H. Snippe,* Measurement of the Humoral Immune Response Against *Streptococcus pneumoniae* Type 14-Derived Antigens by an ELISA and ELISPOT Assay Based on Biotin-Avidin Technology, J. Immunol. Methods *126,* 79–87 (1990).

[52] *B. Schliebs, H. Gattner, K. Naithani, M. Fabry, A. N. Khalaf, L. Kerp, K. G. Petersen,* The Detection of Single Cells Forming Antibodies to Defined Epitopes on Insulin, J. Immunol. Methods *126,* 169–175 (1990).

[53] *S. Avrameas, T. Ternynk,* Peroxidase Labelled Antibody and Fab Conjugates with Enhanced Intracellular Penetration, Immunochemistry 8, 1175–1183 (1973).

[54] *P. K. Nakane, A. Kawaoi,* Peroxidase-Labelled Antibody. A New Method of Conjugation, J. Histochem. Cytochem. *22,* 1084–1091 (1974).

[55] *L. A. Sternberger, P. H. Hardy Jr., J. J. Coculin, H. G. Meyer,* The Unlabelled Enzyme Method of Immuno-Histochemistry: Preparation of Antigen-Antibody Complex (Peroxidase-Anti-Peroxidase) in Identification of Spirochetes, J. Histochem. Cytochem. *18,* 315–327 (1970).

[56] *H. Hertzman, R. M. Richards,* Use of Avidin-Complex for Staining of Biological Membranes in Electron Microscopy, Proc. Natl. Acad. Sci. USA *71,* 3537–3541 (1974).

[57] *L. A. Herzenberg, S. J. Black, T. Tokuhisa, L. Herzenberg,* Memory B Cells at Successive Stages of Differentiation: Affinity Maturation and the Role of IgD Receptors, J. Exp. Med. *151,* 1071–1078 (1980).

[58] *J. W. Kelly,* An Evaluation of the Metachromasy of Anionic Dyes. I. Visual Detection on Tissue Sections, Stain. Technol. *31,* 275–283 (1956).

7.2   Cytokine Analysis in Cells

Anthony R. Mire-Sluis, Meenu Wadhwa, Christopher R. Bird, M. Gisella Cavallo, Lisa A. Randall and Robin Thorpe

Cytokines are small or medium-sized proteins or glycoproteins which mediate a number of biological functions. They play an integral role in the regulation of many important biological and physiological processes which control the immune system, neuroendocrine function and the inflammatory response. About forty individual cytokines have been positively identified and discovery of new molecules is progressing very rapidly.

Cytokines are be secreted by many cell types, often following some form of activation stimulus. Activation of a single cell type generally results in the production of several cytokines, dependent upon the cell type and activation signal, and each cytokine may in turn exert pleiotropic biological effects on target cells. They may, for example, stimulate or inhibit the production of other cytokines; effect the modulation of cytokine receptor levels; display synergistic, antagonistic or additive effects on cell function and influence the regulation of cell proliferation and differentiation.

A number of approaches have been employed to analyse the production of cytokines by cells, perhaps the most common being the use of bioassays and immunoassays to quantify cytokines in biological fluids. Valuable information can be obtained by the use of these methods. However, due to the inherent limitations of the systems, caution has to be exercised when interpreting data obtained from complex biological fluids.

The most common approach to quantify cytokines in a complex milieu, such as body fluids or supernatants of cultured cells, has been to use bioassays.

Bioassays which use primary cultures of cells obtained from animals, or continuous, cytokine-dependent cell-lines, are rarely entirely specific (e. g., thymocyte assay, assays based on leukaemic cell-lines). In these assays, specificity for a particular cytokine must be established by using a monospecific neutralizing antibody [1], this approach being crucial for confirming the presence of individual cytokines in biological samples. In certain circumstances (assaying tissue fluids or blood samples), a bioassay can underestimate cytokine content due to the presence of binding proteins or other antagonistic molecules, e. g., the IL-1 receptor antagonist or other cytokines such as transforming growth factor β (TGFβ) or interferon γ (IFNγ) which exert an inhibitory effect and in turn mask the biological activity. In addition, bioassays may not distinguish between different molecular species of some cytokines, e. g. IL-1α and β, which, although structurally different, cannot be discriminated because of virtually identical biological effects (at least, on homologous cells). These problems have led to use of immunochemical methods for detection and quantitation of cytokines.

Immunochemical methods are usually easier to perform than classical bioassays and are often quicker and more reproducible. However, they can detect biologically inactive cytokine molecules resulting in a false impression of the possible physiological/clinical significance of cytokine levels detected. The procedures are also limited by the quality of the cytokine antibodies used, as a good antibody can produce high sensitivity and specificity whereas poor antibodies/antisera can cause artefacts and may be useless for most practical applications. Such limitations demand that a cautious approach be taken in the selection of appropriate techniques for a precise measurement of cytokine levels.

7.2.1 Analysis of Cell Extracts

Immunoassays often used for measurement of cytokines are radioimmunoassay (RIA), immunoradiometric assay (IRMA), and enzyme-linked immunoabsorbent assay (ELISA). A basic requirement of each is properly characterized specific antibodies which only recognize the particular cytokine to be quantified. A careful validation of the immunoassays to eliminate nonspecific artefacts is imperative, particularly if they are to be used for assaying clinical samples.

Before analysis it is necessary to extract the intracellular protein by an appropriate method. For detection of cytokines by bioassays, repeated freeze-thawing or hypotonic lysis is generally adequate. However, for some immunochemical methods and immunological assays, a lysis step as detailed below may be required:

1. Pellet cells by centrifugation and discard supernatant.
2. Add 200 μl lysis solution (2% (v/v) Nonidet P40; phenyl methyl sulphonyl fluoride, 1 mmol/l; EDTA, 60 mmol/l; Hepes, 40 mmol/l, pH 7.4; Aprotinin, 1 I.U./ml; Leupeptin, 20 μmol/l) at 4 °C.
3. Mix and centrifuge cells at 1500 × g for 5 min at 4 °C.
4. Remove supernatant and freeze until required for further analysis.

7.2.1.1   Radioimmunoassays (RIA)

In setting up these assays it is essential to radiolabel a relatively pure preparation of the cytokine with ^{125}I to a high specific activity using a method which does not denature the cytokine in any manner [2]. Various methods are employed for iodination of cytokines [3]; however, the suitability of these for a particular cytokine should be carefully determined. A detailed protocol for a RIA is given below.

Method

1. Add cytokine standard or sample in serial dilutions in 100 μl of assay diluent (PBS/0.5% w/v BSA) to a dilution of sheep polyclonal anti-cytokine (in 300 μl of assay diluent) in plastic tubes and incubate for 24–28 h at 4 °C.
2. Add ^{125}I-cytokine tracer (10000 cpm; 100–150 μCi/μg) in 100 μl assay diluent and incubate for a further 48–72 h at 4 °C.
3. Separate the bound antibody-cytokine complexes from the free cytokine by an anti-sheep second antibody. Incubate for 4 h at room temperature.
4. Add PEG 6000 (4% v/v) and centrifuge at 1000 × g for 30 min.
5. Discard the supernatant from each tube and count the bound radioactivity in the precipitate using a gamma counter. Calculate the percentage of counts bound (correct for nonspecific binding).
6. Plot a dose-response curve of bound counts against the logarithm of the ligand concentration. Bound counts are maximal in the absence of any cytokine and fall towards zero with increasing concentration of the unlabelled cytokine, giving a sigmoidal curve. Estimate activity of an unknown sample by comparison with the standard curve.

7.2.1.2   IRMA and ELISA

In these assays, the ligand reacts with an excess of labelled antibody. For the measurement of cytokines, a two-site IRMA, which employs solid-phase antibody and liquid-phase ^{125}I-labelled antibodies directed to distinct antigenic epitopes on the ligand, is often used. A combination of two anti-cytokine mAbs can be particularly effective although pAbs can be just as effective in many cases.

For use in an IRMA, both antibodies require purification [3]. The detecting antibody also needs to be radiolabelled with ^{125}I using a method which does not denature the antibody [3]. As a typical example, a detailed protocol of the immunoassay used for measurement of human IL-1α is described [4].

Method

1. Coat wells of flexible 96-well microtitre plates with purified capture antibody at a concentration of 5–10 µg/ml (200 µl/well diluted in PBS containing azide 0.02% w/v) by incubation either overnight at 4 °C or for at least 3 h at 37 °C.
2. Wash plates with 3 changes of PBS azide containing haemoglobin (3% w/v) (Hb-PBS) and block the remaining protein-binding sides by incubation with Hb-PBS for 30 min at room temperature.
3. Following another wash with Hb-PBS, incubate wells with test samples or dilutions of the cytokine standard (200 µl/well diluted in Hb-PBS) for 3 h at room temperature or overnight at 4 °C.
4. Wash plates 4 times with Hb-PBS and incubate for 2 h at room temperature with the second anti-cytokine antibody (either a mAb or a pAb) radiolabelled with ^{125}I to serve as a detecting reagent (200 µl/well containing approximately 250 000 cpm).
5. Wash the plates 5 times with Hb-PBS. Cut out individual wells with a hot-wire plate cutter and estimate the radioactivity bound to the wells by counting in a gamma counter.
6. Plot the data as cpm bound (eliminate the nonspecific binding obtained with the control) against the concentration of the cytokine in I.U./ml to obtain a standard curve or dose-response curve. Estimate activity of cytokine in test samples by interpolation in the standard curve.

A similar strategy has been used for measuring human IL-3 and IL-4 [5]. For measurement of human G-CSF, however, a slightly different design of two-site assay has been used [6]. Instead of adding antigen directly to the wells as in step 3, antigen is complexed with the antibody (mAb to G-CSF) in separate 96-well plates for 1.5 h at 37 °C. This complex is subsequently transferred to a plate coated with a different antibody (purified sheep anti-G-CSF) and incubated for 2 h at 37 °C. Finally, the plate is washed and the bound G-CSF-complex detected using ^{125}I-sheep anti-mouse IgG.

Extensive characterization of the antibodies (using different recombinant forms of the cytokine) is essential prior to their use in immunoassays, particularly if recombinant products containing sequence modifications have been used to generate hybridomas.

This protects against the possibility of preferential recognition of a particular recombinant form of the molecule.

Enzyme-linked immunosorbent assays (ELISA) for cytokines in principle are essentially the same as IRMA, the difference being that the detecting antibody is conjugated to an enzyme, e. g., POD (EC 1.11.1.7), or AP (EC 3.1.3.1) or others. Various types of ELISA have been described for cytokines and several are commercially available (e. g. *R&D Systems*).

7.2.1.3   Detection by Immunoblotting

Standard immunoblotting procedures can be used to detect cytokines [7] in cell lysates. Advantages of the procedure are that no purification of cytokine protein from homogenates is necessary and, as cell homogenates can be run in several tracks of the same gel, probing for several cytokines in a particular cell preparation can be carried out simultaneously and *directly* compared. Some antigenic determinants do not survive the electrophoresis conditions (especially if reducing SDS-PAGE is used) and this can be a particular problem for mAbs. The method can be very sensitive but the very small amounts of cytokine protein present in some cells can be a limitation. For example, it is difficult to detect IL-2 in lectin-stimulated human T-cells but IL-1 is detectable in monocyte lysates (Fig. 1). Most methods can be applied to cytokine detection but the choice of antibody is very important and blocking reagents should be protein-based, e. g., haemoglobin or milk protein solutions; detergents alone can cause problems due

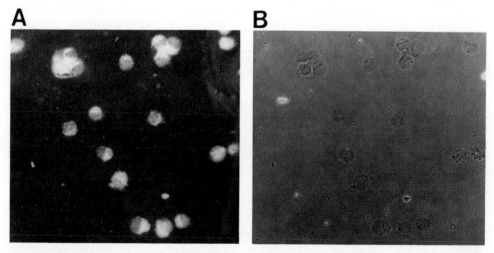

Fig. 1. Immunoblot of a lysate from activated human monocytes probed with an anti-IL-1β sheep pAb reagent. Most of the IL-1β is present as an approximate 31,000 M_r precursor. Various lower molecular weight processed forms can also be detected. Results from two different cell donors are illustrated.

to inefficient inhibition of nonspecific antigen-antibody interactions [8]. A generally applicable procedure is described below (cf. Volume 1, 3.6.4).

Method

1. Run the cell extract/sample on a SDS-PAGE gel (other gel systems e.g. isoelectric focusing can be used).
2. Fill the immunoblot electrophoresis tank with transfer buffer. Fold a piece of filter-paper twice the size of the internal cassette in half, soak in transfer buffer and place on the cathodal side of the cassette.
3. Unfold the filter-paper and place the gel on the half of the filter-paper covering the cathode (or on the cathodal side of the cassette). Immediately soak the nitrocellulose sheet in transfer buffer and place it on the gel, expelling any trapped air bubbles. Do not move the nitrocellulose once it has been positioned.
4. Fold over the other half of the filter-paper and overlay with another sheet of filter-paper soaked in transfer buffer. Fill the remaining space in the cassette with scouring pads soaked in transfer buffer, ensuring that the gel is pressed firmly against the nitrocellulose. Secure the cassette tightly.
5. Place the cassette in the tank and fit the lid. If apparatus has the facility for buffer recirculation, turn on the recirculating pump. If not, use a magnetic stirrer to agitate the transfer buffer.
6. Electrophorese for 1–4 h at 0.45 A.
7. Turn off power and remove nitrocellulose sheet and gel from the cassette. The gel can be stained if required.
8. Shake nitrocellulose sheet for 30 min in 50–200 ml of Hb-PBS (3% w/v bovine Hb in PBS) at room temperature.
9. Shake sheet for 2–16 h with 20–40 ml Hb-PBS containing antibody (about 1–100 µl antiserum or ascites fluid or 50 µl – 1 ml hybridoma culture fluid).
10. Wash for 0.5–1 h (6 to 7 changes, 20–200 ml each) with Hb-PBS. Use brisk agitation on an orbital shaker.
11. Shake for 2–6 h with 20–50 ml Hb-PBS containing ^{125}I-labelled anti-Ig. Use 5×10^5–10^6 cpm/track (approximately 20–50 ng IgG) or 5×10^6 cpm/gel.
12. Wash for 0.5–1 h (6 to 8 changes, 20–200 ml each) with PBS.
13. Pin blots to a suitable support so that they hang freely in air. Dry at room temperature, or in an oven at 56 °C or by using a hair-dryer. When completely dry, carry out autoradiography using X-ray film, e.g. *Kodak* X-OMAT.

7.2.2   Analysis of Individual Cells

7.2.2.1   Reverse Haemolytic Plaque Assay

Since the discovery of an intricate network of cytokine production, actions and interactions, characterization of cytokines on an individual basis has become important. Recently, a reverse haemolytic plaque assay (RHPA) modified from the classical plaque-forming cell assay [9] has been adapted to measure cytokine production by individual cells. The secretion of a selected cytokine in the presence of an appropriate antiserum results in a haemolytic plaque from which quantitative data can be obtained [10].

Conjugation of protein-A to ovine erythrocytes

Method

1. Prepare ovine erythrocytes carefully by centrifugation at $400 \times g$ for 25 min using Ficoll-Hypaque according to manufacturer's instructions (*Sigma*) for removal of leucocytes (cf. 2.2). Wash pellet several times in 0.9% (w/v) NaCl solution (saline) by further centrifugation at $400 \times g$ for 5–10 min.
2. Add 1 ml protein-A (0.5 mg/ml in saline) to the cell pellet and mix with 10 ml chromium chloride (0.1 mg/ml in saline). (N. B. the $CrCl_3$ solution should be made up and stored for at least one week at 4 °C in the dark before use. This solution can be used for up to 6 months).
3. Resuspend and incubate the cells for 1 h at 30 °C.
4. Wash cells several times with saline or with *Dulbecco's* Modified *Eagle* Medium (DMEM) containing 0.1% (w/v) BSA.
5. Resuspend as a 2% suspension (v/v) in DMEM containing 0.1% BSA and antibiotics.
6. Store the cells at 4 °C and use 1–5 days after conjugation to achieve the best monolayers in the RHPA.

Reverse haemolytic plaque assay

Method

1. Immerse glass slides in acid alcohol for 5 min.
2. Rinse 4 times in doubly distilled water and immerse in 1% (v/v) DMSO for 5 min. Wash slides extensively again in water and air-dry.
3. Place slides in a solution of poly-L-lysine, 0.05 mg/ml, for 10 min, then rinse in water and air-dry.

4. Construct *Cunningham* chambers [11].
5. Spin down 10 ml of 2% (v/v) protein-A-conjugated ovine erythrocytes at $300 \times g$ for 5 min.
6. Resuspend pellet to yield a 40% suspension (v/v) of the conjugated erythrocytes in DMEM containing 0.1% BSA (w/v) and antibiotics.
7. Add test cells ($1–10 \times 10^6$ cells/ml) to the erythrocytes at a 1:1 ratio (v/v). Mix well and apply 100 µl to each chamber.
8. Leave the cell mixture to settle on glass slides by incubating for 30–45 min in a 5% CO_2 humidified atmosphere. This allows formation of a confluent monolayer of cells.
9. Rinse chamber 4 times with warm (37 °C) assay medium (RPMI 1640 supplemented with 0.1% (w/v) BSA and antibiotics).
10. Add 90–100 µl of appropriate anti-cytokine antibody (for pAb, 1/50–1/100 dilution is adequate) in assay medium and incubate the slides at 37 °C in a 5% CO_2 humidified atmosphere for 6–16 h. For a negative control, use an equivalent concentration of an irrelevant antibody or the IgG fraction of pre-immune serum from the donor animal. Rinse slides to remove unbound antibody.
11. Infuse guinea-pig complement ($^{1}/_{50}$ dilution; Gibco) in warm assay medium to initiate plaque formation and incubate for a further 20–30 min. If needed, assess viability (by incubation with 0.2% (w/v) trypan blue for 5 mins at 37 °C) (cf. section 2.1) or go to fixation step directly).
12. Fix the slides with 2% (v/v) glutaraldehyde in phosphate buffer and store at 4 °C (for up to 2 weeks) for later analysis.
13. Analyse the area for haemolytic plaques using a forward projection microscope systematically to scan each entire chamber of cells.

A particular advantage of using the RHPA over other methods for analysing cytokines secreted by individual cells is that the size of the plaque relates directly to the amount of cytokine secreted and can therefore produce quantitative data [12]. In addition, the cells remain viable throughout the assay and can be used for further studies, such as phenotype analysis [12]. The assay can be simplified for routine analysis by conjugating an anti-cytokine antibody directly to ovine erythrocytes [13]. It must be remembered, however, that the RPHA isolates cells from the complex cytokine network and therefore may not reflect the true pattern of cytokine production *in vivo*.

7.2.2.2 Immunocytochemical Analysis

Intracellular cytokines can be identified in the cells that make them at the microscopic level using immunocytochemical techniques. These are rapid and specific enabling the identification and visualization of cytokine-producing cells. Immunostaining is not quantitative and the precise amount of cytokine produced by each individual cell cannot be accurately determined using this method.

Both pAbs and mAbs are suitable for immunostaining cytokines. mAbs have the advantage of giving less background staining but polyclonal antisera usually recognise different molecular forms of the cytokine and may increase the sensitivity of the method. The background produced by polyclonal antisera can sometimes be reduced by affinity-purifying the antibodies.

The indirect binding technique using unlabelled anti-cytokine antibodies and labelled anti-Ig antibodies is usually preferred because it avoids the need to label several different specific antibodies.

Immunostaining can detect cytokines in either individual cells or tissue sections. Cells need to be fixed and permeabilized prior to staining to allow the antibodies to penetrate cells and bind to intracellular cytokine proteins. Pre-immune sera or mAbs with irrelevant specificities should always be included as controls to determine nonspecific binding. It is essential to ensure that the conjugated antibodies do not bind to proteins of the target structure; in particular a cross-reactivity of such antibodies with endogenous immunoglobulins may cause problems. Cells or sections should therefore be incubated with labelled second-step antibodies alone as a control.

General Methods

The procedure described below can be applied to tissue sections and cells dried onto microscope slides and can be adapted for detecting different cyctokines. Extensive discussion of the procedures is given in Sections 5.2. and 5.5 The appropriate dilution for each cytokine-specific antibody should be determined empirically: in general a dilution of 1:50–1:100 is suitable for most pAbs, whilst the optimal concentration for mAbs is 10–20 μg/ml.

Fixation and permeabilization

1. Fix 5–6 μm tissue sections or cytocentrifuge smears by soaking slides in 4% paraformaldehyde (PFA) in PBS, pH 7.6, for 20 min at room temperature. Wash twice with PBS containing 4% sodium azide for 5 min each.
2. Permeabilize cells by treatment with 0.2% Triton X-100 in PBS for 5 min at 4 °C. Wash twice with PBS azide for 5 min each.

Such preparations can be stored at 4 °C in PBS/azide for up to one month before use.

Immunofluorescence (IF) staining

1. Dip slides in PBS containing 0.1% BSA before staining in order to reduce the background.
2. Add 100 μl of appropriate dilution of cytokine-specific antibodies and control antibodies (pre-immune sera or mAbs with irrelevant specificity, at the concentra-

tion chosen for the test antibody) in PBS containing 5% (v/v) normal serum and incubate 1 h at room temperature in a moist chamber (ideally, the normal serum should be from the species in which the second antibody was raised). Wash 4 times with PBS azide containing 5% normal serum for 5 min each time.

3. Add 100 μl of appropriate dilution of FITC-labelled anti-Ig antibodies in PBS and incubate 30–45 min at room temperature in a moist chamber (antibodies should be centrifuged before use in order to remove aggregates). Wash 4 times with PBS azide, 5 min each time.

4. Incubate sections with 4% paraformaldehyde in PBS for 5 min at room temperature to fix staining. Wash briefly with PBS.

5. Mount slides with 10 μl of mounting medium (PBS:Glycerol 1:9 containing 1,4-diazabicyclo-(2,2,2)-octane (DABCO), 0.22 mol/l, pH 8.6) on the top of the tissue area and cover with a glass coverslip.

6. View the slides using a fluorescence microscope (Fig. 2).

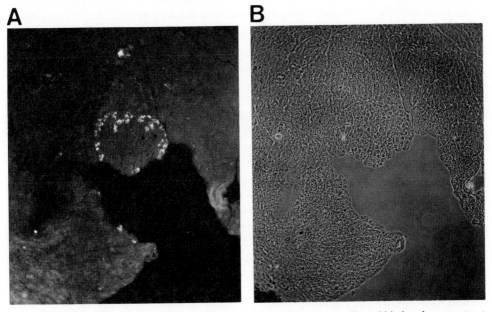

Fig. 2. a) Immunofluorescence staining of mouse GM-CSF in β islet cells and b) the phase contrast microscopy of the field in (a). Murine GM-CSF in (a) was detected by using a specific anti-murine GM-CSF antibody (Magnification × 280).

Immunoperoxidase staining

Fixation can be carried out as for IF staining, but this should not contain sodium azide. To inhibit endogenous peroxidase, sections can be pre-treated with 0.01% (v/v) H_2O_2 (cf. 5.6.1.5).

1. Dip slides in PBS containing 0.1% BSA before staining.
2. Pre-incubate sections with PBS containing 10% normal serum for 10 min at room temperature to reduce nonspecific antibody binding. The normal serum should be from the species in which the second antibody (POD-conjugated) was raised.
3. Add 100 µl of appropriate dilution of cytokine-specific antibodies and control antibodies (pre-immune sera or mAbs with irrelevant specificity, at the same concentration of the test antibody) in PBS containing 5% (v/v) normal serum and incubate for 1 h at room temperature in a moist chamber. Wash 4 times with PBS containing 5% normal serum for 5 min each time.
4. Add 100 µl of appropriate dilution of POD-labelled anti-Ig antibodies in PBS and incubate 30–45 min at room temperature in a moist chamber. Make up a solution of the substrate by dissolving DAB in Tris-HCl (0.5 mg/ml). Wash 4 times with PBS, 5 min each time.
5. Add 10 µl/ml of 1% (v/v) H_2O_2 to the substrate solution and incubate sections with substrate for 10 min and wash briefly with PBS.
6. Counterstain with haematoxylin for 5 min, wash with tap water and dehydrate sections with 70% ethanol, twice with absolute ethanol and 3 times with xylene.
7. Mount in DPX mountant and view using a light microscope.

Alkaline phosphatase (AP) staining

1. Fix sections in ice-cold acetone for 10 min. Wash twice with Tris-buffered saline (NaCl 0.15 mol/l in Tris-HCl, 10 mmol/l, pH 7.3) for 5 min.
2. Incubate with anti-cytokine antibodies at appropriate dilution and with control antibodies for 60 min at room temperature in a moist chamber. Wash 4 times with TBS for 5 min.
3. Incubate sections with AP-conjugated anti-Ig antibody for 30–45 min at room temperature in a moist chamber. Wash 4 times with TBS for 5 min.
4. Make up substrate solution by dissolving a) naphthol AS-BI phosphate, 25 mg/ml, in dimethylformamide and b) Fast Red TR salt, 0.5 mg/ml, in barbitone-acetate buffer. Mix 1 vol. solution (a) with 100 vol. solution (b) and add levamisole to 25 mg/ml to block endogenous phosphatase.
5. Incubate sections with fresh substrate solution for 10–15 min at room temperature and wash twice with TBS for 5 min.
6. Counterstain with haematoxylin for 5 min and wash with tap water.
7. Mount with glycerine jelly and view with a light microscope.

Staining cells in suspension

1. Wash cells 3 times in 4 ml V-bottomed tubes.
2. Fix by adding 0.5 ml 4% paraformaldehyde in PBS to the cell pellets and incubate for 5 min at 4 °C.

3. Add PBS to the tubes and centrifuge at 1,300 rpm at $400 \times g$ and wash twice with PBS.
4. Permeabilize cells by adding 0.5 ml 0.1% Triton X-100 in PBS and incubate for 5 min at 4 °C, wash twice with PBS.
5. Add 100 µl of cytokine-specific antibody at appropriate dilution and incubate for 1 h at 4 °C, wash twice with PBS.
6. Add 100 µl of FITC-labelled anti-Ig antibody at appropriate dilution and incubate 30–45 min at 4 °C. Wash 4 times with PBS.
7. Put a drop of the cell suspension on a glass slide and allow to dry.
8. Mount by adding a drop of DABCO onto the cell area. Cover with a glass coverslip and view with a fluorescence microscope (Fig. 3).

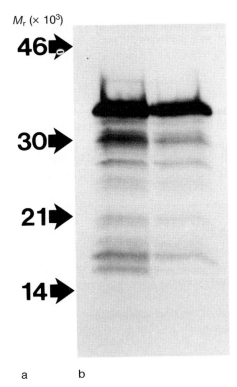

M_r (× 10^3)

46

30

21

14

a   b

Fig. 3. a) Immunofluorescence staining of mouse IL-1β and b) the corresponding phase contrast photo-micrograph showing the morphology of LPS-activated P388D1 cells. The intracellular accumulation of IL-1β in a) observed as amorphous staining was obtained using a specific anti-mouse IL-1β antibody (Magnification × 820).

With the above procedure, it is essential to use a fairly large number of cells since loss of fixed cells during washing is quite high. When a limited number of cells is available it is preferable to use cytospreads for immunofluorescence staining.

7.2.2.3   Flow-Cytometric Analysis of Intracellular Cytokines

The technique allows both the analysis of larger numbers of cells in a short period and also the quantitation of results. The method is also less subjective than immunocyto-chemical procedures. However, flow cytometry has been limited to the analysis of cell surface antigens since many methods of cell membrane permeabilization which would permit the detection of intracellular antigens often lead to morphological damage, cell aggregation or loss of intracellular antigenicity [14–16]. These problems have now largely been overcome by a combination of fixation and permeabilization techniques that stabilize cell membranes and preserve cell morphology [17]. It should be noted that permeabilization without fixation reduces forward scattered light through the loss of cytoplasmic material. The procedure below outlines a chemical membrane permeabil-ization method using lysolecithin which, because of its applicability to routine analysis and combination with acidic sodium acetate buffer and PFA fixation, proves to be particularly suitable for the detection of intracellular antigens [18]. For full discussion cf. 5.11.

Method

1. Wash cells twice in ice-cold PBS, 0.15 mol/l, pH 7.4 and resuspend the cells in ice-cold PBS to a concentration of 2×10^6 cells/ml.
2. Take 100 µl aliquots of this cell suspension and add to each 1 ml of a 5 µg/ml solution of lysolecithin (lysophosphatidylcholine, *Sigma*) in sodium acetate buffer, 20 mmol/l, pH 4.5 at 4 °C for 2 min.
3. Stop permeabilization by adding 250 µl of 4% paraformaldehyde in PBS, 0.15 mol/l, pH 7.4.
4. Wash cells twice in 4 ml PBS containing 1% (w/v) BSA and sodium azide, 20 mmol/l.
5. Incubate cells with an appropriate anti-cytokine antibody for 30 min at 4 °C (steps 5–6 should be omitted for samples of cells to act as a control for nonspecific staining).
6. Wash cells twice in ice-cold PBS/BSA/azide.
7. Incubate cells with an appropriately conjugated second layer antibody for 30 min at 4 °C.
8. Wash cells twice in ice-cold PBS/BSA/azide.
9. Analyse cells by flow cytometry.

mAbs usually produce less nonspecific staining than pAbs and controls should be stained with a mAb of identical isotype and at the same concentration. Optimization of flow cytometric analysis can be achieved using phycoerythrin-conjugated subclass-specific second step antibodies and linear, not logarithmic, amplification for cytoplas-mic antigen detection [19].

7.2.3   Detection of Cytokine mRNA

As an alternative to the quantitative analysis of cytokines produced by cells, cytokine gene expression can be measured by determining cytokine mRNA levels using hybridization techniques such as dot-blot, northern analysis or *in situ* hybridization [20, 21]. Detection of mRNA by hybridization to a complementary probe (e.g., synthetic oligonucleotide, cDNA or cRNA) requires the incorporation of a detectable molecule into the applied nucleic acid probe. This has generally consisted of a radioactive label which is detected by autoradiography, however, a number of alternative, non-isotopic techniques are commonly used. The enzymatic introduction of a hapten as an immunochemical marker or, alternatively, the chemical modification of a probe have been used successfully [22, 23]. The interaction between the probe and the target may be visualized by means of a specific antibody directed against the hapten, or the chemically modified nucleic acid, which can be coupled to an enzyme (e.g. POD or AP) so that a colour precipitate is formed at the site of hybridization in the presence of an appropriate chromogenic substrate. FITC-conjugated antibodies can also be used and the site of hybridization detected by flow cytometry [24].

The enzymatic introduction of biotin into nucleotides has had widespread applications. Biotinylated probes can be detected with conjugated anti-biotin antibodies or with avidin and streptavidin conjugates. A more recent development has been the incorporation of the steroid hapten digoxigenin into synthetic oligonucleotide probes using digoxigenin-dUTP and 3' tail-labelling using terminal transferase. Digoxigenin can also be incorporated into cDNAs by random priming methods using *Klenow* polymerase, or by direct labelling using photodigoxigenin. These techniques have produced both sensitive and stable probes which may be detected by means of anti-digoxigenin antibodies [25, 26]. With the use of haptenated or modified probes, the signal can be localized clearly through a coloured precipitate, which allows for subsequent identification of cell morphology and detection of multiple mRNAs within a cell, or tissue section. In addition, the long exposure time required with low energy radionucleotides (e.g. ^{3}H. ^{35}S) is eliminated.

The use of digoxigenin-labelled probes in combination with anti-digoxigenin-conjugated antibodies provides a highly sensitive method for detecting nucleotide sequences, and one which has been used successfully for detection of cytokine mRNA transcripts at the single cell level by *in situ* hybridization [27]. A number of protocols detailing the theoretical and practical considerations of hybridization techniques have been described [20, 21, 26]. The methods may have to be adjusted for each application to optimize tissue preparation, probe hybridization conditions, selection of probe, and the signal-to-noise ratio. Essentially, the steps involved can be divided into a) tissue preparation (according to the use of tissue sections or intact cells) e.g., rapid fixing/freezing of tissue and cryotome sectioning; b) pre-hybridization treatments to decrease background interactions between probe and cell/tissue components and to optimize the access of the probe for the target mRNA; c) probe hybridization, the time and temperature for optimal hybridization varying for different applications; d) post-hybridization, to remove unbound probe and reduce background, and e) detection of bound probe, e. g., by immunological detection with a conjugated antibody. Outlines of the methods for probe labelling and immunological detection of probe are given below.

Labelling of oligonucleotide probes with digoxigenin-11 dUTP

Method

3′ tail-labelling of oligonucleotides can be performed with digoxigenin-11 dUTP by means of terminal deoxynucleotidyl transferase *(Boehringer Mannheim)*. The labelling reaction is performed as follows:

1. Into a 1.5 ml sterile *Eppendorf* tube on ice add 2.5 µl of 10x reaction buffer (potassium cacodylate 1.4 mmol/l, Tris base, 0.3 mol/l, pH 7.2, cobalt chloride, 10 mmol/l, dithiothreitol, 2 mmol/l). 2.5 µl of digoxigenin-11 dUTP, 1 mmol/l *(Boehringer Mannheim)*, 25 U of terminal transferase *(Boehringer Mannheim)*, 200 ng of probe in 5 µl distilled water, 12 µl of DEPC-treated water.
2. Incubate the reaction mixture at 37 °C for 90 min and then store at −20 °C in 5 µl aliquots.

The procedures for *in situ* hybridization are detailed in the technical data sheets accompanying the Genius™ non-radioactive nucleic acid labelling and detection system from *Boehringer Mannheim*.

Immunological detection

Method

1. Wash slides in Tris-HCl, 0.1 mol/l, NaCl, 0.15 mol/l, pH 7.5 (Tris-saline).
2. Block slides with 2% (v/v) normal sheep serum plus 0.3% Triton X-100 for 30 min at room temperature.
3. Dilute polyclonal sheep anti-digoxigenin antiserum conjugated to AP (1:500) in Tris-saline containing 1% (v/v) normal sheep serum and 0.3% Triton X-100.
4. Incubate slides with diluted antibody enzyme conjugate (100 µl/section) for 2 h at room temperature.
5. Wash slides for 15 min in 200 ml Tris-saline.
6. Incubate slides for 2 min in 200 ml Tris-HCl, 0.1 mol/l, NaCl, 0.1 mol/l, MgCl$_2$, 0.05 mol/l, pH 9.5.
7. Develop slides by incubation for 2 h at room temperature with colour solution; 45 µl nitroblue tetrazolium and 35 µl of X-phosphate solution *(Boehringer Mannheim)* and 2.4 mg levamisole *(Sigma)* in 10 ml of Tris-HCl, 0.1 mol/l, NaCl, 0.1 mol/l, MgCl$_2$ 0.05 mol/l, pH 9.5 (500 µl/slide).

8. Stop the colour reaction with Tris-HCl, 0.1 mol/l containing EDTA, 1 mmol/l, pH 8.5.
9. Mount the tissue sections in glycerol-PBS (9:1), cover with a glass coverslip and examine under a microscope.

It should be understood that the presence of mRNA for a particular cytokine is not necessarily an indication that the protein is translated and secreted by the cell. The evidence for the existence of human IL-3, for instance, appears to be based solely on the presence of transcripts in activated T-cells [28], the protein product of this gene being apparently undetectable. The combination of immunocytochemistry with *in situ* hybridization makes this technique an extremely powerful tool for studying cytokine gene expression, as analysis of mRNA expression as well as the phenotypic expression of the cytokine protein *in situ* may be achieved.

References

[1] *M. Wadhwa, C. Bird, A. Tinker, A. Mire-Sluis, R. Thorpe*, Quantitative Biological Assays for Individual Cytokines, in: *F. R. Balkwill* (ed.), Cytokines: A Practical Approach, IRL Press, Oxford 1991, pp. 309–330.

[2] *S. Poole, A. F. Bristow, S. Selkirk, B. Rafferty*, Development and Application of Radioimmunoassays for Interleukin-1α and Interleukin-1β, J. Immunol. Methods *115*, 259–264 (1989).

[3] *A. P. Johnstone, R. Thorpe*, Immunochemistry in Practice, 2nd Edition, Blackwell Scientific Publications, London 1987.

[4] *R. Thorpe, M. Wadhwa, A. J. H. Gearing, B. Mahon, S. Poole*, Sensitive and Specific Immunoradiometric Assays for Human Interleukin-1 Alpha, Lymphokine Res. 7, 119–127 (1988).

[5] *C. Bird, M. Wadhwa, R. Thorpe*, Development of Immunoassays for Human IL-3 and IL-4 Some of which Discriminate between Different Recombinant DNA Derived Molecules, Cytokine 3, 562–567 (1991).

[6] *M. Wadhwa, R. Thorpe, C. R. Bird, A. J. H. Gearing*, Production of Polyclonal and Monoclonal Antibodies to Granulocyte Colony-Stimulating Factor (G-CSF) and Development of Immunoassays, J. Immunol. Methods *128*, 211–217 (1990).

[7] *H. Towbin, J. Gordon*, Immunoblotting and Dot Immunobinding – Current Status and Outlook, J. Immunol. Methods 73, 313–318.

[8] *C. R. Bird, A. J. H. Gearing, R. Thorpe*, The Use of Tween 20 Alone as a Blocking Agent for Immunoblotting can Cause Artefactual Results, J. Immunol. Methods *106*, 175–179 (1988).

[9] *N. K. Jerne, A. A. Nordin*, Plaque Formation in Agar by Single Antibody-producing Cells, Science 140, 405–409 (1963).

[10] *C. E. Lewis, S. P. McCarthy, P. S. Richards, P. Lorenzen, E. Harak, J. O'D McGee*, Measurement of Cytokine Release by Human Cells: A Quantitative Analysis at the Single Cell Level Using the Reverse Haemolytic Plaque Assay, J. Immunol. Methods *127*, 51–59 (1990).

[11] *A. J. Cunningham, A. Szenberg*, Further Improvements in the Plaque Technique for Detecting Single Antibody-forming Cells, Immunology 14, 599–602 (1968).

[12] *C. E. Lewis, D. McCracken, R. Ling, P. S. Richards, S. P. McCarthy, J. O'D McGee*, Cytokine Release by Single, Immunophenotyped Human Cells: Use of the Reverse Hemolytic Plaque Assay. Immunol. Rev. *119*, 23–39 (1991).

[13] *G. A. Molinaro, S. Dray,* Antibody Coated Erythrocytes as Manifold Probe Antigens, Nature *248,* 515–517 (1974).
[14] *U. Andersson, G. Halldén, U. Persson, J. Hed, G. Möller, M. Deley,* Enumeration of IFN-γ-Producing Cells by Flow Cytometry. Comparison with Fluorescence Microscopy, J. Immunol. Methods *112,* 139–142 (1988).
[15] *E. Hofsli, O. Bakke, U. Nonstad, T. Espevik,* A Flow Cytometric and Immunofluorescence Microscopic Study of Tumour Necrosis Factor Production and Localization in Human Monocytes, Cell Immunol. *122,* 405–415 (1989).
[16] *R. W. Schroff, C. D. Bucana, R. A. Klein, M. M. Farrell, A. C. Morgan Jr,* Detection of Intracytoplasmic Antigens by Flow Cytometry, J. Immunol. Methods *70,* 167–177 (1984).
[17] *G. Halldén, U. Andersson, J. Hed, S. G. O. Johansson,* A New Membrane Permeabilisation Method for the Detection of Intracellular Antigens by Flow Cytometry, J. Immunol. Methods *124,* 103–109 (1989).
[18] *M. Labalette-Houache, G. Torpier, A. Capron, J. P. Dessaint,* Improved Permeabilisation Procedure for Flow Cytometric Detection of Internal Antigens. Analysis of Interleukin-2 Production, J. Immunol. Methods *138,* 143–153 (1991).
[19] *B. Sander, J. Andersson, U. Andersson,* Assessment of Cytokines by Immunofluorescence and the Paraformaldehyde-saponin Procedure, Immunol. Rev. *119,* 65–93 (1991).
[20] *M. S. Naylor, F. R. Balkwill,* Northern Analysis and *in situ* Hybridization of Cytokine Messenger RNA, in: *F. R. Balkwill* (ed.), Cytokines: A Practical Approach: IRL Press, Oxford 1991, pp. 31–50.
[21] *M. J. Dallman, R. A. Montgomery, C. P. Larsen, A. Wanders, A. F. Wells,* Cytokine Gene Expression: Analysis Using Northern Blotting, Polymerase Chain Reaction and *in situ* Hybridization, Immunol. Rev. *119,* 163–179 (1991).
[22] *P. Tohen, P. P. R. Fuchs, E. Sage, M. Leng,* Chemically Modified Nucleic Acids as Immunodetectable Probes in Hybridization Experiments, Proc. Natl. Acad. Sci. USA *81,* 3466–3470 (1984).
[23] *R. Q. H. Zheng, E. Abney, C. Q. Chu, M. Field, B. Grubeck-Loebenstein, R. N. Maini, M. Feldmann,* Detection of Interleukin-6 and Interleukin-1 Production in Human Thyroid Epithelial Cells by Non-radioactive *in situ* Hybridization and Immunohistochemical Methods, Clin. Exp. Immunol. *83,* 314–319 (1991).
[24] *J. A. Bayer, J. G. J. Bauman,* Flow Cytometric Detection of β-Globin mRNA in Murine Haemopoietic Tissues Using Fluorescent *in situ* Hybridization, Cytometry *11,* 132–143 (1990).
[25] *R. Martin, C. Hoover, S. Grimme, C. Grogan, J. Höltke, C. Kessler,* A Highly Sensitive, Nonradioactive DNA Labelling and Detection System, BioTechniques *9,* 762–768 (1990).
[26] *F. Baldino, M. E. Lewis,* Nonradioactive in situ Hybridization Histochemistry with Digoxigenin-deoxyuridine 5′-triphosphate Labelled Oligonucleotides, in: *P. M. Conn* (ed.), Methods of Neuroscience, Gene Probes, Academic Press, New York 1989, pp. 282–292.
[27] *M. Samoszuk, L. Nansen,* Detection of Interleukin-5 Messenger RNA in *Reed-Sternberg* Cells of *Hodgkin's* Disease with Eosinophilia, Blood *75,* 13–16 (1990).
[28] *C. M. Niemeyer, C. A. Sieff, B. Mathey-Prevot, J. Z. Wimperis, B. E. Bierer, S. C. Clark, D. G. Nathan,* Expression of Human Interleukin-3 (multi-CSF) is Restricted to Human Lymphocytes and T-Cell Tumour Lines, Blood *73,* 945–951 (1989).

8 Analysis of Immune Cell Function

8.1   The Nature of Immunocytes

Frank Emmrich and Andreas H. Guse*

Over the last 20 years, an ever-increasing number of assays has been developed for dissecting the complex interactions involved in the generation of an immune response. Without discussing experimental details, this chapter aims to display the whole spectrum of methods applied in analysis of immune cell function together with some general considerations. More detailed information can be found in this volume on various procedures of isolation and purification of cells (cf. 2), cell culture (cf. 3) and phenotyping (cf. 5 and 6). Some assays for evaluation of antibody and cytokine production are outlined in 7.

A brief account of the nature and characteristics of the cells concerned in the immune response is followed by a discussion of immune cell isolation and phenotyping, since precise results of cellular assays or *in-vivo* experiments, including cell transfer, critically depend on purity of the cells investigated. Then an outline of some basic procedures to study signal transduction in immune cells after receptor triggering will be followed by assays for determination of effector functions of isolated cells. Finally, consideration will be given to cellular interactions which can be studied only partly *in vitro* and may require more complex systems such as organ culture or *in-vivo* experiments.

The T and B lymphocytes are the specific cellular elements unique to the immune system. However, for many years it has been evident that many other cell types, including dendritic cells, monocytes and macrophages, not only contribute as accessory cells to immune cell functions, but also are recruited and armed to exert a variety of effects even beyond the pathways of the immune system. Some of these cells are not easily distinguished morphologically from lymphocytes, as in NK-cells. However, there is one denominator which clearly differentiates between the specific and non-specific cells of the immune system and this is the presence of the antigen receptors of T- and B-cells. These receptors confer the unique diversity of antigen recognition and the capability to respond selectively to foreign invaders by multiplying T- or B-cells and antibodies. The immune response to foreign structures (antigens) results in rapid expansion of lymphocytes with specificity for the inducing antigens and the development of effector functions. T-cells depend on the thymus (T) for their maturation and B-cells are so designated since they are derived from bone marrow (B) precursor cells. Birds have developed a specialized organ, the *bursa fabricii* for B-cell differentiation.

The antigen receptors on B-cells consist of immunoglobulin heavy and light chains distributed into variable and constant portions, with the variable portion constituting the antigen binding site. Interaction of cell surface immunoglobulin with antigen induces B-cell activation and differentiation into plasma cells, provided that appro-

---

* Entire Section 8

priate help is contributed by T-cells. B-cells and plasma cells produce immunoglobulins which appear as circulating antibodies. Plasma cells are the most differentiated stage in B-cell development and secrete large amounts of antibodies.

Nursing of B-cells, i.e. help for B-cell differentiation and proliferation, is one of the major functions of T-cells and is mediated through the production of lymphokines. T-cell-derived lymphokines are involved in stimulating or inhibiting a great variety of functions. Some T-cells, referred to as cytotoxic T-cells, kill target cells that express foreign antigenic structures. According to a differential expression of certain cell surface proteins, T-cells are divided into two major subsets: $CD4^+$ and $CD8^+$ T-cells. Most of the $CD4^+$ T-cells are helper cells and recognize antigen in association with cell surface molecules on antigen presenting cells which are encoded by the Class II genes of the major histocompatibility complex (MHC), while $CD8^+$ T-cells recognize antigen in association with MHC class I gene products and comprise mainly cytotoxic T-cells.

The antigen receptor of T-cells (TCR) is composed of a set of invariant polypeptide chains collectively called the CD3 complex which is associated with a heterodimer forming the antigen binding site. The latter is divided into constant and variable parts, like the immunoglobulins. In humans more than 95% of T-cells use a combination of α- and β-chains, while a minority of less than 3%, which usually do not express CD4 or CD8 antigens, make use of a different heterodimer composed of γ- and δ-chains.

T-cells are not able to interact with foreign antigen that is free in solution but recognize antigenic peptides in conjunction with MHC glycoproteins on other cell surfaces. This process is called antigen presentation and requires uptake and processing of protein antigens by specialized accessory or antigen presenting cells (APC). In addition to presentation and processing of antigen, the APC or distinct third-party accessory cells have to provide further signals in order to activate a T-cell. These second signals are incompletely defined but may include cytokines such as IL-1 and IL-6 and other differentiation factors, or even contact with certain surface molecules on activated cells. Potential accessory cells include dendritic cells, monocytes, macrophages, B-cells, and endothelial cells. Antigen processing and presentation is traditionally thought of in the context of the activation of CD4 T-cells restricted by MHC Class II molecules. However, it must be remembered that CD8 T-cells, restricted by Class I MHC molecules, also require antigen processing and presentation. However, CD8 T-cells appear not to have obligatory requirements for help from other T-cells: rather they are autostimulatory in the sense that they provide their own cytokines for growth and differentiation.

There is another T-cell distinction with potential functional implications. It has been demonstrated that subsets of $CD4^+$ T-cells produce only a selection of cytokines. The so-called Th1 cells secrete IL-2 and IFNγ while Th2 cells produce IL-4 and IL-5. Since, for example, IL-4 differentially stimulates the production of IgG4 and IgE, a different ratio of activated Th1/Th2 cells will have selective regulatory influences.

8.2   Cell Isolation, Phenotyping and Culture

The majority of analytical procedures for immune cell function require isolation of cells from blood, body fluids or tissues followed by phenotyping before the experiments begin. It is recommended to perform these phenotypic analyses as carefully as possible. Under certain circumstances even small numbers of contaminating cells may have dramatic influences on subsequent experiments. For example, some cell functions are very sensitive to cytokines that may be produced by a few cells. It is known that monocyte contamination of even less than 1% may influence *in-vitro* assays of T-cell functions. Since routine cytofluorimetry has a sensitivity threshold of about 1%, it is recommended in this situation to choose another method for control of cell purity. This could be a highly specific histochemical staining procedure or a very sensitive functional assay.

Most cell separation protocols start with simple separation procedures based on different physical properties of cell populations, such as the ability of monocytes and B-cells, but not T-cells, to adhere to nylon wool. For human lymphoid cells, nearly all separation procedures begin with gradient centrifugation in inert media of adjusted density such as metrizoate (cf. 2.2). This procedure allows one to separate in a very simple and reproducible way human mononuclear cells including T-cells, B-cells, monocytes and NK cells. Rosetting with sheep erythrocytes stabilized by neuramini-dase or AET allows for positive selection of human T-cells [1]. The procedure is based on the interaction of LFA3 on the erythrocyte surface membrane with CD2 on the T-cells. Rosette formation alters the density of the erythrocyte T-cell complex which can be used for differential centrifugation in a density gradient.

More sophisticated separation techniques may depend on binding of antibodies to cell surface antigens that are differentially expressed on a particular cell population. In processes of negative selection, unwanted cells can be removed by specific antibodies which can activate complement [2]. Complement sources are fresh rabbit or guinea pig sera which have to be titrated before use to find the optimal concentration between efficacy and toxicity. A problem is that disintegrated cells, i.e. cell fragments coated with the cytolytic antibodies, cannot always be removed if they are attached to other cells and so may interfere with subsequent procedures.

Except for antibody- and complement-mediated cytolysis, all other methods can be used for positive as well as negative selection of cell subpopulations. The term "panning" describes procedures in which antibody-coated cells are selectively bound to plastic plate surfaces precoated with anti-immunoglobulin antibodies from which cells can be collected after removal of uncoated, i.e. negative, cells by gentle washing (cf. 4.2). The method is simple and inexpensive but depends on good reproduction of the washing procedures and is not precise or quantitative. The most precise separation technique is cell sorting with a flow cytometer (cf. 4.2.2). However, this requires expensive equipment and because of the limited flow rate not more than a few million cells can be separated.

Thus rosetting procedures represent a good compromise between reproducibility, cell yields and costs. The first such rosetting techniques were based on ox erythrocytes coated with anti-mouse immunoglobulin *via* chromium chloride [3]. Guided by the first antibody which is directed to a defined cell marker, the target cells become surrounded by a layer of erythrocytes, forming a rosette and thereby increasing the density of the target for gradient centrifugation. Another variation of this technique is the use of magnetic particles of different sizes which are directly coated with either primary antibodies or with anti-species immunoglobulin antibodies [4]. Cells are separated by simply applying a magnetic field to the cell suspension to retain cells together with the magnetic particles. The anti-cell antibodies can be directly coupled to the magnetic beads or used for precoating of the cells followed by incubation with anti-mouse immunoglobulin antibodies on the beads. The latter gives more precise results.

Removal of positively selected cells from erythrocytes, magnetobeads or plastic surfaces often generates problems of unwanted cell destruction and contamination with cell fragments and antibodies. Contamination with antibodies used for separation may interfere with subsequent phenotypic analysis normally performed to monitor the purification process. Moreover, inadvertent activation of cells may result, especially if conditions allow cross-linking of cell surface molecules. This has been described for anti-MHC class II antibodies in B-cells and for anti-CD3 and anti-CD4 antibodies in T-cells. This possibility must be considered when interpreting the results of functional assays performed with positive selection procedures. Therefore, in most experiments negatively selected cell populations are preferred.

It is important that expression of a certain cell marker does not necessarily correlate with a particular function. For example, not only dendritic cells, monocytes and macrophages but also some B-cells are able to present antigen; cytotoxic T-cell function is not an exclusive property of CD8 T-cells but can also be exerted by some CD4 T-cells; and, for some functionally indistinct subpopulations such as Th1 and Th2 cells, no cell membrane marker molecules that allow physical separation have yet been described.

Some experimental designs require multi-step cell purification procedures which are sometimes difficult to perform in one day. Storage of cells at 4°C normally does not interfere with cell function. Most, but not all, assays can also be performed with cells that have been cryopreserved.

To examine the fine specificities of B- and T-cells, for example by epitope mapping, or the features of antigen-specific cell activation it is essential to have homogeneous cell populations that consequently bear the same antigen receptor (cf. 3.3).

A procedure widely used to obtain long-term human B-cell lines is cell transformation by *Epstein-Barr* virus (EBV). EBV-transformed B-cell lines are relatively stable but fixed with regard to their level of differentiation; thus they are not suitable to study the effects of various stimuli on B-cell development. Most EBV-transformed lines produce IgM in low quantities and can be used, with some restrictions, as antigen-presenting cells.

Long-term T-cell lines can be established by repeated stimulation with antigen and appropriate antigen-presenting cells. It is possible to obtain single T-cell clones by *in-vitro* expansion stimulated by antigen, antigen-presenting cells and IL-2 after single cell cloning. These T-cell clones can keep their antigenic specificity for months or even years. T-cell hybridomas that grow autonomously without restimulation are easier to handle and are generated by cell fusion with T-cell lines. Antigenic specificity can be checked by cytokine release upon appropriate stimulation. Unfortunately, human T-cell hybridomas are rather unstable and the best fusion partners are mouse T-cells (reviewed in [5]). B- and T-cell clones with well-characterized specificity can be used together with other cells in order to investigate antigen-induced cell interactions and effector functions.

8.3   Signal Transduction

The analysis of early intracellular events in activated T- and B-cells requires a broad range of methods to study processes such as protein phosphorylation, phospholipid decomposition, second messenger (inositol phosphate) metabolism and Ca^{2+} mobilization. To achieve methodological access to such processes, a number of biochemical techniques should be available, including protein biochemistry, HPLC and TLC, as well as fluorimetric analyses. In addition, electrophysiological and immunological methods such as the patch-clamp technique or cytofluorimetry may be helpful to study certain aspects of signal transduction in lymphocytes. Several standard methods are available as outlined below.

8.3.1   Protein Phosphorylation

Protein phosphorylation occurs at least during two stages of the cellular activation process (Fig. 1). Firstly, a T- or B-cell-specific tyrosine kinase is activated which in turn phosphorylates specific substrates at tyrosine residues [6]. One important substrate is the phosphoinositol-specific phospholipase C (see below). Secondly, a serine/threonine protein kinase named protein kinase C, PLC phosphorylates a different set of substrates [7]. A basic approach to address protein phosphorylation during cell activation is to label intact cells metabolically with $^{32}PO_4^{3-}$, to prepare lysates from stimulated and

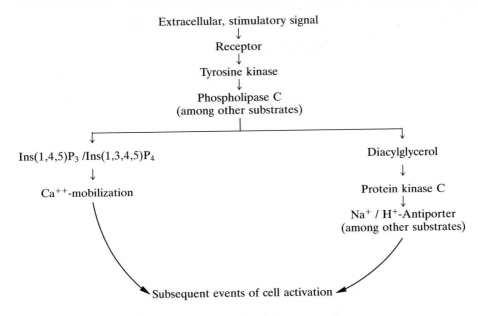

Fig. 1. The routes of second messenger generation in immune cells.

non-stimulated cells and to analyse them on SDS-PAGE. Phosphorylated bands are made visible by autoradiography or, alternatively, by directly counting small pieces of the chopped gel. This method, however, does not discriminate between phosphorylation on tyrosine or serine/threonine residues respectively. Recently-developed antibodies recognizing specifically phosphotyrosine residues of protein can be used in western blot experiments for specific staining. In such experiments, lysates from stimulated and non-stimulated cells are run on SDS-PAGE, proteins are transferred to nitrocellulose sheets and stained with the specific anti-phosphotyrosine antibody. The first antibody is then made visible by a second antibody (either radiolabelled or linked to an enzyme) or by radiolabelled protein A.

A different approach is to measure the protein kinase activity directly in lysates using exogenous substrates. In the case of protein kinase C, the kinase activity in the membrane fraction can also be measured, since protein kinase C is translocated from the cytosol to the plasma membrane during activation.

8.3.2   Metabolism of Phosphoinositides and Inositol Phosphates

Phosphoinositides such as phosphatidylinositol, phosphaditylinositol 4-monophosphate and phosphatidylinositol 4,5-bisphosphate serve as substrates for the phosphoinositol-specific phospholipase C. Activation of the enzyme results in decreases of the lipids and increases of the corresponding inositol phosphates; e. g., $Ins(1)P_1$, $Ins(1,4)P_2$ and $Ins(1,4,5)P_3$. $Ins(1,4,5)P_3$ and its phosphorylation product $Ins(1,3,4,5)P_4$ are important for cell activation by regulating Ca^{2+} release from intracellular stores [8] as well as Ca^{2+} entry from the extracellular space [9].

To measure receptor-activated changes in phosphoinositides or inositol phosphates a basic strategy is to label intact cells with myo-[^{3}H]inositol and to extract water-soluble or organic-solvent-soluble material under conditions in which no further metabolism takes place. Phosphoinositides are then separated by TLC or as the corresponding deacylated glycerophosphoinositols on HPLC. Inositol phosphates can be separated on gravity-fed columns or on HPLC columns in order to obtain isomeric separation. Detection can be performed by liquid scintillation counting of individual HPLC fractions or by collecting bands from TLC plates for subsequent liquid scintillation counting.

The data obtained by these methods describe relative differences between resting and activated cells. The stability of the method and the relatively low cell number needed per sample are advantages. However, a significant disadvantage is the lack of precise concentrations for the intracellular second messengers. This is of particular importance when time courses of, e. g., $Ins(1,4,5)P_3$ are compared with the potency of $Ins(1,4,5)P_3$ to release Ca^{2+} from internal stores in permeabilized cells. To overcome these problems, a novel approach using a complexometric post-column dye system has been introduced for monitoring phosphorylated components directly [10]. At present, the sensitivity of this method cannot compete with radio-tracer methods and its use is therefore restricted to cell lines or mass cell preparations. However, the method has already been shown to give new insights into immune cell activation [11, 10]. As already pointed out for the radio-tracer methods, the post-column dye system is applicable also to lipid analysis when the phosphoinositides are deacylated to the corresponding glycerophosphoinositols prior to analysis.

8.3.3   Free Cytosolic Calcium Concentration

Activation of immune cells, e. g. *via* the T-cell receptor, leads to an increase of $[Ca^{2+}]_i$ [13]. This can be monitored directly and easily in intact cells using intracellularly trapped fluorescent Ca^{2+} chelators such as quin-2 or fura-2. The fluorescence of these compounds at a certain wavelength is increased after Ca^{2+} binding. To monitor $[Ca^{2+}]_i$, the cells are loaded with the membrane-permeable acetoxymethylesters (e. g. fura-2/AM, quin-2/AM) which are cleaved in the cytosol to free acid (fura-2, quin-2) by nonspecific esterases. Thereby, the chelator loses its ability to penetrate membranes. Since esterases are not present in intracellular organelles such as mitochondria or endoplasmic reticulum, the measurements refer to $[Ca^{2+}]$ in the cytosol only. After washing or rinsing off the excess of ester in the incubation buffer, $[Ca^{2+}]_i$ can be monitored fluorimetrically. Addition of stimulators such as antibodies to the TCR results in rapidly increasing fluorescence. The calculation of molarity of $[Ca^{2+}]_i$ is possible when the maximal fluorescence (by addition of the Ca^{2+}-ionophore ionomycin and Ca^{2+}) and the minimal fluorescence (by addition of EGTA) are determined.

A sophisticated development of the method is the measurement of $[Ca^{2+}]_i$ in single cells using fluorescence microscopy with digital imaging. In contrast to the technique described above, fura-2-loaded cells are monitored with a fluorescence microscope equipped with facilities to record fluorescence in single cells. Results from such experiments show that certain cell types respond to stimulation with periodic oscillations of $[Ca^{2+}]_i$.

The technique of monitoring ions by intracellularly trapped fluorescence indicators has been applied also to other ions. For cells of the immune system, the cytosolic alkalinization has been measured as a decrease of $[H^+]$ in the cytosol by using the dye BCECF/AM [14].

8.4   Effector Function

Once the cascade of second messengers and intracellular signals has reached the nucleus, transcription and translation of newly synthesized proteins initiate complex programmes of cell activation, proliferation and differentiation. Moreover, stimulated cells change their functional capabilities and begin producing effector proteins such as antibodies or cytokines. They may express newly synthesized interaction molecules on their surfaces or acquire new functions as, for instance, cytolytic potential. Table 1 shows assays for frequently analysed effector functions.

Stimulated cells typically increase in size, an effect which can be measured by flow cytometry using forward light scatter (cf. 5.11). Flow cytometry also offers the possibility to perform cell cycle analyses. Increased expression of cell surface molecules, such as MHC class II molecules on human T-cells, which are expressed upon activation can also be measured by flow cytometry using directly labelled mAbs or sandwich

Table 1. Lymphocyte effector functions upon stimulation

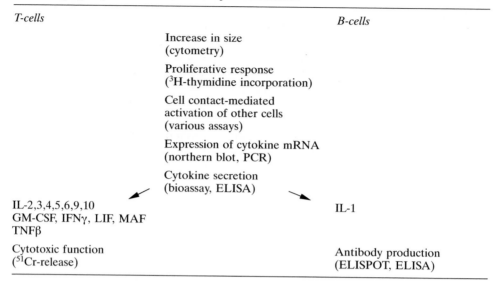

T-cells		*B-cells*
	Increase in size (cytometry)	
	Proliferative response (^{3}H-thymidine incorporation)	
	Cell contact-mediated activation of other cells (various assays)	
	Expression of cytokine mRNA (northern blot, PCR)	
	Cytokine secretion (bioassay, ELISA)	
IL-2,3,4,5,6,9,10 GM-CSF, IFNγ, LIF, MAF TNFβ		IL-1
Cytotoxic function (^{51}Cr-release)		Antibody production (ELISPOT, ELISA)

GM-CSF – granulocyte monocyte-colony stimulating factor; IFN – interferon; IL – Interleukin; LIF – leucocyte inhibition factor; MAF – macrophage activating factor; TNF – tumour necrosis factor

techniques. Simultaneous detection of two or three different cell surface molecules by the use of fluorescent dyes with different emission wavelengths allows the determination of marker molecules and thus makes studies on the expression of cell surface molecules possible, even in mixed cell populations that cannot be differentiated by their size alone.

8.4.1   Polyclonal *versus* Antigen-Specific Stimulation

Polyclonal stimulants are mitogens or antibodies that can activate all or most B-cells or T-cells in an antigen independent and nonspecific manner. They are used more frequently with human cells than for the analysis of animal immune cell functions. Preimmunization of animals increases the frequency of differentiated B- or T-cells with a particular antigenic specificity in all lymphoid organs from which they can be obtained for cell isolation and *in-vitro* experiments. On the other hand, immunization of humans is restricted to certain vaccinations performed for medical reasons (e.g., tetanus toxoid): thus, the antigen-specific cell populations available from human blood or tissues are often too small for adequate analyses. Polyclonal stimulation circumvents this problem by addressing a larger number of cells but it is not equivalent to antigenic stimulation. This is even true when anti-receptor antibodies such as anti-CD3 for T-cells or anti-Ig for B-cells are used as stimulants, since physiological activation of T-cells and B-cells by antigen involves additional accessory molecules and cytokine-mediated signals. Thus, it is important to verify results obtained with polyclonal activators by antigen-specific assays as far as possible. Since *in-vitro* immunization (priming) is rather difficult to achieve, the human starting material is usually cells from individuals who have been recently immunized with the antigen to be used (for instance tetanus toxoid), so that a sufficient number of antigen-reactive cells become available.

8.4.2   B-Cell Functions

B-cell functions can be studied by using polyclonal stimulants such as staphylococcal protein A or anti-Ig, which cross-link B-cell surface immunoglobulin thereby inducing B-cell proliferation, differentiation and immunoglobulin production. Antigen-specific stimulation requires a sufficient number of antigen-reactive cells as mentioned above.

It should be known whether the antigen used is a T-cell-dependent or independent antigen. This determines the requirement for helper signals. Most protein antigens are T-cell-dependent antigens and require the presence of T-cells which support B-cell proliferation and differentiation upon activation. The helper function of T-cells is mediated by various cytokines. Only some T-cell-dependent antigens such as SRBC do not require the physical presence of T-cells, and are able to stimulate primed B-cells if the appropriate T-cell cytokines are added.

T-cell-independent antigens stimulate B-cells *in vitro* in the absence of T-cells. The so-called type I antigens act as polyclonal activators while type II antigens do not. It has been demonstrated that type I antigens such as trinitrophenylated lipopolysaccharide (LPS) can stimulate responses in both mature and immature (neonatal) B-cells, whereas type II antigens such as trinitrophenylated Ficoll and dextran are able to stimulate responses only in immature B-cells (reviewed in [15]).

It should be noted that a given protein antigen displays a series of epitopes for B-cells as well as epitopes for T-cells and these are different in most cases. Well-defined low molecular-weight B-cell epitopes (haptens) can be attached to larger protein molecules (carriers) displaying T-cell epitopes. The hapten can be placed on various carriers and this allows the precise measurement of the T-cell dependence of a given B-cell response.

A very direct approach to measurement of B-cell function is enumeration of immunoglobulin-producing B-cells by the haemolytic plaque assay [16, 17] or by the ELISPOT technique [18] which is particularly recommended for the assessment of human B-cells (cf. 7.1). In this assay, antibodies produced by single B-cells recognize their antigen on the plastic surface of culture wells upon which the cells sit. By the use of enzyme-coupled anti-immunoglobulin antibodies together with substrates that become insoluble after reaction with the enzyme, antibody production is assessed by measuring and counting coloured spots on the bottom of the culture vessel. Each spot represents antibody production by a single B-cell. Assay variations allow assessment of B-cells producing either total immunoglobulin, a certain isotype, or antigen-specific antibodies.

Another possibility is quantitation of immunoglobulin production be measuring various types of antibodies in the supernatants of cell cultures by an ELISA. With the help of limiting dilution techniques (cf. 8.5), frequency analyses of B-cells become possible. While nowadays the more direct ELISPOT assay will be the method of choice with regard to frequency analyses of B-cells, a measurement of antibody production in culture supernatants remains of value. It does not require as many microcultures as the ELISPOT assay and estimates the total amount of antibody produced in a cell culture.

8.4.3   T-Cell Functions

Polyclonal stimulation of human T-cells can be achieved by various mitogens such as PHA or Con A, or anti-CD3 antibodies, or more artificially by phorbol ester and calcium ionophore. Besides measuring proliferation, these stimuli are used to stimulate secretion of lymphokines into the culture medium or expression of lymphokine message. T-cell activators such as PHA, but also anti-CD3, normally require accessory cells to be effective. Antigen-specific stimulation requires a sufficient number of corresponding precursor cells equipped with a functional T-cell receptor.

Determination of the proliferative potential (usually of CD4 T-cells) as indicated by DNA synthesis and incorporation of ^{3}H-thymidine is the most widely used functional assay [19]. Procedures for assessing cytotoxic lymphocytes (CTL) are also used frequently by release of ^{51}Cr from antigen-expressing target cells [20]. Another parameter of cytotoxic activity is the release of serine esterases into the medium upon activation [21]. Esterases are released from cytoplasmic granules of CTL and can easily be measured with synthetic substrates. This assay solely measures CTL activity regardless of the target cells used. Cytolytic potential can be measured nonspecifically by using mitogens such as PHA; the so-called PHA-dependent kill.

Antigen-specific stimulation requires sufficient numbers of T-cells expressing the appropriate antigen receptor. About one in two hundred T-cells normally responds to allogeneic cells while the frequency of T-cells reactive to a xenogeneic protein antigen is much lower. Therefore, specific T-cell proliferation in bulk culture requires about five to seven days before cell expansion becomes measurable. This is in contrast to polyclonal activation which causes a significant proliferation detectable after two days. The same considerations apply if antigen-specific cytokine production is to be measured. Information on cytokine and lymphokine assays at the cell level can be obtained from 7.2.

The ELISPOT assay has also been used for determination of the number of cytokine-producing T-cells. Since T-cell proliferation is not required in this assay, it is a very valuable contribution to the arsenal of available T-cell tests.

8.5   **Regulatory Interactions**

Some of the effector functions mentioned above require interaction of two different cell types, for instance antigen-presenting cells and T-cells. A sufficient cell number and a certain differentiation stage is normally required for a good read-out system. More complex interactions resembling those that take place during immunization *in vivo* include multicellular interaction at specialized tissue sites, such as the germinal centres of lymphoid organs. It is appropriate to mention that even the most sophisticated *in-vitro* system for examining cell function and interaction cannot model exactly the condition under which cells normally function *in vivo*. It is commonplace to find discrepancies between the apparent activity of lymphocytes *in vitro* and the observable immune status of the whole animal. For example, animals functionally unresponive to, e.g., a tolerated allotransplant may have T-cells that are alloreactive *in vitro*. Explanations for such phenomena are elusive, but it may be assumed that it is difficult if not impossible to recreate the regulatory systems that function in ordered micro-environments *in vivo*. However, the limitation of current technology demands that the use and value of *in-vitro* methods are maximized.

It is difficult to achieve a significant *in-vitro* expansion of cells with a particular specificity. Nonetheless, a few systems for priming *in vitro* have been described with animal cells [22]. They are restricted to certain complex antigens such as sheep erythrocytes (SRBC), and these work effectively because they contain immunogenic epitopes that cross-react with those present in environmental antigens, so that the number of specific precursor cells is large enough even in lymphoid organs of non-immunized animals. Only IgM antibody responses are induced in these animals, while IgG anti-SRBC responses can be seen only with cells taken from SRBC-primed animals. Only limited information is available on *in-vitro* priming with human cells.

The growth of specific immune cells and their differentiation to effector cells is regulated normally by T-cells that exert helper or suppressor functions. These regulatory cells stimulate or inhibit proliferation, differentiation and protein secretion of immune cells. A major development in the late 1970s was the so-called limiting dilution technique for investigation and quantification of regulatory cell interactions (for details see [23]). This method takes into account the fact that there is no simple way to identify individual cells of a defined specificity and function among large populations of lymphocytes. These cells are rare and morphologically indistinguishable from the silent majority of resting lymphocytes. However, limiting dilution analysis allows the calculation of precursor frequencies based on the measurement of active cell clones generated by clonal expansion within a given population of cells. As each active clone is derived from one precursor, one can estimate retrospectively the frequency of precursors that gave rise to those clones. Beyond estimation of the precursor frequency, the system can be used for analysing complex cellular interactions at a clonal level. The method makes use of *Poisson* statistics. A straight line is generated if cultures with different densities are analysed and conditions are similar for clonal expansion and development of cell function in every microculture. Curves deviating from linearity are generated if the conditions become discontinuous and other cell types with different frequencies begin to interfere.

Another approach to mimic the complex *in-vitro* situation is the use of culture systems with two compartments in which cells are separated from each other by a membrane which allows only penetration by soluble molecules such as cytokines or antibodies [24]. By means of these double chamber culture systems it becomes possible to determine whether a certain function is critically dependent upon either direct cell-to-cell contact or soluble mediators.

In recent years new methods have been developed for work with organ cultures, especially with thymus cultures. Mouse thymic lobes are cultured on membranes floating on nutrient medium [25]. Stimulants are easy to add under these conditions and for a few days these thymic organ cultures develop in a normal way.

However, as stressed already many functions of the immune system are far too complex to be dissected *in vitro*. Cell diversity at a certain location and the multitude of soluble factors cannot be reconstituted *in vitro*. Therefore, animal experiments are needed. They are of particular importance for such complex functions as graft-versus-host disease, graft rejection or delayed-type hypersensitivity. No *in-vitro* cell systems or organ cultures are available for the comprehensive modelling of these functions. Historically, *in-vivo* systems were nearly exclusively used to investigate the benefit of immunomodulatory treatments, but now many *in-vivo* models have contributed to our understanding of mechanistic aspects of the immune system.

Novel methods can dissect more carefully than before immune cell functions *in vivo*. It is possible, with specific antibodies, to ablate certain cell populations or to induce redistribution of cells within an animal [26]. Most effective is treatment from birth, for instance with anti-μ antibodies, which causes B-cell depletion, or with antibodies to CD4 or CD8 causing depletion of the respective cell populations. In this way selective depletion allows one to determine the contribution of a particular cell population to a particular immune function.

Another way is to study animals with genetic defects which either occur naturally or are introduced by "knocking-out" (homologous recombination) the corresponding genes [27]. Many such animals have been produced lacking one or another cytokine. The development of transgenic and "gene knock-out" animals is a major contribution to our understanding of the immune system. With the ever-increasing description of cell surface molecules and soluble mediators important for interaction there seems to be no way to determine the particular importance of each of the elements other than to manipulate its expression under carefully defined conditions, leaving all other elements in their natural environment.

References

[1] F. Indiveri, J. Huddlestone, M. A. Pellegrino, S. Ferrone, Isolation of Human T Lymphocytes: Comparison between Wool Filtration and Rosetting with Neuraminidase (VcN) and 2-Aminoethylisothiouronium Bromide (AET) Treated Sheep Blood Cells, J. Immunol. Methods *34*, 107–115 (1980).

[2] A. Marshak-Rothstein, P. Fink, T. Gridley, D. H. Raulet, M. J. Bevan, M. L. Gefter, Properties and Applications of Monoclonal Antibodies Directed against Determinants of the Thy-1 Locus, J. Immunol. *122*, 2491–2499 (1979).

[3] P. E. Bigazzi, C. L. Burek, N. R. Rose, Antibodies to Tissue-specific Endocrine Gastrointestinal, and Neurological Antigens, in: N. Rose, H. Friedman, J. L. Fahey (eds.), Manual of Clinical Laboratory Immunology, 3rd. ed., American Society for Microbiology, Washington D. C. 1986, pp. 762–763.

[4] S. Funderud, K. Nustad, T. Lea, F. Vartdal, G. Gaudernack, P. Stensted, J. Ugelstad, Fractionation of Lymphocytes by Immunomagnetic Beads, in: G. G. B. Klaus (ed.), Lymphocytes: A Practical Approach, Oxford University Press, N. Y. 1987, pp. 55–61.

[5] W. Born, J. White, R. O'Brien, R. Kubo, Development of T Cell Receptor Expression: Studies Using T Cell Hybridomas, Res. Immunol. *7*, 279–291 (1988).

[6] M. J. Trevillyan, A. Nordstrom, T. J. Linna, High Tyrosin Protein Kinase Activity in Normal Peripheral Blood Lymphocytes, Biochim. Biophys. Acta *845*, 1–9 (1985).

[7] Y. Nishizuka, The Role of Protein Kinase C in Cell Surface Signal Transduction and Tumor Promotion, Nature *308*, 693–698 (1984).

[8] H. Streb, R. F. Irvine, M. J. Berridge, J. Schulz, Release of Ca^{2+} from a Non-Mitochondrial Intracellular Store in Pancreatic Acinar Cells by Inositol 1,4,5-Trisphosphate, Nature *306*, 67–68 (1983).

[9] A. H. Guse, E. Roth, F. Emmrich, D-Myo-Inositol 1,3,4,5-Tetrakisphosphate Releases Ca^{2+} from Crude Microsomes and Enriched, Vesicular Plasma Membranes but not from Intracellular Stores of Permeabilized T-lymphocytes and Monocytes, Biochem. J., *288*, 489–495 (1992)

[10] G. W. Mayr, A Novel Metal-Dye Detection System Permits Picomolar-Range H.P.L.C. Analysis of Inositol Polyphosphates from Non-radioctively Labelled Cells or Tissue Specimens, Biochem. J. *254*, 585–591 (1988).

[11] A. H. Guse, F. Emmrich, T Cell Receptor-mediated Metabolism of Inositol Polyphosphates in *Jurkat* T Lymphocytes. Identification of a D-myo-inositol 1,2,3,4,6-pentakisphosphate-2-Phosphomonoesterase Activity, a D-Myo-Inositol 1,3,4,5,6-Pentakisphosphate-1/3-phosphatase Activity and a D/L-Myo-Inositol 1,2,4,5,6-Pentakisphosphate-1/3-Kinase Activity, J. Biol. Chem. *266*, 24498–24502 (1991).

[12] *A. H. Guse, F. Emmrich,* Determination of Inositol Polyphosphates from Human T Lymphocyte Cell Lines by Anion-Exchange High-performance Liquid Chromatography and Post-Column Derivatization, J. Chromatogr. *593,* 157–163 (1992).

[13] *R. Y. Tsien, T. Pozzan, T. J. Rink,* Calcium Homeostasis in Intact Lymphocytes: Cytoplasmic Free Ca^{2+} Monitored with a New, Intracellularly-Trapped Fluorescent Indicator, J. Cell. Biol. *94,* 325–334 (1982).

[14] *P. M. Rosoff, L. C. Cantley,* Stimulation of the T3-T Cell Receptor-Associated Ca^{2+}-Influx Enhances the Activity of the Na^+/H^+ Exchanger in a Leukemic Human T Cell Line, J. Biol. Chem. *260,* 14053–14059 (1985).

[15] *I. Scher,* The CBA/N Mouse Strain: an Experimental Model Illustrating the Influence of the X-Chromosome on Immunity, Adv. Immunol. *33,* 1–71 (1982).

[16] *N. K. Jerne, A. A. Nordin,* Plaque Formation in Agar by Single Antibody Producing Cells, Science *140,* 405–408 (1963).

[17] *A. J. Cunningham, A. Szenberg,* Further Improvements in the Plaque Technique for Detecting Single Antibody Forming Cells, Immunology *14,* 599–600 (1968).

[18] *C. Czerkinsky, L. A. Nilsson, A. Tarkowski, W. J. Koopman, J. Mestecky, O. Ouchterlony,* The Enzyme-Linked Immunospot Assay for Detection of Specific Antibody-Secreting Cells: Methodology and Applicability, in: *D. M. Kemeny, S. J. Challacombe* (eds.), Theoretical and Technical Aspects of ELISA and Other Solid Phase Immunoassays, John Wiley & Sons, N.Y. 1988, pp. 217–239.

[19] *G. Corradin, H. M. Etlinger, M. Chiller,* Lymphocyte Specificity to Protein Antigens. I. Characterization of the Antigen-Induced *in vitro* T Cell Dependent Proliferative Response with Lymph Node Cells from Primed Mice, J. Immunol. *119,* 1048–1055 (1977).

[20] *E. Simpson, P. Chandler,* Analysis of Cytotoxic T Cell Responses, in: *D. M. Weir, L. A. Herzenberg, C. Blackwell* (eds.), Cellular Immunology, Vol. 2, 4. Blackwell Scientific, Oxford 1986, pp. 68.1–68.16.

[21] *H. Takayama, G. Trenn, M. V. Sikovsky,* A Novel Cytotoxic T Lymphocyte Activation Assay: Optimized Conditions for Antigen Receptor Triggered Granule Enzyme Secretion, J. Immunol. Methods *104,* 183–190 (1987).

[22] *R. I. Mishell, R. W. Dutton,* Immunization of Dissociated Spleen Cell Cultures from Mice, J. Exp. Med. *126,* 423–442 (1967).

[23] *I. Lefkovits, H. Waldmann,* Limiting Dilution Analysis of Cells in the Immune System, Cambridge University Press, Cambridge 1979.

[24] *S. Howie, In vitro* Production and Testing of Antigen-Induced Mediators of Helper T Cell Function, in: *I. Lefkovits, B. Pernis* (eds.), Immunological Methods Vol. II, Academic Press, N.Y. 1981, pp. 199–211.

[25] *E. J. Jenkinson, R. Kingston, J. J. T. Owen,* Importance of IL-2 Receptors in Intra-thymic Generation of Cells Expressing T Cell Receptors, Nature *329,* 160–162 (1987).

[26] *A. M. Kruisbeek, In vivo* Depletion of CD4- and CD8-Specific T Cells, in: *J. E. Coligan, A. M. Kruisbeek* et al. (eds.), Current Protocols in Immunology, John Wiley & Sons 1990, pp. 4.1.1–4.1.5.

[27] *B. H. Koller, O. Smithies,* Altering Genes in Animals by Gene Targetting, Annu. Rev. Immunol. *10,* 705–730 (1992).

Appendix

I Symbols, Quantities, Units and Constants

Symbol	Name	Unit
A	absorbance	1
b	catalytic activity concentration	$U \cdot l^{-1}$, $kat \cdot l^{-1}$
Bq	becquerel	s^{-1}
c	substance concentration	$mol \cdot l^{-1}$
c	speed of light in a medium	$m \cdot s^{-1}$
c_0	speed of light *in vacuo*	$m \cdot s^{-1}$
cpm	counts per minute	$N \cdot min^{-1}$
C	counting rate of the radioactive product	$N \cdot min^{-1}$
C	electric capacitance	F or $C \cdot V^{-1}$
d	light path	mm
dpm	disintegrations per min	$N \cdot min^{-1}$
D	electric displacement	$C \cdot m^{-2}$
D	diffusion coefficient	$m^2 \cdot s^{-1}$
E	electromotive force	V
F	Faraday constant	96485 $C \cdot mol^{-1}$
g	acceleration due to gravity	9.806 $m \cdot s^{-2}$
g	gram	
h	*Planck's* constant	$1.0546 \cdot 10^{-34} Js$
h	hour	
I	light intensity	cd
I.U.**	international unit (for others than enzymes)	
J	Joule	$m^2 \cdot kg \cdot s^{-2}$
k_a	kinetic association rate constant (for hapten-Ab interaction)	$l \cdot mol^{-1} \cdot s^{-1}$
k_d	kinetic dissociation rate constant (for hapten-Ab interaction)	s^{-1}
kat	katal	$mol \cdot s^{-1}$
K	equilibrium constant for hapten-Ab interaction	$l \cdot mol^{-1}$
K	Kelvin	
K_m	*Michaelis* constant	$mol \cdot l^{-1}$
l	litre	$m^3 \cdot 10^{-3}$
m	metre	
m_s	mass of substance	g

Symbol	Name	Unit
min	minute	
M_r	molecular weight, relative molecular mass	1
n	refractive index	1
n_c	amount of substance	mol
n_c/m_s	substance content	$mol \cdot kg^{-1}$
pH	negative logarithm of the hydrogen ion concentration	1
pK	negative logarithm of the dissociation constant	1
Pa	pascal	$N \cdot m^{-2}$
Q	electric charge	C
rad	radiation absorbed dose	Gy or $0.01 \; J \cdot kg^{-1}$
rpm	rotations per minute	$N \cdot min^{-1}$
R	gas constant	$8.312 \; J \cdot mol^{-1} \cdot K^{-1}$
RSD	relative standard deviation (or coefficient of variation)	
s, SD	standard deviation	
s	second	
sp.gr.	specific gravity at 20° C relative to water at 4° C	1
T	temperature	°C
t	time	s (h, min)
$\varDelta t$	time interval between measurements	s (h, min)
T	temperature	K
U*	international unit (for enzymes)	$\mu mol \cdot min^{-1}$
v	volume (usually volume of sample in assay mixture)	ml
v	rate of reaction	$mol \cdot l^{-1} \cdot s^{-1}$
V	maximum rate of reaction	$mol \cdot l^{-1} \cdot s^{-1}$
V	volume (usually volume of assay mixture)	ml
w	mass fraction	
$\bar{x}$	mean value	
X	specific radioactivity	$Bq \cdot mol^{-1}$
Y	number of counts measured	
z	catalytic activity	U or kat
z_c/m_s	catalytic activity content (specific catalytic activity)	$U \cdot g^{-1}$ or $kat \cdot kg^{-1}$
Z	decay rate, disintegrations per minute	$N \cdot min^{-1}$

Symbol	Name	Unit
α_e	electric polarizability	$C \cdot m^2 \cdot V^{-1}$
ε	linear molar absorption coefficient	$l \cdot mol^{-1} \cdot mm^{-1}$
ε_0	permittivity of vacuum	$F \cdot m^{-1}$
ε_r	relative permittivity	1
η	counting efficiency	1
λ	wavelength	nm
μ	ionic strength (often represented by I)	$mol \cdot kg^{-1}$
ν	kinematic viscosity	$m^2 \cdot s^{-1}$
ν	frequency of emitted light	Hz
ξ	rate of conversion	$mol \cdot s^{-1}$ $(\mu mol \cdot min^{-1})$
ϱ	mass concentration	$g \cdot l^{-1}$
φ	volume fraction (of sample in assay mixture)	
%	percentage	
% (v/v)	percentage, volume related to volume	
% (v/w)	percentage, volume related to weight	
% (w/v)	percentage, weight related to volume	
% (w/w)	percentage, weight related to weight	

* There is no abbreviation used for arbitrary unit, it is expressed as "unit" in this series.

** In general defined by WHO or other authorities for antigens.

Prefixes for unit symbols

Prefix	Symbol	Factor
exa	E	10^{18}
peta	P	10^{15}
tera	T	10^{12}
giga	G	10^9
mega	M	10^6
kilo	k	10^3
milli	m	10^{-3}
micro	μ	10^{-6}
nano	n	10^{-9}
pico	p	10^{-12}
femto	f	10^{-15}
atto	a	10^{-18}

II   List of Abbreviations

AEC   Aminoethyl carbazole
AET   2-Aminoethylisothiouronium
ALL   Acute lymphoblastic leukemia
AML   Acute myeloid leukemia
AP   Alkaline phosphatase
APC   Antigen-presenting cells
ASC   Antibody-secreting cells

BAL   Bronchoalveolar lavage
BCIP   Bromo-chloro indolyl phosphate
BCL   EBV transformed B-cell line

CD(s)   Cluster(s) of differentiation
CLL   Chronic lymphocytic leukemia
CR   Complement receptor
CTL   CD8+ cytotoxic T-lymphocyte

DC   Dendritic cells

E   Erythrocyte
EA   Erythrocyte coated with anti-E antibody
EAC   Erythrocyte coated with IgM anti-E and complement
ECM   Extracellular matrix
ELISA   Enzyme-linked immunoabsorbent assay
ELISPOT   Enzyme-linked immunospot

FBS   Foetal bovine serum
FCM   Flow cytometry
FcR   Fc receptor
FCS   Foetal calf serum
FMLP   Formylmethinyl-leucyl-phenylalanine
FSC   Forward scatter

g   Generation time (h)
GMB   Glomerular basement membrane
GM-CSF   Granulocyte monocyte-colony stimulating factor

HA   Hyaluronan
HES   Hydroxy-ethyl starch
HRP   Horseradish peroxidase
HS-PG   Heparan sulphate proteoglycan

IF	Immunofluorescence
IFN	Interferon
IFs	Intermediate filaments
IL	Interleukin
ISP 42	Import site protein M_r 42,000
KLH	Keyhole limpet haemocyanin
K_s	Monod saturation constant (mg/l)
LCMV	Lymphocytic choriomeningitis virus
LIF	Leucocyte inhibition factor
LP1	Protease resistant central domain of laminin
MAb(s)	Monoclonal antibodies
MACS	Magnetic cell sorter
MAF	Macrophage activating factor
MCMV	Mouse cytomegalovirus
MFs	Microfilaments
MNC	Mononuclear cells
MOM 72 and MOM 19	Mitochondrial outer membrane proteins with M_r values 72,000 and 19,000 respectively
MTs	Microtubules
N	Number of cells at the time t
n	Number of cell divisions
μ	Specific growth rate (h^{-1})
μ_{max}	Maximum specific growth rate (h^{-1})
NBT	Nitroblue tetrazolium
NC1	Carboxyterminal domain of type IV collagen
ND	Nycodenz
NHL	Non-Hodgkin lymphoma
NK	Natural killer (cell)
N_0	Initial number of cells
N_S	Speed number of the stirrer (min^{-1})
OGDC	2-Oxoglutarate dehydrogenase complex
ORBC	Ox red blood cells
P	Product
p	Pressure (kPa)
PBMC	Peripheral blood mononuclear cells
PDC	Pyruvate dehydrogenase complex
PFC	Plaque-forming cell
PHA	Phytohaemaglutinin A
PICB	Type I collagen carboxypeptide

PMA	Phorbol myristate acetate
PMN	Polymorphonuclear neutrophil(s)
P_O	External power from the agitator (g · cm/s)
POD	Peroxidase
PIIINP	Type III collagen aminopeptide
QIFI	Quantitative immuno-fluorescence indirect assay
Rcpt	Receptor
RIA	Radioimmunoassay
RT	Room temperature
R10 +	RPMI 1640 + 10% FCS
S	Substrate (g/l)
7S-collagen	Protease resistant crosslinked domain of type IV collagen
SFC	Spot-forming cell
SSC	Side scatter
TNF	Tumour necrosis factor
TNFα	Tumour necrosis factor alpha
URFs	Unidentified reading frames
vvm	Volume per volume per minute
X	Biomass concentration (g dry weight/l)

* indicates labelled compound

III   List of Symbols used for the Figures

Basic antibody

Antibodies corresponding to different epitopes on antigens

Antibodies against other immunoglobulins

Fab fragment

Antigens with different epitopes

Hapten

Avidin or streptavidin

Biotin

Metal particles like gold or silver

Latex particle, small-sized

Latex particle, large-sized

Enzyme

Enzyme bound to an anti-enzyme antibody

Label (unspecified or other than enzyme)

Carrier protein

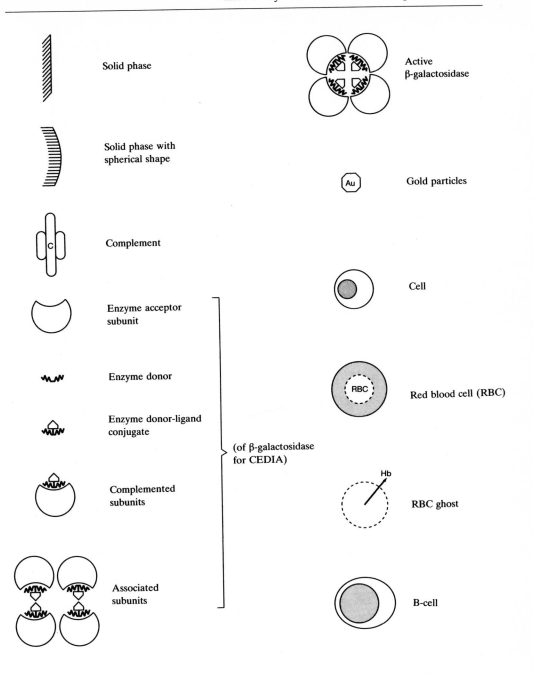

Solid phase

Solid phase with
spherical shape

Complement

Enzyme acceptor
subunit

Enzyme donor

Enzyme donor-ligand
conjugate

Complemented
subunits

Associated
subunits

(of β-galactosidase
for CEDIA)

Active
β-galactosidase

Gold particles

Cell

Red blood cell (RBC)

RBC ghost

B-cell

Index

ABAP immunostaining 528
– ELISPOT assay 526 f.
ABC complex 271, 273, 275
– autoradiography 259
ABC staining (avidin-biotin complex) 234,
  271 f., 286, 527
– ELISPOT assay 525 f.
– protocol 294
Absorption
– absolute 340
– control 307 f., 333
– relative 340
Accessory cell 128
Acetone 321
Acetoxymethylester 565
Acetylation 436, 457
Acousto-optic deflector, see AOD
Acrylic resin 213, 323
– gold labelling protocol for EM 329 f.
Activation of T- and B-cells 562 f.
Active adherence 167
Active gene 444, 446 f.
AD (analogue-to-digital) converter 349
– hardware 349
Adenine nucleotide translocase 472
Adherence, see Cell adherence
AEC (3-amino-9-ethyl carbazole) 232, 247
Aedes aegypti 73
AER (albumin excretion rate) 488
AET 176
Affinity chromatography 169
– for subcellular fractionation 198
Ag blot 309
Aggregated Ig 303
AIDS 129
– phenotype analysis 396 f.
Albumin 57
Albumin excretion rate, see AER
Alcohol fixation 383
Alcoholic hepatitis 485 f.
Aldehyde group 302
Alkaline phosphatase 225, 232 f., 240, 275,
  508, 519
– antigen localization 341
– chromogen/substrate solution 514
– double direct staining 282
– endogenous reaction 302
– immunostaining of cytokines 550
– phosphate-precipitation method 342
– visualization 253 ff.

Allogeneic cell 128
Allogeneic chimaera 427
Alveolar cells 52
– BAL 52
AMCA 231, 238, 282
3-Amino-9-ethyl carbazole, see AEC
Amplification
– of immunostaining signal 275
– – for ELISPOT assay 521 f.
– of signals 266
Androgenesis 150
Animal experiments 570
Ante-natal diagnosis 405
Antibody 565
– affinity chromatography 198
– against chromatin 443
– against chromosomal proteins 442
– against fusion proteins 434 f.
– against nuclear proteins 440
– against peptides 435, 471
– against type I collagen 480
– aggregated Ig 303
– as probe of function 8 f.
– biotinylated 271, 525, 537
– clonal analysis 504
– contaminating lymphocyte
  preparations 561
– control 380
– coupling to SRBC 178 f.
– cytokine-specific 548
– cytophilic 534
– detection of genetic defects 469
– dilution 286, 290, 310 f.
– for cell separation 171 ff.
– for cytoskeleton characterization 431 ff.
– in immunoanalysis 3 ff.
– in immunocytochemistry 204 ff.
– labelling 206 f., 237 ff.
– – bridging label 236 f.
– – colloidal gold 234 f.
– – enzymes 207, 231 ff.
– – fluorescent 229 f., 372
– – radioactive 234
– microinjection 447
– monoclonal, see Monoclonal antibody
– production 307
– – partially purified protein as antigen 434
– quantification 504
– – secreting cell, see ASC
– specificity 223, 300 f., 307, 382, 443

– storage   311
– technology   388
– use in differential diagnosis   485f.
Anti-Fab antibody   169, 182
Anti-foam   159
Anti-freeze   322
Antigen
– accessibility   441
– after microwave treatment   297
– antibody complex
– – nonspecific binding   308
– binding site   558
– concentration   286, 357f.
– cytological localization   341, 346, 393
– – chromosomal   440
– – intracellular   383
– – kinetochore-associated-   454
– – surface   388f., 401
– density   390, 393, 395
– for ELISPOT assay
– – coating   506, 510, 516
– fusion protein   434f.
– GLAD   275
– *in-situ* detection   418
– labelling   275
– level of expression   394
– neo-antigen   398
– peptide   435
– presentation   559
– presenting cell, see APC
– preservation by freeze-drying   219
– quantification   392
– receptor   134, 556ff.
– reference range   482, 487, 493
– relative availability   444
– RICH   275
– SDS-PAGE band   434
– soluble-   506
– specificity   133
– study of enzymatic cleavage   394
– type I   567
– type II   567
Antigenic stimulation   123, 567
Anti-hapten antibody   236
Anti-idiotype antibody   465
Anti-Ig antibody   173
Anti-peroxidase antibody   526
Anti-species antibody   317
– specificity   266
AOD (acousto-optic deflector)   370f.
AP, see Alkaline phosphatase
APAAP
– complex   240, 277
– technique   232f., 277, 285, 292
– protocol   292

APC (antigen-presenting cell)   559
Araldite®   213
Arbovirus   145
Archimedian spiral   371
Arcton   218
Area measurement in image analysis   357
Arsanilic acid   236
Arthritis   492
Arthropod
– cell culture   71, 139ff.
– – culture parameters   144
– cell lines
– – growth conditions   141
– – SF9-cells   143
– characteristics   69
– hormones   140
– preparation of tissues   69ff.
– – for sectioning   75
– PTTH   74
– purification of brain   71
– shock-freezing   69
– vitellogenin
ASC (antibody-secreting cell)   506ff., 533
Astrocyte   373
ATP synthase   472
Attached cell line   106
Authentication
– cytogenetic analysis   117
– DNA fingerprinting   117
– isoenzyme analysis   116
Authentikit System   116
Autoantibody, see Autoimmune
   disease   432, 506
Autoclaving   92
Autofluorescence   57
Autoimmune disease   399, 432, 506
– phenotype analysis   399
Autologous cell   128
Automated immunostaining   312
Automatic enzyme analyser   200
Automatic zonal centrifuge   197
Autoradiography   234, 259f., 278, 389
Average optical density   358f.
Avian model   419f.
Avidin   185, see also ABC complex, ABC
   staining   237, 274, 282
– background binding   303
– labelled-   272
Avidin-biotin complex, see ABC complex
– immunostaining, see ABC staining
Axial setting accuracy   363

Background   229, 235, 300ff.
– in image processing   352
– in immunocytochemical reaction   209

Back-scattered electron image, see BEI
Bacteria
– as contamination 111
Bacterial cell, see Prokaryotic cell
Bacterial growth 89
Baculovirus expression system 72, 145
BAL (bronchoalveolar lavage) 52 ff.
– cell yield 55 ff.
– – standardization 57
– in humans 52, 56
– in rodents 54
– in dogs 53
– in sheep 54
Balbiani ring 446
Banding, see Chromosome banding
Bank, see Cell bank
Batch culture 156, 160
– feeding 160
BCECF/AM 565
B-cell 63, 65, 173, 420, 558 f., 566
– activation 562 ff.
– differential adherence 169
– EBV-transformed, see EBV-transformed
  B-cell line
– function 567
– phosphorylation 562 f.
– transformation 124
B5-medium 151
BCG 44
BCIG (5-bromo-4-chloro-indolyl-β-D-
  galactoside) 256
BCIP (5-bromo-4-chloro-3-indolyl
  phosphate) 255, 509, 514
Bean disruption 80
BEI (back-scattered electron image) 329 f.
Bernard-Soulier syndrome 401
Bichromatic ELISPOT assay 529 f.
Binary image 347, 353
Binding level 393
Bioassay of cytokine content 541
Biogel 44
Biohazard
– handling regulations 97 f.
Biomass 160
Biopsy 190 f.
– -based cell separation 190 ff.
Bioreactor 154, 156 ff. see also Fermenter
Biotin, see also ABC complex, ABC staining
– endogenous 237, 271, 302, 327, 525
– -labelled nucleotides 553
Biotinylation 241, 537
Bird
– developmental biology 419
Bit 347
Blocking 382

Blood cell recognition 356
Blood cells
– erythrocytes 35
– granulocytes 25 ff.
– lymphocytes 33
– MNC 25 ff.
– monocytes 34
– platelets 36 f.
– preparation of leucocytes 66 f.
– reticulocytes 36
– separation of 22 f.
– unfractionated leucocytes 24
Bone marrow 60
– preparation of cells 62
Bouin's fluid 211, 226
Boundary
– in image analysis 353
Brewers' complete thioglycollate broth 43
Bridging label 237
Bronchoalveolar lavage, see BAL
Bronchoscope 52 f.
Brush border 196
BSA 311
Build-up immunostaining 275
– ELISPOT assay 521 ff.
Bursa of *Fabricius* 420, 558
– colonization 421

Cacodylate buffer 320
Ca^{2+} concentration after cell activation 565
Callus 148
– culture 150
Cancer 401 f.
CAPD (Continuous Ambulatory Perfusion
  Dialysis) 42
Capping 223
Capture reaction 342
Capture reagent 179
Carbonate buffer 514
Carnoy's fixative 112, 210, 227
Carrier-free electrophoresis 199
Cathode ray tube, see CRT
CD (cluster of differentiation) 393
CD4+ 398
CD4+ T-cell line 121 ff., 131, 396 f.
– cloning 126 ff.
– hybridoma 125
– *Jurkat* line 125
CD8+ T-cell line 121, 129 ff., 183, 397 f.,
  559
cdc2 452
cDNA library 394
– expression library 418, 432
Cell adherence
– differential 167

– matrix   167
– sequential   167 ff.
– use in immunocytochemistry   221 f.
Cell bank   107
– preparation   108
– quality control   117
Cell counting   13 ff., 107, 221
– electronic   15
– in BAL fluid   55
– with haemocytometer   13 f.
Cell culture   96 ff., 105
– adherence, see Cell adherence
– agarose substrate for ELISPOT assay   536
– cell line authentication   116 ff.
– cloning   144
– contamination   111 ff.
– double chamber system   570
– ELISPOT assay   511, 516, 520
– finite   103
– freezing   100, 107 ff.
– general principles   96
– growth factor   104
– handling regulations   97 f.
– haploid   150
– incubator   98
– insect cells   139 ff.
– long-term culture   103
– lyophilized stock   92
– medium   104 f., 142, 151
– of arthropod tissue   71
– on coverslips   222
– open culture system   99
– plant cells   148 ff.
– primary, see Primary culture
– prokaryotic cells   92 f., 156 ff.
– quality control   110
– SOP   101
– stock   107
– storage   100
– subculture   105 f.
Cell cycle   444
– analysis   384
– yeast conditional lethal mutant   458
Cell growth
– log phase   105
Cell line   103, 541
– age   107
– arthropod   139 ff.
– arthropod growth medium   142
– attached-   106
– authentication   116 ff.
– cytokine-dependent   541
– establishment   72
– mycoplasma-free   112
– suspension   106

– T-cell   123
– types   103 f.
– transformation   103
Cell-lineage   393
Cell-mediated cytotoxicity   389
– immunity, see CMI
Cell membrane   343
– preparation   85
Cell phenotype   388
Cell preparation on slides   224 f.
Cell proliferation   384
Cell quantitation   4
– flow cytometry   5
– within tissues   5
Cell separation   5, 12, 15, 166 ff., 394
– adherence to surfaces   19, 167 ff.
– – macrophages   46
– alveolar cell
– antibody-based methods   171 ff.
– arthropod cells   68 ff.
– biopsy-based methods   190 ff.
– blood cells   22 ff.
– cells from peritoneal lavage   46 f.
– centrifugation   19
– estimation of cell viability   15 ff.
– from lymphoid tissue   60 ff.
– immunocyte   560
– lymphocytes   122
– plant cells   79 ff.
– prokaryotic cells   89 ff.
– serous cavity cells   39 ff.
– single cell suspension   535
– tissue samples   19
Cell sorting   560
– flow cytometry   185
– magnetic   183
Cell stain   13, 15 ff.
Cellular matrix   455
Cell viability   381
– dye exclusion and-   15
– dye uptake and-   17
– handling conditions and-   18 ff.
– – handling medium   18
– – sterility   19
– – temperature   20
– nitrogen storage   100
Cell wall
– preparation   83
– primary   79
– secondary   79
CENP (Centromere Protein)   454 f.
Central vacuole   79
Centrifugation   196 f.
– automatic zonal   197
– cell separation   19